THE IMMUNOLOGICAL
BASIS OF ASTHMA

LUNG BIOLOGY IN HEALTH AND DISEASE

Executive Editor

Claude Lenfant
Director, National Heart, Lung, and Blood Institute
National Institutes of Health
Bethesda, Maryland

176. Non-Neoplastic Advanced Lung Disease, *edited by J. Maurer*

ADDITIONAL VOLUMES IN PREPARATION

Therapeutic Targets in Airway Inflammation, *edited by N. T. Eissa and D. Huston*

Respiratory Infections in Asthma and Allergy, *edited by S. Johnston and N. Papadopoulos*

Acute Respiratory Distress Syndrome, *edited by M. A. Matthay*

Upper and Lower Respiratory Disease, *edited by J. Corren, A. Togias, and J. Bousquet*

Venous Thromboembolism, *edited by J. E. Dalen*

Acute Exacerbations of Chronic Obstructive Pulmonary Disease, *edited by N. Siafakas, N. Anthonisen, and D. Georgopolous*

Lung Volume Reduction Surgery for Emphysema, *edited by H. E. Fessler, J. J. Reilly, Jr., and D. J. Sugarbaker*

The opinions expressed in these volumes do not necessarily represent the views of the National Institutes of Health.

THE IMMUNOLOGICAL BASIS OF ASTHMA

Edited by

Bart N. Lambrecht
Henk C. Hoogsteden
Zuzana Diamant
Erasmus University Medical Centre
Rotterdam, The Netherlands

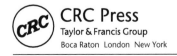
CRC Press
Taylor & Francis Group
Boca Raton London New York

CRC Press is an imprint of the
Taylor & Francis Group, an **informa** business

CRC Press
Taylor & Francis Group
6000 Broken Sound Parkway NW, Suite 300
Boca Raton, FL 33487-2742

First issued in paperback 2019

© 2003 by Taylor & Francis Group, LLC
CRC Press is an imprint of Taylor & Francis Group, an Informa business

No claim to original U.S. Government works

ISBN-13: 978-0-8247-0882-5 (hbk)
ISBN-13: 978-0-367-39542-1 (pbk)

Library of Congress Cataloging-in-Publication Data
A catalog record for this book is available from the Library of Congress.

Visit the Taylor & Francis Web site at
http://www.taylorandfrancis.com

and the CRC Press Web site at
http://www.crcpress.com

To my wife, Tine [BL]
To my wife, Gerrie, and to my mentor, Prof. Chris Hilvering [HCH]
To my husband, Peter, and my daughters, Sharon and Lauren [ZD]

INTRODUCTION

The editors of this volume begin their Preface by saying "Our thinking on the pathogenesis of asthma has changed substantially over the last two decades." No statement could be more true! Not only has our thinking about pathogenesis changed, but the scientific, medical, and public health interest in this disease has led to remarkable progress in both our knowledge and our ability to care for patients. These successes, however, should not make us forget the long route that preceded these last 20 years in our odyssey to understand and manage asthma.

Although descriptions resembling asthma may be traced as far back as the 28th century B.C., it was Aretaeus, a Greek physician, who gave the first observation of asthma as we know it today in the 2nd century B.C. Well · · · more or less! Yet, it is noteworthy that Aretaeus did not mention allergy or a humoral mechanism. These concepts had been developed two centuries earlier by Hippocrates. Their omission from Aretaeus' comments is due to the fact that Hippocrates described these concepts not in relation to respiratory disorders, but in relation to food intolerance:

> Cheese does not harm all men alike, some can eat their fill of it without the slightest hurt, nay, those it agrees with are wonderfully strengthened thereby. Others come off badly. So the constitution of these men differ, and the difference lies in the constituent of the body which is hostile to cheese, and is roused and stirred to action under its influence.

Hippocrates did not know it, but actually he was telling us that atopy and the immune response are programmed from birth.

Of course, since that time, and especially in the last decades of the twentieth century, extraordinary knowledge and understanding of the immune process have been gained. How this process relates and leads to inflammation and then to clinical manifestations of asthma is also well understood. In fact, we can be sure that any volume or article about asthma will include sections on immune response and inflammation and their relationship to asthma. However, this new volume is unique because it brings it all together. The interactions between allergen, antigens, immune responses at the cellular and humoral level, and genetic determinants are all presented, discussed, and integrated with the goal of exploring new therapeutic approaches.

The editors reached out for contributors in many countries to develop a most comprehensive volume. This Lung Biology in Health and Disease series of monographs has presented many, many volumes on asthma, and this volume is a noteworthy and timely addition. I am grateful to Drs. Lambrecht, Hoogsteden, and Diamant and to all their contributors for their valuable contributions.

Claude Lenfant, M.D.
Bethesda, Maryland, U.S.A.

PREFACE

Our thinking on the pathogenesis of asthma has changed substantially over the last two decades, in large part because of the progress in invasive and noninvasive measurements of airway inflammation and lung function as well as in the fields of immunology and cell biology. It is currently believed that a dysregulated cellular and humoral immune response to allergen might be the basis for atopy. This immune response is already programmed in early life and is influenced by the genetic background of the individual as well as by environmental factors such as lifestyle, infections, and pollution. All these factors seem to influence the various cells and regulatory processes of the immune system in a complex and interrelated manner. Although atopy is a risk factor for the development of asthma, not all atopics develop bronchial hyperreactivity and symptoms of asthma. Additional factors, such as those derived from airway epithelial cells and tissue resident cells, may be of critical importance for the regulation of immune responses in the lung and the development of chronic self-perpetuating airway inflammation that leads to functional changes and, ultimately, to irreversible airway remodeling.

Along with this increasing knowledge about the natural evolution of asthma, there has been an explosion of research in which animal models of eosinophilic airway inflammation have been used to draw conclusions about the role of a particular cell or mediator in the pathogenesis of asthma. Although these models can only partly address the complex regulatory mechanisms in human asthma, they have elucidated the important functional roles of antigen-presenting cells, T lymphocytes, cytokines, chemokines, and neuropeptides and, at the same time, have cast some doubt on the most classic paradigms of allergy, such as the contribution of mast cells, IgE, and eosinophils to certain aspects of chronic airway inflammation and bronchial hyperreactivity.

In this book, data on the immunology of asthma obtained from human studies are presented in light of data obtained from animal models of the disease. In Part One, the various cells of the pulmonary immune system as well as the products they secrete will be discussed briefly. This will provide the nonimmunologist with the basic knowledge about these cells necessary to understand the subsequent chapters of this volume. In Part Two, the steady-state regulatory processes that operate within the immune system of the lung are discussed. The fundamental outcome of a first exposure to antigen can be tolerance or immunity. Tolerance to inhaled allergen can be the result of ignorance, anergy, or suppression, but is generally thought to be the result of an active, proliferative immune response to allergen. The induction of immunity results from a complex interaction between antigen-presenting cells and naive T cells that initially occurs in the central lymphoid organs. However, naive T cells eventually differentiate to become migratory memory/effector T cells that migrate through the lung and produce polarized sets of cytokines upon encounter with antigen. Part Three discusses the immunological aspects of airway inflammation and remodeling in atopic and nonatopic asthma. Whereas human biopsy studies only allow associations to be made between an observed cell or mediator and the asthmatic phenotype, animal models show cause and effect. Animal models of allergen- or virally induced eosinophilic airway inflammation have intensively highlighted the functional importance of dendritic cells, T cells, cytokines, and chemokines to the induction and maintenance of eosinophilic airway inflammation and bronchial hyperreactivity. In vitro studies of human material also show cause and effect of an immunological mediator on the pathophysiology of asthma.

The eventual goal for increasing our knowledge of the immunology of asthma is to devise new strategies aimed at reversing the spontaneous evolution and symptoms of asthma. In Part Four, the manner in which our current therapies already affect many of the immune cells and their regulatory processes within the lung is discussed. Newer, specifically designed therapeutics exploit the immune system more selectively to intervene in asthma. Increasing knowledge of the epidemiology of asthma also suggests that exploiting bacterial motifs to stimulate the innate immune system may hold promise for devising a preventive vaccine. Finally, newer techniques to screen the expression of immune-related genes in healthy and diseased tissues may allow identification of novel genes that interfere with asthma pathogenesis, with the ultimate goal of devising antagonists to block a disease-causing gene product or to introduce a novel gene (product) to protect against asthma.

This book will provide a guide to scientists, clinicians, and clinical pharmacologists who wish to understand the origins of asthma in greater detail and to devise new therapies for asthma based on immunological interventions that ultimately change the natural course of the disease. It has been an honor to be able to collaborate with the contributors to this volume and we would like to take this opportunity to thank them for their fine efforts. We would also like to acknowledge the interest and support of the staff at Marcel Dekker, Inc., and Dr. Claude Lenfant, Executive Editor of this series, which have made this volume possible.

Bart N. Lambrecht
Henk C. Hoogsteden
Zuzana Diamant

CONTRIBUTORS

David Alvarez, B.Sc. Department of Pathology and Molecular Medicine, McMaster University, Hamilton, Ontario, Canada

Peter J. Barnes, D.M., D.Sc., F.R.C.P. Professor, Department of Thoracic Medicine, National Heart and Lung Institute, Imperial College School of Medicine, London, England

Jean Bousquet, M.D., Ph.D. Clinique de Maladies Respiratoires and INSERM U454, Montpellier, France

Armin Braun, Ph.D. Fraunhofer Institute for Toxicology and Aerosol Investigation, Hannover, Germany

Paul J. Coffer, Ph.D. Associate Professor, Department of Pulmonary Diseases, University Medical Center, Utrecht, The Netherlands

Anthony J. Coyle, Ph.D. Department of Biology, Millennium Pharmaceuticals, Cambridge, Massachusetts, U.S.A.

Esther C. De Jong, Ph.D. Department of Cell Biology and Histology, Academic Medical Centre, University of Amsterdam, Amsterdam, The Netherlands

Zuzana Diamant, M.D., Ph.D. Chest Physician, Department of Pulmonary and Critical Care Medicine, Erasmus University Medical Centre, Rotterdam, The Netherlands

Klaus J. Erb, Ph.D. Centre for Infectious Diseases, University of Würzburg, Würzburg, Germany

Anthony J. Frew, M.A., M.D., F.R.C.P. Professor, University of Southampton School of Medicine, and Department of Medical Specialties, Southampton General Hospital, Southampton, England

Jose-Carlos Gutierrez-Ramos, Ph.D. Department of Biology, Millennium Pharmaceuticals, Cambridge, Massachusetts, U.S.A.

Hamida Hammad, Ph.D. Department of Pulmonary and Critical Care Medicine, Erasmus University Medical Centre, Rotterdam, The Netherlands

Stephen T. Holgate, M.D., D.Sc., F.R.C.P., F.R.C.Path., F.Med.Sci. Professor, Department of Respiratory Cell and Molecular Biology, University of Southampton, Southampton, England

Henk C. Hoogsteden, M.D., Ph.D. Professor, Department of Pulmonary and Critical Care Medicine, Erasmus University Medical Centre, Rotterdam, The Netherlands

Gerard F. Hoyne, Ph.D. Genome Center, Australian National University, Canberra, Australia

Marc Humbert, M.D., Ph.D. Professor, Department of Respiratory Medicine, Hôpital Antoine Béclère, Assistance Publique–Hôpitaux de Paris, Clamart, France

Elizabeth R. Jarman, Ph.D. MRC Centre for Inflammation Research and Respiratory Medicine Unit, University of Edinburgh Medical School, Edinburgh, Scotland

Manel Jordana, M.D., Ph.D. Professor, Department of Pathology and Molecular Medicine, McMaster University, Hamilton, Ontario, Canada

Pawel Kalinski, M.D., Ph.D. Department of Cell Biology and Histology, Academic Medical Centre, University of Amsterdam, Amsterdam, The Netherlands

Martien L. Kapsenberg, Ph.D. Professor, Department of Cell Biology and Histology, Academic Medical Centre, University of Amsterdam, Amsterdam, The Netherlands

A. Barry Kay, M.D., Ph.D. Department of Allergy and Clinical Immunology, National Heart and Lung Institute, Imperial College School of Medicine, London, England

Johan C. Kips, M.D., Ph.D. Professor, Department of Respiratory Diseases, Ghent University Hospital, Ghent, Belgium

Leo Koenderman, Ph.D. Professor, Department of Pulmonary Diseases, University Medical Center, Utrecht, The Netherlands

Harmjan Kuipers, M.Sc. Department of Pulmonary and Critical Care Medicine, Erasmus University Medical Centre, Rotterdam, The Netherlands

Jonathan R. Lamb, Ph.D., D.Sc., F.R.C.Path., F.Med.Sci., F.R.S.E. Professor, Respiratory Medicine Unit, University of Edinburgh Medical School, Edinburgh, Scotland

Bart N. Lambrecht, M.D., Ph.D. Department of Pulmonary and Critical Care Medicine, Erasmus University Medical Centre, Rotterdam, The Netherlands

Mark Larché, Ph.D. Department of Allergy and Clinical Immunology, National Heart and Lung Institute, Imperial College School of Medicine, London, England

Clare M. Lloyd, Ph.D. Leukocyte Biology, Faculty of Medicine, Imperial College, London, England

Stephen Manning, Ph.D. Department of Biology, Millennium Pharmaceuticals, Cambridge, Massachusetts, U.S.A.

Marco A. Martins, Ph.D. Senior Lecturer, Department of Physiology and Pharmacodynamics, Oswaldo Cruz Foundation, Rio de Janeiro, Brazil

Laurent P. Nicod, M.D. Division of Pneumology, University Hospital of Geneva, Geneva, Switzerland

Wolfgang A. Nockher, Ph.D. Department of Clinical Chemistry and Molecular Diagnostics, University of Marburg, Marburg, Germany

Wieslawa Olszewska National Heart and Lung Institute, Imperial College School of Medicine, London, England

Peter J. M. Openshaw, Ph.D., F.R.C.P. Department of Respiratory Medicine, National Heart and Lung Institute, Imperial College School of Medicine, London, England

Reinhard Pabst, M.D. Professor, Department of Functional and Applied Anatomy, Hannover Medical School, Hannover, Germany

Clive Page, B.Sc., Ph.D. Professor, Sackler Institute of Pulmonary Pharmacology, King's College London, London, England

Romain A. Pauwels, M.D., Ph.D. Professor, Department of Respiratory Diseases, Ghent University Hospital, Ghent, Belgium

Martin J. Plummeridge, M.B., M.R.C.P. Department of Respiratory Medicine, Frenchay Hospital, Bristol, England

Susan L. Prescott, M.B.B.S., B.Med.Sci.(Hons), F.R.A.C.P., Ph.D. Associate Professor, Department of Pediatrics, University of Western Australia, Perth, Western Australia, Australia

Harald Renz, M.D., Ph.D. Professor, Department of Clinical Chemistry and Molecular Diagnostics, University of Marburg, Marburg, Germany

Douglas S. Robinson, M.D. Department of Allergy and Clinical Immunology, National Heart and Lung Institute, Imperial College School of Medicine, London, England

Sarbjit S. Saini, M.D. Assistant Professor, Division of Clinical Immunology, Johns Hopkins University School of Medicine, Baltimore, Maryland, U.S.A.

Sundeep S. Salvi, M.D., D.N.B., Ph.D. Department of Respiratory Cell and Molecular Biology, University of Southampton, Southampton, England

Anthony P. Sampson, Ph.D. Director, Division of Respiratory Cell and Molecular Biology, University of Southampton School of Medicine, Southampton General Hospital, Southampton, England

Patricia M. R. e Silva, Ph.D. Senior Researcher, Department of Physiology and Pharmacodynamics, Oswaldo Cruz Foundation, Rio de Janeiro, Brazil

Domenico Spina, Ph.D. Sackler Institute of Pulmonary Pharmacology, King's College London, London, England

Thomas Tschernig, M.D. Department of Functional and Applied Anatomy, Hannover Medical School, Hannover, Germany

Leonie S. Van Rijt, M.Sc. Department of Pulmonary and Critical Care Medicine, Erasmus University Medical Centre, Rotterdam, The Netherlands

Antonio M. Vignola, M.D., Ph.D. Istituto di Medicina Generale e Pneumologia, University of Palermo, Palermo, Italy

Eddy A. Wierenga, Ph.D. Department of Cell Biology and Histology, Academic Medical Centre, University of Amsterdam, Amsterdam, The Netherlands

Ryan E. Wiley, B.ArtsSci. Department of Pathology and Molecular Medicine, McMaster University, Hamilton, Ontario, Canada

Gisela Wohlleben, Ph.D. Centre for Infectious Diseases, University of Würzburg, Würzburg, Germany

Sun Ying, M.D., Ph.D. Department of Allergy and Clinical Immunology, National Heart and Lung Institute, Imperial College School of Medicine, London, England

CONTENTS

THE IMMUNOLOGICAL
BASIS OF ASTHMA

1

Overview of the Pulmonary Immune Response

LAURENT P. NICOD

University Hospital of Geneva
Geneva, Switzerland

I. Introduction

The upper and lower airways together represent the largest epithelial surface exposed to the outside environment. The inspired air is a source of the necessary oxygen for the body, but also introduces numerous particles, toxic gases, and microorganisms inside the body. In addition, the lungs are inoculated repeatedly with bacteria which are aspirated from the nasooropharynx. In order to allow for gas exchange, foreign substances and microorganisms must be stopped and removed without undue inflammation.

Schematically, the components of the pulmonary immune responses are framed by the requirements of lung defense. The mechanisms can be divided into those located in the airways and those in the alveoli (Table 1). The upper airways protect the lungs with the anatomical barriers they represent. These are associated with the cough reflex, the mucociliary apparatus, and the production of secretory immunoglobulin A (IgA). The superficial layers of the respiratory mucosa in the nose and conducting airways contain a tight network of dendritic cells (DCs) that will sense and catch any invading organisms and bring them to the draining lymph nodes around the main airways or in the hilum of the lung. In the respiratory units beyond the respiratory bronchioles particles will be caught by alveolar macrophages (AMs) in a milieu that is rich in nonspecific defense elements, such as IgG, complement, surfactant, and fibronectin. In these distal respiratory units, various amounts of inflammatory cells will be recruited when there is an inflammatory stimulus, such as a bacterial infection.

Several innate immune processes can take place either in the central or in the more distal airways. The inflammatory mediators released during the recognition of antigen by the innate immune system have the potential to

1

Table 1 Constituents of the Immune Response

I. Airways and the mucociliary apparatus
Anatomical barriers
Mucociliary clearance
Secretory IgA
Lysozyme, lactoferrin, etc.

II. The mucosa and submucosa
Epithelial barrier
Epithelial cell mediators (cf. Table 2)
Immature (mature) dendritic cells (cf. Table 3)
Lymphocytes
Eosinophils

III. Alveolar spaces
Pneumocytes types I and II
Alveolar macrophages
Lymphocytes
Neutrophils
Eosinophils
Immunoglobulins and opsonins

IV. Mast cells and basophils

---

recruit inflammatory cells and favor the generation of a long-lived and adaptive immune response. The activation or maturation of DCs by interleukin-1 (IL-1) or tumor necrosis factor-α (TNF-α) is perhaps the best illustration of the influence of innate immunity on the adaptive immunity. DC activation is followed by migration to the regional lymph node and the priming of T- and B-cell responses, the major components of adaptive immunity. Lymphoid structures are usually poorly developed in humans, except during some inflammatory processes when more or less developed bronchus-associated lymphoid tissue (BALT) can appear.

II. The Airways and the Mucociliary Apparatus

A. Nonspecific Defense Mechanisms

The airways are protected by the anatomical barriers, the cough reflex, the mucociliary apparatus, and the airway epithelium. The nasopharyngeal anatomical barriers are important to prevent the penetration of particles or organisms bigger than 2–3 μm into the lower airways. Particles and microbes from the inhaled air will be stopped by impaction on the mucosal surface.

Cough is generated by a forced expiration against a closed glottis, which opens suddenly to produce an expulsive phase. This allows enough turbulence and shearing forces to be produced in the major bronchi and trachea to extrude material such as debris, infected mucus, or products of epithelial damage. The cough is triggered by a wide variety of stimuli, mechanical or chemical, such as several inflammatory mediators (1).

B. Mucociliary Transport and Enzymes Carried Within It

More than 90% of inhaled particles with a diameter greater than 2–3 μm are deposited on the mucus overlying the ciliated epithelium of bronchi. The particles are transported from the terminal bronchioles to the trachea by the ciliary beats in the mucus. This motion occurs at a speed varying between 100 and 300 μm/s. The airway mucus is composed of a sole phase, or periciliary liquid about 5–10 μm deep allowing the cilia to beat, and a gel phase on the surface of the cilia whose thickness varies between 2 and 20 μm. The flow of the gel is referred to as the mucociliary transport. The physical properties of mucus are provided mainly by mucins, which are mucoglycoproteins and proteoglycans secreted from the surface of epithelial cells and from the glands. Phospholipids are also secreted by the epithelial cells and submucosal glands of the airways, weakening the adhesion of the mucus and altering its physical properties. The mucus gel acts as a barrier for bacteria that adhere to it but can also allow growth under certain conditions (2). Secretory IgA, lysozyme, lactoferrin, or peroxide is carried within the mucus. These substances participate in the nonspecific first line of defense to invasion by microorganisms. Thus, the lysozyme is a muramidase that degrades a glycosidic linkage of bacterial membrane peptidoglycans. It is regularly found in the lung secretions and, when purified, demonstrates bactericidal properties (3). Epithelial cells, serous cells of submucosal glands, macrophages, and neutrophils can be a source of lysozyme. Lactoferrin is an iron-binding protein that reduces the availability of elemental iron, an obligatory cofactor for bacterial replication. Lactoferrin may also be bactericidal by binding to endotoxin (4). The secretory peroxides (lactoperoxidases) or those from leukocytes (myeloperoxidases) act on thiocyanate ions or produce oxygen radicals that are bacteriostatic or bactericidal. Many of these active plasma components extravasate from the blood vessels to the mucosa during airways inflammation. Immunoglobulins and complement factors take part then in the defense mechanism as well as in the inflammatory cascade. Others, such as the protease inhibitors, may protect the airways (5).

C. Secretory IgA

The IgA released by the epithelial cells is the first line of defense formed by the adaptive immune system. IgA antibodies synthesized in the lamina propria are secreted as IgA dimeric molecules associated with a single J chain of 23,000 daltons. This polymeric form of IgA binds specifically to a molecule called the "poly-Ig receptor" or the "secretory component" expressed on the basolateral surfaces of the overlying epithelial cells. The complex is internalized and carried through the cytoplasm of the epithelial cells in a transport vesicle to its apical surface and released in the airways. IgAs are particularly important as they neutralize toxins and viruses and block the entry of bacteria across the epithelium. IgAs are poor activators of the classical pathway of complement but can activate the alternate pathway allowing a better opsonization of bacteria (6). The role of the airway epithelium in regulation of IgA synthesis is discussed in Chapter 7.

III. The Mucosa and Submucosa

A. Epithelial Cells

Epithelial cells form the lining of the luminal surface of the airways and are attached to neighboring cells by several structures: tight junctions, intermediate junctions, gap junctions, and desmosomes (7). These structures form a barrier between the luminal space and the pulmonary parenchyma. Desmosomes mediate mechanical adhesion of cells to their neighbors, and tight junctions completely obliterate the intercellular space just below the luminal surface (8). The gap junctions provide cell–cell communications for small molecules to travel between airway epithelial cells. Communication via gap junctions is believed to help maintain the uniform beating of the cilia (9,10), and transport through gap junctions may be a means for the cells to provide their neighbors with defense molecules such as antioxidants (11). This organization of epithelial cells, on one hand, creates an effective mechanical barrier and, on the other hand, allows for polarity in function, thus maintaining an ionic gradient for directional secretion of many substances.

Epithelial cells are key cells in inflammatory processes (Table 2). They are capable of up-regulating the expression of adhesion molecules such as intercellular adhesion molecule 1 (ICAM-1) in response to inflammatory stimuli that will favor the binding of neutrophils or monocytes to an inflamed area. In addition, epithelial cells are capable of expressing the major histocompatibility complex (MHC) of class I and II when exposed to cytokines such as interferon-γ (IFN-γ). Epithelial cells have a certain capacity for presenting antigens to lymphocytes and potentially to amplify an antigen-driven lymphocyte response (12).

Epithelial cells recruit inflammatory cells by releasing several chemoattractants. They release the arachidonic acid derivate 15-HETE, an active neutrophil chemoattractant that can also modulate immune cells (13). They release IL-8 in a bidirectional manner with preferential secretion into the lumen (14). A variety of stimuli have been demonstrated to induce the release of IL-8. These include cigarette smoke, endotoxin and other bacterial products (15), viral infections (16), and a variety of cytokines including IL-1, TNF-α, and IFN-γ (17). Other chemokines include GROα, GROβ, thymus and activation regulated chemokine (TARC), and monocyte chemotactic protein-1 (MCP-1). Epithelial cells also release "lymphocyte chemoattractant factor" or IL-16 (18). IL-16 is also an activating factor for CD4 T cells. Epithelial cells also produce

Table 2 Epithelial Cell Mediators

Chemokines
α (CXC) Chemokines
    IL-8
    GROα
    GROβ
    etc.
β (CC) Chemokines

Colony-stimulating factors (CSF)
GM-CSF, G-CSF, M-CSF, CSF-1

Growth factors (GF)
EGF; PDGF; β-FGF; TGFα and β; IGF-1

Pleiotrophic cytokines
IL-1; TNF-α
IL-6, IL-11, IL-15, IL-16, etc.

Inducible enzymes
15-Lipoxygenase; cyclooxygenase 2
Nitric oxide synthetase type 2

---

the epithelial or β-defensins in response to stimulation by bacterial stimuli or TNF-α. These factors have direct bactericidal activity and attract more inflammatory cells through signaling via the CCR6 chemokine receptor (see Chap. 2).

Overall, epithelial cells are capable of producing and responding to a variety of eicosanoids, cytokines, and growth factors which form a complex network regulating inflammatory responses. They also express cell surface receptors that can interact directly with inflammatory cells.

B. Dendritic Cells

A tight network of DCs lies above and below the basement membrane in a resting or "immature" state. These cells extend their dendrites between the intercellular channels formed by the epithelial cells. They form a network optimally situated to sample inhaled antigens (19,20). The intimate association of DCs with epithelial basal cells is reminiscent of the interaction between Langerhans cells and keratinocytes of the skin. There are 1400 ± 140 cells/mm^2 in the rat trachea, including these located above and below the lamina propria. Recent evidence indicates that airway DCs constitute a highly reactive population, whose numbers and MHC content change rapidly under (experimental) phathological conditions. For example, DCs become more numerous in response to inhaled antigens (21) and rapidly decrease in number after treatment with glucocorticoids (22). Lung DCs, like "immature" DCs derived from blood, are characterized by a high endocytic activity that can be measured with fluorescent isothiocyanate (FITC) dextran incorporation (23), but show only limited expression of CD40, CD80, and CD86 (23) (Table 3). Inflammatory stimuli on DCs result in a loss of the antigen-capturing machinery and in an increase in T-cell stimulatory function, a process referred to as *maturation*. Once activated lung DCs migrate to lymphoid structures they acquire the CCR7 receptor described in other systems, at the same time down-regulating the CCR1 and CCR5 receptors (23,24). In this way, they direct their interest away from the site of inflammation toward the T-cell zone in the lymph nodes.

It is possible that the rupture of epithelial tight junctions is not a prerequisite for DCs to sample foreign particles or organisms. Indeed, it has been showed in the gut that DCs can extend processes through epithelial tight junctions into the lumen, to sample luminal content, which might include bacteria. During this process DCs seem even to express tight junction proteins so as to preserve the epithelial barrier permeability (26). DCs can also phagocytose apoptotic cells after viral infections. Activated by these cells and their content, they will be able to induce cytotoxic T cells (26).

After antigen uptake, airway DCs migrate to the paracortical T-cell zone of the draining lymph nodes of the lung, where they interact with naive T cells

Table 3 Phenotype and Function of Macrophages and Dendritic Cells in the Lungs

	Macrophages	Dendritic cells	
		Immature	Mature
Location	Alveoli (Tissue)	Tissue network (around airways and vessels)	Nodes (around major bronchi)
Functions			
Immunity	Innate immunity	Acquired immunity	
Phagocytosis			
Particles	+++	+	−
Pathogens	+++	+++	±
Cytokines			
TNF-α, IL-1, IL-8	+++	++	+
T-cell activation	+	++	++++
Phenotype			
MHC class I	++	+++	++++
MHC class II	++++	+++	++++
CD14	++	+++	−
CD40	± +	+	+++
CD80	±	+	+++
CD86	±	+	+++
CD83	±	+	+++

(27).When labeling DCs with green fluorescent protein, labeled DCs injected in the trachea of mice were traced in the draining mediastinal lymph nodes 24 hours after injection, but not in nondraining lymph nodes or spleen (28). However, activated memory T cells migrate other lymphoid structures and also to nonlymphoid structures of the body (28). Indeed, organs such as the lung have even been shown to be preferentially colonized by these memory CD4 and CD8 T cells (29).

C. Effector Cells

γδ T cells and natural killer (NK) cells are part of the innate immunity, independent of DCs. They are likely to play a crucial role in lung immunity, in that they react to pathogens in the absence of preliminary priming. Recent studies indicate that γδ T-cell clones can also be segregated into "T1" or "T2" cytokine patterns, with a bias toward production of T1 cytokines (30). However, they might represent less than 1% of T cells (31).

Eosinophils are bone marrow–derived granulocytes, and granulocyte-macrophage colony-stimulating factor (GM-CSF), IL-3, and IL-5 promote their differentiation from myeloid precursors. Eosinophils are present in low numbers in peripheral tissues, especially mucosal linings. Their numbers can increase by recruitment in pathological processes, especially allergic diseases. Cytokines produced by Th2 cells promote their recruitment and activation. Eosinophils release numerous mediators that are toxic to parasitic organisms and may injure normal tissue. Some of these mediators will be discussed later. The functional role of these cells is dealt with in great detail in Chapter 6.

IV. Immune Response in the Alveolar Spaces

The major components of inflammation and immunity which can be found in the alveolar milieu will be briefly reviewed. The importance of type I epithelial cells and of their precursors, the type II pneumocytes, will only be eluded to in the present chapter. However, their importance in the homeostasis of alveoli should not be underscored. We will focus our interest on cells retrieved by bronchoalveolar lavage.

A. Alveolar Macrophages

Alveolar macrophages (AMs) represent 85% of the cells retrieved from the alveoli by bronchoalveolar lavage. They are the most important population of phagocytic cells in the lower respiratory tract. They avidly phagocytose inhaled particles. They must neutralize the invading pathogens or will recruit neutrophils and mononuclear cells acutely. Once the infection or inflammatory process has been controlled, cell debris and exudate must be removed in order to recover the alveolar architecture.

The ability of macrophages to interact with pathogens is mediated by surface receptors capable of binding to specific ligands, including toxins, polysaccharides, lipopolysaccharides, complement proteins, and immunoglobulins. The ability to recognize surface lipopolysaccharides, peptidoglycans, or bacterial DNA appears to be related to the presence of Toll-like receptor (TLR)-2, TLR4, or TLR9 on monocytes/macrophages (32). The modulation of these receptors may be linked to the capacity of mononuclear cells to release IL-12 instead of IL-10 (33). The capacity of CR3 to bind directly to microbes in the absence of an opsonin may represent another mechanism whereby macrophages recognize potential pathogens (34). The mannose receptor mediates phagocytosis of yeast, *Pneumocystis carinii*, and many organisms containing carbohydrate recognition–like domains (35).

Alveolar macrophages have multiple functions through the release of numerous mediators with the following properties.

Initiation of Inflammation

The release of IL-1α and IL-1β or TNF-α induces a cascade of events in the alveolar milieu, such as the appearance of adhesion molecules on endothelial cells or epithelial cells or the release of chemokines (IL-8, MIP-1α/β, RANTES, MCP-1/3), and growth factors such as GM-CSF, G-CSF, or M-CSF. Inflammatory cytokines will favor the activation of neighboring cells and attract several inflammatory elements from the blood. In addition, bioactive lipids, mostly derived from cyclooxygenase products of arachidonic acid such as thromboxane A_2, LTB$_4$, 5-HETE, prostaglandin E_2 (PGE$_2$), and PGD$_2$, will influence vasoactive mechanisms, as well as the function of T and B lymphocytes and of macrophages, in an autocrine manner.

Control of Inflammation

AM release inhibitors of IL-1 or TNF-α in the form of IL-1 receptor antagonist or TNF-soluble receptors (TNFSR55 or TNFSR75) (36). Macrophages have the capacity to markedly reduce IL-1 or TNF synthesis by their own release of IL-10 (37).

Lung Remodeling

Macrophages are involved in lung remodeling and repair. Indeed, they produce macrophage metalloelastase, collagenase, metalloproteases (MMP1, MMP9) and their inhibitors tissue inhibitor of metalloproteases (TIMPs) under the tight regulation of cytokines (38) and surface proteins of activated T cells, among which is surface TNF (39). Macrophages also remodel matrix constituents by their own production of urokinase to remove fibrin deposition. Meanwhile they can also release fibroblast growth factors such as transforming growth factor-β or platelet-derived growth factor.

Bactericidal Activity

The bactericidal properties of macrophages are realized by the production of lysozyme. Defensins are cationic proteins capable of killing a wide variety of bacteria, including mycobacteria or fungi (40). Reactive oxygen intermediates (superoxide anion, hydrogen peroxide, hydroxyl radicals) or reactive nitrogen intermediates (nitric oxide, nitrites, or nitrates) are also involved in killing microorganisms and, eventually, tumor cells.

Several components of complement are produced by macrophages as well as the C1q inhibitor (41). Complement promotes the clearance of immune complexes, an important means of eliminating antibody-coated bacteria. If, however, immune complexes cannot be eliminated, then complement becomes chronically activated and can incite inflammation. Complement also bind to cells that have undergone apoptosis and helps to eliminate these cells from tissue (42). Complement that is activated at sites of tissue injury can cause damage through the deposition of the membrane-attack complex and cell-bound ligands, including C4b and C3b, that activate leukocytes bearing complement receptors. Complement can also amplify injury by means of the anaphylatoxins C5a and C3a, which cause the influx and activation of inflammatory cells.

Antigen Presentation

AMs can, under yet poorly understood circumstances, acquire some characteristics of DCs and may thus be able to activate T cells (43). This is in contrast to the common knowledge that they do prevent T-cell activation in normal subjects (44,45). This capacity to enhance or inhibit T-cell immunity remains a matter of major interest as their production of IL-10, which tightly controls their IL-12 release, may favor a milieu leading to a Th1 or Th2 response. Macrophages, such as dendritic cells, can indeed produce IL-12 when stimulated by bacterial lipopolysaccharides and IFN-γ or during the interaction of CD40-CD40L on T cells and macrophages (46).

B. Lymphocytes

Alveoli contain about 10% lymphocytes of which 50% are CD4, 30% CD8, 10–15% killer or NK cells, and 5% B lymphocytes. The CD4/CD8 lymphocyte ratio is 1.5 and thus similar to that of peripheral blood. In the alveolar milieu, lymphocytes may have a slightly altered phenotype and function. For instance, NK lymphocytes are Leu 7 positive in the alveoli and their cytotoxic function is altered compared to interstitial Leu 11–positive NK cells (47). In addition, most T lymphocytes that are present in the BAL fluid have a memory phenotype, although it is unclear whether these cells have seen antigen. Both humoral and cellular immunity require initially the presentation of antigens to T and B lymphocytes which will be sensitized essentially in structures such as lymph nodes. Once they are primed, T lymphocytes may be reactivated by DCs around the vessels or around the airways or by less professional antigen-presenting cells (APCs). In theory, all those cells on which MHC class I or II cells are present or inducible can present antigen to primed T cells. The real importance of epithelial cells, endothelial cells, or fibroblasts for these purposes relay mostly on *in vitro* studies in which endothelial cells appear potentially the most efficient APCs (48).

C. Neutrophils

Neutrophils are also known as polymorphonuclear neutrophils (PMNs) because of their characteristic multilobed nuclei. They are the most abundant type of leukocytes in the body. Their maturation process takes about 2 weeks in the marrow; then they are released into the blood where about half are believed to be "marginated," that is, pooled on the wall of the vessels. Their half-life is 8 h. In the BAL they normally represent less than 2% of the cells. However, if cells residing in the alveoli are unable to control infectious agents, a massive flux of neutrophils occurs. Thus in an experimental model, if only 4×10^5 *Staphylococcus aureus* are inoculated, they will be neutralized by macrophages only. But if 10^7 *S. aureus* are applied, a massive flux of PMNs occurs that is able to control the infection. With an inoculation of 10^8 *S. aureus* mice do not survive, despite or because of an even more important influx of PMNs (49). PMNs have been shown to be essential in the early clearance of many bacteria such as *P. aeruginosa, Klebsiella pneumoniae*, and *H. influenzae* (50).

The migration of PMNs into the lungs first involves their weak binding to the vascular endothelium through interactions between carbohydrate ligands on the PMNs and selectins on the endothelium. Sialyl Lewis-x moiety on the surface of PMNs recognizes the TNF-α induced P-selectins and E-selectins, whose expression appears after a few hours. This allows for their "rolling," the loose connection of PMNs on the endothelium facilitating this process. The leukocyte migration depends on the interaction of ICAM-1 (LFA-1) on the surface of PMNs. The extravasation of PMNs involves LFA-1 and endothelial cell adhesion molecules, expressed on the leukocytes and at the junction of endothelial cells. PMNs will then migrate toward chemotactic gradients (51). Chemotactic factors include C5 fragments generated by the activation of the alternative pathway by bacteria or cleaved by proteases from alveolar macrophages. Alveolar macrophages generate products of arachidonic acid such as 5- or 11-monohydroxyeicosatetraenoic acid and LTB_4 (52). Chemokines are small polypeptides also critically involved in PMN recruitment. The C-X-C chemokines include IL-8, GROα, and GROβ; promote migration of neutrophils; and are found in BAL of patients with various types of pneumonias (53). Mononuclear phagocytes, endothelial cells, and epithelial cells have the ability to generate chemokines in response to microbial products such as lipopolysaccharide. In addition, TNF-α and IL-1 are produced by the cells of the host and are required for the production of chemokines by fibroblasts and smooth muscle cells. Chemokines bind to proteoglycan molecules both in the extra-cellular matrix and on parenchymal cells. Chemokines are thus displayed on a solid substrate along which leukocytes migrate.

Activated neutrophils eliminate microorganisms by means of a range of mechanisms, which involve phagocytosis, release of oxygen radicals, and production of cytotoxic peptides or proteins. Their granules contain compo-nents able to kill and degrade microorganisms. Carbohydrate residues of bac-teria are attacked by enzymes such as sialidase, x-mannosidase, β-glucurone, N-acetyl-β-glucosoaminidase, and lysozyme. "Cytotoxic protein," such as α- or neutrophil defensins and serine proteinases, damage bacterial membranes by still only partially understood mechanisms (54).

Not surprisingly, defects in neutrophil function lead to severe disorders. In Chediak-Higaschi disease, a congenital immunological defect known to be accompanied by severe pyogenic infections, the granules cannot package the protein elastase or the cathepsin-G superfamily (55). In chronic granulomatous disease, affected individuals are susceptible to bacterial infections because their phagocytic cells are unable to generate the products of respiratory bursts (56). Neutrophil migration itself is impaired in leukocyte adhesion deficiencies (LAD); thus, in LAD-II, a defect in the expression of sialyl Lewis-x, the coun-tereceptor for E-selectin and P-selectin has been demonstrated (57).

D. Eosinophils

Eosinophils are granulated cells characterized by their unique crystalloid granules, which contain four basic proteins: major basic protein, eosinophil peroxidase, eosinophil cationic protein, and eosinophil-derived neurotoxin. Eosinophils develop in the bone marrow, and after maturation they circulate in the blood to migrate into tissues. GM-CSF, IL-3, and IL-5 all promote eosino-phil differentiation from myeloid precursors (58).

Eosinophils are abundant in the infiltrates of late-phase reactions and contribute to many of the pathological processes in allergic diseases. Cytokines produced by Th2 cells promote the activation of eosinophils and their recruit-ment to the late-phase reaction at inflammatory sites. Eosinophil recruitment and infiltration into tissues depends on various chemoattractants, including chemokines such as eotaxin and monocyte chemotactic protein-5, the comple-ment product C5a, and the lipid mediators platelet-activating factor (PAF) and LTB_4 (59).

Activated eosinophils, like mast cells and basophils, produce and release lipid mediators with proinflammatory properties. Many of the lipid mediators have vasoactive properties that may augment the effects of mediators produced by mast cells and basophils. In particular, eosinophils use the 5- and 15-lipox-ygenase pathways to synthesize lipid mediators, including LTC_4 and its deri-vatives LTD_4 and LTE_4. These molecules are potent stimulators of vasomotor activity, bronchial constriction, and mucus secretion. Eosinophils also produce a variety of cytokines, including GM-CSF, IL-3, IL-5, RANTES, MIP-1α, eotaxin, TNF-α, IL-1α, IL-6, IL-4, and IL-10.

E.   Immunoglobulins and Opsonins

Several components in normal bronchoalveolar lavage fluid have the capacity of coating, in a nonspecific manner, certain bacteria that will enhance phagocytic uptake by AMs, thus qualifying as nonimmune opsonins. Surfactant (60), fibronectin (61) and C-reactive protein may have opsonic activities. IgG, which constitutes 5% of the total protein content of normal BAL fluid (62), seems to be the predominant immunoglobulin with the strongest opsonic activity in the alveoli, contrary to IgA. Secretory IgA does not have obvious secretory mechanisms to be delivered in the alveoli. IgG_1 and IgG_2 are present in greatest concentrations (65% and 28%, respectively), whereas IgG_3 and IgG_4 together account for less than 10% (63). In terms of host defense, IgG_1 and IgG_3 are considered to be the most important as only these two antibodies fix complement. IgG_2 is a type-specific antibody against pathogens such as *Streptococcus pneumoniae* or *Haemophilus influenzae* (64). IgG_4 acts as a reaginic antibody in allergic disease, and increased IgG_4 may lead to hypersensitivity pneumonitis. In the absence of IgG_4, there is a predisposition to sinopulmonary infections and bronchiectasis (65).

Most complement components can be produced by monocytes or macrophages *in vitro*. However, most of them are produced by the liver and carried to the lung via the blood. Activation of the entire complement pathway in the presence of microbes can result in their lysis and killing. When bacteria activate the alternate pathway, C3b is released allowing a good opsonization of bacteria for neutrophils or macrophages. C5a has proinflammatory properties and exerts a powerful chemoattractant effect for PMNs. The complement pathway is under the tight control of C1q released by AMs or released from blood exudation. Complement and, in particular, the alternative complement pathway are likely to play an important role as the first line of defense against many extracellular microbes as part of the innate immune defenses (65,66).

V.   Mast Cells and Basophils

Mast cells, basophils, and eosinophils are the effector cells of immediate hypersensitivity reactions and allergic diseases. Mature mast cells are found throughtout the body, predominantly located near blood vessels, nerves, and beneath epithelia. Basophils are inflammatory granulocytes with structural and functional similarities to mast cells but are derived from a different cell lineage. Basophils are derived from bone marrow and circulate in their differentiated form. Basophils constitute less than 1% of the total blood leukocytes. Although normally not present in tissues, basophils are recruited to some inflammatory sites, usually together with eosinophils (60).

Activation of mast cells (and basophils) results in three types of biological response: secretion of the preformed contents of their granules by a regulated exocytosis; synthesis and secretion of lipid mediators; synthesis and secretion of cytokines. Preformed mediators include biogenic amines and granule macromolecules. In human mast cells the major biogenic amine is histamine. Neutral serine proteases, including tryptase and chymase, are the most abundant protein constituent of mast cell secretory granules.

The major arachidonic acid–derived mediator produced by the cyclooxygenase pathway in mast cells is PGD_2. The most important arachidonic acid–derived mediators produced by the lipoxygenase pathway in mast cells and basophils are the leukotrienes, especially leukotriene C4 (LTC_4) and its degradation products LTC_4 and LTE_4. A third type of lipid mediator produced by mast cells is PAF. Mast cells and basophils produce many different cytokines that may contribute to allergic inflammation. These cytokines include TNF-α, IL-1, IL-4, IL-5, IL-6, IL-13, MIP-α, MIP-β, and various colony-stimulating factors such as IL-3 and GM-CSF.

The biogenic amines and lipid mediators induce vascular leakage and bronchoconstriction, all components of the immediate response. Cytokines and lipid mediators both contribute to inflammation, which is part of the late-phase reaction. Enzymes probably contribute to tissue remodeling (61).

References

1. Widdicombe JG. Relationship among the composition of mucus, epithelial lining liquid, and adhesion of micro-organisms. Am J Respir Crit Care Med 1995; 151:2088–2093.

2. Puchelle E, Girod-de-Bentzmann S, Jacquot J. Airway defence mechanisms in relation to biochemical and physical properties of mucus. Eur Respir Rev 1992; 2:259–263.

3. Jacquot J, Puchelle E, Zahm JM, Beck G, Plotkowski MC. Effect of human airway lysozyme on the in vitro growth or type 1. *Streptococcus pneumoniae.* Eur J Respir Dis 1987; 71:295–305.

4. Ellison RT III, Giehl TJ. Killing of gram-negative bacteria by lactoferrin and lysozyme. J Clin Invest 1991; 88:1080–1091.

5. Persson CG. Plasma exudation from tracheobronchial microvessels in health and disease. In Butler J, ed. The Bronchial Circulation. New York: Marcel Dekker, 1992: 443–473.

6. Underdown BJ, Schiff JM. Immunoglobulin A: strategic defense at the mucosal surface. Annu Rev Immunol 1986; 4:389–417.

7. Mercer RR, Russell ML, Roggli VL, Crapo JD. Cell number and distribution in human and rat airways. Am J Respir Cell Mol Biol 1994; 10:613–624.

8. Plopper CG, Mariassy AT, Wilson DW, Alley JL, Nishio SJ, Nettesheim P. Comparison of nonciliated tracheal epithelial cells in six mammalian species: ultrastructure and population densities. Exp Lung Res 1983; 5:281–294.

9. Sanderson MJ, Chow I, Dirksen ER. Intercellular communication between ciliated cells in culture. Am J Physiol 1988; 254:C63–C74.

10. Sanderson MJ, Charles AC, Boitano S, Dirksen ER. Mechanisms and function of intercellular calcium signaling. Mol Cell Endocrinol 1994; 98:173–187.

11. Barhoumi R, Bowen JA, Stein LS, Echols J, Burghardt RC. Concurrent analysis of intracellular glutathione content and gap junctional communication. Cytometry 1993; 14:747–756.

12. Rossi GA, Sacco O, Balbi B Oddera S, Mattioni T, Corte G, Ravazzoni C, Allegra L. Human ciliated bronchial epithelial cells. Expression of the HLA-DR alpha gene, modulation of the HLA-DR antigens by gamma-interferon and antigen-presenting function in the mixed leukocyte reaction. Am J Respir Cell Mol Biol 1990; 3:431–439.

13. Holtzman MJ. Arachidonic acid metabolism in airway epithelial cells. Annu Rev Physiol 1992; 54:303–329.

14. Bedard M, McClure CD, Schiller NL, Francoeur C, Cantin A, Denis M. Release of interleukin-8, interleukin-6 and colony-stimulating factors by upper airway epithelial cells: Implications for cystic fibrosis. Am J Respir Cell Mol Biol 1993; 9:455–462.

15. Massion PP, Inoue H, Richman-Eisenstat J, Grunberger D, Jorens PG, Housset B, Pittet JF. Novel pseudomonas product stimulates interleukin-8 production in airway epithelial cells in vitro. J Clin Invest 1994; 93:26–32.

16. Choi AM, Jacoby DB. Influenza virus A infection induces interleukin-8 gene expression in human airway epithelial cells. FEBS Lett 1992; 309:327–329.

17. Adler KB, Fischer BM, Wright DT, Cohn LA, Becker S. Interactions between respiratory epithelial cells and cytokines: relationships to lung inflammation. Ann NY Acad Sci 1994; 725:128–145.

18. Center DM, Kornfeld H, Cruikshank W. Interleukin 16 and its function as a CD4 ligand. Immunol Today 1996; 17:476–481.

19. Sertl K, Takemura T, Tschachler E, Ferrans VJ, Kaliner MA, Shevach EM. Dendritic cells with antigen presenting capability reside in airway epithelium, lung parenchyma and visceral pleura. J Exp Med 1986; 163:436–451.

20. Holt PG, Haining S, Nelson DJ, Sedgwick JD. Origin and steady-state turnover of class II MCH-bearing dendritic cells in the epithelium of the conduction airways. J Immunol 1994; 153:256–261.

21. McWilliam AS, Nelson D, Thomas JA, Holt PG. Rapid dendritic cell recruitment is a hallmark of the acture inflammatory response at mucosal surfaces. J Exp Med 1994; 179:1331–1336.

22. Brokaw JJ, White GW, Baluk P, Anderson GP, Umemoto EY, McDonald DM. Glucocorticoid-induced apoptosis of dendritic cells in the rat tracheal mucosa. Am J Respir Cell Mol Biol 1998; 19:598–605.

23. Cochand L, Isler P, Songeon F, Nicod LP. Human lung dendritic cells have an immature phenotype with efficient mannose receptors. Am J Respir Cell Mol Biol 1999; 21:547–554.

24. Sallusto F, Schaerli P, Loetscher P, Schaniel C, Lenig D, Mackay CR, Qin S, Lanzavecchia. Rapid and coordinated switch in chemokine receptor expression during dendritic cell maturation. Eur J Immunol 1998; 28:2760–2769.

25. Rescigno M, Urbano M, Valzasina B, Francolini M, Rotta G, Bonasio R, Granucci F, Kraehenbuhl JP, Ricciardi-Castagnoli P. Dendritic cells express tight

junction proteins and penetrate gut epithelial monolayers to sample bacteria. Nat Immunol 2001; 2:361–367.

26. Albert ML, Sauter B, Bhardwaj N. Dendritic cells acquire antigen from apoptotic cells and induce class I-restricted CTLs. Nature 1998; 392:86–89.

27. Nicod LP, Cochand L, Dreher D. Antigen presentation in the lung: dendritic çells and macrophages. Sarcoidosis Vasc Diffuse Lung Dis 2000; 17:246–255.

28. Vermaelen KY, Carro-Muino I, Lambrecht BN, Pauwels RA. Specific migratory dendritic cells rapidly transport antigen from the airways to the thoracic lymph nodes. J Exp Med 2001; 193:51–60.

29. Masopust D, Vezys V, Marzo AL, Lefrançois L. Preferential localization of effector memory cells in nonlymphoid tissue. Science 2001; 291:2413–2417.

30. Spada FM, Grant EP, Peters PJ, Sugita M, Melian A, Leslie DS, Lee HK, Van Donselaar E, Hanson DA, Krensky AM, Majdic O, Porcelli SA, Morita CT, Brenner MB. Self-recognition of CD1 by gamma/delta T Cells: implications for innate immunity. J Exp Med 2000; 191:937–948.

31. Reynolds HY. Integrated host defense against infections. In: Crystal RG, West JB, Weibel ER, Barnes P, eds. The Lung: Scientific Foundations, 2nd ed. Philadelphia: Lippincott–Raven, 1997.

32. Krutzik SR, Sieling PA, Modlin RL. The role of Toll-like receptors in host defense against microbial infection. Curr Opin Immunol 2001; 13:104–108.

33. Thoma-Uszynski S, Kiertscher SM, Ochoa MT, Bouis DA, Norgard MV, Miyake K, Godowski PJ, Roth MD, Modlin RL. Activation of toll-like receptor 2 on human dendritic cells triggers induction of IL-12, but not IL-10. J Immunol 2000; 165:3804–3810.

34. Brown EJ. Complement receptors and phagocytosis. Curr Opin Immunol 1991; 3:76–82.

35. Ezekowitz RA, Williams DJ, Koziel H, Armstrong MY, Warner A, Richards FF, Rose RM. Uptake of *Pneumocystis carinii* mediated by the macrophage mannose receptor. Nature 1991; 351:155–158.

36. Galve-de Rochemonteix B, Nicod LP, Dayer JM. Tumor necrosis soluble receptor 75: The principal receptor form released by human alveolar macrophages and monocytes in the presence of interferon gamma. Am J Respir Cell Mol Biol 1996; 14:279–287.

37. Nicod LP, El Habre F, Dayer JM, Boehringer N. Interleukin-10 decreases tumor necrosis factor alpha and beta in alloreactions induced by human lung dendritic cells and macrophages. Am J Respir Cell Biol 1995; 13:83–90.

38. Lacraz S, Nicod L, Galve-de-Rochemonteix B, Baumberger C, Dayer JM, Welgus HG. Suppression of metalloproteinase biosynthesis in human alveolar macrophages by interleukin-4. J Clin Invest 1992; 90:382–388.

39. Ferrari-Lacraz S, Nicod LP, Chicheportiche R, Welgus HG, Dayer JM. Human lung tissue macrophages, but not alveolar macrophages, express matrix metalloproteinases after direct contact with activated T lymphocytes. Am J Respir Cell Mol Biol 2001; 24:442–451.

40. Kisich KO, Heifets L, Higgins M, Diamond G. Antimycobacterial agent based on mRNA encoding human beta-defensin 2 enables primary macrophages to restrict growth of Mycobacterium tuberculosis. Infect Immun 2001; 69:2692–2699.

41. Hamacher J, Sadallah S, Schifferli JA, Villard J, Nicod LP. Soluble complement receptor type 1 (CD35) in bronchoalveolar lavage of inflammatory lung diseases. Eur Respir J 1998; 11:112–119.

42. Walport MJ. Complement at the interface between innate and adaptive immunity. N Eng J Med 2001; 334:1140–1144.

43. Nicod LP, Isler P. Alveolar macrophages in sarcoidosis coexpress high levels of CD86 (B7.2) CD40 and CD30L. Am J Respir Cell Mol Biol 1997; 17:91–96.

44. Toews GB, Vial WC, Dunn MM, Guzzetta P, Nunez G, Stastny P, Lipscomb MF. The accessory cell function of human alveolar macrophages in specific T cell proliferation. J Immunol 1984; 132:181–186.

45. Metzeger ZVI, Hoffeld JT, Oppenheim JJ. Macrophage-mediated suppression. J Immunol 1980; 124:983–988.

46. Isler P, Galve-de-Rochemonteix B, Songeon F, Boehringer N, Nicod P. Interleukin-12 production by human alveolar macrophages is controlled by the autocrine production of interleukin-10. Am J Respir Cell Mol Biol 1999; 20:270–278.

47. Weissler JC, Nicod LP, Lipscomb MF, Toews GB. Natural killer cell function in human lung is compartmentalized. Am Rev Respir Dis 1987; 135:941–949.

48. Geppert TD, Lipsky PE. Dissection of the antigen presenting function of tissue cells induced to express HLA-DR by gamma interferon. J Rheumatol 1987; 14:59–62.

49. Onofrio JM, Toews GB, Lipscomb MF, Pierce A. Granulocyte-alveolar macrophage interaction in the pulmonary clearance of *Staphylococcus aureus*. Am Rev Respir Dis 1983; 127:335–341.

50. Toews GB, Vial WC, Hansen EJ. Role of C5 and recruited neutrophils in early clearance of nontypable *Haemophilus influenzae* from murine lungs. Infect Immun 1985; 50:207–212.

51. Albelda SM, Smith CW, Ward PA. Adhesion molecules and inflammatory injury. FASEB J 1994; 8:504–512.

52. Valone FH, Franklin M, Sun FF, Goetzl EJ. Alveolar macrophage lipoxygenase products of arachidonic acid. Isolation and recognition as the predominant consituents of the neutrophil chemotactic activity elaborated by alveolar macrophages. Cell Immunol 1985; 54:390–401.

53. Villard J, Dayer-Pastore F, Hamacher J, Aubert JD, Schelegel-Haueter S, Nicod LP. GRO alpha and interleukin-8 in *Pneumocystis carinii* or bacterial pneumonia and adult respiratory distress syndrome. Am J Respir Crit Care Med 1995; 152:1549–1554.

54. Burnett D. Neutrophils. Pulmonary Defences. Chichester: Wiley, 1997.

55. Barbosa MD, Barrat FJ, Tchernev VT, Nguyen QA, Mishra VS, Colman Sd, Pastural E, Dufourcq-Lagelouse R, Fischer A, Holcombe RF, Wallace MR, Brandt SJ, de Saint Basile G, Kingsmore S. Identification of mutations in two major mRNA isoforms of the Chediak-Higashi syndrome gene in human and mouse. Hum Mol Genet 1997; 6:1091–1098.

56. Curnette JT, Whitten DM, Babior BM. Defective superoxide production by granulocytes from patients with chronic granulomatous disease. N Engl J Med 1974; 290:593–597.

57. Von Adrian UH, Berger EM, Ramezani L, Chambers JD, Ochs HD, Harlan JM, Paulson JC, Etzioni A, Arfors K. In vivo behavior of neutrophils from two patients

with distinct inherited leukocyte adhesion deficiency syndromes. J Clin Invest 1993; 91:2893–2897.

58. Walsh GM, Wardlaw AJ. Eosinophils. Pulmonary Defences. Chichester: Wiley, 1997.

59. Wardlaw AJ, Moqbel R, Kay AB. Eosinophils: biology and role in disease. Adv Immunol 1995; 60:151–266.

60. O'Neil SJ, Lesperance E, Klass DJ. Human lung lavage surfactant enhances staphylococcal phagocytosis by alveolar macrophages. Am Rev Respir Dis 1984; 130:1177–1179.

61. Laurenzi GA, Potter RT, Kass EH. Bacteriologic flora of the lower respiratory tract. N Engl J Med 1961; 265:1273–1278.

62. Reynolds HY, Newball HH. Analysis of proteins and respiratory cells obtained from human lungs by bronchial lavage. J Lab Clin Med 1974; 84:559–573.

63. Merrill WW, Naegel GP, Olchowski JJ, Reynolds HY. Immunoglobulin G subclass proteins in serum and lavage fluid of normal subjects: quantitation and comparison with immunoglobulins A and E. Am Rev Respir Dis 1985; 131:584–587.

64. Siber GR, Schur Ph, Aisenberg AC, Weitzman SA, Schiffman G. Correlation between serum IgG-2 concentrations and the antibody response to bacterial polysaccharide antigens. N Engl J Med 1980; 303:178–182.

65. Gross GN, Rehm Sr, Pierce AK. The effect of complement depletion on lung clearance of bacteria. J Clin Invest 1978; 62:373–378.

66. Robertson J, Goldwell JR, Castle JR, Waldman RH. Evidence for the presence of components of the alternative (properdin) pathway of complement activation in respiratory secretions. J Immunol 1976; 117:900–903.

67. Abraham SN, Arock M. Mast cells and basophils in innate immunity. Semin Immunol 1998; 10:373–381.

68. Galli SJ, Maurer M, Lantz CS. Mast cells as sentinels of innate immunity. Curr Opin Immunol 1999; 11:53–59.

2

Antigen-Presenting Cells

**HENK C. HOOGSTEDEN, HAMIDA HAMMAD, and
BART N. LAMBRECHT**

Erasmus University Medical Centre
Rotterdam, The Netherlands

I. Introduction

Allergic diseases, such as atopic dermatitis (AD), rhinitis (AR), and asthma (AA), are thought to result from a dysregulated immune response to commonly encountered antigens in genetically predisposed individuals. Immunological research into the mechanisms of allergy has identified cytokine production by T-helper 2 (Th2) effector lymphocytes as being critical for orchestrating allergic inflammation rich in eosinophils. Upon recognition of their cognate antigen, Th2 lymphocytes produce cytokines that regulate IgE synthesis, growth and activation of eosinophils and mast cells, and expression of endothelial cell adhesion molecules. Despite the wealth of experimental data implying allergen-specific Th2 cells as critical effector cells in the allergic response, less information is available on the generation of these cells from naive Th0 precursors. The first step in the allergic immune response is the uptake and presentation of allergen by professional antigen-presenting cells (APCs) such as dendritic cells (DCs), macrophages, and B lymphocytes. Immature DCs reside in the epithelia of the skin, upper and lower airways, and gut and have the potential to sense foreign antigens and nonspecific inflammatory tissue damage. Following recognition and uptake of Ag, mature DCs migrate to the T-cell-rich area of draining lymph nodes, display an array of Ag-derived peptides on the surface of major histocompatibility complex (MHC) molecules, and acquire the cellular specialization to select and activate naive Ag-specific T cells. Alveolar macrophages (Ams) are exposed to inhaled antigens but normally suppress immune responses in the lung. This chapter deals with the role of DCs and AMs in the generation of the immune response to inhaled allergens.

19

II. Dendritic Cells

A. Origin of Dendritic Cells

Human Studies

There are two subsets of DCs that originate from $CD34^+$ hematopoietic stem cells (HSCs) obtained from bone marrow or peripheral blood. Myeloid DCs or DC1s have a lineage relationship with monocytes and macrophages, whereas plasmacytoid DCs or DC2s have a lineage relationship with T cells (Fig. 1). Caux et al. showed that cord blood $CD34^+$ HSCs cultured in granulocyte-macrophage colony-stimulating factor (GM-CSF), stem cell factor, and tumor necrosis factor-α (TNF-α) differentiate along two myeloid DC pathways: the

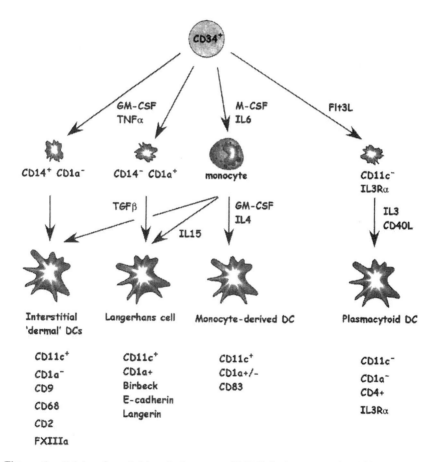

Figure 1 Origin of myeloid and plasmacytoid DCs in humans. The different growth factors that stimulate the development of a particular differentiation pathway are indicated. See text for further explanation.

Langerhans cell (LC) pathway in which $CD14^-CD1a^+$ DC precursors differentiated into $CD1A^+$, Lag^+, E cadherin$^+$, Birbeck granule$^+$ LCs; and the dermal DC pathway in which $CD14^+CD1a^-$ DC precursors differentiate into dermal DCs lacking those markers [1]. Transforming growth factor-β (TGF-β) can induce the formation of $CD1a^+$ LCs in these cultures. Alternatively, $CD34^+$ HSCs can differentiate into common lymphoid progenitors [giving rise to T cells, B cells, natural killer (NK) cells, and DCs] and plasmacytoid DCs (preDC2s) in a cytokine cocktail of Flt-3 ligand and stem cell factor [2].

Two distinct populations of DC precursors exist in the blood. Sallusto and Lanzavecchia have very elegantly shown that blood monocytes (preDC1s) can be induced to become myeloid DCs (DC1s) by culturing them for 7 days in GM-CSF and IL-4 or IL-13 [3]. This process also occurs spontaneously as blood monocytes leave the bloodstream through the endothelium and enter the extracellular matrix [4]. The addition of GM-CSF and IL-15 promotes the differentiation of blood monocytes into LCs [5]. Upon CD40 ligand activation, immature myeloid DC1s undergo maturation and produce large amounts of IL-12. The mature DC1s induced by CD40 ligand are able to polarize naive $CD4^+$ T cells into Th1 cells.

The second type of DC precursor cell, preDC2s (previously known as plasmacytoid T cell/monocyte), are characterized by a unique surface phenotype ($CD4^+IL-3R\alpha^{2+}CD45RA^+HLA-DR^+$ lineage marker-negative and $CD11C^-$) and at the ultrastructural level resemble Ig-secreting plasma cells. Several lines of evidence suggest that preDC2s are of lymphoid origin: (1) preDC2 lack expression of the myeloid antigens CD11c, CD13, CD33, and mannose receptor; (2) preDC2s isolated from the thymus express the lymphoid markers CD2, CD5, and CD7; (3) preDC2s have little phagocytic activity; (4) preDC2s do not differentiate into macrophages after culture with GM-CSF and M-CSF; (5) preDC2s express pre-TCR-α transcripts. PreDC2s differentiate into immature DC2s, when cultured with monocyte-conditioned medium, IL-3, interferon-α/β (IFN-α/β), and TNF-α, or viruses like herpes simplex virus or influenza virus [6]. Upon CD40 ligand activation, immature DC2s undergo maturation but produce low levels of IL-12. Mature DC2s are able to polarize naive $CD4^+$ T cells into a Th2 phenotype. Recent studies showed that the preDC2s are the elusive natural IFN-producing cells (IPCs), capable of producing high amounts of IFN-α/β upon viral stimulation. Taken together, preDC2/IPCs represent a unique hematopoietic lineage, capable of performing crucial functions both in innate and in adapted immunity.

Mouse Studies

In the mouse, three major DCs have been described. Lymphoid DCs are $CD8\alpha^+$ $CD11b^- CD11C^+$ cells that are found in the lymph nodes and spleen and induce Th1 responses by producing IL-12. Myeloid DCs are $CD8\alpha^- CD11b^+ CD11c^+$

that are found in peripheral tissues, lymph nodes, and spleen and induce Th2 responses (7). Recently, the murine counterpart of human plasmacytoid DCs (preDC2s) has been described in lymph nodes, spleen, and bone marrow as a $CD11b^-$ $CD8\alpha^-$ $CD11c^{dim}$ $B220^+$ $GR-1^+$ population that produces large amounts of IFN-α upon viral infection (8). The precise lineage relationship between these three forms of DCs is far from clear at present (9).

B. Immature DCs Reside in the Periphery to Take Up Antigen

The skin and mucosae of the body are continuously exposed to foreign antigens. Dendritic cells represent a significant proportion of cells lining these barriers. Even though it has been estimated that (LCs) represent only 1–3% of epidermal cells, the extension of cellular processes in between keratinocytes ensures that 25–30% of the skin barrier area is covered by LCs. Similarly, the mucosa of the nose and airway is covered with an extensive network of DCs that reside in the para- and intercellular channels surrounding the basal epithelial cells (Fig. 2). In the lung, the lateral intercellular space is sealed from the outside environment by epithelial tight junctions (10). To interact with DCs, potential aero-allergens must cross the lung epithelium and gain access to this space. In confluent airway epithelial cells, the cysteine proteinase enzymatic activity of

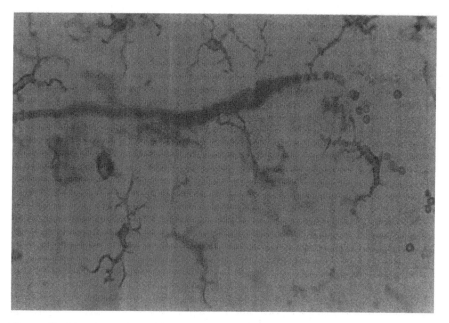

Figure 2 Mouse trachea stained with an antibody directed against MHC class II molecules demonstrating the network of DCs that is located in the upper layers of the airway epithelium. Occasional red blood cells can be seen.

Der p1—one of the major allergens of house dust mite (HDM)—led to cleavage of the tight junction protein occludin and to effective breakdown of the epithelial barrier function (11). In addition, DCs can direct their cell processes to the outer limits of the airway epithelium, without disrupting the integrity of the airway barrier by formation of tight junctions between their processes and epithelial cells.

In all nonlymphoid tissues, DCs are in a resting so-called immature state that is specialized for antigen uptake by three dominant mechanisms. First, antigenic material can be acquired via receptor-mediated endocytosis involving clathrin-coated pits. Immature DCs express a plethora of specialized cell receptors for patterns associated with foreign antigens, such as the C-type lectin carbohydrate receptors (langerin, DC-SIGN, dectin, BDCA-2, macrophage mannose receptor, and the unique carhobydrate receptor DEC-205) (12–16). Lectin receptor–mediated uptake by DCs results in a approximately 100-fold more efficient presentation to T cells, as compared to antigens internalized via fluid phase (16,17). Interestingly, langerin is a C-type lectin displaying mannose binding specificity and is exclusively expressed by DCs that display Birbeck granules (BGs), such as lung DCs and skin LCs. Pollen starch granules were shown to bind to C-type lectin receptors on AMs and DCs, although internalization occurred only in macrophages (18). Also, Pestel et al. recently demonstrated that Der p1 uptake into cultured DCs involves mannose receptor–mediated endocytosis and that this process is more efficient in DCs obtained from allergic donors. A second mechanism of antigen uptake is constitutive macropinocytosis that involves the actin skeleton–driven engulfment of large amounts of fluid and solutes (about one cell volume per hour) by the ruffling membrane of the DC followed by concentration of soluble antigen in the endocytic compartment (19). Macropinocytosis seems to be a dominant mechanism involved in the uptake of recombinant Bet v 1 and Phl p 1 pollen allergens by LCs and of Der p1 by cultured DCs, and can be inhibited by cytochalasin D and amiloride (20). Third, immature LCs and cultured DCs have been shown to phagocytose particulate antigens, such as latex beads and even whole bacteria, as well as apoptotic cells, and could be the dominant mechanism of uptake of particulate allergens (21).

The antigens that are taken up by any of the above mechanisms accumulate in the endocytic compartment, where they are loaded on newly synthesized and recycling MHC class II molecules but may also be transported into the cytosol, where they become accessible to the class I antigen presentation pathway (Fig. 3) (19,22,23). Within the endocytic compartment, antigen is cleaved into short immunogenic peptides by proteolytic enzymes of the cathepsin family. Antigen loading on MHC class II molecules occurs in an acidic cellular compartment rich in newly synthesized MHC class II molecules, called the MIIC compartment (24). This multivesicular complex is located at the intersection of the biosynthetic (ER, Golgi complex, secretory granules) and endocytic pathway of vesicle transport within the cell and contains

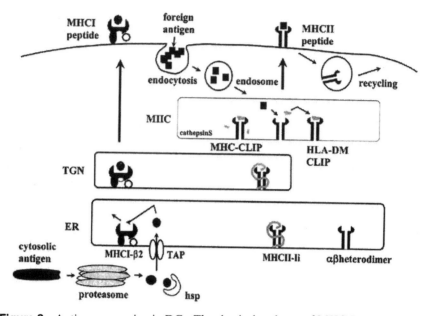

Figure 3 Antigen processing in DCs. The classical pathway of MHC-I presentation is initiated by the cytosolic degradation of protein antigen by the proteasome, a complex multicatalytic protease. This ubiquitin-dependent protein degradation generates peptide fragments of defined length ("molecular rule" function). These fragments bind to heat-shock proteins and target to an ATPase-dependent TAP transporter (*t*ransporter associated with *a*ntigen *p*resentation) on the endoplasmic reticulum (ER) membrane. The TAP transporter transports peptides (8–12 amino acids) to the lumen of the ER. Inside the ER, peptides are loaded onto newly synthesized MHC-I (α-chain and β_2-microglobulin) molecules. Chaperone molecules (tapasin, calnexin) prevent immature MHC-I molecules from being loaded with irrelevant endogenous ER proteins and disengage after high-affinity binding of cytosolic peptides. Peptide-loaded complexes are transported to the cell membrane after passing through the Golgi and *trans*-Golgi network (TGN). For successful expression of MHC-II–peptide complexes on the cell surface, endocytosed and partly digested antigen needs to be efficiently mixed with newly synthesized or recycling MHC-II molecules in a specialized subcellular compartment called MIIC. The highly polymorphic MHC-II molecules consist of an $\alpha\beta$ heterodimer that assembles in the ER with a third molecule, the invariant chain (Ii). After transport to the TGN, the MHC-II-Ii complex is targeted to the endocytic MIIC pathway, via a signal sequence on the Ii chain. In addition, some $\alpha\beta$–Ii complexes are directly targeted to the cell membrane, followed by recycling to the endocytic compartment. In the endocytic pathway invariant chain proteolysis by cathepsin-S generates the CLIP (*c*lass II associated *i*nvariant chain *p*eptide) fragment, which binds to the peptide-loading groove of the $\alpha\beta$ heterodimer. Binding of CLIP protects the peptide-binding groove from interacting with irrelevant ER peptides (generated for MHC-I loading). The CLIP fragment is then exchanged for immunogenic peptides, generated in the endocytic/lysosomal pathway by proteolysis of intact protein antigen into peptides 12–20 amino acids long. The exchange is catalyzed by HLA-DM. The binding of high-affinity antigenic peptide stabilizes the

the MHC II–related HLA-DM peptide exchanger that is essential for loading high-affinity antigenic peptides on MHC II (16,25,26). Alternatively, there is a pathway of peptide loading onto preformed MHC II molecules that have been internalized into mildly acidic endosomal vesicles after being expressed on the cell surface (16,27,28). Surprisingly, proteolysis of antigen by immature DCs can also occur extracellularly through secreted proteases, generating peptides that can be loaded onto empty cell surface–expressed MHC class II (29).

It is at present unclear how allergens are loaded onto MHC class II molecules by DCs. In sensitized individuals, internalization of allergens via receptor-mediated endocytosis by multivalent cross-linking of the high-affinity IgE receptor (FcεRI) on immature DCs targets the antigen to the MIIC compartment (30–32). In contrast, the generation of peptide–MHC complexes derived from macropinocytosis of Bet v 1 and Phl p 1 pollen allergens was shown to be inhibited only partly when the pH of the endosomes was altered, suggesting that part of the molecules were not metabolized in the lysosomal MIIC compartment (20).

C. DCs Migrate to the Draining Lymph Nodes to Stimulate Naive T Cells

The differential expression of chemokine receptors explains the complicated migration behavior of DCs (Fig. 4). Immature DCs express CC chemokine receptor-1 (CCR-1), CCR5, and most importantly CCR6, and are attracted to sites where inflammatory chemokines are expressed. (MIP) 3α is the CCR6 ligand that is expressed in normal skin keratinocytes and venular endothelial cells, the epithelium overlaying tonsil and Peyers' patch crypts, and probably lung epithelium, where it is involved in constitutive trafficking of CCR6$^+$ DCs (33–37). More importantly, MIP3α is strongly up-regulated in keratinocytes of inflamed skin and inflammatory tonsil crypts, and is the determining chemokine attracting immature LCs to these sites of inflammation (38). Another CCR6 ligand that is induced by lipopolysaccharide (LPS) and TNF-α is the epithelial β-defensin HBD-2 which can attract immature DCs in vitro (39).

A critical event in the induction of cellular immunity is for DCs to migrate from the infected peripheral tissues to the draining lymphoid organ, bearing antigens from the infecting agent (40). This migration has to occur against the chemotactic gradient that attracts immature DCs. As part of the maturation program that is induced by contact with pathogens or tissue damage, the

---

Figure 3 Continued. αβ heterodimer; HLA-DM binds the released CLIP fragment and physically disengages. Due to the loss of association with the intact invariant chain, stabilized αβ–peptide complexes are targeted to the cell membrane and are transiently expressed before being recycled via the endocytic pathway.

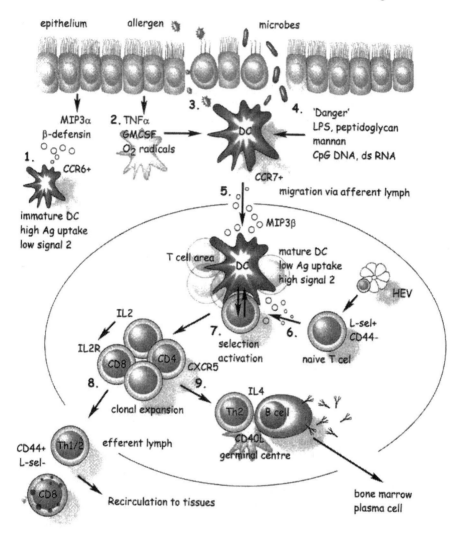

Figure 4 Induction of the primary immune response by DCs. **1.** Under baseline conditions and upon exposure to foreign antigens, epithelia produce *m*acrophage *in*-flammatory *p*rotein (MIP) 3α and β-defensin to attract CCR6+ immature DCs from the bloodstream. **2.** Resident cell types produce inflammatory mediators and growth factors that attract and activate the recently recruited DC. **3.** DCs capture allergens and other foreign antigens such as bacteria and viruses. **4.** DCs can discriminate between "dangerous" antigens, and nonpathogenic antigens such as self-antigens and probably most allergens, by recognizing certain viral and bacterial patterns. **5.** The recognition of infection and tissue damage up-regulates the CCR7 and CXCR4 and DCs migrate to the T-cell area of draining lymph nodes where the ligand MIP3β and SDF-1 is constitutively expressed. During this migration, DCs lose the capacity to take up antigen but become strong stimulators of naive T cells by their strong expression of signal 2. **6.** In the T-cell

expression of CCR6 is shut down whereas that of CCR7 and CXCR4 is increased, explaining why maturing DCs direct their interest to afferent lymphatics and T-cell area of draining lymph nodes where the CCR7 ligands SLC (secondary lymphoid chemokine, 6C-kine) and MIP3-β and the CXCR4 ligand SDF-1 (stromal cell–derived factor) are expressed (36,40). The stimulation of the CCR7 is crucial for entry of LCs into skin lymphatic vessels, migration to the draining lymph nodes, and for generation of contact hypersensitivity and delayed-type hypersensitivity reactions, as illustrated in mice with a targeted deletion of CCR7 or treated with antibodies against SLC (41–43).

D. Mature DCs Interact with Naive T Cells in the Lymph Node to Induce T-Cell Activation

When DCs have reached the T-cell area of draining lymph nodes, the antigen uptake capacity has been shut down completely and cellular specializations to stimulate naive T cells are acquired. This process involves attraction of naive T cells, provision of peptide-MHC to the T-cell receptor (TCR) (signal 1), and costimulation to T cells (signal 2; see Fig. 5). In the T-cell area, DCs produce chemokines for naive T cells (MIP3-β, DCCK-1) and resting T cells [monocyte-derived chemokine (MDC), thymus and activation-regulated chemokine (TARC)] that make up the scent of the T-cell zone (40). Attraction of naive T cells may help to ensure that DCs interact rapidly with multiple T cells, allowing efficient scanning for cells that recognize the antigen. Naive T cells repeatedly engage and disengage contact with antigen-bearing DCs via interaction of adhesion molecules such as DC-SIGN and CD54 interacting with ICAM-3 and CD11a/CD18 (13,44). This initial contact between DCs and T cells is not dependent on recognition of peptide-MHC by the TCR of the responding T cells yet allows partial activation of the T cell (45). The major function of these nonspecific interactions is to approximate the two cell types and allow the initial screening and serial triggering of the low-affinity TCR for recognition

---

Figure 4 Continued. area, DCs produce chemokines to attract naive T cells that continuously leave the bloodstream via the *h*igh *e*ndothelial *v*enules (HEV). 7. Naive T cells are first arrested and then selected for antigen specificity. The recognition of the correct peptide-MHC induces the activation of naive T cell, which will lead to further terminal differentiation of DC function. **8.** The activation of T cells leads to autocrine production of IL-2 and to clonal expansion of Ag-specific CD4$^+$ and CD8$^+$ T cells. These cells differentiate into effector cells that leave the lymph node via the efferent lymphatic. These effector cells are poised to migrate to peripheral tissues, especially to inflamed areas. **9.** Upon contact with DCs, some Ag-specific CD4$^+$ T cells up-regulate CXCR5 receptor and migrate to the B-cell follicles of the draining lymph node. Here they further interact with germinal center DCs to induce CD40L-dependent B-cell immunoglobulin switching and affinity maturation (germinal center reaction). Most high-affinity B cells go to the bone marrow to become Ig-producing plasma cells.

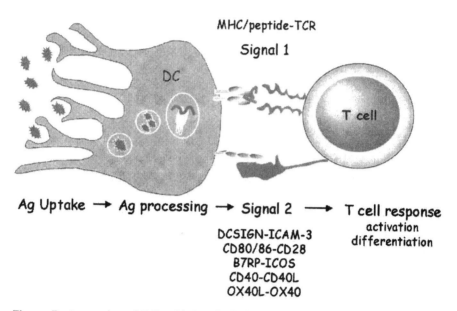

MHC/peptide-TCR

Signal 1

Ag Uptake → Ag processing → Signal 2 → T cell response

DCSIGN-ICAM-3   activation
CD80/86-CD28   differentiation
B7RP-ICOS
CD40-CD40L
OX40L-OX40

Figure 5 Interaction of DCs with T cells during the formation of the immunological synapse. See text for explanation.

of its specific peptide-MHC (46). As part of their maturation program, DCs that have migrated from the periphery express surface MHC II–peptide complexes and costimulatory molecules such as CD80 and CD86 for CD28 on the naive T cell (26,28). In T cells, a successful and sustained peptide–MHC/TCR interaction together with CD28 ligation induces supramolecular activation complexes (SMACs) consisting of concentric rings of lipid rafts that efficiently polarize and concentrate triggered TCRs, CD28, and signal transduction machinery toward the site of interaction with the DC—the immunological synapse (47). The TCR and engaged CD28 are selectively concentrated toward the central part of the immunological synapse, to react to peptide-MHC and costimulation, whereas integrins such as LFA-1 are selectively clustered toward the outer part of the immunological synapse. Similarly, DCs concentrate CD86 and peptide–MHC complexes in lipid rafts or tetraspan microdomains on their membrane surface, toward sites of T-cell contant (26,48,49). Triggered by these mechanisms, activated T cells express CD40L and TRANCE that lead to increased survival and terminal maturation of DCs by up-regulating CD80, CD86, and cytokine production, further sustaining the cognate interaction (21). The end result is that the induction of T-cell division by antigen-loaded DCs is very rapid in vivo and that 2 days after injection of DCs some antigen-specific T cells have already divided twice. Another 24–48 h later, divided cells have acquired effector phenotype and migrate from the draining node to the periphery (50).

E. Dendritic Cells Determine Th-Cell Polarization

As DCs are the vehicle of immunity after exposure to foreign antigens, not surprisingly they also determine the polarization of Th responses after arrival in the draining nodes. This issue has received considerable attention in the most recent literature and is reviewed in Chapter 11 (51–53). Various pathways of regulation are operative to induce an optimal T-cell response. Immature DCs can be instructed by the characteristics of the antigen or its accompanying adjuvant to induce a Th1, a Th2, or an undifferentiated Th0 response. The microbe-derived pattern molecules inducing Th1 responses do so by enhancing the production of bioactive IL-12 p70 in DCs, via triggering of ancient innate immune receptors expressed on DCs (54). The Toll-like receptors (TLRs) are widely expressed on DCs and mediate LPS-induced IL-12 production by enhancing the cellular levels of NF-κB transcription factors (55). Liu et al. demonstrated that monocytes preferentially express TLR 1, 2, 4, 5, and 8, and that plasmacytoid preDC2s strongly express TLR 7 and 9. In accordance with these TLR expression profiles, monocytes respond to the known microbial ligands for TLR2 (peptidoglycan, lipoteichoic acid) and TLR4 (lipopolysaccharide), by producing TNF-α and IL-6. Monocyte-derived DC1s preferentially express TLR 1, 2, and 3 and respond to TLR 2–ligand PGN by producing large amounts of TNF-α, and to viral double-stranded RNA by producing IFN-α and IL-12. In contrast, plasmacytoid preDC2s only respond to the microbial TLR9-ligand, CpG-ODNs (oligodeoxynucleotides containing unmethylated CpG motifs), by producing IFN-α. The expression of distinct sets of TLRs and the corresponding difference in reactivity to microbial molecules among subsets of DCs support the concept that they have developed through distinct evolutionary pathways to recognize different microbial antigens (56).

However, the paradigm that DCs exposed to microbial factors are stable inducers of Th1 immunity is gradually shifting. Indeed, microbial products need additional host-derived microenvironmental instruction (in the form of IFN-γ or even IL-4) to induce stable IL-12 production in DCs (57). Moreover, after activation by LPS, monocyte-derived human DCs produce IL-12 only transiently and become refractory to further IL-12 production upon interaction with CD40L$^+$ T cells. Soon after stimulation DCs prime strong Th1 responses, whereas at later time points the same cells preferentially prime Th2 and nonpolarized T cells (58). Not only does the production of IL-12 go down, but there is also a gradual decrease in the number of DCs reaching the draining lymph nodes. When DCs stimulate naive T cells at low stimulator/responder ratios, Th2 polarization is favored despite the presence of IL-12 (59). Recently, it was proposed that the developmental lineage of DCs can determine either Th1 or Th2 polarization; hence, the terminology DC1 or DC2 (53,60). In the original description, monocyte-derived DC1s (i.e., myeloid DCs) induced IL-12-dependent Th1 responses, whereas DC2s derived from IL3Rα$^+$ CD4$^+$ CD3$^-$ CD11c$^-$ plasmacytoid precursor cells (i.e., lymphoid DCs) induced IL-4-independent Th2 responses pre-ferentially (60,61). However, follow-up studies have shown that additional levels of regulation determine the outcome of Th differentiation by mo-DCs. Also, it was shown that mo-DCs could be separated into a CD1a$^+$ or CD1a$^-$ subpopulation, inducing Th1 or Th2 responses, respectively. Although both subsets express similar levels of constimulatory molecules, IL-12 production is completely lacking in CD1a$^-$ mo-DCs, even after stimualtion with anti-CD40, LPS, and IFN-γ (62). In conclusion, priming of Th responses by DCs is very flexible, allowing the simultaneous generation of Th1, Th2, and Th0 responses.

F. Phenotype of Human Lung DCs

Holt was the first to demonstrate the network of HLA-DR-positive DCs in human central airways (63). We have studied the phenotype of lung DCs. Macro-phages, identified as large, rounded, acid phosphatase–positive cells, were mainly detected in the alveolar spaces, in the lumen of the bronch(iol)us, and in the bronchoalveolar lavage (BAL). They were positive for MHC class II anti-gens (DR, DQ), CD68, RFD7, RFD9, and partly positive for RFD1. Irregularly shaped cells with a marker pattern comparable to that of blood-derived DC (positive for DR, DQ, L25, RFD1, and CD68) were predominantly observed in the epithelium and subepithelial tissue of the bronch(iol)us and in the bronchus-associated lymphoid tissue. In the epithelium, approximately 30% of these cells were positive for CD1a (OKT6). In the subepithelial tissue, these DC formed characteristic small clusters with T cells. The BAL, the alveolar spaces, and the alveolar walls contained only a small number of DC. These immuno-histological data suggest that the bronch(iol)us is well equipped to initiate immune responses (64). Subsequent studies demonstrated that CD1a$^+$ DCs expressed the LC marker S100 and were better APCs than the CD1a$^-$ DCs in the lung (65). Nicod's group has extensively studied lung DCs as well. Lung DCs were shown to express some characteristics of in vitro immature DC. These are (1) low expression of the costimulatory molecules CD40, CD80, and CD86; (2) poor expression of the differentiation marker CD83 and no CD1a; and (3) good capacity to incorporate dextran due to expression of the macrophage mannose receptor. Lung DCs express moderate levels of CCR1 and CCR5, and carry mRNA for CCR6. However, lung DCs, like in vitro mature DCs, express high levels of MHC class II molecules, show low expression of CD14 and CD64, and are characterized by their high capacity to stimulate allogeneic T cells to proliferate during mixed leukocyte reactions (MLRs). Although lung DC express low levels of CD80 and CD86, the important role of these costimu-latory molecules in inducing high MLRs was demonstrated by using blocking antibodies. Therefore, while lung DCs have overall a phenotype and an endo-cytic capacity close to in vitro immature DCs, they share, like in vitro mature DCs, a powerful capacity to stimulate T cells (15). These studies have been performed mainly in BAL fluid and interstitial DCs. By contrast, few data are available on the phenotype of bronchial wall DCs. They have been shown to be HLA-DR$^+$, CD1a$^+$ (30%), L25$^+$, and langerin$^+$ (66).

G. Dendritic Cells in Animal Models of Allergy

It is only recently that DCs have been studied in murine models of allergy, such as the rodent asthma model of ovalbumin (OVA)–induced eosinophilic airway inflammation. In early studies, Holt et al. demonstrated that rat airway DCs can be rapidly recruited to sites of inflammation, capture inhaled OVA, and process it into an immunogenic form on MHC class II molecules. The function of lung DCs is suppressed by secreted products of alveolar macrophages (e.g., nitric oxide) that keep them in an immature antigen capture mode (67). These immature myeloid DCs do not produce IL-12 and induce Th2-dependent immunoglobulin production after intravenous transfer into naive rats (68). After transfer of OVA-pulsed bone marrow–derived DCs into the trachea, we have recently shown that mice and rats can be sensitized to develop eosinophilic airway inflammation and goblet cell hyperplasia, controlled by IL-4 and IL-5–producing Th2 CD4$^+$ cells (69,70). The sensitization process occurred after migration of immature DCs into the draining mediastinal lymph nodes (50). Primary exposure to OVA via the respiratory route is normally a tolerogenic event. However, when endogenous airway DCs were activated by transgenic expression of GM-CSF or by concomitant viral infection with influenza virus, tolerance was avoided and eosinophilic airway inflammation ensured (71,72). From these models, it appears that DCs are responsible for sensitization to inhaled allergen. More importantly, DCs are also attracted from the bone marrow and the bloodstream to sites of eosinophilic airway inflammation during the secondary immune response to OVA and are functionally important for the maintenance of eosinophilic airway inflammation and IgE synthesis in sensitized mice, identifying the DC as a target for therapeutic intervention (73–75).

H. Dendritic Cells in Human Allergy

Dendritic Cells and the Hygiene Hypothesis

From the above discussion it seems likely that human DCs are also implicated in Th2 sensitization to common allergens in genetically predisposed individuals. It has been proposed that during the neonatal period and early infancy—the peak period of sensitization—DCs are functionally immature, failing to counterbalance the default Th0/Th2 priming to common allergens at this age (76). A failure of proper education of the immune system by reduced exposure to environmental microbial load—a consequence of the western lifestyle—could explain why DCs are not instructed to produce IL-12 and fail to counteract Th2 responses. Alternatively, an intrinsic deficiency in

IL-12 production has been described in blood monocytes (i.e., precursors of DCs) of AD and AA patients, although this could be the consequence of the allergic phenotype rather than its origin and recent data suggest that there is no difference in IL-12 production in mo-DCs between atopics and non-atopics (77,78). Another explanation could be the nature of the allergen exposure. Chronic low-level exposure to inhaled allergens could lead to low levels of DCs continuously migrating to the lymph nodes and inducing sustained TCR ligation at low stimulator/responder ratios, conditions known to bias toward Th2 responses (58,59). Administration of allergen-pulsed DCs to humans to prove that they elicit sensitization is is unethical. However, DCs have been used as therapeutic vaccines in immunotherapy for melanoma and other cancers. There has been one report of induction of novel Th2-dependent sensitization to bovine serum albumin—used in the autologous DC preparation—after repeated injection of DCs, which led to anti-bovine albumin IgE and anaphylactic reactions (79).

Dendritic Cells Accumulate at Sites of Allergic Inflammation

The function of DCs in patients with established allergic disease is more relevant from a therapeutic perspective. Increased numbers of CD1a$^+$ DCs can be found in the nose of AR patients, in lesional skin of AD patients, and in the bronchial epithelium of stable AA patients (80–85). The DCs in the airways of AA patients were found in close proximity of IL-4 and GM-CSF-producing cell types, suggesting that local differentiation of monocytes into DCs could be behind the observed increase (83). Out-of-season topical allergen challenge to the nose of AR patients is accompanied by a further recruitment of intra-epithelial CD1a$^+$ DCs as well as recruitment of distinct lamina propria CD4$^+$ IL3Rα^+ (CD123$^+$) CD11c$^-$ CD1a$^-$ plasmacytoid DCs (precursor DC2s, see above) (86,87). The latter cells expressed high levels of L-selectin and were shown to accumulate together with naive T cells at endothelial venules expressing the L-selectin ligand peripheral node addressin (PNAd). Recently, it was shown that allergen challenge of atopic asthmatics induced an increase in CD1a$^+$ HLA-DR$^+$ myeloid—but not plasmacytoid—DCs 4 h after allergen challenge (88). This increase was accompanied by a decrease in circulating myeloid DCs, suggesting direct recruitment of DCs from the bloodstream (89). The question as to what role the plasmacytoid DCs (preDC2s) have to play in asthma is less clear. It was shown that the percentage of these cells in peripheral blood is enhanced in atopic patients, correlating well with IgE and circulating eosinophil levels. In atopic patients, IL-4 enhances the survival of DC2 cells, whereas in nonatopics it induces apoptosis (60,90). Interestingly, IL3Rα^+ plasmacytoid DC2s did not accumulate in nasal polyps or other mucosal inflammatory lesions, suggesting that they are specifically associated with AR (87).

Functional Comparison of DCs from Atopic and Nonatopic Individuals

The function of DCs of patients with or without atopic diseases has been compared in vitro. It was shown that immature mo-DCs from AA have an enhanced allostimulatory function and higher levels of CD11b and HLA-DR compared with non-atopic patients, although others have refuted this idea (78,91). When mo-DCs were pulsed with relevant allergen (Der p1 and 2, Bet v1) and cultured with autologous naive or memory T cells, they induced both Th1 and Th2 cytokines—but predominantly Th2 when atopic donors were used—despite similar IL-2 production (78,92–94). The addition of rIL-12 induced a separate IFN-γ producing subset without decreasing the IL-5 producing subset, whereas addition of anti-IL-12 reduced bulk IFN-γ production without affecting IL-4 production. Interestingly, culture of DCs on collagen type I could strongly enhance IL-12 production in DCs and induce IFN-γ and reduce IL-5 in allergen specific T cells (95). These data confirm that DCs can efficiently stimulate human allergen-specific memory Th2 cells to produce Th2 cytokines and maybe contribute to ongoing allergic inflammation (74, 96).

Dendritic Cells Are Uniquely Sensitive to the Enzymatic Effect of Der p1

The interaction between aeroallergens and lung DCs is allowed only if these allergens cross the barrier function of the lung epithelium. Der p1, one of the major allergens of the HDM *Dermatophagoides pteronyssinus*, displays a cysteine protease enzymatic activity responsible for the cleavage of the tight junction protein occludin, thus increasing the accessibility of DCs residing beneath the epithelial barrier (11). Der p 1 has direct effects on DCs as well (Fig. 6). The effect of Der p1 on monocyte-derived DCs of HDM-sensitive patients and healthy donors was compared. It was shown that Der p1 could induce the maturation of DCs obtained from HDM allergic patients by increasing the expression of the costimulatory molecule CD86 and of CCR7, the receptor for the chemokines SLC and MIP 3β expressed in afferent lymphatic vessels (94 and unpublished). Der p 1 also enhanced the release of IL-10 and of the Th2 chemokines TARC and MDC [96a]. The enzymatic activity of Der p1 was necessary for these observed effects as pro Der p1 did not induce any of these changes. In contrast, Der p1 enhanced the production of the pro-Th1 cytokine IL-12 and of the Th1-attracting chemokine IP-10 by DCs from healthy donors (94). Moreover, the allergic state per se was not responsible for the observed effect of Der p1 in HDM-sensitive patients as Der p1 induced changes similar to healthy controls in pollen-sensitive allergic patients. Additional data confirmed that DCs from HDM allergic patients exposed to Der p1 favored the recruitment and the stimulation of allergen-specific memory Th2 cells, whereas DCs from healthy donors exposed to Der p1 promoted recruitment and stimulation of Th1 cells. Consistent with the in vitro data, we were able

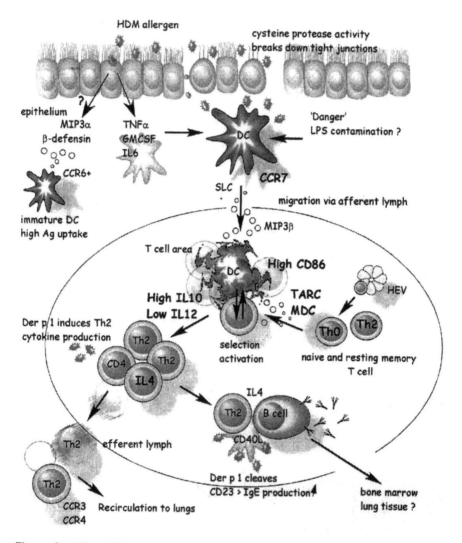

Figure 6 Effect of Der p1 on the immune response induced by DCs. Der p1 activates the bronchial epithelium to release inflammatory chemokines. It also cleaves tight junction proteins to gain access to the epithelial DCs. Upon recognition of Der p1, the expression of the CCR7 chemokine receptor is enhanced, leading to the migration of DCs toward the draining lymph nodes, where the ligands SLC and MIP3β are expressed. Here, Der p1 exposed DCs lead to preferential activation of Th2 cells by expression of CD86 and by production of IL-10 in the absence of IL-12. Moreover, Der p1 exposed DCs selectively attract Th2 cells by production of MDC and TARC. Der p1 also stimulates B-cell IgE synthesis by cleavage of CD23 into soluble CD23.

to show in a humanized SCID mouse model that monocyte-derived DCs from HDM patients pulsed with Der p1 migrated strongly to the draining lymph nodes and significantly enhanced the cellular infiltration of human allergen-specific T cells in the lungs of challenged mice and boosted the formation of allergen-specific IgE (96a, 97).

I. Possible Role of DCs in Perpetuating Allergic Inflammation

From the above paragraphs it is clear that DCs have roles in the generation of allergic inflammation that are far beyond their role in sensitization. Why would DCs be such important cells in ongoing allergic inflammation (Fig. 7)?

Provision of Costimulation to Memory T Cells Depends on DCs

It is possible that memory T cells in vivo are more dependent on costimulation than can be appreciated from in vitro data, and therefore rely on a professional APC that can provide these stimuli. Indeed, allergen-induced IL-4 and IL-13 production in bronchial explants and in peripheral blood cells from asthmatics is dependent on delivery of costimulation via the CD80/CD86 pathway (98). Similarly, animal models have shown that eosinophilic airway inflammation in sensitized mice can be suppressed by blocking the CD80/CD86-CD28 pathway. As airway DCs are the predominant cells expressing costimulatory molecules, proper activation of resting Th2 cells to become effector cells may depend on these cells.

Airway DCs Target Allergens via IgE

Alternatively, DCs may be critical for the recognition of allergen via specific IgE bound to the high-affinity or low-affinity (CD23) receptor for IgE. In this regard, an interesting study by Coyle et al. demonstrated that memory Th2 lymphocytes of sensitized mice failed to produce Th2 cytokines upon recognition of inhaled allergen when allergen-specific IgE was captured by a non-anaphylactogenic anti-IgE antibody (99). The CD1a$^+$ LCs in the skin of AD patients and DCs in the nose and bronchi of AR and AA patients contain the high-affinity IgE receptor Fcε RI (84,100). Despite the fact that the α chain of this receptor is expressed intracellularly on most LCs of controls and atopics, the surface expression is highly up-regulated in atopic patients and correlates with the level of serum IgE (32,100). Recently, the expression of this receptor on blood DCs of atopic asthmatic patients was studied. The total expression of FcεRI on the surface of DCs from healthy and asthmatic subjects was not significantly different. However, in vivo, DCs from AA subjects had higher levels of receptor occupancy by IgE and bound exogenous IgE in vitro more efficiently than DCs from healthy subjects, suggesting a higher affinity or longer stability of IgE binding to its receptor. At least in AD and AR patients, the LCs are covered with monomeric IgE which suggests that FcεRI functions as an allergen-focusing molecule and that allergens are more efficiently taken up, processed,

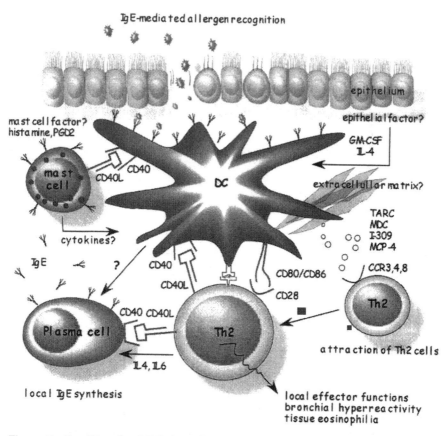

Figure 7 Possible role of DCs in maintaining chronic eosinophilic airway inflammation. Allergen targeting to the DCs occurs via membrane-bound IgE, leading to efficient uptake of allergens. During chronic inflammation, DCs interact with many cell types, including mast cells, epithelial cells, and fibroblasts. Mediators released by these cells can activate the DC so that it is induced to mature and to attract memory Th2 cells through release of Th2-selective chemokines. MDC, *m*onocyte-*d*erived *c*hemokine; TARC, *t*hymus and *a*ctivation-*r*egulated *c*hemokine.

and presented to T cells following targeting via FcεRI (81,86). Critically lowering atopic individuals' threshold to mount allergen-specific T-cell responses would result in the perpetuation of allergen-specific IgE production (type I reactions) and perhaps even in the occurrence of T-cell-mediated delayed-type hypersensitivity reactions in allergen-exposed tissues. It was recently reported that only those atopic patients having IgE on their LCs develop eczematous skin lesions upon epicutaneous application of aeroallergens (101). Therefore, reducing the levels of allergen-specific IgE, either by non-anaphylactogenic anti-IgE monoclonals (E25) or by allergen avoidance, can be seen as a therapeutic strategy that extends beyond its effects on IgE-mediated effector mechanisms (i.e., mast cell degranulation).

Allergic Inflammation Promotes Local Antigen Presentation by DCs

Finally, DCs could be critical for maintaining a chronic localized immune response in the airways (Fig. 8). Much emphasis has been put forward that chronic asthma is a localized disease, as evidenced by the transfer of the disease by lung transplantation into nonasthmatic patients. It is tempting to speculate that the presence of chronic inflammation and airway structural changes leads to local maturation of DCs and to antigen presentation occurring in the

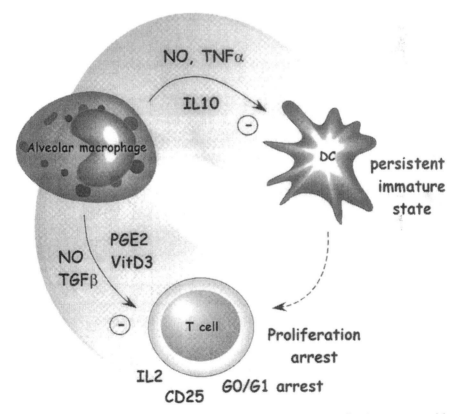

Figure 8 Immune regulation in the alveolar compartment. Following contact with activated T cells, alveolar macrophages directly suppress the proliferation of T cells, so that they are arrested into the G_0/G_1 phase of the cell cycle. In addition, AM also suppress the function of resident DCs to keep these in an immature state, unable to activate T cells. This mechanism protects the alveolus from overt damage.

airways. The cytokines TNF-α, GM-CSF, and IL-4 are expressed in asthmatic epithelium and have the potential to up-regulate the costimulatory capacity and survival of DCs. Abnormal responses of the epithelium in asthma have been clearly demonstrated (Chap. 8) and DCs could well form the link between these epithelial changes and chronic changes in the T-cell response to allergens. Alternatively, DCs might communicate with mast cells to perpetuate allergic inflammation. Mast cells in asthmatic airways express CD40L and produce cytokines that can activate DCs and prolong their survival in tissues (102). Upon activation by cross-linking of membrane-bound IgE during the early response to allergens, mast cells release mediators such as histamine, PGD$_2$, and leukotrienes. Histamine has profound effects on DCs in vitro through the histamine H$_1$ and H$_2$ receptor. It reduces the production of IL-12, at the same time boosting IL-10 synthesis, and modifies the behavior of DCs so as to become a Th2 polarizing cell type (103,104). Leukotrienes influence the migration of DCs toward the draining lymph nodes and could be responsible for keeping DCs immobilized within sites of allergic inflammation (105). The process of airway remodeling leads to the deposition of extracellular matrix components (collagens, fibronectin, heparan sulfate) that have the capacity to enhance DC differentiation and costimulatory function.

In addition to their potential to activate T cells in the airways, myeloid DCs produce chemokines that preferentially attract recently activated Th2 cells. In this regard, monocyte-derived DCs have been shown to produce the CC chemokines *m*onocyte-*d*erived *c*hemokine (MDC) and *t*hymus and *a*ctivation-*r*egulated *c*hemokine (TARC), which attract recently activated Th2 cells expressing CCR4 (106). Activation of DCs induces the mRNA for *m*onocyte *c*hemotactic *p*rotein MCP-4 and I-309, the ligands for CCR3 and CCR8 receptors, also expressed on Th2 cells (107,108). In this way, DCs ensure that the recently activated effector cells are attracted and retained in the airways and do not migrate back to the draining lymph nodes. Moreover, it has been shown that chronic antigen presentation by DCs leads to neoformation of organized lymphoid structures within peripheral tissues, such as the pancreas (109). These organized follicles contain high endothelial venules, specialized for the extravasation of lymphocytes, and are the sites of local immunoglobulin production. It is speculative that repetitive presentation of antigen to Th2 cells by DCs in the airways would also lead to formation of these aggregates and to local production of IgE. At least in rodents, repetitive inhalation of allergen in sensitized animals leads to the formation of organized lymphoid tissues in the airways.

It is challenging to suggest that studying local presentation by DCs might offer some answers to the mysteries surrounding atopic disease. It could be the reason why some atopic individuals develop chronic eosinophilic airway inflammation and airway remodeling, whereas others do not. Moreover, the presence of ongoing airway inflammation in asthmatic patients who have avoided allergen exposure for years (e.g., baker's asthma) could be explained by ongoing local activation of DCs induced by the structural changes of the airways, followed by sustained nonspecific activation of Th2 cells and perpetuation of the disease. Finally, modulation of the localized DC-driven immune response by tissue-specific factors (e.g., derived from epithelial cells or keratinocytes) might also be the answer for the individual tissue-specific manifestation of allergic disease, which can occur either separately or simultaneously in the skin, nose, or lung.

J. Targeting DCs as a Therapeutic Strategy for Asthma

Studies in mice with an inducible depletion of airway DCs have clearly shown that reduction of airway DC function leads to a complete absence of airway inflammation upon challenge with relevant allergen in sensitized animals (74). Therefore, DCs are clearly novel targets for intervention in asthma. Our current standard therapy of allergic diseases—the regular use of corticosteroids—has profound effects on the function of DCs in inflamed tissues. It was shown that regular use of inhaled corticosteroids reduces the number of DCs in the airways and nose of AA and AR patients (82,110,111). Systemic and inhaled steroids inhibit the differentiation and maturation process of DCs and induce the apoptosis of lung DCs (112–114). Interestingly, exposure of immature mouse and human DCs to steroids leads to a phenotype that induces T-suppressor cells that could down-regulate Th1-mediated inflammation (115,116). Systemic steroids also reduce the numbers of circulating plasmacytoid DCs (preDC2), although the significance of these findings is less clear (117). More studies are needed to address the effects of current and future therapeutics on human DCs in vivo.

III. Macrophages

The lung contains a large variety of macrophages of which the phenotype and function varies considerably in baseline and inflammatory conditions. However, the vast majority in the lung are alveolar macrophages (AMs) and interstitial macrophages (IMs).

A. Origin of Alveolar Macrophages

AMs also originate from a $CD34^+$ HSC and differentiate along the myeloid pathway under the influence of M-CSF and IL-6. These cells have therefore a lineage relationship with DCs. The immediate precursors of lung macrophages are blood monocytes, which have the potential to differentiate into macrophages upon arrival in the lung tissues and alveolar compartment. Apart from a bone marrow supply, it has been demonstrated by bone marrow irradiation experiments that alveolar macrophages derive also from a local proliferating pool of precursor macrophages that respond to M-CSF (118).

B. Function of AM in Baseline Conditions

Phagocytosis of Inhaled Particulate Antigens

The predominant function of AMs is to phagocytose inhaled particulate antigens and to effectively sequester these antigens from the immune system. Therefore, AMs are endowed with many receptors, such as CR1 and CR3 complement receptors, Fc receptors for opsonized antigens, macrophage mannose receptor, as well as scavenger receptors. A very efficient system of phagolysosomes fuses with endocytosed particles to neutralize the ingested material. Kradin has very elegantly demonstrated that AMs sequester inhaled particulate antigens to shield them from the specific immune system induced by DCs. A pulmonary cellular immune response is generated to an inhaled particulate antigen when the protective phagocytic capacities of the lung are exceeded and antigen can interact directly with interstitial DCs. The diversion of particulate antigens by pulmonary phagocytes may help to limit undesirable pulmonary inflammation while allowing the generation of antigen-specific immune lymphocytes in vivo (119).

Suppression of T-Cell Activation in the Lung

The lung is continually exposed to the outside world and thus is a portal of entry for microbial invasion to which a defense reaction must be mounted. At the same time it has a delicate gas-exchange mechanism that should be protected from overtly distorting inflammatory responses. It has been estimated that as many as half of the total pool of lymphocytes ($\cong 10 \times 10^9$ lymphocytes) as well as a large number of nonspecific immune cells are continuously located in the pulmonary vascular bed, interstitium, and BAL fluid (120). More than 90% of T cells in human and animal lung express the phenotype of memory cells, which suggests previous encounter with antigen (121). Despite this enormous potential for antigen reactivity and T-cell-mediated pathology, the lung is protected from mounting an immune response to harmless antigens by a variety of nonspecific barriers (mucociliary transport, bacteriostatic molecules, etc.), while allowing the induction of adaptive immunity when these barriers are breached by pathogenic antigens. Dendritic cells and macrophages are at the focal point of the control mechanisms that maintain immunological homeostasis in the lung and airways (Fig. 8).

Although AMs are ideally exposed to inhaled antigen, numerous studies have demonstrated that these cells are weak APCs for lymphocyte responses and even actively suppress the activation of T cells (122). T cells stimulated in the presence of AMs are only partially activated and fail to divide because of IL-2 unresponsiveness (123–125). This could be caused in part by the absence of signal 2 (CD80) on AMs or the production of suppressive molecules such as TGF-β, NO, IL-1 receptor antagonist, or PGE$_2$ (126–128.) Moreover, AMs actively suppress the function of airway and interstitial DC (129). The strongest evidence for a suppressive role in vivo comes from experiments in which AMs were depleted by instillation of liposomes filled with the toxic molecules dichloromethylene diphosphonate. The primary immune response to inhaled antigen is not affected, but secondary responses in primed animals are characterized by increased T-cell activation, tissue inflammation, and Th2-dependent IgE production (130–132).

C. Function of AM in Inflammatory Conditions and Asthma

Under inflammatory conditions, fresh monocytes and DCs are recruited to the airways and these cells "dilute" the immunosuppressive AMs, allowing a window phase in which T-cell responses can be induced. Freshly recruited monocytes and alveolar macrophages produce a variety of inflammatory mediators (Fig. 9). The local production of GM-CSF in these conditions can also switch the immunosuppressive AMs into a stimulatory cell (133). In humans, the recently recruited AMs can be discriminated from the resident AMs by means of staining with the combination of RFD1/RFD7, initially described by Spiteri and Poulter. Using these antibodies, it was shown that $RFD1^+/RFD7^-$ AMs have a stimulating function, whereas the $RFD1^+/RFD7^+$ and $RFD1^-/RFD7^+$ subsets have a suppressive function on T cells. Strikingly, the RFD1 marker is also expressed on lung DCs (64,134). The airways of AA patients and of sarcoidosis patients contain increased amounts of $RFD1^+$ AMs.

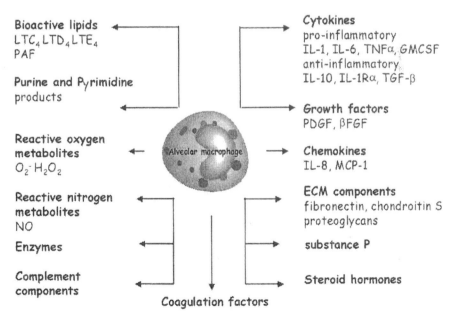

Bioactive lipids
LTC_4 LTD_4 LTE_4
PAF

Purine and Pyrimidine products

Reactive oxygen metabolites
O_2^- H_2O_2

Reactive nitrogen metabolites
NO

Enzymes

Complement components

Alveolar macrophage

Cytokines
pro-inflammatory
IL-1, IL-6, TNFα, GMCSF
anti-inflammatory
IL-10, IL-1Rα, TGF-β

Growth factors
PDGF, βFGF

Chemokines
IL-8, MCP-1

ECM components
fibronectin, chondroitin S proteoglycans

substance P

Steroid hormones

Coagulation factors

Figure 9 Secretory products of alveolar macrophages.

Numerous studies have demonstrated that the phenotype and function of AMs in patients with asthma are fundamentally different from those in healthy controls. Most notably has been the increased expression of CD80 and/or CD86, CD1a, ICAM-1, and LFA-1 and of the low-affinity receptor for IgE on AMs from patients with AA (135–138). Conversely, the expression of CD40 is lower in the AMs of asthma patients (139). When compared with healthy controls, the AMs of patients with AA produce more IL-1, IL-6, TNF-α, and IL-10, and less IL-12, explaining their preferential induction of Th2 responses (140,141). When AMs of AA patients were cocultured with syngeneic $CD4^+$ T cells, they induced the production of IL-5. In the same experiments, the AMs of healthy controls suppressed IL-5 production. In some experiments, the production of IL-5 could be inhibited by blocking antibodies against CD80 and/or CD86, IL-1, IL-6, or TNF-α (142–144). Conversely, antibodies to CD40 enhanced the AM-induced IL-5 production by T cells (139). These studies suggest that AMs from AA patients can activate effector function in Th2 cells, at least in vitro.

IV. Conclusion

Recent advances in immunology, cell biology, and in animal models of allergy have identified DCs as the principal APCs involved in the induction and maintenance of Th2 allergic responses and AMs as suppressors of T-cell activation. In human asthma, however, it is clear that AMs can have an activated phenotype that contributes to T-cell stimulation. It can be foreseen that in the near future studies on the functional role of these cells in humans will lead to an increased insight in the pathogenesis of allergic diseases and hopefully to better strategies for preventing and managing these conditions.

References

1. Caux C, Dezutter Dambuyant C, Schmitt D, Banchereau J. GM-CSF and TNF-alfa cooperate in the generation of dendritic Langerhans cells. Nature 1992; 360:258–261.
2. Blom B, Ho S, Antonenko S, Liu YJ. Generation of interferon alpha-producing predendritic cell (Pre-DC)2 from human CD34(+) hematopoietic stem cells. J Exp Med 2000; 192:1785–1796.
3. Sallusto F, Lanzavecchia A. Efficient presentation of soluble antigen by cultured human dendritic cells is maintained by granulocyte/macrophage colony-stimulating factor plus interleukin 4 and downregulated by tumor necrosis factor alfa. J Exp Med 1994; 179:1109–1118.
4. Randolph GJ, Beaulieu S, Lebecque S, Steinman RM, Muller WA. Differentiation of monocytes into dendritic cells in a model of transendothelial trafficking. Science 1998; 282:480–483.

5. Mohamadzadeh M, Berard F, Essert G, Chalouni C, Pulendran B, Davoust J, Bridges G, Palucka AK, Banchereau J. Interleukin 15 skews monocyte differentiation into dendritic cells with features of Langerhans cells. J Exp Med 2001; 194:1013–1020.

6. Grouard G, Rissoan MC, Filgueira L, Durand I, Banchereau J, Liu YJ. The enigmatic plasmacytoid T cells develop into dendritic cells with interleukin (IL)-3 and CD40-ligand. J Exp Med 1997; 185:1101–1111.

7. Maldonado-Lopez R, De Smedt T, Michel P, Godfroid J, Pajak B, Heirman C, Thielemans K, Leo O, Urbain J, Moser M. CD8alpha+ and CD8alpha− Subclasses of dendritic cells direct the development of distinct T helper cells in vivo. J Exp Med 1999; 189:587–592.

8. Asselin-Paturel C, Boonstra A, Dalod M, Durand I, Yessaad N, Dezutter-Dambuyant C, Vicari A, O'Garra A, Biron C, Briere F, Trinchieri G. Mouse type I IFN-producing cells are immature APCs with plasmacytoid morphology. Nat Immunol 2001; 2:1144–1150.

9. del Hoyo GM, Martin P, Arias CF, Marin AR, Ardavin C. CD8alpha(+) dendritic cells originate from the CD8alpha(−) dendritic cell subset by a maturation process involving CD8alpha, DEC-205, and CD24 up-regulation. Blood 2002; 99:999–1004.

10. Evans MJ, Van Winkle LS, Fnucchi MV, Hyde D, Plopper CG, Davis CA. Lateral intercellular space of tracheal epithelium of house dust mite sensitized Rhesus monkeys. Am J Respir Crit Care Med 2000; 161:778.

11. Wan H, Winton HL, Soeller C, Tovey ER, Gruenert DC, Thompson PJ, Stewart GA, Taylor GW, Garrod DR, Cannell MB, Robinson C. Der P 1 facilitates transepithelial allergen delivery by disruption of tight junctions. J Clin Invest 1999; 104:123–133.

12. Valladeau J, Ravel O, Dezutter-Dambuyant C, Moore K, Kleijmeer M, Liu Y, Duvert-Frances V, Vincent C, Schmitt D, Davoust J, Caux C, Lebecque S, Saeland S. Langerin, a novel C-type lectin specific to Langerhans cells, is an endocytic receptor that induces the formation of Birbeck granules. Immunity 2000; 12:71–81.

13. Geijtenbeek TBH, Torensma R, van Vliet SJ, van Duijnhoven GCF, Adema GJ, van Kooyk Y, Figdor CG. Identification of DC-SIGN, a novel dendritic cell-specific ICAM-3 receptor that supports primary immune responses. Cell 2000; 100:575–585.

14. Ariizumi K, Shen GL, Shikano S, Xu S, Ritter R, 3rd, Kumamoto T, Edelbaum D, Morita A, Bergstresser PR, Takashima A. Identification of a novel, dendritic cell-associated molecule, dectin-1, by subtractive cDNA cloning. J Biol Chem 2000; 275:20157–20167.

15. Cochand L, Isler P, Songeon F, Nicod LP. Human lung dendritic cells have an immature phenotype with efficient mannose receptors. Am J Respir Cell Mol Biol 1999; 21:547–554.

16. Mahnke K, Guo M, Lee S, Sepulveda H, Swain SL, Nussenzweig M, Steinman RM. The Dendritic Cell Receptor for Endocytosis, DEC-205, Can Recycle and Enhance Antigen Presentation via Major Histocompatibility Complex Class II-positive Lysosomal Compartments. J Cell Biol 2000; 151:673–684.

17. Engering A, Cella M, Fluitsma DM, Brockhaus M, Hoefsmit ECM, Lanzavecchia A, Pieters J. The mannose receptor functions as a high capacity and broad

specificity antigen receptor in human dendritic cells. Eur J Immunol 1997; 27:2417–2425.

18. Currie AJ, Stewart GA, McWilliam AS. Alveolar macrophages bind and phagocytose allergen-containing pollen starch granules via C-type lectin and integrin receptors: implications for airway inflammatory disease. J Immunol 2000; 164:3878–3886.

19. de Baey A, Lanzavecchia A. The role of aquaporins in dendritic cell macropinocytosis. J Exp Med 2000; 191:743–748.

20. Noirey N, Rougier N, Andre C, Schmitt D, Vincent C. Langerhans-like dendritic cells generated from cord blood progenitors internalize pollen allergens by macropinocytosis, and part of the molecules are processed and can activate autologous naive T lymphocytes. J Allergy Clin Immunol 2000; 105:1194–1201.

21. Banchereau J, Briere F, Caux C, Davoust J, Lebecque S, Liu Y-J, Pulendran B, Palucka KA. Immunobiology of dendritic cells. Annu Rev Immunol 2000; 18:767–811.

22. Rodriguez A, Regnault A, Kleijmeer M, Ricciardi-Castagnoli P, Amigorena S. Selective transport of internalized antigens to the cytosol for MHC class I presentation in dendritic cells. Nat Cell Biol 1999; 1:362–368.

23. Li M, Davey GM, Sutherland RM, Kurts C, Lew AM, Hirst C, Carbone FR, Heath WR. Cell-associated ovalbumin is cross-presented much more efficiently than soluble ovalbumin in vivo. J Immunol 2001; 166:6099–6103.

24. Nijman HW, Kleijmeer MJ, Ossevoort MA, Oorschot VMJ, Vierboom MPM, Vandekeur M, Kenemans P, Kast WM, Geuze HJ, Melief CJM. Antigen capture and major histocompatibility class II compartments of freshly isolated and cultured human blood dendritic cells. J Exp Med 1995; 182:163–174.

25. Denzin LK, Cresswell P. HLA-DM induces CLIP dissociation from MHC class II alpha beta dimers and facilitates peptide loading. Cell 1995; 82:155–165.

26. Turley SJ, Inaba K, Garrett WS, Ebersold M, Unternaehrer J, Steinman RM, Mellman I. Transport of peptide-MHC Class II complexes in developing dendritic cells. Science 2000; 288:522–527.

27. Pinet VM, Long EO. Peptide loading onto recycling HLA-DR molecules occurs in early endosomes. Eur J Immunol 1998; 28:799–804.

28. Cella M, Engering A, Pinet V, Pieters J, Lanzavecchia A. Inflammatory stimuli induce accumulation of MHC class II complexes on dendritic cells. Nature 1997; 388:782–787.

29. Santambrogio L, Sato AK, Carven GJ, Belyanskaya SL, Strominger JL, Stern LJ. Extracellular antigen processing and presentation by immature dendritic cells. Proc Natl Acad Sci USA 1999; 96:15056–15061.

30. Van der Heijden FL, Van Neerven RJ, Van Katwijk M, Bos JD, Kapsenberg ML. Serum-IgE-facilitated allergen presentation in atopic disease. J Immunol 1993; 150:3643–3650.

31. Maurer D, Fiebiger E, Reininger B, Ebner C, Petzelbauer P, Shi GP, Chapman HA, Stingl G. Fc epsilon receptor I on dendritic cells delivers IgE-bound multivalent antigens into a cathepsin S-dependent pathway of MHC class II presentation. J Immunol 1998; 161:2731–2739.

32. Geiger E, Magerstaedt R, Wessendorf JH, Kraft S, Hanau D, Bieber T. IL-4 induces the intracellular expression of the alpha chain of the high-affinity receptor for IgE in in vitro-generated dendritic cells. J Allergy Clin Immunol 2000; 105:150–156.

33. Charbonnier AS, Kohrgruber N, Kriehuber E, Stingl G, Rot A, Maurer D. Macrophage inflammatory protein 3alpha is involved in the constitutive trafficking of epidermal langerhans cells. J Exp Med 1999; 190:1755–1768.

34. Iwasaki A, Kelsall BL. Localization of distinct Peyer's patch dendritic cell subsets and their recruitment by chemokines macrophage inflammatory protein (MIP)-3alpha, MIP-3beta, and secondary lymphoid organ chemokine. J Exp Med 2000; 191:1381–1394.

35. Power CA, Church DJ, Meyer A, Alouani S, Proudfoot AEI, ClarkLewis I, Sozzani S, Mantovani A, Wells TNC. Cloning and characterization of a specific receptor for the novel CC chemokine MIP-3 alpha from lung dendritic cells. J Exp Med 1997; 186:825–835.

36. Dieu MC, Vanbervliet B, Vicari A, Bridon JM, Oldham E, Ait-Yahia S, Briere F, Zlotnik A, Lebecque S, Caux C. Selective recruitment of immature and mature dendritic cells by distinct chemokines expressed in different anatomic sites. J Exp Med 1998; 188:373–386.

37. Cook DN, Prosser DM, Forster R, Zhang J, Kuklin NA, Abbondanzo SJ, Niu XD, Chen SC, Manfra DJ, Wiekowski MT, Sullivan LM, Smith SR, Greenberg HB, Narula SK, Lipp M, Lira SA. CCR6 mediates dendritic cell localization, lymphocyte homeostasis, and immune responses in mucosal tissue. Immunity 2000; 12:495–503.

38. Dieu-Nosjean MC, Massacrier C, Homey B, Vanbervliet B, Pin JJ, Vicari A, Lebecque S, Dezutter-Dambuyant C, Schmitt D, Zlotnik A, Caux C. Macrophage inflammatory protein 3alpha is expressed at inflamed epithelial surfaces and is the most potent chemokine known in attracting Langerhans cell precursors. J Exp Med 2000; 192:705–718.

39. Yang D, Chertov O, Bykovskaia SN, Chen Q, Buffo MJ, Shogan J, Anderson M, Schroder JM, Wang JM, Howard OM, Oppenheim JJ. Beta-defensins: linking innate and adaptive immunity through dendritic and T cell CCR6. Science 1999; 286:525–528.

40. Cyster JG. Chemokines and cell migration in secondary lymphoid organs. Science 1999; 286:2098–2102.

41. Forster R, Schubel A, Breitfeld D, Kremmer E, Renner-Muller I, Wolf E, Lipp M. CCR7 coordinates the primary immune response by establishing functional microenvironments in secondary lymphoid organs. Cell 1999; 99:23–33.

42. Saeki H, Moore AM, Brown MJ, Hwang ST. Cutting edge: secondary lymphoid-tissue chemokine (SLC) and CC chemokine receptor 7 (CCR7) participate in the emigration pathway of mature dendritic cells from the skin to regional lymph nodes. J Immunol 1999; 162:2472–2475.

43. Engeman TM, Gorbachev AV, Glaude RP, Heeger PS, Fairchild RL. Inhibition of functional T cell priming and contact hypersensitivity responses by treatment with anti-secondary lymphoid chemokine antibody during hapten sensitization. J Immunol 2000; 164:5207–5214.

44. Gunzer M, Schafer A, Borgmann S, Grabbe S, Zanker KS, Brocker EB, Kampgen E, Friedl P. Antigen presentation in extracellular matrix: interactions of T cells with dendritic cells are dynamic, short lived, and sequential. Immunity 2000; 13:323–332.

45. Revy P, Sospedra M, Barbour B, Trautmann A. Functional antigen-independent synapses formed between T cells and dendritic cells. Nat Immunol 2001; 2:925–931.

46. Lanzavecchia A, Sallusto F. Dynamics of T lymphocyte responses: intermediates, effectors, and memory cells. Science 2000; 290:92–97.
47. Dustin ML. Membrane domains and the immunological synapse: keeping T cells resting and ready. J Clin Invest 2002; 109:155–160.
48. Anderson HA, Hiltbold EM, Roche PA. Concentration of MHC class II molecules in lipid rafts facilitates antigen presentation. Nat Immunol 2000; 1:156–162.
49. Kropshofer H, Spindeldreher S, Rohn TA, Platania N, Grygar C, Daniel N, Wolpl A, Langen H, Horejsi V, Vogt AB. Tetraspan microdomains distinct from lipid rafts enrich select peptide-MHC class II complexes. Nat Immunol 2002; 3:61–68.
50. Lambrecht BN, Pauwels RA, Fazekas De St Groth B. Induction of rapid T cell activation, division, and recirculation by intratracheal injection of dendritic cells in a TCR transgenic model. J Immunol 2000; 164:2937–2946.
51. Moser M, Murphy KM. Dendritic cell regulation of Th1-Th2 development. Nat Immunol 2000; 1:199–205.
52. Kalinski P, Hilkens CM, Wierenga EA, Kapsenberg ML. T-cell priming by type-1 and type-2 polarized dendritic cells: the concept of a third signal. Immunology Today 1999; 20:561–567.
53. Reid SD, Penna G, Adorini L. The control of T cell responses by dendritic cell subsets. Curr Opin Immunol 2000; 12:114–121.
54. Hilkens CMU, Kalinski P, deBoer M, Kapsenberg ML. Human dendritic cells require exogenous interleukin-12- inducing factors to direct the development of naive T-helper cells toward the Th1 phenotype. Blood 1997; 90:1920–1926.
55. Thoma-Uszynski S, Kiertscher SM, Ochoa M, Bouis DA, Norgard MV, Miyake K, Godowski PJ, Roth MD, Modlin RL. Activation of Toll-like receptor 2 on human dendritic cells triggers induction of IL-12, but not IL-10. J Immunol 2000; 165:3804–3810.
56. Kadowaki N, Ho S, Antonenko S, Malefyt RW, Kastelein RA, Bazan F, Liu YJ. Subsets of human dendritic cell precursors express different toll-like receptors and respond to different microbial antigens. J Exp Med 2001; 194:863–869.
57. Vieira PL, de Jong EC, Wierenga EA, Kapsenberg ML, Kalinski P. Development of Th1-inducing capacity in myeloid dendritic cells requires environmental instruction. J Immunol 2000; 164:4507–4512.
58. Langenkamp A, Messi M, Lanzavecchia A, Sallusto F. Kinetics of dendritic cell activation: impact on priming of Th1, Th2 and nonpolarized T cells. Nat Immunol 2000; 1:311–316.
59. Tanaka H, Demeure C, Rubio M, Delespesse G, Sarfati M. Human monocyte-derived dendritic cells induce naive T cell differentiation into T helper cell type 2 (Th2) or Th1/Th2 effectors: role of stimulator/responder ratio. J Exp Med 2000; 192:405–411.
60. Rissoan MC, Soumelis V, Kadowaki N, Grouard G, Briere F, de Waal Malefyt R, Liu YJ. Reciprocal control of T helper cell and dendritic cell differentiation. Science 1999; 283:1183–1186.
61. Cella M, Jarrossay D, Facchetti F, Alebardi O, Nakajima H, Lanzavecchia A, Colonna M. Plasmacytoid monocytes migrate to inflamed lymph nodes and produce large amounts of type I interferon. Nature Med 1999; 5:919–923.

62. Chang CC, Wright A, Punnonen J. Monocyte-derived CD1a+ and CD1a− dendritic cell subsets differ in their cytokine production profiles, susceptibilities to transfection, and capacities to direct Th cell differentiation. J Immunol 2000; 165:3584–3591.

63. Holt PG, Schon-Hegrad MA, Phillips MJ, McMenamin PG, Ia-positive dendritic cells form a tightly meshed network within the human airway epithelium. Clin Exp Allergy 1989; 19:597.

64. Van Haarst JMW, de Wit HJ, Drexhage HA, Hoogsteden HC. Distribution and immunophenotype of mononuclear phagocytes and dendritic cells in the human lung. Am J Respir Cell Mol Biol 1994; 10:487–492.

65. van Haarst JM, Verhoeven GT, de Wit HJ, Hoogsteden HC, Debets R, Drexhage HA. CD1a+ and CD1a− accessory cells from human bronchoalveolar lavage differ in allostimulatory potential and cytokine production. Am J Respir Cell Mol Biol 1996; 15:752–759.

66. Valladeau J, Duvert-Frances V, Pin JJ, Dezutter-Dambuyant C, Vincent C, Massacrier C, Vincent J, Yoneda K, Banchereau J, Caux C, Davoust J, Saeland S. The monoclonal antibody DCGM4 recognizes Langerin, a protein specific of Langerhans cells, and is rapidly internalized from the cell surface. Eur J Immunol 1999; 29:2695–2704.

67. Holt PG, Stumbles PA. Regulation of immunologic homeostasis in peripheral tissues by dendritic cells: the respiratory tract as a paradigm. J Allergy Clin Immunol 2000; 105:421–429.

68. Stumbles PA, Thomas JA, Pimm CL, Lee PT, Venaille TJ, Proksch S, Holt PG. Resting respiratory tract dendritic cells preferentially stimulate T helper cell type 2 (Th2) responses and require obligatory cytokine signals for induction of Th1 immunity. J Exp Med 1998; 188:2019–2031.

69. Lambrecht BN, De Veerman M, Coyle AJ, Gutierrez-Ramos J, Thielemans K, Pauwels RA. Dendritic cells induce Th2 responses to inhaled antigen leading to eosinophilic airway inflammation. J Clin Invest 2000; 106:551–559.

70. Lambrecht BN, Peleman RA, Bullock GR, Pauwels RA. Sensitization to inhaled antigen by intratracheal instillation of dendritic cells. Clin Exp Allergy 2000; 30:214–224.

71. Stampfli MR, Wiley RE, Scott Neigh G, Gajewska BU, Lei XF, Snider DP, Xing Z, Jordana M. GM-CSF transgene expression in the airway allows aerosolized ovalbumin to induce allergic sensitization in mice. J Clin Invest 1998; 102:1704–1714.

72. Yamamoto N, Suzuki S, Shirai A, Suzuki M, Nakazawa M, Nagashima Y, Okubo T. Dendritic cells are associated with augmentation of antigen sensitization by influenza A virus infection in mice. Eur J Immunol 2000; 30:316–326.

73. Lambrecht BN, Carro-Muino I, Vermaelen K, Pauwels RA. Allergen-induced changes in bone-marrow progenitor and airway dendritic cells in sensitized rats. Am J Respir Cell Mol Biol 1999; 20:1165–1174.

74. Lambrecht BN, Salomon B, Klatzmann D, Pauwels RA. Dendritic cells are required for the development of chronic eosinophilic airway inflammation in response to inhaled antigen in sensitized mice. J Immunol 1998; 160:4090–4097.

75. McWilliam AS, Napoli S, Marsh AM, Pemper FL, Nelson DJ, Pimm CL, Stumbles PA, Wells TNC, Holt PG. Dendritic cells are recruited into the airway

epithelium during the inflammatory response to a broad spectrum of stimuli. J Exp Med 1996; 184:2429–2432.

76. Holt PG, Macaubas C, Stumbles PA, Sly PD. The role of allergy in the development of asthma. Nature 1999; 402:B12–17.

77. van der Pouw Kraan TC, Boeije LC, de Groot ER, Stapel SO, Snijders A, Kapsenberg ML, van der Zee JS, Aarden LA. Reduced production of IL-12 and IL-12-dependent IFN-gamma release in patients with allergic asthma. J Immunol 1997; 158:5560–5565.

78. Bellinghausen I, Brand U, Knop J, Saloga J. Comparison of allergen-stimulated dendritic cells from atopic and nonatopic donors dissecting their effect on autologous naive and memory T helper cells of such donors. J Allergy Clin Immunol 2000; 105:988–996.

79. Mackensen A, Drager R, Schlesier M, Mertelsmann R, Lindemann A. Presence of IgE antibodies to bovine serum albumin in a patient developing anaphylaxis after vaccination with human peptide- pulsed dendritic cells. Cancer Immunol Immunother 2000; 49:152–156.

80. Holm AF, Fokkens WJ, Godthelp T, Mulder PG, Vroom TM, Rijntjes E. Effect of 3 months' nasal steroid therapy on nasal T cells and Langerhans cells in patients suffering from allergic rhinitis. Allergy 1995; 50:204–209.

81. Wollenberg A, Wen S, Bieber T. Langerhans cell phenotyping: a new tool for differential diagnosis of inflammatory skin diseases [letter]. Lancet 1995; 346:1626–1627.

82. Moller GM, Overbeek SE, VanHeldenMeeuwsen CG, VanHaarst JMW, Prens EP, Mulder PG, Postma DS, Hoogsteden HC. Increased numbers of dendritic cells in the bronchial mucosa of atopic asthmatic patients: Downregulation by inhaled corticosteroids. Clin Exp Allergy 1996; 26:517–524.

83. Bertorelli G, Bocchino V, Zhou X, Zanini A, Bernini MV, Damia R, Di Comite V, Grima P, Olivieri D. Dendritic cell number is related to IL-4 expression in the airways of atopic asthmatic subjects. Allergy 2000; 55:449–454.

84. Tunon de Lara JM, Redington AE, Bradding P, Church MK, Hartley JA, Semper AE, Holgate ST. Dendritic cells in normal and asthmatic airways: expression of the alfa subunit of the high affinity immunoglobulin E receptor. Clin Exp Allergy 1996; 26:648–655.

85. Bellini A, Vittori E, Marini M, Ackerman V, Mattoli S. Intraepithelial dendritic cells and selective activation of Th2-like lymphocytes in patients with atopic asthma. Chest 1993; 103:997–1005.

86. Godthelp T, Fokkens WJ, Kleinjan A, Holm AF, Mulder PG, Prens EP, Rijntes E. Antigen presenting cells in the nasal mucosa of patients with allergic rhinitis during allergen provocation. Clin Exp Allergy 1996; 26:677–688.

87. Jahnsen FL, Lund-Johansen F, Dunne JF, Farkas L, Haye R, Brandtzaeg P. Experimentally induced recruitment of plasmacytoid (CD123high) dendritic cells in human nasal allergy. J Immunol 2000; 165:4062–4068.

88. Jahnsen FL, Moloney ED, Hogan T, Upham JW, Burke CM, Holt PG. Rapid dendritic cell recruitment to the bronchial mucosa of patients with atopic asthma in response to local allergen challenge. Thorax 2001; 56:823–826.

89. Upham JW, Wood L, Denburg JA, O'Byrne PM. Circulating dendritic cells and asthma: rapid response to inhaled allergen. Am J Respir Crit Care Med 1999; 159:B93(A).

90. Uchida Y, Kurasawa K, Nakajima H, Nakagawa N, Tanabe E, Sueishi M, Saito Y, Iwamoto I. Increase of dendritic cells of type 2 (DC2) by altered response to IL-4 in atopic patients. J Allergy Clin Immunol 2001; 108:1005–1011.

91. van den Heuvel MM, Vanhee DD, Postmus PE, Hoefsmit EC, Beelen RH. Functional and phenotypic differences of monocyte-derived dendritic cells from allergic and nonallergic patients. J Allergy Clin Immunol 1998; 101:90–95.

92. Sung SJ, Taketomi EA, Smith AM, Platts-Mills TA, Fu SM. Efficient presentation of house dust mite allergen Der p 2 by monocyte-derived dendritic cells and the role of beta 2 integrins. Scand J Immunol 1999; 49:96–105.

93. De Wit D, Amraoui Z, Vincart B, Michel O, Michils A, Van Overvelt L, Willems F, Goldman M. Helper T-cell responses elicited by Der p 1-pulsed dendritic cells and recombinant IL-12 in atopic and healthy subjects. J Allergy Clin Immunol 2000; 105:346–352.

94. Hammad H, Charbonnier AS, Duez C, Jacquet A, Stewart GA, Tonnel AB, Pestel J. Th2 polarization by Der p 1–pulsed monocyte-derived dendritic cells is due to the allergic status of the donors. Blood 2001; 98:1135–1141.

95. Brand U, Bellinghausen I, Enk AH, Jonuleit H, Becker D, Knop J, Saloga J. Allergen-specific immune deviation from a TH2 to a TH1 response induced by dendritic cells and collagen type I. J Allergy Clin Immunol 1999; 104:1052–1059.

96. Lambrecht BN. The dendritic cell in allergic airway diseases: a new player to the game. Clin Exp Allergy 2001; 31:206–218.

96a. Hammad H, Lambrecht BN, Pochard P, et al. Monocyte-derived dendritic cells induce a house dust mite–specific TH2 allergic inflammation in the lung of humanized SCID mice: Involvement of CCR7. J Immunol 2002; 169:1524–1534.

97. Hammad H, Duez C, Fahy O, Tsicopoulos A, Andre C, Wallaert B, Lebecque S, Tonnel AB, Pestel J. Human dendritic cells in the severe combined immunodeficiency mouse model: their potentiating role in the allergic reaction. Lab Invest 2000; 80:605–614.

98. Jaffar ZH, Roberts K, Pandit A, Linsley P, Djukanovic R, Holgate ST. B7 costimulation is required for IL-5 and IL-13 secretion by bronchial biopsy tissue of atopic asthmatic subjects in response to allergen stimulation. Am J Respir Cell Mol Biol 1999; 20:153–162.

99. Coyle AJ, Wagner K, Bertrand C, Tsuyuki S, Bews J, Heusser C. Central role of immunoglobulin (Ig) E in the induction of lung eosinophil infiltration and T helper 2 cell cytokine production: inhibition by a non-anaphylactogenic anti-IgE antibody. J Exp Med 1996; 183:1303–1310.

100. Jurgens M, Wollenberg A, Hanau D, de la Salle H, Bieber T. Activation of human epidermal Langerhans cells by engagement of the high affinity receptor for IgE, Fc epsilon RI. J Immunol 1995; 155:5184–5189.

101. Leung DY. Atopic dermatitis: new insights and opportunities for therapeutic intervention. J Allergy Clin Immunol 2000; 105:860–876.

102. Caux C, Massacrier C, Vanbervliet B, Dubois B, Van Kooten C, Durand I, Banchereau J. Activation of human dendritic cells through CD40 cross-linking. J Exp Med 1994; 180:1263–1272.

103. Mazzoni A, Young HA, Spitzer JH, Visintin A, Segal DM. Histamine regulates cytokine production in maturing dendritic cells, resulting in altered T cell polarization. J Clin Invest 2001; 108:1865–1873.

104. Caron G, Delneste Y, Roelandts E, Duez C, Bonnefoy JY, Pestel J, Jeannin P. Histamine Polarizes Human Dendritic Cells into Th2 Cell-Promoting Effector Dendritic Cells. J Immunol 2001; 167:3682–3686.

105. Robbiani DF, Finch RA, Jager D, Muller WA, Sartorelli AC, Randolph GJ. The leukotriene C(4) transporter MRP1 regulates CCL19 (MIP-3beta, ELC)-dependent mobilization of dendritic cells to lymph nodes. Cell 2000; 103:757–768.

106. Imai T, Nagira M, Takagi S, Kakizaki M, Nishimura M, Wang J, Gray PW, Matsushima K, Yoshie O. Selective recruitment of CCR4-bearing Th2 cells toward antigen-presenting cells by the CC chemokines thymus and activation-regulated chemokine and macrophage-derived chemokine. Int Immunol 1999; 11:81–88.

107. Hashimoto S, Suzuki T, Dong HY, Nagai S, Yamazaki N, Matsushima K. Serial analysis of gene expression in human monocyte-derived dendritic cells. Blood 1999; 94:845–852.

108. Kikuchi T, Crystal RG. Antigen-pulsed dendritic cells expressing macrophage-derived chemokine elicit Th2 responses and promote specific humoral immunity. J Clin Invest 2001; 108:917–927.

109. Ludewig B, Odermatt B, Landmann S, Hengartner H, Zinkernagel RM. Dendritic cells induce autoimmune diabetes and maintain disease via de novo formation of local lymphoid tissue. J Exp Med 1998; 188:1493–1501.

110. Hoogsteden HC, Verhoeven GT, Lambrecht BN, Prins J. Airway inflammation in asthma and chronic obstructive pulmonary disease with special emphasis on the antigen-presenting dendritic cell: influence of treatment with fluticasone propionate. Clin Exp Allergy 1999; 29 S2:116–124.

111. Holm AF, Godthelp T, Fokkens WJ, Severijnen EA, Mulder PG, Vroom TM, Rijntjes E. Long-term effects of corticosteroid nasal spray on nasal inflammatory cells in patients with perennial allergic rhinitis. Clin Exp Allergy 1999; 29:1356–1366.

112. Woltman AM, de Fijter JW, Kamerling SW, Paul LC, Daha MR, van Kooten C. The effect of calcineurin inhibitors and corticosteroids on the differentiation of human dendritic cells. Eur J Immunol 2000; 30:1807–1812.

113. Brokaw JJ, White GW, Baluk P, Anderson GP, Umemoto EY, McDonald DM. Glucocorticoid-induced apoptosis of dendritic cells in the rat tracheal mucosa. Am J Respir Cell Mol Biol 1998; 19:598–605.

114. van den Heuvel MM, van Beek NM, Broug-Holub E, Postmus PE, Hoefsmit EC, Beelen RH, Kraal G. Glucocorticoids modulate the development of dendritic cells from blood precursors. Clin Exp Immunol 1999; 115:577–583.

115. Matyszak MK, Citterio S, Rescigno M, Ricciardi-Castagnoli P. Differential effects of corticosteroids during different stages of dendritic cell maturation. Eur J Immunol 2000; 30:1233–1242.

116. de Jong EC, Vieira PL, Kalinski P, Kapsenberg ML. Corticosteroids inhibit the production of inflammatory mediators in immature monocyte-derived DC and induce the development of tolerogenic DC3. J Leukoc Biol 1999; 66:201–204.

117. Shodell M, Siegal FP. Corticosteroids depress IFN-alpha-producing plasmacytoid dendritic cells in human blood. J Allergy Clin Immunol 2001; 108:446–448.

118. Godleski JJ, Brain JD. The origin of alveolar macrophages in mouse radiation chimeras. J Exp Med 1972; 136:630–643.

119. MacLean JA, Xia WJ, Pinto CE, Zhao LH, Liu HW, Kradin RL. Sequestration of inhaled particulate antigens by lung phagocytes: A mechanism for the effective inhibition of pulmonary cell-mediated immunity. Am J Pathol 1996; 148:657–666.

120. Krug N, Tschernig T, Holgate ST, Pabst R. How do lymphocytes get into the asthmatic airways? Lymphocyte traffic into and within the lung in asthma. Clin Exp Allergy 1998; 28:10–18.

121. Marathias KP, Preffer FI, Pinto C, Kradin RL. Most human pulmonary infiltrating lymphocytes display the surface immune phenotype and functional responses of sensitized T cells. Am J Respir Cell Mol Biol 1991; 5:470–476.

122. Holt PG. Regulation of antigen-presenting cell function(s) in lung and airway tissues. Eur Respir J 1993; 6:120–129.

123. Upham JW, Strickland DH, Bilyk N, Robinson BWS, Holt PG. Alveolar macrophages from humans and rodents selectively inhibit T-cell proliferation but permit T-cell activation and cytokine secretion. Immunology 1995; 84:142–147.

124. Upham JW, Strickland DH, Robinson BWS, Holt PG. Selective inhibition of T cell proliferation but not expression of effector function by human alveolar macrophages. Thorax 1997; 52:786–795.

125. Strickland D, Kees UR, Holt PG. Regulation of T-cell activation in the lung: Alveolar macrophages induce reversible T-cell anergy in vitro associated with inhibition of interleuk in-2 receptor signal transduction. Immunology 1996; 87:250–258.

126. Chelen CJ, Fang Y, Freeman GJ, Secrist H, Marshall JD, Hwang PT, Frankel LR, Dekruyff RH, Umetsu DT. Human alveolar macrophages present antigen ineffectively due to defective expression of B7 costimulatory cell surface molecules. J Clin Invest 1995; 95:1415–1421.

127. Bilyk N, Holt PG. Cytokine modulation of the immunosuppressive phenotype of pulmonary alveolar macrophage populations. Immunology 1995; 86:231–237.

128. Lipscomb MF, Pollard AM, Yates JL. A role for TGF-beta in the suppression by murine bronchoalveolar cells of lung dendritic cell initiated immune responses. Reg Immunol 1993; 5:151–157.

129. Holt PG, Oliver J, Bilyk N, McMenamin C, McMenamin PG, Kraal G, Thepen T. Downregulation of the antigen presenting cell function(s) of pulmonary dendritic cells in vivo by resident alveolar macrophages. J Exp Med 1993; 177:397–407.

130. Thepen T, Van Rooijen N, Krall G. Alveolar macrophage elimination in vivo is associated in vivo with an increase in pulmonary immune responses in mice. J Exp Med 1989; 170:494–509.

131. Thepen T, McMenamin C, Oliver J, Kraal G, Holt PG. Regulation of immune responses to inhaled antigen by alveolar macrophages (AM): differential effects of AM elimination in vivo on the induction of tolerance versus immunity. Eur J Immunol 1991; 21:2845–2850.

132. Thepen T, McMenamin C, Girn B, Kraal G, Holt PG. Regulation of IgE production in pre-sensitized animals: in vivo elimination of alveolar macrophages preferentially increases IgE responses to inhaled allergen. Clin Exp Allergy 1992; 22:1107–1114.

133. Bilyk N, Holt PG. Inhibition of the immunosuppressive activity of resident pulmonary alveolar macrophages by granulocyte/macrophage colony-stimulating factor. J Exp Med 1993; 177:1773–1777.

134. Spiteri MA, Poulter LW. Characterization of immune inducer and suppressor macrophages from the normal human lung. Clin Exp Immunol 1991; 83:157–162.

135. Agea E, Forenza N, Piattoni S, Russano A, Monaco A, Flenghi L, Bistoni O, Gillies DA, Azuma M, Bertotto A, Spinozzi F. Expression of B7 co-stimulatory molecules and CD1a antigen by alveolar macrophages in allergic bronchial asthma. Clin Exp Allergy 1998; 28:1359–1367.

136. Burastero SE, Magnani Z, Confetti C, Abbruzzese L, Oddera S, Balbo P, Rossi GA, Crimi E. Increased expression of the CD80 accessory molecule by alveolar macrophages in asthmatic subjects and its functional involvement in allergen presentation to autologous TH2 lymphocytes. J Allergy Clin Immunol 1999; 103:1136–1142.

137. Chanez P, Vignola AM, Lacoste P, Michel FB, Godard P, Bousquet J. Increased expression of adhesion molecules (ICAM-1 and LFA-1) on alveolar macrophages from asthmatic patients. Allergy 1993; 48:576–580.

138. Williams J, Johnson S, Mascali JJ, Smith H, Rosenwasser LJ, Borish L. Regulation of low affinity IgE receptor (CD23) expression on mononuclear phagocytes in normal and asthmatic subjects. J Immunol 1992; 149:2823–2829.

139. Tang C, Ward C, Reid D, Bish R, O'Byrne PM, Walters EH. Normally suppressing CD40 coregulatory signals delivered by airway macrophages to TH2 lymphocytes are defective in patients with atopic asthma. J Allergy Clin Immunol 2001; 107:863–870.

140. Plummeridge MJ, Armstrong L, Birchall MA, Millar AB. Reduced production of interleukin 12 by interferon gamma primed alveolar macrophages from atopic asthmatic subjects. Thorax 2000; 55:842–847.

141. Magnan A, van Pee D, Bongrand P, Vervloet D. Alveolar macrophage interleukin (IL)-10 and IL-12 production in atopic asthma. Allergy 1998; 53:1092–1095.

142. Tang C, Rolland JM, Ward C, Li X, Bish R, Thien F, Walters EH. Modulatory effects of alveolar macrophages on CD4+ T-cell IL-5 responses correlate with IL-1beta, IL-6, and IL-12 production. Eur Respir J 1999; 14:106–112.

143. Tang C, Rolland JM, Li X, Ward C, Bish R, Walters EH. Alveolar macrophages from atopic asthmatics, but not atopic nonasthmatics, enhance interleukin-5 production by CD4+ T cells. Am J Respir Crit Care Med 1998; 157:1120–1126.

144. Larche M, Till SJ, Haselden BM, North J, Barkans J, Corrigan CJ, Kay AB, Robinson DS. Costimulation through CD86 is involved in airway antigen-presenting cell and T cell responses to allergen in atopic asthmatics. J Immunol 1998; 161:6375–6382.

3

CD4 T Lymphocytes in Allergic Asthma

MARK LARCHÉ and A. BARRY KAY

National Heart and Lung Institute
Imperial College School of Medicine
London, England

I. Introduction

The processes that result in reversible narrowing of the airways in asthma remain partially defined but are clearly associated with chronic inflammation in and around the bronchi. In the majority of cases, these are associated with aberrant immunological responses to otherwise innocuous substances, such as pollens, animal danders, and mite proteins. Both environmental and genetic factors have been implicated in the genesis of allergic hypersensitivity in asthma. In the context of this chapter, these issues will be discussed primarily in relation to their possible roles in the induction of "asthmagenic" T-cell responses.

It is now appreciated that the role of the T lymphocyte, and in particular the $CD4^+$ T cell, in asthma goes beyond that of providing help for the switching of allergen-specific B cells to the epsilon immunoglobulin isotype. For example, direct activation of allergen-specific CD4 T cells in asthmatic subjects following administration of allergen-derived peptides suggests a role for the T cell in the induction of bronchoconstriction that is independent of mast cells and IgE. The precise elucidation of the role of the T cell in the development and maintenance of chronic asthma may eventually lead to a definition of the disease based on immunological principles. Having defined the disease, we may then develop logical approaches toward curative therapeutic intervention.

II. A Historical Perspective of the CD4 T Cell in Asthma

The introduction of the fiberoptic bronchoscope facilitated rapid develop-ments in many areas of medicine and, in particular, those of gastroenterology and pulmonology. In the late 1980s, Corrigan and colleagues described the presence of activated lymphocytes in peripheral blood of severe asthmatics (1). T cells were also demonstrated in increased numbers in bronchial mucosal biopsies obtained following episodes of fatal asthma (2). Robinson and co-workers went on to define the T-helper 2 (Th2) nature of CD2 cells in the lung (3), thus linking the earlier observations of Wierenga (4) and Romagnani (5,6) both of whom had described the association of Th2-type T-cell phenotypes with atopic responses.

The presence of increased numbers of CD4 T cells in the bronchial mucosa at baseline and their subsequent increase following allergen challenge provides circumstantial evidence that these cells have a role in pathogenesis but provides no functional connection between the cell and the disease. Hamid and colleagues attempted to establish a more direct link by quantify-ing numbers of interleukin-5 (IL-5) mRNA expressing cells in the bronchial mucosa of asthmatic subjects and comparing these findings to levels in con-trols (7). Numbers of $CD25^+$ T cells in the lung were found to correlate posi-tively with levels of mRNA for IL-5. Furthermore, IL-5 mRNA expression was shown to correlate with numbers of $EG2^+$ eosinophils. A relationship between numbers of activated T cells and eosinophils was also demonstrated by Virchow and colleagues using a segmental allergen challenge model (8). In a study directly comparing normal, non-atopic control subjects with asth-matics, Bentley demonstrated that cells obtained from alveolar lavage of asthmatic airways contained increased numbers of cells expressing mRNA for Th2 cytokines [IL-3, IL-4, IL-5, and granulocyte-macrophage colony-stimulating factor (GM-CSF)] (9). In contrast, no difference was observed between asthma and control lavage cells with respect to the expression of mRNA encoding IL-2 and interferon-γ (IFN-γ). Furthermore, expression of Th2 cytokine mRNA was localized to T cells within the lavage cell population. Subsequent studies (10,11) demonstrated the sensitivity of Th2 cytokine pro-duction to glucocorticosteroids, reflecting the efficacy of this form of treat-ment in asthma and providing insight into the mechanism of action of this class of therapeutic. In addition, asthma symptom scores and bronchial hyperactivity were shown to correlate with numbers of cells expressing Th2 cytokines (12).

The interpretation of these observations was that allergen-specific T cells were present in increased numbers in the lung in asthma and that production by these cells of relatively high concentrations of the eosinophil-active cytokine IL-5 leads to enhanced eosinophil maturation, survival, and release from the bone marrow (13,14). Identification and characterization of eosinophil che-moattractants, in the form of chemokine ligands of the CCR3 receptor, has provided a link in the series of events that begins with production of IL-5 by allergen-specific T cells and results in eosinophil accumulation in the lung (15,16). Subsequent activation of eosinophils in the lung results in the release of leukotrienes, giving rise to bronchoconstriction, and the release of charged proteins such as major basic protein (MBP), eosinophil cationic protein (ECP), and others, leading to epithelial damage, airway remodeling, and further airway obstruction.

III. Antigen Recognition by T Cells

T-cell receptors (TcRs) occur in membrane-bound form and, unlike B-cell receptors, are not secreted. Recognition of antigen by TcR differs from BcR in that T-cell receptors recognize small fragments of antigen presented by molecules encoded by the class I and II regions of the major histocompatibility complex (MHC). In general, TcRs recognize peptide fragments of antigen coupled to MHC (although in some cases they may be able to interact with glycolipids bound to nonclassical MHC molecules such as the CD1 family (17). In addition to MHC-restricted recognition of peptides and glycolipids, MHC-independent recognition of carbohydrate moieties from pollen allergens has also recently been suggested (18).

The response of B lymphocytes to the majority of antigens is T lymphocyte dependent, requiring interaction between cell surface structures such as CD40 on the surface of B cells and its ligand on activated T cells. In addition, soluble factors secreted by T cells act on B cells, directing their choice of immunoglobulin heavy-chain gene segments and thus the ultimate class of Ig produced. The repertoire of cytokines produced by T lymphocytes has been used to identify separate populations of cells whose products promote qualitatively different effector responses to antigen encounter. Cell-mediated immunity is generated primarily through interferon-γ (IFN-γ) secreting cells known as T-helper 1 (Th1) cells. Induction of Th1 responses has been demonstrated to be dependent on IL-12 produced by monocytic and dendritic antigen-presenting cells (APCs). The apparent specificity of IL-12 action on Th1 cells may be explaned by the observation of Rogge and colleagues that the β_2 subunit of the IL-12 receptor is expressed by Th1 but not Th2 cells (19). However, Varga and colleagues have demonstrated the presence of mRNA encoding the IL-12Rβ2 subunit in T cells from both alveolar lavage and peripheral blood following inhaled allergen challenge in asthmatic subjects (20). Production of IL-5 in response to specific allergen could be modulated by IL-12, indicating that cells from atopic subjects may remain responsive to IL-12 by virtue of expression of the β_2 chain of the receptor. In addition, reduced production of IL-12 and IL-12-dependent IFN-γ has been demonstrated in patients with allergic asthma (21). Humoral immunity has been ascribed to Th2 cells that produce cytokines characteristic of those found in allergic inflammation such as IL-4 and IL-5. It is clear, however, that switching to certain antibody isotypes (IgA and IgG) may be elicited by Th1 cytokines. Induction of Th2 cells has been demonstrated to be dependent on the presence of IL-4 during priming of naive cells. Although absolute divisions between Th1 and Th2 responses may be more demonstrable in vitro than in vivo, it is clear that in general terms allergic inflammation is driven by Th2-type cytokines, notably IL-4 and IL-5.

IV. Effect of Allergen Dose and Genetic Background on the Development of T-Cell Responses

Data from a number of animal models has led to the conclusion that almost any protein antigen can be allergenic but that the induction of Th1 vs. Th2 T-cell responses may be more related to the genetic background of the host and to dose of antigen administered. Furthermore, dose, as related to affinity of TcR interaction and numbers of receptor ligated, may be the primary determining factor in which cytokine phenotype is generated. Murray analyzed the response of inbred strains of mice to immunization with the same peptide. The same peptide was capable of inducing Th1 responses in certain strains and Th2 responses in others (22). These observations emphasize the importance of the genetic contribution of allergic diseases in humans where familial associations with asthma have been observed.

Several investigators have addressed the issue of dose by immunizing mice with varying amounts of antigen and observing the subsequent effect on T-cell maturation into Th1 or Th2 subsets. Immunization of peptide determinants from human collagen was shown to lead to Th1 responses at high dose and Th2 responses at low dose (23). Hosken and colleagues (24) used mice carrying a transgenic TcR specific for ovalbumin peptide to analyze the effect of antigen dose in T-cell priming for Th1 and Th2 responses. At very low ($<0.05 \mu M$) and very high ($>10 \mu M$) doses of peptide, Th2 responses were observed whereas midrange concentrations ($0.3-0.6 \mu M$) led to Th0/Th1 responses. Guery and colleagues used a miniosmotic pump to administer low doses of soluble antigen continuously (25). Proliferative responses were inhibited and correlated with suppression of Th1-type responses and a strong Th2 response with high levels of IL-4 and IL-5 production. The effect of the genetic background of the mice was also analyzed, with BALB/c mice demonstrating enhanced Th2 responses compared to other strains such as DBA/2, C3H, and C57BL/6. Interestingly, the inhibition of IFN-γ responses was found to occur equally in all strains analyzed. These observations suggest that the ability to inhibit Th1 responses with soluble antigen can be regulated independently from the ability of certain genetic backgrounds to promote Th2 responses. A consistent finding in murine models of Th2 induction is that blockade of IL-4 during priming of naive cells abrogates Th2 development. The issue of why both very low and very high doses of antigen give rise to Th2-type responses remains unclear. However, it has been suggested (26) that increased sensitivity of Th1 cells to activation-induced apoptosis at high antigen dose may result in lower numbers of Th1 cells surviving in cultures, allowing outgrowth of Th2 cells in the absence of inhibitory cytokines such as IFN-γ.

V. Effects of Affinity on the Development of T-Cell Responses

Altering the affinity of interaction between antigenic peptide and MHC or TcR molecules may have profound effects on both the proliferative capacity and the cytokine production profile of T cells. By altering peptide residues that interact with either the TcR or the MHC, changes in proliferative capacity and cytokine production have been observed in several systems. The initial demonstration that amino acid substitution in peptide antigen can lead to dissociation between production of cytokines (IL-4 in this example) and the ability to proliferate was provided by Evavold and Allen (27). Altered peptide ligands have been employed to investigate the role of affinity in terms of the ability of peptides to induce cytokine and proliferative responses. Kumar (28) analyzed several peptides derived from the myelin basic protein peptide (Ac1-9). Substituted peptides were assayed for binding to I-A^u and for their ability to induce proliferation and cytokine expression. Peptide binding to I-A^u varied dramatically. The ability of the analogues to induce proliferative responses correlated with peptide-MHC affinity, with higher affinity peptides inducing the strongest proliferation. Furthermore, cytokine production also correlated with peptide affinity. High-affinity peptides could be shown to induce fivefold more IFN-γ production. In contrast, the frequency of IL-4 and IL-5 producing cells was similar between high- and low-affinity peptides. In order to assess the combined effects of dose and affinity, the authors increased the dose of low-affinity peptide by 50- to 100-fold and found that the frequency of IL-5-producing cells increased by 10-fold in the absence of a concomitant increase in IFN-γ producing cells.

The conclusions to be drawn from these and many other studies regarding the effects of antigen dose, affinity of T-cell receptor interaction with peptide antigen, and, finally, genetic background may be that in genetically susceptible individuals, low-dose chronic exposure to allergen gives rise to Th2-type responses and ultimately to atopy. Observations such as the induction of Th1 responses by increasing the affinity of peptide ligands may hold promise for future therapy in allergic diseases, although caution should be exercised in view of the association of Th1 responses with autoimmunity.

VI. Factors Influencing T-Helper-Cell Differentiation

Studies from our own group have addressed differences in the way T cells
from clinically defined groups of patients respond to allergen at the level of
individual epitopes (29). Proliferative and cytokine responses to overlapping sets of peptides spanning chain one of the major cat allergen Fel
d1 were assayed in four clinical groups; cat-allergic asthmatics, non-cat-
allergic asthmatics, cat-allergic rhinitics, and normal, non-atopic controls.
Large numbers of replicate cultures were performed with each peptide and
at least two different doses of peptide compared in order to derive robust
datasets.

The first observation to be made was that all four groups of subjects
mounted approximately equivalent proliferative responses to each of the peptides. The magnitude of the proliferative response to each peptide varied both
within individuals and within groups but no clear differences were observed. It
appeared, therefore, that in the case of Fel d1, allergic individuals were not
allergic simply because they recognize a protein that is not recognized by nonallergic individuals.

The second observation was that the cytokine profile (IL-5 and IFN-γ) of
each group was different. Of interest was the fact that in all groups, equivalent
IFN-γ responses were observed and these responses were predominantly
restricted to the amino terminus of the molecule. These data indicated that
certain parts of a molecule may be more likely to induce IFN-γ responses, perhaps by virtue of being high-affinity binders to commonly expressed MHC
molecules. However, there was no obvious difference in the ability of each
individual clinical group to make IFN-γ in response to allergen-derived
epitopes.

The third observations arising from this study was that asthmatics in
general, i.e., cat-allergic asthmatics and non-cat-allergic asthmatics, had a
propensity to secrete IL-5 in response to the Fel d1 peptides. This response
was more pronounced in the cat-allergic subjects and was approximately
equivalent throughout the molecule, in contrast to the amino terminal pattern observed with IFN-γ. Clearly, at the protein level, these results are in
keeping with previous observations that asthmatics make IL-5 in response
to allergen. However, at the submolecular level it is clear that there are
regions of the allergen molecule that may elicit qualitatively different
responses from T cells. Indeed, it appears that there are epitopes in an
allergen that can induce both IFN-γ and IL-5 in asthmatics (Th0 phenotype) and other areas that induce a predominantly IL-5 response (Th2
phenotype). Given the outbred nature of the human population, it is possible that severity of disease may be linked to regions of the molecules that
an individual, by virtue of MHC expression, is capable of recognizing,
coupled to the propensity of that epitope to elicit a Th0 or Th2 response
(29).

VII. T-Cell Homing to the Lung

T lymphocytes traffic between the peripheral circulation, lymphatics, and tissues in response to chemoattractants and complex pattern of expression of adhesion molecules such as integrins and selectins. Expression of both chemoattractants and adhesion molecules is under the partial control of Th1 and Th2 cytokines, and release of the latter determines the quality of the ensuing response. Th2 cytokines such as IL-4 and IL-13 selectively up-regulate expression of chemokines such as eotaxin, eotaxin-2, monocyte chemoattractant protein-1 (MCP-1), thymus and activation-regulated chemokine (TARC), and macrophage-derived chemokine (MDC) (30–36). Receptors for these chemokines include CCR3 (eotaxin, eotaxin-2), CCR4 (TARC, MDC), and CCR8 (TARC). Th2-associated chemokine receptor–ligand combinations have been shown to be up-regulated in allergic inflammation. For example, Ying and colleagues demonstrated increased levels of eotaxin and CCR3 protein and mRNA expression in bronchial biopsies from asthmatic subjects when compared to normal individuals (37). Increased expression of CCR4 has been observed in the asthmatic lung (38), together with enhanced expression of the CCR4 ligand TARC in asthmatic versus normal bronchial mucosa. Furthermore, expression of TARC was induced with IL-4 and TNF-α (mast cell and T-cell products) and induction was inhibited with glucocorticosteroids (39).

The chemokine receptors described above are expressed selectively on Th2 cells (40–43) and have been demonstrated to play a crucial role in the accumulation of such cells at the site of allergic inflammation. Indeed, Lloyd and colleagues demonstrated a sequential dependence on CCR3 coupled with eotaxin and CCR4 coupled with MDC, in the recruitment of murine Th2 cells into the lung (44).

IL-16 is a T-cell chemoattractant that binds CD4 (45). Recent studies have implicated IL-16 in T-cell accumulation at sites of allergic inflammation, particularly in the lung. IL-16 was found to be overexpressed in the bronchial mucosa of asthmatics when compared with normal controls (46). Furthermore, expression of IL-16 was found to be up-regulated following segmental allergen challenge in asthmatic subjects (47).

It appears, therefore, that T cells may accumulate in the airways in response to Th2-specific chemokine/chemokine receptor induction in addition to other molecules, such as IL-16. Sequential dependence on chemokines and their receptors provides a mechanistic basis for homeostasis, suggesting that encounter with allergen results in release of mast cell products such as IL-4, IL-13, and TNF-α, leading to up-regulation of Th2-specific (and nonspecific) chemokines and chemokine receptors. Th2-associated adhesion molecules such as VLA-4 are induced, providing a tissue localization signal for trafficking leukocytes (48). Shortly after mast cell activation, eosinophils and Th2 cells begin to accumulate. Allergen-specific T cells become activated in response to allergen-derived peptides presented in the context of MHC molecules, and release cytokines such as IL-4 and IL-13, which further amplify the expression of chemokines and their receptors, resulting in further accumulation of T cells and eosinophils and ultimately giving rise to the characteristic patterns of cellular accumulation observed in numerous biopsy studies from the challenged lung.

VIII. Th2 Cytokines in Asthma

A. Interleukins 4 and 13 in Isotype Switching to IgE

Interleukin-4 is a pleiotropic cytokine produced by a variety of cell types, including T cells, mast cells, and bone marrow stromal cells. In the context of allergic responses including asthma, IL-4 is involved in the switching of anti-body isotype to the IgE subclass. Production of sterile germline transcripts of the epsilon heavy-chain gene segment can be demonstrated in B cells following incubation with IL-4 and also with the related cytokine IL-13. Concomitant signals via the CD40/CD40L pathway and IL-4 (IL-13) are required for IgE production (49). Studies in atopic individuals have revealed a direct correlation between serum IgE concentrations and the quantity of IL-4 produced by T cells from the peripheral blood. Interestingly, in the context of allergic disease, recent data suggest that mast cells, which synthesize IL-4 and express CD40L, may also have the capacity to effect isotype switching of B cells to the IgE sub-class providing a T-cell-independent mechanism for amplification of the aller-gic response (50,51).

B. Interleukin-5 and GM-CSF

The actions of IL-5 are primarily confined to eosinophils and basophils. This cytokine, of which the T cell is an important source, promotes terminal differ-entiation of the committed eosinophil precursor, releases mature eosinophils from the bone marrow, and enhances the effector capacity of the mature eosi-nophil (52). IL-5 also prolongs the survival of eosinophils in vitro, and anti-IL-5 inhibits allergen-induced bronchial hyperresponsiveness and eosinophilia in both a guinea pig model (53) and a primate model as asthma (54). Elevated numbers of IL-5 mRNA[+] cells were found in endobronchial mucosal biopsies from asthmatics compared with controls (7). Within the subjects who demon-strated detectable IL-5 mRNA there was a correlation between IL-5 mRNA expression and the number of CD25[+] and EG2[+] cells and total eosinophil counts.

In studies examining cytokine profiles in atopic asthma, Robinson demonstrated that there were increased numbers of BAL cells encoding mRNA[+] for IL-3, IL-4, IL-5, and GM-CSF, when non-atopic controls were compared to asthmatics (3). Messenger RNA for IL-4 and IL-5 was localized to T cells within the BAL cell population. Spontaneous expression of mRNA for Th2-type cytokines localized to CD4, but not $CD8^+$, cells was observed in asthmatic subjects but not in controls and was accompanied by elaboration of the eosinophil-active cytokines IL-3, IL-5, and GM-CSF. These results were confirmed in part by Kamei and colleagues who observed allergen-induced release of IL-5 and GM-CSF protein from blood T cells of asthmatics (55). Similarly, Del Prete and colleagues found that T-cell clones raised in vitro from bronchial mucosal biopsies of asthmatics had predominantly the Th2 cytokine profile (56).

Subsequent studies demonstrated that atopic asthma provoked by allergen inhalation was associated with local increases in activated T cells, eosinophils, and cells expressing mRNA for IL-4, IL-5, and GM-CSF (9,57), supporting the hypothesis that allergen-induced late asthmatic responses are accompanied by T-cell activation. Furthermore, increased expression of cytokines such as IL-5 and GM-CSF leads to local recruitment and activation of eosinophils in the bronchial mucosa.

Significant associations between the numbers of cells expressing mRNA for IL-4, IL-5, and GM-CSF and airflow restriction, bronchial hyperresponsiveness, and an asthma symptom score have been demonstrated using the technique of in situ hybridization (58). The use of semiquantitative reverse-transcriptase polymerase chain reaction (RT-PCR) technique has confirmed these findings (59). Moreover, Virchow (8), using segmental allergen challenge, found a correlation between IL-5 concentrations, eosinophil numbers, and activated T cells, supporting the hypothesis that T-cell-derived IL-5 is involved in tissue eosinophilia in allergic asthma.

Glucocorticosteroid treatment in asthmatic subjects was associated with reduction of cells expressing mRNA for IL-4 and IL-5 in bronchoalveolar lavage (BAL) fluid (60,61), a decrease in BAL eosinophils, and clinical improvement, as shown by an increase in the methacholine PC_{20}. Furthermore, there was an increase in the number of cells expressing mRNA for IFN-γ, indicating that prednisolone treatment may favor expression of a cytokine that down-regulates IgE production.

Despite the clear association of IL-5 and eosinophils with asthma, early clinical trials of a monoclonal anti-IL-5 antibody in human have failed to improve symptoms and responses to allergen challenge, perhaps due to insufficient dose (62). Preclinical models have suggested dissociation between the ability of antibodies to IL-5 to remove eosinophils from the circulation, on the one hand, and to modify nonspecific bronchial hyperreactivity, on the other. Thus, it appears that IL-5 may regulate eosinophil accumulation and function in the bronchial mucosa of asthmatics. However, the precise role of eosinophils in establishing and maintaining bronchial hyperreactivity remains to be defined.

C. T Cells as a Source of Th2 Cytokines

Although there has been some debate as to the principal cellular source of IL-4 and IL-5, using the technique of double in situ hybridization/ immunohistochemistry, T cells were shown to be the major source of mRNA encoding IL-4 and IL-5 in bronchial biopsies obtained from asthmatics at baseline (63). Eosinophils and mast cells also contribute to the overall cytokine profile, although the numbers of mRNA[+] cells were fivefold lower than the number of CD3[+] T cells. Furthermore, using a combination of semiquantitative PCR, in situ hybridization, and immunohistochemistry, IL-4 and IL-5 expression appeared similar in bronchial biopsies taken from atopic and non-atopic asthmatics, with IL-5 being significantly higher in asthmatics compared with atopic nonasthmatic normal controls, whereas IL-4 was elevated in asthma and atopic nonasthmatics compared to normal non-atopic controls (59).

The detection of elevated IL-4 mRNA bearing cells in atopic nonasthmatic bronchial mucosal biopsies by RT-PCR raises the possibility that, in general, IL-5 is related more closely to clinical expression of asthma, whereas IL-4 is related to overproduction of IgE. In both atopic and non-atopic asthmatics mRNA for IL-4 and IL-5 colocalized predominantly to CD4[+] but also to CD8[+] T cells, MBP[+] eosinophils, and tryptase[+] mast cells (64). These findings are in agreement with those of Till and colleagues who found that CD8[+] as well as CD4[+] T-cell lines from BAL from asthmatics elaborated the IL-5 protein (65). Cytotoxic type 2 lymphocyte (Tc2) cells may, therefore, also play a role in allergic inflammation at mucosal surfaces.

Maestrelli and colleagues isolated and cloned T cells from bronchial biopsies taken from patients with asthma induced by toluene diisocyanate (66). The majority of clones secreted IL-5 and IFN-γ and were of the CD8[+] phenotype. Whether these findings are related specifically to this form of occupational asthma or to the method of cloning is unclear. Thus, the relative contributions of CD4 and CD8 T cells and the precise cytokine profile of different forms of asthma remain to be firmly established.

IL-4 and IL-5 protein product proved difficult to detect in bronchial biopsies from atopic and non-atopic asthmatics due to the high rate of turnover of cytokines, via secretion, in these cells (64). Detection of these cytokines in other cell types where cytokines are stored in granules has proven more effective (67,68). Having considered the limitations of immunocytochemical detection of cytokines, it is apparent that T cells are an important source of IL-4 and IL-5 in asthma, although the relative contribution of the different cell types to the overall cytokine profile remains uncertain.

D. Interleukin-13 as an Effector Cytokine in Asthma

Interleukin-13 has been implicated as an effector molecule in allergic diseases, particularly allergic asthma. Increased IL-13 responses were observed following antigen challenge of peripheral blood mononuclear cells from atopic allergic subjects when compared to non-atopic subjects (69). IL-13 responses correlated with IL-5 but not IL-4 production. Two important studies investigated the effect of IL-13 blockade in vivo in murine models of asthma (70–72). Soluble fragments of the IL-13 receptor (sIL-13α2) were administered to mice prior to allergen challenge, resulting in a marked reduction in airway hyperresponsiveness, eosinophil recruitment, and mucus hypersecretion. Ablation of IL-4 failed to achieve similar results although a dependence on the IL-4Rα chain was demonstrated. Similarly, Cohn and colleagues identified a role for IL-13, produced by IL-4 knockout Th2 cells, in mucus hypersecretion in an ovalbumin (OVA) peptide-specific murine model of asthma (73). A greater understanding of the role of IL-13 in induction of airways eosinophilia may be provided by the observation that IL-13 is a potent inducer of the eosinophil-active chemokine eotaxin (74). The role of IL-13 and other soluble mediators has been extensively investigated in animal models of asthma.

IX. Exploring the Role of T Cells in Asthma Using Animal Models

A number of murine models of "asthma" have been developed in which either mice or rats of various strains are primed with antigen and adjuvant followed by inhalation challenge, which results in airway hyperresponsiveness (AHR), eosinophil infiltration, and antigen-specific IgE synthesis. Results obtained vary considerably and are often contradictory. Such discrepancies may be due, at least in part, to the different sensitization protocols adopted and to the differing genetic backgrounds employed.

A. Role of T Cells in the Induction of Bronchial Hyperreactivity in Animal Models

Murine models have allowed the demonstration that depletion of CD4 T cells abolishes antigen-induced AHR and that AHR to inhaled antigen can be transferred by adoptive transfer of CD4 T cells (75). Although the majority of investigators have focused on Th2 responses, Randolph and colleagues have also demonstrated a role for allergen-specific Th1 cells in the inflammatory response (76). In this study and another from Hansen and colleagues (77), passive transfer of Th1 cells not only failed to protect from Th2-dependent inflammation but resulted in more severe responses. In support of these findings, Tsitoura and colleagues compared nasal administration of allergen in the presence or absence of IL-12 in a mouse model of allergic sensitization (78). In both cases, the protocol employed resulted in a loss of bronchial hyperactivity in primed mice when subsequently rechallenged with aerosolized allergen. Intranasal administration of OVA alone was shown to induce tolerance in the T-cell compartment and a subsequent failure to initiate a pathogenic Th2 response. The combined allergen challenge with OVA and IL-12, however, gave rise to a Th1 response that, while protective in terms of bronchial hyperreactivity, proved histologically to contribute to airways inflammation. The authors conclude that the currently popular therapeutic strategy of attempting to drive Th2 responses toward a Th1 phenotype may be ineffective and in some cases counterproductive, with significant pathological sequelae.

B.   Role of Antigen Presentation and Costimulation in Asthma

Approaches that induce "tolerance" in the T-cell compartment may hold the key to switching off allergic inflammation in the lung and other target organs. Recently, Lambrecht and colleagues transferred 10^6 bone marrow–derived myeloid dendritic cells that had been pulsed overnight with OVA, intratracheally into C57BL/6 mice (79). Dendritic cells migrated to draining lymph nodes (mediastinal) within a few hours. Subsequent aerosol challenge with allergen resulted in profound airways eosinophilia with cells detected in lavage fluid and also visible by histology as perivascular and peribronchial infiltrates. Transfer of pulsed dendritic cells into gene targeted knockout animals in which either the IL-4 gene or the CD28 gene had been deleted failed to induce comparable responses, implying a critical role in the process for these molecules. Furthermore, blockade of T-cell costimulation through the Th2 cell marker T1/ST2 using a monoclonal antibody directed against the T1/ST2 molecule or a T1/ST2-Ig fusion protein (blocking the as-yet-unidentified receptor), resulted in marked attenuation of airways eosinophilia. Animal models have also allowed testing of potential therapeutic strategies, such as blocking anti-IL-5 antibodies (53,80,81), blocking T-cell costimulation (82,83), and T-cell-directed peptide therapy (84,85). Although animal models have been useful for establishing the principles of immunological intervention, they are some way from the clinical setting in humans.

C.   Neurogenic Inflammation in Asthma

Animal models have also recently been used to explore the role of neurogenic inflammation in asthma. In particular, specific neurokinin receptor antagonists have been employed in order to dissect the early and late asthmatic reaction. Maghni and colleagues (86) used a model of allergen-induced early and late airways response in Brown Norway rats. NK receptor antagonists (NK-1; CP-99,994 and NK-2; SR-48968) were employed to block receptor-dependent events following allergen challenge. Neither antagonist was able to block early airway responses to allergen but both inhibited late responses. Interestingly, only the NK-2 receptor antagonist reduced eosinophil numbers and Th1/Th2 cytokines, suggesting that NK-1 and 2 receptors may activate distinct pathways, all of which result in airway narrowing but through different pathways.

Schuiling and colleagues observed similarly distinct responses to NK receptor antagonists (NK-1; SR-140333 and NK-2; SR-48968) although the outcomes in their guinea pig model differed from those of Maghni (87,88). In the guinea pig, allergen inhalation resulted in both early and late reactions that induced airways hyperresponsiveness to histamine. Neither antagonist affected the severity of the early airway response whereas the NK-2 receptor antagonist, but not the NK-1 antagonist, inhibited the late airway reaction. Furthermore, the NK-1 receptor–specific compound blocked accumulation of eosinophils, neutrophils, and lymphocytes whereas the NK-2 receptor antagonist inhibited the accumulation of neutrophils and lymphocytes only. Both models demonstrate a role for neurokinins in both early and late asthmatic reactions and imply a role for T-cell products in the induction of late-phase responses. Subsequent studies should clarify the role of neurogenic inflammation in asthma.

X. Pharmacological Intervention as a Tool for Defining the Role of the T Cell in Asthma

Therapeutic intervention in humans using modulators of T-cell function has provided further evidence for the role of the T cell in the pathogenesis of asthma. Cyclosporin A, an inhibitor of T-cell activation and mast cell degranulation, was administered to patients with severe, steroid-dependent asthma and was shown to reduce sypmtomatology in baseline asthma (89) and to facilitate the reduction of corticosteriod use (90,91). In a subsequent placebo-controlled, double-blind, crossover study, cyclosporin was shown to reduce the magnitude of the late, but not the early, asthmatic reaction induced by allergen challenge (92). The apparent inability of cyclosporin to modulate mast cell responses in the early-phase reaction may have been related to dose and implies that the reduction in exacerbations and steroid-sparing effects of cyclosporin observed in earlier studies was likely due to effects primarily on T cells. However, it was possible, based on the pleiotropic actions of cyclosporin, that the observed improvements in clinical outcomes were, at least in part, dependent on cells other than T cells.

In order to target the CD4 T cell, Kon and colleagues gave a single infusion of a primatized monoclonal antibody directed at the human CD4 molecule to a group of subjects with steroid-dependent asthma (93). Two dose groups were compared with placebo in a double-blind controlled study. The highest dose (3 mg/kg) was found to improve both morning and evening peak flow measurements for 14 days following a single infusion. Thus, based on the ability to inhibit T-cell function and improve surrogate markers of disease, it may be concluded that T cells play an active role in human asthma.

In more recent studies, peptide fragments corresponding to T-cell epitopes have been administered to allergic asthmatics in order to induce T-cell hyporesponsiveness. In an attempt to desensitize individuals allergic to cats, peptides were administered, by injection, to sensitized subjects. Peptide vaccines were designed based on the amino acid sequence of the major cat allergen Fel dl for cat-allergic individuals and Amb al for subjects allergic to ragweed. In the Fel dl preparation, two relatively large (27 amino acid residues each) peptides were employed. Some individuals developed immediate hypersensitivity reactions that were likely to be the result of IgE cross-linking by the peptides. Moreover, delayed symptoms of breathlessness and wheeze were reported in a percentage of patients. These symptoms occurred 1 h or more after peptide administration and typically presented 2–6 h postinjection (94,95). Since the majority of those experiencing late-onset allergic symptoms did not experience immediate reactions, we postulated that these reactions were due to direct activation of allergen-specific T cells.

In an attempt to directly activate T cells in the absence of IgE- and mast cell-dependent events, we synthesized short allergen-derived peptides and administered them, by intradermal injection, to cat-allergic asthmatic subjects. Epitope mapping studies were performed with peripheral blood cells from cat-allergic and non-cat-allergic subjects in order to determine the region of the Fel dl molecule that induced T-cell responses in the largest percentage of individuals. Peptides of 16 to 17 amino acids were chemically synthesized and purified by HPLC. Three peptides, termed FC1P (Fel d Chain 1 Peptides) were selected from chain 1 of the Fel dl molecule. In vitro histamine release assays were performed in which the peptides were evaluated together with whole cat dander allergen for their ability to release histamine from enriched basophils isolated from peripheral blood of sensitized cat-allergic subjects. Titration of increasing concentrations of whole cat dander extract resulted in increasing histamine release. In contrast, increasing concentrations of a mixture of the three peptides (FC1P) induced no significant histamine release. Thus, FC1P did not appear to cross-link adjacent IgE molecules in the representative individuals studied.

XI.   Induction of Isolated Late Asthmatic Reactions with Allergen Peptides

For safety reasons, in vivo studies were initiated at doses of peptide that were not expected to give rise to late asthmatic reactions (LARs). A dose-finding study was performed in which small numbers of allergic asthmatic individuals were injected intradermally with a mixture of the three peptides containing either 10, 20, 40, or 80 μg of each peptide. Injections were given in the volar aspect of the forearm. In the group receiving the highest dose, a proportion of subjects experienced a late-onset fall in FEV_1 of greater than 20% of baseline that was accompanied by wheezing. The magnitude of the response varied among those who developed reactions, with certain individuals experiencing a fall in FEV_1 of up to 65%. Subjects experiencing isolated (LARs) reported the reaction as being similar to natural exposure to cats since the reduction in airway caliber occurred gradually (unlike an IgE-mediated early reaction). All subjects receiving peptide injection were monitored in the clinic for a minimum of 6 h after injection. Reversal of airway narrowing was achieved in all individuals experiencing LAR with the use of short-acting β_2 agonists, suggesting that the mechanism of bronchoconstriction involved airway smooth muscle contraction. An example of an isolated, peptide-induced LAR is shown in Fig. 1.

XII. MHC Restriction of Peptide-Induced LAR

A total of 40 cat-allergic asthmatic subjects of mild to moderate severity were challenged with 80 µg of FC1P. Nine of the 40 developed isolated LARs. The

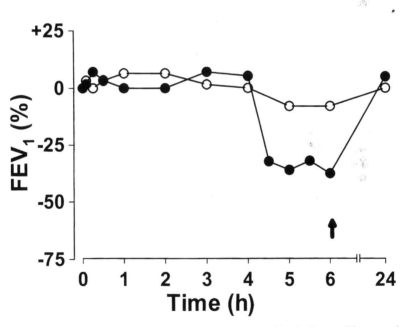

Figure 1 **Isolated late asthmatic reaction following peptide challenge.** Three synthetic overlapping peptides (closed circles; 80 µg or each peptide) corresponding to a region of the major cat allergen, Fel d1, or (or diluent control; open circles) were administered by intradermal injection in the volar aspect aspect of the forearm at time zero. Spirometry was performed at 15-min intervals for the first hour and hourly thereafter. At the 4-h time point, FEV_1 (forced expiratory volume in 1 s) was reduced. FEV_1 remained constant at approximately 70% of baseline for 2 h, prior to reversal with inhaled β_2 against. No early changes in lung function corresponding to mast cell activation were observed.

response to the peptide mixture was believed to be T-cell mediated. T cells recognize peptide epitopes in an MHC-restricted fashion (96). Tissue typing was performed on all individuals to determine HLA class II expression. The results revealed that four of the nine subjects developing LAR expressed an HLA-DR13 allele, three expressed a DR1 allele, and three expressed a DR4 allele. Although there is considerable variation in estimates of the percentage of a given population that express a particular MHC allele, these frequencies (particularly DR13) appeared to be higher than that expected in a random sample of the population, despite the small numbers of individuals analyzed.

In order to test the hypothesis that one or more of these three DR molecules was capable of restricting the T-cell response to one or more of the FC1P peptides, presentation experiments were performed in vitro. The three FC1P peptides were incubated overnight with fibroblast cell lines transfected with the genes encoding the HLA-DR molecules of interest. Thus, one cell line expressed the HLA-DRB1*1301 chain together with the invariant HLA-DRA chain. Another cell line expressed a further variant of DR13 (DRB1*1302), and similar lines were available expressing DR1 and DR4 molecules. Peptide-pulsed fibroblasts were placed in culture together with cells from a cat allergen–specific T-cell line from an individual expressing the appropriate MHC allele who had experienced a LAR. All T-cell lines were generated from study subjects before peptide administration. Individuals who expressed DR13 and had experienced an isolated LAR were assayed with murine fibroblasts expressing human DR13 molecules. Proliferative and cytokine responses of the T-cell lines were measured 48 h later. The results demonstrated that the responses to the second of the FC1P peptides was restricted by DR4 alleles and that the responses to the third peptide could be restricted by DR1 and DR13 alleles, indicating promiscuous peptide–MHC associations.

Based on the MHC restriction observed in these experiments it was concluded that isolated LAR occur as a direct result of T-cell activation in an MHC-restricted fashion, following intradermal administration of allergen-derived peptide sequences.

XIII. Mechanisms Underlying Isolated LAR

Bronchial whole-allergen challenge in atopic asthmatic individuals is characterized by a cellular infiltrate consisting primarily of increased numbers of eosinophils in both the bronchial mucosa and in BAL fluid. Studies with endobronchial biopsies have shown accumulation of eosinophils in the bronchial mucosa 3, 4, and 24 h postchallenge (9,97,98). Furthermore, eosinophils have been demonstrated in BAL at 4, 6, and 24 h (3,98,99). Accumulation of eosinophils is believed to occur as a result of the actions of IL-5 and eotaxin (100), although, at present, the source of IL-5 (mast cell or T cell) remains unclear. The role of the eosinophil in the induction of late-phase reactions, particularly LARs, remains an important issue, which has yet to be resolved.

The ability to induce IgE-independent LARs by directly activating allergen-specific T cells has provided in ideal opportunity to address both the source of IL-5 for eosinophil accumulation and the role of the eosinophil in bronchoconstriction. Thus, eight cat-allergic asthmatic subjects underwent bronchoscopic investigation 6 h after a randomized (crossover design) intradermal injection of either 80 μg of FC1P or diluent control (101). Bronchial mucosal biopsies were taken for analysis of cellular infiltrate and mRNA expression by immunohistochemistry. BAL provided fluid for analysis of soluble mediators and cellular infiltrate.

In contrast to bronchial whole-allergen challenge, peptide-induced LARs did not appear to be accompanied by increased numbers of eosinophils, neutrophils, basocphils, or lymphocytes 6 h after challenge. Eosinophils were not observed in lavage fluid. Thus, the results of intradermal challenge with peptides indicate that eosinophilic infiltration is not a characteristic of the T-cell component of the LAR and suggest that in models of whole-allergen challenge, eosinophil accumulation during the early stages of the LAR may be dependent on IL-5 released from mast cells during the EAR.

However, it should be borne in mind that there are substantial differences in the route of challenge employed in whole (inhaled)–allergen challenge and peptide (intradermal) challenge. In the case of peptide-induced late asthmatic reactions, it is important to note that the peptide challenge was via the intradermal route and was, therefore, assumed to be blood-borne in the sense that peptides reaching the lung would do so via the vasculature rather than via a mucosal surface. Thus, eosinophils and other cells present in the mucosa following conventional allergen challenge may have been localized deeper in the tissue, in the proximity of blood vessels. Studies involving inhalation of nebulized peptides are currently underway to address this issue.

XIV. T Cells as Mediators of Bronchial Hyperreactivity

A central role for the T cell in the development and maintenance of bronchial hyperreactivity (BHR) has been suggested in many studies in experimental animals, many of which have been described earlier in this chapter. For example, DeSanctis and colleagues adoptively transferred allergen-specific Th2 cells into naive recipients and challenged them, via the inhaled route, with aerosolized allergen. The mice displayed hallmark features characteristic of BHR (75).

Hogan and colleagues induced BHR in mice following priming and inhaled challenge with OVA. In an attempt to isolate the factors responsible for BHR, the authors administered monoclonal antibodies directed against IL-4, IL-5, or CD4 to mice deficient in IL-4 or IL-5. BHR was still observed after removal of IL-4 and/or IL-5. While deficiency in IL-5 reduced the accumulation

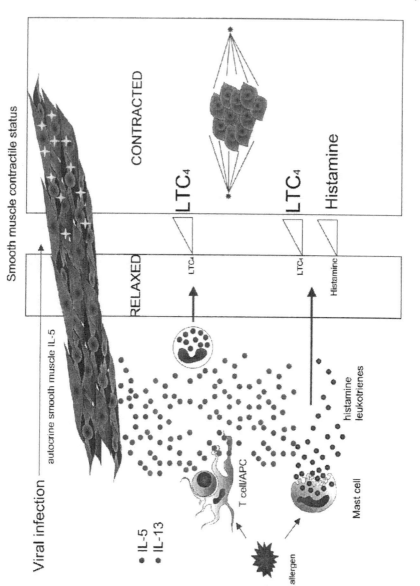

of pulmonary eosinophils, it was only the infusion of anti-CD4 antibodies that resulted in an abrogation of BHR, suggesting a T-cell-dependent mechanism for the induction of BHR that was not entirely dependent on IL-4 and/or IL-5 (102).

The failure to resolve BHR using antibodies to IL-4 and IL-5 in this model suggested that there may be contributions other than Th2 cytokines that are required from T cells to elicit the hyperreactive phenotype. However, a number of recent observations in a variety of models may clarify the role of both the T-cell and Th2 cytokines in the generation and maintenance of enhanced smooth muscle reactivity to nonspecific stimuli such as methacholine, histamine, and other bronchoconstrictors. (Fig. 2).

Grunig and colleagues and Wills-Karp and colleagues established the ability of IL-13 to induce BHR (70,71). Administration of soluble IL-13 receptor–Ig chimeric molecules resulted in blockade of IL-13 resulting in a reversal of sensitivity to inhaled methacholine.

In more recent studies, Grunstein and colleagues have described the ability of IL-5 (via IL-1β) but non IL-4 to enhance the ability of cultured smooth muscle cells to respond to acetylcholine and to suppress the ability of these cells to relax in the presence of isoproterenol (103). Similarly, studies of Laporte and colleagues have ascribed a similar function to IL-13. Cultured smooth muscle cells were incubated with either IL-4 or IL-13. Both cytokines induced phosphorylation of STAT-6 but with differing kinetics. However, only IL-13 was able to reduce isoproterenol-induced increases in intracellular cAMP formation and hence muscle relaxation (104). Grunstein and colleagues reported the observation that infection of airway smooth muscle cells with rhinovirus resulted in autocrine production of IL-5 (105). This finding provides a plausible explanation for the association of wheeze and asthma exacerbation with viral infection.

Figure 2   Th2 cytokines in the induction and maintenance of bronchial hyperreactivity. Allergen activates both mast cells (via IgE cross-linking) and T cells (following allergen processing and presentation by APC) resulting in the release of Th2 cytokines such as IL-4 and IL-5, and IL-13. Histamine and leukotrienes released from mast cells raise the local concentrations of bronchoconstrictor mediators. IL-5 and IL-13 act directly on airway smooth muscle cells and enhance their ability to respond to histamine, leukotrienes, and other mediators. IL-5 releases eosinophils from the bone marrow. Eosinophils migrate to the lung in response to chemokines such as eotaxin induced by the action of Th2 cytokines on smooth muscle cells that produce large quantities of the mediator. In the lung parenchyma, eosinophils become activated and release large quantities of leukotrienes, further increasing the local levels of mediators and increasing the chance of contraction of the potentiated smooth muscle. Eosinophil granules are released and toxic basic proteins liberated, resulting in damage to airway epithelium. Damaged epithelium reduces the integrity of the physical barrier to allergen and creates a positive-feedback cycle resulting in more inflammation and bronchial hyperreactivity.

In the light of these data one may wonder why the initial studies in humans with monoclonal antibodies to IL-5 failed to improve outcomes related to BHR (62). The answer to the apparent paradox may lie in the fact that the dose of anti-IL-5 administered to humans was primarily designed to reduce eosinophilia. Animal studies had previously shown that higher doses of antibody were required in some preclinical models to block the induction of BHR despite the effective reduction of circulating eosinophils.

The possibility that the eosinophil is guilty by association rather than cause is becoming increasing considered. Allergen impacting a mucosal surface cross-links mast cell–bound IgE and activates the cell. The resultant granule release liberates vasoactive compounds, but also a multitude of cytokines including IL-5 and IL-13. Subsequent activation of allergen-specific T cells following antigen processing and presentation then results in further, more sustained release of IL-5 and IL-13 into the system. Undoubtedly, some IL-5 will reach the bone marrow and result in the release of eosinophils that traffic to the lung. The function of such eosinophils may be to effect repair.

The primary outcome of the release of Th2 cytokines such as IL-5 and IL-13 from both mast cells and T cells may be to lower the activation threshold of airway smooth muscle cells by potentiating their ability to respond to the prevailing milieu of histamine, prostanoids, neuropeptides, and other smooth muscle–contracting compounds. Indeed, it is not necessary to postulate anything other than smooth muscle potentiation to explain most findings that relate to the induction and maintenance of BHR.

That the constriction of bronchial smooth muscle is not dependent the presence of IgE or, indeed, mast cells has been described in a number of animal models (described earlier in this chapter). Furthermore, our own work with T-cell peptide epitopes from the Fel d1 molecule provides support for the concept that T cells, when sufficiently activated by allergen, can provide a signal of sufficient magnitude to smooth muscle cells to result in the potentiation of the ability of these cells to respond to physiological levels of mediators in their immediate environment. Similarly, activation of resident mucosal Th2 cells in intrinsic asthma (by viruses or unidentified endogenous or exogenous proteins) may provide an IgE-independent mechanism for bronchoconstriction in so-called nonallergic individuals.

The inability of an infusion of antibodies against individual cytokines such as IL-5 to inhibit BHR-related outcomes in both human and murine models may lie in the fact that an insufficient dose was administered. A higher dose may be required to block the intimate release and uptake of mediators along the mast cell, T-cell, and smooth muscle axis. The fact that several cytokines and perhaps many more mediators (such as neurotrophins) have the ability to potentiate smooth muscle in this way argues against the effective use of a compound that merely reduces the levels of one disease-relevant cytokine.

XV. Conclusions

Data from animal models of asthma, and more recently from studies with human cells and volunteers, have provided compelling evidence to support the notion that CD4$^+$ T cells are critical to pathogenesis. Th2 cytokines can be produced by T cells, basophils, mast cells, and eosinophils. It is likely that these cytokines, particularly IL-5 and IL-13, play a major role in the induction and maintenance of bronchial hyperreactivity by potentiating the ability of bronchial smooth muscle cells to respond to the surrounding milieu of mediators. Although both mast cells and eosinophils may contribute substantially to local concentrations of mediators capable of contracting smooth muscle cells, it is likely that T cells are necessary (and in certain conditions sufficient; peptide-induced LAR) for the induction of bronchoconstriction. Combined with early results from clinical studies aimed at sequestering single mediators in the allergic cascade, it appears than an effective strategy for the management of allergic asthma may hinge on modulation of the responses of antigen-specific CD4 T cells with agents such as synthetic peptides.

Acknowledgments

ML is a National Asthma Campaign Senior Research Fellow. Funding for some of the studies described in this chapter was provided by the National Asthma Campaign (UK) and the Medical Research Council (MRC). Allergen extracts were provided by ALK Abéllo, Cophenhagen, Denmark and C.B.F. LETI, Spain.

The authors thank the following individuals who contributed in various ways to this chapter: Drs. B. M. Haselden, W. L. Oldfield, D. S. Robinson, S. Ying, Q. Meng; Professors R. I. Lechler, J. R. Lamb, M. Church; Ms. K. Shirley and J. R. Barkans.

References

1. Corrigan CJ, Hartnell A, Kay AB. T lymphocyte activation in acute severe asthma. Lancet 1988; 1(8595):1129–1132.
2. Azzawi M, Johnston PW, Majumdar S, Kay AB, Jeffery PK. T lymphocytes and activated eosinophils in airway mucosa in fatal asthma and cystic fibrosis. Am Rev Respir Dis 1992; 145(6):1477–1482.
3. Robinson DS, Hamid Q, Ying S, Tsicopoulos A, Barkans, J Bentley AM, et al. Predominant TH2-like bronchoalveolar T-lymphocyte population in atopic asthma. N Engl J Med 1992; 326(5):298–304.
4. Wierenga EA, Snoek M, Jansen HM, Bos JD, van Lier RA, Kapsenberg ML. Human atopen-specific types 1 and 2 T helper cell clones. J Immunol 1991; 147(9):2942–2949.

5. Parronchi P, Macchia D, Piccinni MP, Biswas P, Simonelli C, Maggi E, et al. Allergen- and bacterial antigen-specific T-cell clones established from atopic donors show a different profile of cytokine production. Proc Natl Acad Sci USA 1991; 88(10):4538–4542.
6. Romagnani S. Human TH1 and TH2 subsets: doubt no more. Immunol Today 1991; 12(8):256–257.
7. Hamid Q, Azzawi M, Ying S, Moqbel R, Wardlaw AJ, Corrigan CJ et al. Expression of mRNA for interleukin-5 in mucosal bronchial biopsies from asthma. J Clin Invest 1991; 87(5):1541–1546.
8. Virchow JC, Jr., Walker C, Hafner D, Kortsik C, Werner P, Matthys H, et al. T cells and cytokines in bronchoalveolar lavage fluid after segmental allergen provocation in atopic asthma. Am J Respir Crit Care Med 1995: 151(4):960–968.
9. Bentley AM, Meng Q, Robinson DS, Hamid Q, Kay AB, Durham SR. Increases in activated T lymphocytes, eosinophils, and cytokine mRNA expression for interleukin-5 and granulocyte/macrophage colony-stimulating factor in bronchial biopsies after allergen inhalation challenge in atopic asthmatics. Am J Respir Cell Mol Biol 1993; 8(1):35–42.
10. Alexander AG, Barkans J, Moqbel R, Barnes NC, Kay AB, Corrigan CJ. Serum interleukin 5 concentrations in atopic and non-atopic patients with glucocorticoid-dependent chronic severe asthma. Thorax 1994; 49(12):1231–1233.
11. Corrigan CJ, Haczku A, Gemou-Engesaeth V, Doi S, Kikuchi Y, Takatsu K, et al. CD4 T-lymphocyte activation in asthma is accompanied by increased serum concentrations of interleukin-5. Effect of glucocorticoid therapy. Am Rev Respir Dis 1993; 147(3):540–547.
12. Humbert M, Corrigan CJ, Kimmitt P, Till SJ, Kay AB, Durham SR. Relationship between IL-4 and IL-5 mRNA expression and disease severity in atopic asthma. Am J Respir Crit Care Med 1997; 156(3 Pt 1):704–708.
13. Palframan RT, Collins PD, Severs NJ, Rothery S, Williams TJ, Rankin SM. Mechanisms of acute eosinophil mobilization from the bone marrow stimulated by interleukin 5: the role of specific adhesion molecules and phosphatidylinositol 3-kinase. J Exp Med 1998; 188(9):1621–1632.
14. Palframan RT, Collins PD, Williams TJ, Rankin SM. Eotaxin induces a rapid release of eosinophils and their progenitors from the bone marrow. Blood 1998; 91(7):2240–2248.
15. Kay AB. Allergy and allergic diseases. Second of two parts. N Engl J Med 2001; 344(2):109–113.
16. Kay AB. Allergy and allergic diseases. First of two parts. N Engl J Med 2001; 344(1):30–37.
17. Prigozy TI, Naidenko O, Qasba P, Elewaut D, Brossay L, Khurana A, et al. Glycolipid antigen processing for presentation by CD1d molecules. Science 2001; 291(5504):664–667.
18. Corinti S, De Palma RD, Fontana A, Gagliardi C, Pini C, Sallusto F. Major histocompatibility complex–independent recognition of a distinctive pollen antigen, most likely a carbohydrate, by human CD8+ alpha/beta T cells. J Exp Med 1997; 186(6):899–908.

19. Rogge L, Barberis-Maino L, Biffi M, Passini N, Presky DH, Gubler U, et al. Selective expression of an interleukin-12 receptor component by human T helper 1 cells. J Exp Med 1997; 185(5):825–831.

20. Varga EM, Wachholz P, Nouri-Aria KT, Verhoef A, Corrigan CJ, Till SJ, et al. T cells from human allergen-induced late asthmatic responses express IL-12 receptor beta 2 subunit mRNA and respond to IL-12 in vitro. J Immunol 2000; 165(5):2877–2885.

21. van der Pouw Kraan TC, Boeije LC, de Groot ER, Stapel SO, Snijders A, Kapsenberg ML, et al. Reduced production of IL-12 and IL-12 dependent IFN-gamma release in patients with allergic asthma. J Immunol 1997; 158(11):5560–5565.

22. Murray JS, Pfeiffer C, Madri J, Bottomly K. Major histocompatibility complex (MHC) control of CD4 T cell subset activation. II. A single peptide induces either humoral or cell-mediated responses in mice of distinct MHC genotype. Eur J Immunol 1992; 22(2):559–565.

23. Pfeiffer C, Stein J, Southwood S, Ketelaar H, Sette A, Bottomly K. Altered peptide ligands can control CD4 T lymphocyte differentiation in vivo. J Exp Med 1995; 181(4):1569–1574.

24. Hosken NA, Shibuya K, Heath AW, Murphy KM, O'Garra A. The effect of antigen dose on CD4+ T helper cell phenotype development in a T cell receptor-alpha beta-transgenic model. J Exp Med 1995; 182(5):1579–1584.

25. Guery JC, Galbiati F, Smiroldo S, Adorini L. Selective development of T helper (Th)2 cells induced by continuous administration of low dose soluble proteins to normal and beta(2)-microglobulin-deficient BALB/c mice. J Exp Med 1996; 183(2):485–497.

26. Constant SL, Bottomly K. Induction of Th1 and Th2 CD4+ T cell responses: the alternative approaches. Annu Rev Immunol 1997; 15:297–322.

27. Evavold BD, Allen PM. Separation of IL-4 production from Th cell proliferation by an altered T cell receptor ligand. Science 1991; 252(5010):1308–1310.

28. Kumar V, Bhardwaj V, Soares L, Alexander J, Sette A, Sercarz E. Major histocompatibility complex binding affinity of an antigenic determinant is crucial for the differential secretion of interleukin 4/5 or interferon gamma by T cells. Proc Natl Acad Sci U S A 1995; 92(21):9510–9514.

29. Haselden BM, Syrigou E, Jones M, Huston D, Ichikawa K, Chapman MD, et al. Proliferation and release of IL-5 and IFN-γ by peripheral blood mononuclear cells from cat-allergic asthmatics and rhinitics, non-cat allergic asthmatics, and normal controls to peptides derived from Fel d 1 chain 1. J Allergy Clin Immunol 2001; 108:349–356.

30. Mochizuki M, Schroder J, Christophers E, Yamamoto S. IL-4 induces eotaxin in human dermal fibroblasts. Int Arch Allergy Immunol 1999; 120 Suppl 1:19–23.

31. Teran LM, Mochizuki M, Bartels J, Valencia EL, Nakajima T, Hirai K, et al. Th1- and Th2-type cytokines regulate the expression and production of eotaxin and RANTES by human lung fibroblasts. Am J Respir Cell Mol Biol 1999; 20(4):777–786.

32. Mochizuki M, Bartels J, Mallet AI, Christophers E, Schroder JM. IL-4 induces eotaxin: a possible mechanism of selective eosinophil recruitment in helminth infection and atopy. J Immunol 1998; 160(1):60–68.

33. Goebeler M, Schnarr B, Toksoy A, Kunz M, Brocker EB, Duschl A, et al. Interleukin-13 selectively induces monocyte chemoattractant protein-1 synthesis and secretion by human endothelial cells. Involvement of IL-4R alpha and Stat6 phosphorylation. Immunology 1997; 91(3):450–457.

34. Yano S, Yanagawa H, Nishioka Y, Mukaida N, Matsushima K, Sone S. T helper 2 cytokines differently regulate monocyte chemoattractant protein-1 production by human peripheral blood monocytes and alveolar macrophages. J Immunol 1996; 157(6):2660–2665.

35. Matsukura S, Stellato C, Georas SN, Casolaro V, Plitt JR, Miura K, et al. Interleukin-13 upregulates eotaxin expression in airway epithelial cells by a STAT6-dependent mechanism. Am J Respir Cell Mol Biol 2001; 24(6):755–761.

36. Rollins BJ, Pober JS. Interleukin-4 induces the synthesis and secretion of MCP-1/JE by human endothelial cells. Am J Pathol 1991; 138(6): 1315–1319.

37. Ying S, Robinson DS, Meng Q, Rottman J, Kennedy R, Ringler DJ, et al. Enhanced expression of eotaxin and CCR3 mRNA and protein in atopic asthma. Association with airway hyperresponsiveness and predominant co-localization of eotaxin mRNA to bronchial epithelial and endothelial cells. Eur J Immunol 1997; 27(12):3507–3516.

38. Panina-Bordignon P, Papi A, Mariani M, Di Lucia P, Casoni G, Bellettato C, et al. The C-C chemokine receptors CCR4 and CCR8 identify airway T cells of allergen-challenged atopic asthmatics. J Clin Invest 2001; 107(11):1357–1364.

39. Sekiya T, Miyamasu M, Imanishi M, Yamada H, Nakajima T, Yamaguchi M, et al. Inducible expression of a Th2-type CC chemokine thymus- and activation-regulated chemokine by human bronchial epithelial cells. J Immunol 2000; 165(4):2205–2213.

40. Sallusto F, Mackay CR, Lanzavecchia A. Selective expression of the eotaxin receptor CCR3 by human T helper 2 cells. Science 1997; 277(5334):2005–2007.

41. Bonecchi R, Bianchi G, Bordignon PP, D'Ambrosio D, Lang R, Borsatti A, et al. Differential expression of chemokine receptors and chemotactic responsiveness of type 1 T helper cells (Th1s) and Th2s. J Exp Med 1998; 187(1):129–134.

42. D'Ambrosio D, Iellem A, Bonecchi R, Mazzeo D, Sozzani S, Mantovani A, et al. Selective up-regulation of chemokine receptors CCR4 and CCR8 upon activation of polarized human type 2 Th cells. J Immunol 1998; 161(10):5111–5115.

43. Zingoni A, Soto H, Hedrick JA, Stoppacciaro A, Storlazzi CT, Sinigaglia F, et al. The chemokine receptor CCR8 is preferentially expressed in Th2 but not Th1 cells. J Immunol 1998; 161(2):547–551.

44. Lloyd CM, Delaney T, Nguyen T, Tian J, Martinez A, Coyle AJ, et al. CC chemokine receptor (CCR)3/eotaxin is followed by CCR4/monocyte-derived chemokine in mediating pulmonary T helper lymphocyte type 2 recruitment after serial antigen challenge in vivo. J Exp Med 2000; 191(2):265–274.

45. Center DM, Kornfeld H, Cruikshank WW. Interleukin 16 and its function as a CD4 ligand. Immunol Today 1996; 17(10):476–481.

46. Laberge S, Ernst P, Ghaffar O, Cruikshank WW, Kornfeld H, Center DM, et al. Increased expression of interleukin-16 in bronchial mucosa of subjects with atopic asthma. Am J Respir Cell Mol Biol 1997; 17(2):193–202.

47. Laberge S, Pinsonneault S, Varga EM, Till SJ, Nouri-Aria K, Jacobson M, et al. Increased expression of IL-16 immunoreactivity in bronchial mucosa after segmental allergen challenge in patients with asthma. J Allergy Clin Immunol 2000; 106(2):293–301.

48. Bocchino V, Bertorelli G, D'Ippolito R, Castagnaro A, Zhuo X, Grima P, et al. The increased number of very late activation antigen-4-positive cells correlates with eosinophils and severity of disease in the induced sputum of asthmatic patients. J Allergy Clin Immunol 2000; 105(1 Pt 1):65–70.

49. Monticelli S, Vercelli D. Molecular regulation of class switch recombination to IgE through epsilon germline transcription. Allergy 2001; 56(4):270–278.

50. Gordon JR, Burd PR, Galli SJ. Mast cells as a source of multifunctional cytokines. Immunol Today 1990; 11(12):458–464.

51. Burd PR, Thompson WC, Max EE, Mills FC. Activated mast cells produce interleukin 13. J Exp Med 1995; 181(4):1373–1380.

52. Wardlaw AJ, Moqbel R, Kay AB. Eosinophils: biology and role in disease. Adv Immunol 1995; 60:151–266.

53. Mauser PJ, Pitman A, Witt A, Fernandez X, Zurcher J, Kung T, et al. Inhibitory effect of the TRFK-5 anti-IL-5 antibody in a guinea pig model of asthma. Am Rev Respir Dis 1993; 148(6 Pt 1):1623–1627.

54. Mauser PJ, Pitman AM, Fernandez X, Foran SK, Adams GK, III, Kreutner W, et al. Effects of an antibody to interleukin-5 in a monkey model of asthma. Am J Respir Crit Care Med 1995; 152(2):467–472.

55. Kamei T, Ozaki T, Kawaji K, Banno K, Sano T, Azuma M, et al. Production of interleukin-5 and granulocyte/macrophage colony-stimulating factor by T cells of patients with bronchial asthma in response to *Dermatophagoides farinae* and its relation to eosinophil colony-stimulating factor. Am J Respir Cell Mol Biol 1993; 9(4):378–385.

56. Del Prete GF, De Carli M, D'Elios MM, Maestrelli P, Ricci M, Fabbri L, et al. Allergen exposure induces the activation of allergen-specific Th2 cells in the airway mucosa of patients with allergic respiratory disorders. Eur J Immunol 1993; 23(7):1445–1449.

57. Robinson D, Hamid Q, Bentley A, Ying S, Kay AB, Durham SR. Activation of CD4+ T cells, increased TH2-type cytokine mRNA expression, and eosinophil recruitment in bronchoalveolar lavage after allergen inhalation challenge in patients with atopic asthma. J Allergy Clin Immunol 1993; 92(2):313–324.

58. Robinson DS, Ying S, Bentley AM, Meng Q, North J, Durham SR, et al. Relationships among numbers of bronchoalveolar lavage cells expressing messenger ribonucleic acid for cytokines, asthma symptoms, and airway methacholine responsiveness in atopic asthma. J Allergy Clin Immunol 1993; 92(3):397–403.

59. Humbert M, Durham SR, Ying S, Kimmitt P, Barkans J, Assoufi B, et al. IL-4 and IL-5 mRNA and protein in bronchial biopsies from patients with atopic and nonatopic asthma: evidence against "intrinsic" asthma being a distinct immunopathologic entity. Am J Respir Crit Care Med 1996; 154(5):1497–1504.

60. Bentley AM, Hamid Q, Robinson DS, Schotman E, Meng Q, Assoufi B, et al. Prednisolone treatment in asthma. Reduction in the numbers of eosinophils, T cells, tryptase-only positive mast cells, and modulation of IL-4, IL-5, and interferon-gamma cytokine gene expression within the bronchial mucosa. Am J Respir Crit Care Med 1996; 153(2):551–556.

61. Robinson D, Hamid Q, Ying S, Bentley A, Assoufi B, Durham, S, et al. Prednisolone treatment in asthma is associated with modulation of bronchoalveolar lavage cell interleukin-4, interleukin-5, and interferon-gamma cytokine gene expression. Am Rev Respir Dis 1993; 148(2):401–406.

62. Leckie MJ, ten Brinke A, Khan J, Diamant Z, O'Connor BJ, Walls CM, et al. Effects of an interleukin-5 blocking monoclonal antibody on eosinophils, airway hyper-responsiveness, and the late asthmatic response. Lancet 2000; 356(9248):2144–2148.

63. Ying S, Durham SR, Corrigan CJ, Hamid Q, Kay AB. Phenotype of cells expressing mRNA for TH2-type (interleukin 4 and interleukin 5) and TH1-type (interleukin 2 and interferon gamma) cytokines in bronchoalveolar lavage and bronchial biopsies from atopic asthmatic and normal control subjects. Am J Respir Cell Mol Biol 1995; 12(5):477–487.

64. Ying S, Humbert M, Barkans J, Corrigan CJ, Pfister R, Menz G, et al. Expression of IL-4 and IL-5 mRNA and protein product by CD4+ and CD8+ T cells, eosinophils, and mast cells in bronchial biopsies obtained from atopic and nonatopic (intrinsic) asthmatics. J Immunol 1997; 158(7):3539–3544.

65. Till S, Li B, Durham S, Humbert M, Assoufi B, Huston D, et al. Secretion of the eosinophil-active cytokines interleukin-5, granulocyte/macrophage colony-stimulating factor and interleukin-3 by bronchoalveolar lavage CD4+ and CD8+ T cell lines in atopic asthmatics, and atopic and non-atopic controls. Eur J Immunol 1995; 25(10):2727–2731.

66. Maestrelli P, Del Prete GF, De Carli M, D'Elios MM, Saetta M, Di Stefano A, et al. CD8 T-cell clones producing interleukin-5 and interferon-gamma in bronchial mucosa of patients with asthma induced by toluene diisocyanate. Scand J Work Environ Health 1994; 20(5):376–381.

67. Moqbel R, Ying S, Barkans J, Newman TM, Kimmitt P, Wakelin M, et al. Identification of messenger RNA for IL-4 in human eosinophils with granule localization and release of the translated product. J Immunol 1995; 155(10): 4939–4947.

68. Levi-Schaffer F, Lacy P, Severs NJ, Newman TM, North J, Gomperts B, et al. Association of granulocyte-macrophage colony-stimulating factor with the crystalloid granules of human eosinophils. Blood 1995; 85(9):2579–2586.

69. Li Y, Simons FE, HayGlass KT. Environmental antigen-induced IL-13 responses are elevated among subjects with allergic rhinitis, are independent of IL-4, and are inhibited by endogenous IFN-gamma synthesis. J Immunol 1998; 161(12):7007–7014.

70. Grunig G, Warnock M, Wakil AE, Venkayya R, Brombacher F, Rennick DM, et al. Requirement for IL-13 independently of IL-4 in experimental asthma. Science 1998; 282(5397):2261–2263.

71. Wills-Karp M, Luyimbazi J, Xu, X, Schofield B, Neben TY, Karp CL, et al. Interleukin-13: central mediator of allergic asthma. Science 1998; 282(5397):2258–2261.

72. Wills-Karp M. IL-12/IL-13 axis in allergic asthma. J Allergy Clin Immunol 2001; 107(1):9–18.
73. Cohn L, Homer RJ, MacLeod H, Mohrs M, Brombacher F, Bottomly K. Th2-induced airway mucus production is dependent on IL-4Ralpha, but not on eosinophils. J Immunol 1999; 162(10):6178–6183.
74. Li L, Xia Y, Nguyen A, Lai YH, Feng L, Mosmann TR, et al. Effects of Th2 cytokines on chemokine expression in the lung: IL-13 potently induces eotaxin expression by airway epithelial cells. J Immunol 1999; 162(5):2477–2487.
75. De Sanctis GT, Itoh A, Green FH, Qin S, Kimura T, Grobholz JK, et al. T-lymphocytes regulate genetically determined airway hyperresponsiveness in mice. Nat Med 1997; 3(4):460–462.
76. Randolph DA, Carruthers CJ, Szabo SJ, Murphy KM, Chaplin DD. Modulation of airway inflammation by passive transfer of allergen-specific Th1 and Th2 cells in a mouse model of asthma. J Immunol 1999; 162(4):2375–2383.
77. Hansen G, Berry G, DeKruyff RH, Umetsu DT. Allergen-specific Th1 cells fail to counterbalance Th2 cell-induced airway hyperreactivity but cause severe airway inflammation. J Clin Invest 1999; 103(2):175–183.
78. Tsitoura DC, Blumenthal RL, Berry G, DeKruyff RH, Umetsu DT. Mechanisms preventing allergen-induced airways hyperreactivity: role of tolerance and immune deviation. J Allergy Clin Immunol 2000; 106(2):239–246.
79. Lambrecht BN, De Veerman M, Coyle AJ, Gutierrez-Ramos JC, Thielemans K, Pauwels RA. Myeloid dendritic cells induce Th2 responses to inhaled antigen, leading to eosinophilic airway inflammation. J Clin Invest 2000; 106(4):551–559.
80. Hamelmann E, Oshiba A, Loader J, Larsen GL, Gleich G, Lee J, et al. Anti-interleukin-5 antibody prevents airway hyperresponsiveness in a murine model of airway sensitization. Am J Respir Crit Care Med 1997; 155(3):819–825.
81. Hamelmann E, Cieslewicz G, Schwarze J, Ishizuka T, Joetham A, Heusser C, et al. Anti-interleukin 5 but not anti-IgE prevents airway inflammation and airway hyperresponsiveness. Am J Respir Crit Care Med 1999; 160(3):934–941.
82. Haczku A, Takeda K, Redai I, Hamelmann E, Cieslewicz G, Joetham A, et al. Anti-CD86 (B7.2) treatment abolishes allergic airway hyperresponsiveness in mice. Am J Respir Crit Care Med 1999; 159(5 Pt 1):1638–1643.
83. Tsuyuki S, Tsuyuki J, Einsle K, Kopf M, Coyle AJ. Costimulation through B7-2 (CD86) is required for the induction of a lung mucosal T helper cell 2 (TH2) immune response and altered airway responsiveness. J Exp Med 1997; 185(9):1671–1679.
84. Briner TJ, Kuo MC, Keating KM, Rogers BL, Greenstein JL. Peripheral T-cell tolerance induced in naive and primed mice by subcutaneous injection of peptides from the major cat allergen Fel d I. Proc Natl Acad Sci USA 1993; 90(16):7608–7612.
85. Hoyne GF, O'Hehir RE, Wraith DC, Thomas WR, Lamb JR. Inhibition of T cell and antibody responses to house dust mite allergen by inhalation of the dominant T cell epitope in naive and sensitized mice. J Exp Med 1993; 178(5):1783–1788.
86. Maghni K, Taha R, Afif W, Hamid Q, Martin JG. Dichotomy between neurokinin receptor actions in modulating allergic airway responses in an animal model of helper T cell type 2 cytokine-associated inflammation. Am J Respir Crit Care Med 2000; 162(3 Pt 1):1068–1074.

87. Schuiling M, Zuidhof AB, Meurs H, Zaagsma J. Role of tachykinin NK2-receptor activation in the allergen-induced late asthmatic reaction, airway hyperreactivity and airway inflammatory cell influx in conscious, unrestrained guinea-pigs. Br J Pharmacol 1999; 127(4):1030–1038.

88. Schuiling M, Zuidhof AB, Zaagsma J, Meurs H. Role of tachykinin NK 1 and NK 2 receptors in allergen-induced early and late asthmatic reactions, airway hyperresponsiveness, and airway inflammation in conscious, unrestrained guinea pigs. Clin Exp Allergy 1999; 29 Suppl 2:48–52.

89. Alexander AG, Barnes NC, Kay AB, Corrigan CJ. Clinical response to cyclosporin in chronic severe asthma is associated with reduction in serum soluble interleukin-2 receptor concentrations. Eur Respir J 1995; 8(4):574–578.

90. Lock SH, Kay AB, Barnes NC. Double-blind, placebo-controlled study of cyclosporin A as a corticosteriod-sparing agent in corticosteroid-dependent asthma. AM J Respir Crit Care Med 1996; 153(2):509–514.

91. Kay AB. Immunosuppressive agents in chronic severe asthma. Allergy Proc 1994; 15(3):147–150.

92. Sihra BS, Kon OM, Durham SR, Walker S, Barnes NC, Kay AB. Effect of cyclosporin A on the allergen-induced late asthmatic reaction. Thorax 1997; 52(5):447–452.

93. Kon OM, Sihra BS, Compton CH, Leonard TB, Kay AB, Barnes NC. Randomised, dose-ranging, placebo-controlled study of chimeric antibody to CD4 (keliximab) in chronic severe asthma. Lancet 1998; 352(9134):1109–1113.

94. Maguire P, Nicodemus C, Robinson D, Aaronson D, Umetsu DT. The safety and efficacy of ALLERVAX CAT in cat allergic patients. Clin Immunol 1999; 93(3):222–231.

95. Norman PS, Nicodemus CF, Creticos PS, Wood RA, Eggleston PA, Lichtenstein LM, et al. Clinical and immunologic effects of component peptides in Allervax Cat. Int Arch Allergy Immunol 1997; 113(1–3):224–226.

96. Haselden BM, Kay AB, Larche M. Immunoglobulin E-independent major histocompatibility complex-restricted T cell peptide epitope-induced late asthmatic reactions. J Exp Med 1999; 189(12):1885–1894.

97. Aalbers R, de Monchy JG, Kauffman HF, Smith M, Hoekstra Y, Vrugt B, et al. Dynamics of eosinophil infiltration in the bronchial mucosa before and after the late asthmatic reaction. Eur Respir J 1993; 6(6):840–847.

98. Brown JR. Kleimberg J, Marini M, Sun G, Bellini A, Mattoli S. Kinetics of eotaxin expression and its relationship to eosinophil accumulation and activation in bronchial biopsies and bronchoalveolar lavage (BAL) of asthmatic patients after allergen inhalation. Clin Exp Immunol 1998; 114(2):137–146.

99. Diaz P, Gonzalez MC, Galleguillos FR, Ancic P, Cromwell O, Shepherd D, et al. Leukocytes and mediators in bronchoalveolar lavage during allergen-induced late-phase asthmatic reactions. Am Rev Respir Dis 1989; 139(6):1383–1389.

100. Collins PD, Marleau S, Griffiths-Johnson DA, Jose PJ, Williams TJ. Cooperation between interleukin-5 and the chemokine eotaxin to induce eosinophil accumulation in vivo. J Exp Med 1995; 182(4):1169–1174.

101. Haselden BM, Larché M, Meng Q, Shirley K, Dworski R, Kaplan A, et al. Late asthmatic reactions provoked by intradermal injection of T cell peptide epitopes are not associated with bronchial mucosal infiltration of eosinophils or Th2-type

cells or with elevated concentrations of histamine or eicosanoids in bronch-oalveolar fluid. J Allergy Clin Immunol 2001;108:394–401.

102. Hogan SP, Matthaei KI, Young JM, Koskinen A, Young IG, Foster PS. A novel T cell-regulated mechanism modulating allergen-induced airways hyperreactivity in BALB/c mice independently of IL-4 and IL-5. J Immunol 1998; 161(3):1501–1509.

103. Hakonarson H, Maskeri N, Carter C, Chuang S, Grunstein MM. Autocrine interaction between IL-5 and IL-1 beta mediates altered responsiveness of atopic asthmatic sensitized airway smooth muscle. J Clin Invest 1999; 104(5):657–667.

104. Laporte JC, Moore PE, Baraldo S, Jouvin MH, Church TL, Schwartzman IN, et al. Direct effects of interleukin-13 on signaling pathways for physiological responses in cultured human airway smooth muscle cells. Am J Respir Crit Care Med 2001; 164(1):141–148.

105. Grunstein MM, Hakonarson H, Maskeri N, Chuang S. Autocrine cytokine sig-naling mediates effects of rhinovirus on airway responsiveness. Am J Physiol Lung Cell Mol Physiol 2000; 278(6):L1146–L1153.

4

B-Cell Differentiation and IgE Synthesis

HAMIDA HAMMAD and BART N. LAMBRECHT

Erasmus University Medical Centre
Rotterdam, The Netherlands

I. B-Cell Physiology

A. B-Cell Activation and Differentiation

B lymphocytes represent less than 10% of lymphocytes in lung tissue and BAL fluid. The majority of B cells can be found in the bone marrow and lymphoid organs. B lymphocytes originate from the bone marrow and leave as surface IgM- and IgD-positive naive B lymphocytes to secondary lymphoid organs such as the spleen and lymph nodes. Here they recognize antigens through cross-linking of their surface B-cell receptor (BCR) and become activated by dendritic cells (DCs) and T cells in the T-cell area (Fig. 1). As a result of BCR cross-linking, B cells enter into cell cycle, and demonstrate increased survival by expression of anti-apoptotic proteins. The antigen is endocytosed and presented as small peptides on MHC class II molecules, together with CD80 and CD86 molecules to activated T cells. Activated B cells also have increased expression of cytokine receptors for IL-2 and IL-4 and express CD40, so that they become receptive to T-cell-derived cytokines and CD40L. These interactions between T cells and B cells occur in the outer zones of the T-cell area, in close proximity to B-cell follicles. Following activation by BCR cross-linking and T-cell signals in the outer T-cell zone, B cells initiate isotype class switching (1,2). They differentiate into either short-lived marginal zone plasma cells or migrate to the B-cell follicles to proliferate in the germinal center reaction (Fig. 1). In the germinal center, B cells receive activating signals from follicular DCs (FDC) and helper T cells, and isotype switching proceeds further. This process is followed by somatic hypermutation and affinity maturation. Those B cells with the highest affinity for antigen receive survival signals from FDCs to become long-lived high-affinity memory B cells or high-affinity plasma cells

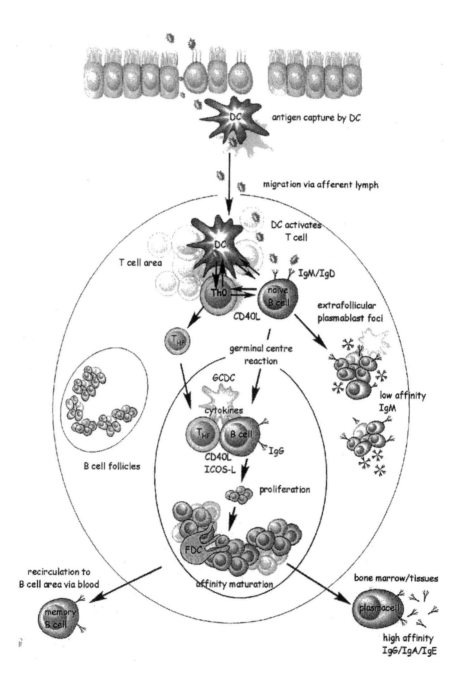

that produce high levels of immunoglobulins. The low-affinity cells die by a process of programmed cell death (apoptosis) and are cleared from the follicles. Plasma cells migrate to the bone marrow, a dominant site of antibody production, whereas memory B cells recirculate throughout the body and become plasma cells upon repeated encounter with antigen.

B. Importance of Chemokine Receptors in T-Cell-Dependent B-Cell Activation

Protein antigens are recognized by specific B and T lymphocytes in peripheral lymphoid organs, and activated cell populations come together in these organs to initiate humoral immune responses. The precursor frequency of B cells or T cells with a particular antigen specificity is very low and in the order of 1 in 10^6 B cells or T cells. Therefore, the chances of these specific cells meeting in vivo are exceedingly small. To solve this problem, evolution has selected a very efficient system of lymphocyte recirculation to increase the chances that these cells physically meet in a specialized zone in the secondary immune organs (lymph nodes and spleen) (1). T and B cells continuously recirculate from blood to lymphoid tissues. This lymphocyte positioning is tightly controlled by chemokine–chemokine receptor interactions (Fig. 2) (3). Genetic experiments have established that B-cell entry to lymphoid B follicles depends on CXCR5 and its ligand CXCL13 (BCA-1/BLC) (4,5), and entry of T cells and DCs to the T zone depends on expression of CCR7 and ligands, CCL19 (SLC), and CCL21 (MIP-3β) (6,7). As a result, naive B cells localize in the B-cell follicles, whereas naive T cells colocalize with DCs in the T-cell area (1). This segregation is important for unprimed T cells to first receive signals from DCs and not from B cells (8). Antigen-specific T cells are first activated by DCs and then migrate to the edge of the T-cell area near the B-cell follicle, where they meet antigen-primed B cells. The two cell types

◄─────────────────────────────────────

Figure 1 B-cell activation by T cells and DCs in the draining lymph nodes of the lung. After antigen transport from the periphery, DCs stimulate naive T cells and naive B cells in the outer T-cell area. B cells that recognize free unprocessed antigen through their surface Ig molecules are activated and present the antigen to activated T cells in the outer T-cell area. T cells provide B cells with essential activation signals such as cytokines and CD40L, leading to the initiation of class switching. Some activated B cells migrate outside the B-cell follicle to become extrafollicular plasmablasts secreting low-affinity IgM. Others migrate to the B-cell follicle and undergo intense proliferation in the germinal center (GC) reaction. Here they are stimulated by specialized T cells called follicular T-helper cells (T_{HF}) that provide help for isotype switching through inducible costimulator (ICOS). The T cells and B cells are also stimulated by germinal center DCs (GCDCs). Proliferating B cells are selected for high affinity on follicular dendritic cells (FDCs) in a process called affinity maturation. Low-affinity cells die by apoptosis. Finally, cells that leave the GC reaction become either recirculating memory B cells or Ig-secreting plasma cells in the bone marrow or tissues.

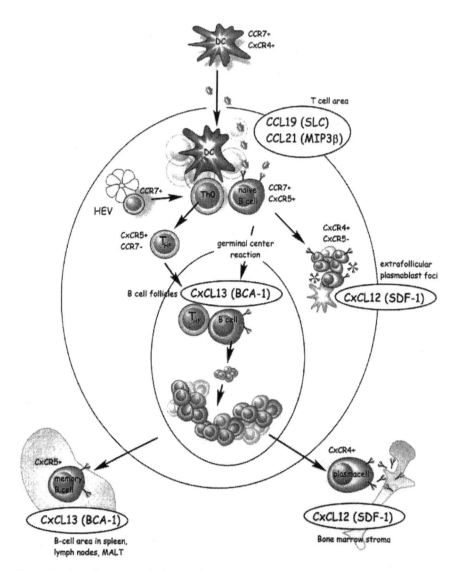

Figure 2 Regulation of cellular traffic of B cells, T cells, and DCs by chemokines and their receptors (cf. Fig. 1). The ultimate fate of these cells in the lymph nodes, tissue, and spleen is dictated by their responsiveness to chemokines expressed at a particular area in the nodes or tissues (chemokine ligands are circled). BCA-1, B-cell chemoattractant 1; CCR, CC chemokine receptor; CXCR, CXC chemokine receptor; HEV, high endothelial venule; MIP3β, macrophage inflammatory protein 3β; SDF-1, stromal cell–derived factor 1.

then physically interact to accomplish CD40-CD40L-dependent B-cell activation. T-cell activation by OX40L on DCs in the T-cell areas results in the loss of responsiveness to "lymphoid" chemokines CCL19 and CCL21 and gain of responsiveness to the chemokine CXCL13 (BCA-1/BLC) (9) that binds to CXCR5. This chemokine receptor is responsible for the homing of a unique subset of T-helper cells to the B-cell follicles for antibody production and induction of the germinal center reaction (10,11). These follicular T-helper cells (T_{FH}) are CXCR5$^+$ T cells and were found to be almost all CD4$^+$ Th2 cells, suggesting a role in immunoglobulin synthesis. Inflamed tonsils, but not blood, contain CXCR5$^+$ T_{FH} cells that were activated and distinct from circulating T cells (10,11). The tonsilar CXCR5$^+$ T cells express CD69 and inducible costimulator (ICOS), and were generally L-selectin negative. Expression of ICOS is particularly noteworthy, as this molecule is a CD28-like family member that facilitates effector functions rather than primary T-cell activation. ICOS probably participates in all effector T-cell responses, particularly T-cell help for antibody production (12–14). CXCR5$^+$ T cells are heterogeneous, and the majority of CXCR5$^+$ T cells are neither capable of nor clearly specialized for providing efficient B-cell help. The efficient B-cell helping effector T cells are a small subset of CXCR5$^+$ T cells that express CD57 (15). Within the germinal center, germinal center DCs (GCDCs) as well as FDCs are a predominant source of CXCL13, attracting both activated B cells and activated T cells for the germinal center reaction. B cells activated by T cells in the follicles differentiate into plasmablasts, which are factories for antibody production, and rapidly leave the follicles. In the spleen, the cells move through marginal zone "bridging channels," and many of them lodge in foci near vessels or collagenous fibers in the red pulp, where they receive survival signals from specialized DCs (16–18). In lymph nodes, plasma cells are found distributed between the lymphatic sinuses of the medullary cords (19). Plasmablasts located at these extrafollicular sites produce mainly low-affinity IgM antibodies for a short period of time. Later in the response, plasma cells that have originated from the germinal center reaction and have class switched start appearing in the bone marrow (20,21). Down-regulation of CXCR5, with its concomitant loss of responsiveness to CXCL13 in the B-cell follicle, and up-regulation of CXCR4 seems likely a part of the mechanism promoting plasma cell movement out of the B-cell area in spleen and lymph node. The ligand for CXCR4 is CXCL12 (SDF-1), which is expressed in the red pulp of the spleen, lymph node medullary cords, and stromal cells of the bone marrow. CXCR4 chemokine receptor seems necessary for the normal distribution of plasma cells near the vessels and fibers in the splenic red pulp and in the bone marrow (22). It is currently unknown which factors determine whether a B cell becomes a plasmablast in the red pulp, a bone marrow plasma cell, or a recirculating memory B cell, although the strength of the T-cell B-cell DC interaction could be important in this decision process (23).

C. Role of Dendritic Cells in Stimulating B-Cell Responses

Dendritic cells are essential to induce primary immune responses in CD4$^+$ and CD8$^+$ T cells. Recently, it has become clear that they can also activate B-cell responses (Table 1). It was shown that DCs can capture Ag in the periphery (e.g., the gut mucosa) and transfer the antigen in an unprocessed form to the B cells in draining lymph nodes (Fig. 1) (24). At the same time, DCs can also process part of the antigen and present it on MHC class II to T cells in the outer T-cell area, in close proximity to the B-cell follicles (25). Therefore, DCs might form a "cellular bridge" to bring together antigen-specific T cells and B cells in the so-called cognate interaction, at the same time providing essential activating signals to T cells and B cells (26,27). The DCs induce the initial activation of naive T cells to become receptive to the B cells presenting cognate antigen. In vitro and in vivo studies have shown that naive B cells fail to activate naive T cells, whereas they can clearly activate primed T cells (8). Moreover, DCs induce the expression of the CXCR5 on T cells by signaling through OX-40, and as a consequence T cells migrate to the germinal center. T-cell area interdigitating DCs induce the formation of plasma cells from naive B cells, and as such could be involved the generation of extrafollicular foci of plasma cells in the red pulp and medullary cords. Extrafollicular plasmablasts receive survival signals from a specialized subset of DCs located in the medullary cords (18,28).

In the germinal center of primary follicles, a specialized GCDC is important for isotype class switching and the germinal center reaction (29–31). It produces Interleukin-12 (IL-12) and IL-6, leading to local production of complement factor 3, an essential cofactor for B-cell activation and germinal center formation (32). It also produces CXCL13 to attract activated T cells and B cells to the GC reaction (33). Moreover, it was shown that DCs can directly induce isotype class switching to IgA$_1$ and IgA$_2$ from CD40-activated naive B

Table 1 Evidence for Stimulation of B Cells by DCs

Animal studies
Rat DCs form clusters with B cells and T cells in vitro and in vivo
Rat DCs transport Ag from periphery to lymph nodes in unprocessed form
Injection of Ag-pulsed mouse DCs primes for IgG$_{2a}$ synthesis after booster of Ag
Mouse spleen DCs induce proliferation and activation of naive B cells
A subset of mouse DCs is associated with extrafollicular plasmablast survival
A subset of mouse DCs enters B-cell follicles and stimulates Ig synthesis
Human studies
Cord-blood derived DCs stimulate IgA$_1$ and IgA$_2$ synthesis in naive B cells
Cord-blood derived DCs stimulate IgG and IgA synthesis from memory
   B cells
Sorted interdigitating tonsillar DCs induce proliferation and IgM synthesis
Germinal center DCs are necessary for the germinal center reaction

cells in the presence of IL-10 and transforming growth factor, β (TGF-β)(34). They also induce proliferation and IgG production from CD40-activated resting memory B cells (35). It was also shown that DCs can express CD40L possibly bypassing some of the T-cell signals for Ig class switching (36).

There is some evidence that the tissue origin of the DC determines the type of Ig class that is produced. When DCs are purified from Peyer's patches of the mouse they induce the formation of IgG_1 and IgA, whereas DCs purified from spleen induce IgG_{2a}. The main explanation is the induction of respectively Th2 and Th1 T-cell responses. When rat lung immature DCs were purified and pulsed with ovalbumin (OVA), they boosted Th2-dependent IgG_1 responses when injected intravenously (37). The role of lung DCs in inducing IgE responses is, however, less clear. In a humanized SCID mouse model of asthma, it was shown that monocyte-derived DCs injected in the lung promote synthesis of human allergen-specific IgE (H.H. and B.L. et al., unpublished, and Ref. 38). Similarly, levels of IgE were reduced to baseline by depleting DCs from the airways of asthmatic mice (39). It is unclear at present whether this is due to the effects of DCs on Th2 cytokine generation by T cells or due to direct effects of DCs on B cells.

II. Immunoglobulin Class Switching

A feature unique to B cells is the sequential production of immunoglobulins of the same antigenic specificity, but distinct biological effector functions due to recombination of the antigen-binding variable domain to particular constant regions such as C_μ, C_δ, C_γ, C_ε, and C_α. The particular type of Ig produced by a particular B cell in response to antigen exposure depends on many factors (Table 2) (40). As an example, IgA is the dominant class of Ig produced at mucosal surfaces in response to bacterial and viral antigens, whereas the same antigens induce IgM or IgG responses when administered systemically. The formation of IgE (and IgG_4) to particular antigens (allergens) is a typical feature of atopic individuals, whereas "normal" individuals generally synthesize other Ig isotypes, such as IgM or IgG_{2a}. However, the production of IgE is not exclusive to the atopic state. Indeed, many infants show short-lived IgE responses to ingested food allergens, and these responses wane as the child grows older (41). Atopic individuals inherit traits that put them at risk for IgE-dependent allergic diseases, but environmental factors (level of allergen exposure, infection rate, lifestyle, bacterial colonization, air pollution) ultimately determine the nature and extent of disease (42,43).

A. Molecular Heavy-Chain Gene Rearrangements Leading to IgE Expression

The production of IgE antibodies by B cells is regulated by a complex network of cytokines and cell surface interactions, followed by molecular

Table 2   Factors Influencing IgE Synthesis

Genetic background of the individual
>   Polymorphism in cytokine (receptor) genes
>   Polymorphism in sCD14 levels
>   Polymorphism in recognition of allergens?

Cytokine balance in the host
>   Th1 cytokines reduce IgE
>   Th2 cytokines stimulate IgE and IgG_4 (or IgG_1 in mouse)

Nature of the antigen
>   Allergens (e.g., house dust mite) stimulate IgE
>   Helminth-derived Ags stimulate IgE
>   Adjuvants, such as diesel exhaust particles, stimulate IgE

Route of antigen administration
>   Airway administration leads to short-lived IgE responses
>   IgA responses at mucosal sites

History of antigen exposure
>   Infant responses to food are IgE biased, later IgG biased
>   Initial high-level exposure at young age stimulates IgE

Level of environmental Ag stimulation
>   Chronic low-level exposure to Ag stimulates IgE
>   Concomitant infection with bacteria reduces IgE
>   Bacterial CpG motifs, Bacille Calmette-Guérin (BCG) reduce IgE

genetic rearrangements at the immunoglobulin heavy-chain locus (IgH)(44,45). Initially, all B cells produce IgD and IgM antibodies. At this point, a $V_H(D)J_H$ cassette of sequences encoding the variable domain is immediately adjacent to the C_μ and C_δ exons, which encode the IgM and IgD constant regions at the 5' end of the IgH locus (Fig. 3). Further downstream in IgH are several widely spaced clusters of exons, $C_\gamma, C_\varepsilon,$ and $C_\alpha,$

Figure 3   Molecular events involved in class switching to IgE. First, transcription at the Iε site is required to provide access for the DNA double-strand break mechanism. RNA splicing of the primary germline transcript is also necessary before deletional class switching can occur. The end result of ε germline transcription is a sterile germline transcript that does not translate protein due to stop codons in every reading frame. Second, DNA intervening between switch (S) regions Sμ and Sε is looped out, followed by double-strand breakage and repair through nonhomologous end joining. Numerous enzymes, such as DNA-protein kinase, activation-induced cytidine deaminase (AID), and proteins such as Nijmegen breakage syndrome 1 (Nbs-1) and γ-histone 2AX are involved in this process. The looped-out DNA still has an active promotor that transcribes circle transcripts for a short period after class switching. These circle transcripts are proof of recent class switching.

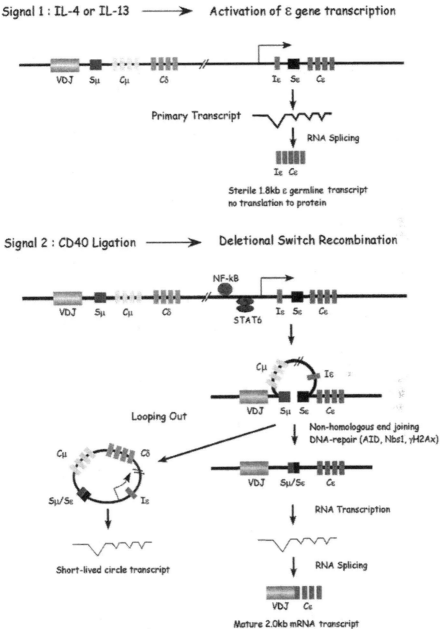

Signal 1 : IL-4 or IL-13 ⟶ Activation of ε gene transcription

VDJ Sμ Cμ Cδ   Iε Sε Cε

Primary Transcript

RNA Splicing

Iε Cε

Sterile 1.8kb ε germline transcript
no translation to protein

Signal 2 : CD40 Ligation ⟶ Deletional Switch Recombination

NF-kB

VDJ Sμ Cμ Cδ   Iε Sε Cε
        STAT6

Cμ   Iε

VDJ Sμ Sε Cε

Looping Out

Non-homologous end joining
DNA-repair (AID, Nbs1, γH2Ax)

VDJ Sμ/Sε Cε

Cμ   Cδ

Sμ/Sε   Iε

RNA Transcription

Short-lived circle transcript

RNA Splicing

VDJ Cε

Mature 2.0kb mRNA transcript
Translation to functional heavy chain

encoding the constant region domains of the IgG, IgE, and IgA heavy-chain isotypes. These heavy-chain genes have introns at their 5' end called switch regions (S), which contain numerous tandem repeats of conserved DNA sequences, which enhance the efficiency of class switching (46). On stimulation by cytokines, together with critical cell–cell interactions with $CD4^+$ T-cell surface accessory molecules, B cells can change the isotype of the antibodies they produce while retaining their original antigenic specificity (44,47). For this process, genomic DNA must be spliced and rejoined at the S regions to move the VDJ elements from their location proximal to C_μ to many kilobases downstream at the target switch region (S_α or S_γ or S_ϵ) of the genes encoding the heavy chains of other isotypes (45,48). A large amount of intervening DNA between the S_μ and target S region is excised and deleted in this irreversible process ("looped out"), and therefore the mechanism is referred to as deletional switch recombination.

Before the initiation of these genomic rearrangements, IL-4/IL-13-stimulated B cells destined to switch from IgM to IgE must first activate RNA transcription at the unrearranged or germline ε-heavy-chain locus (Fig. 3). The RNA produced is referred to as ε-germline transcript and is driven from a promoter 5' of the Iε exon located just upstream of the S_ϵ region and the 4 C_ϵ exon (49). Mature ε-germline RNA includes a 140-bp Iε exon and exons $C_{\epsilon 1}$ to $C_{\epsilon 4}$ (47). Germline transcripts undergo RNA splicing but contain several stop codons in every reading frame. Therefore, these transcripts do not encode a functional protein and are referred to as sterile (49). Germline transcription at the S_ϵ region of the C_ϵ gene followed by RNA splicing of the transcript must occur before deletional switch recombination to IgE can proceed. B cells in which the I_ϵ exon or its promoter have been mutated are unable to undergo isotype switching (50–52). Conversely, the introduction of an active promoter upstream of the I_ϵ exon promotes not only germline transcription but also isotype switching. Germline transcription at the S_ϵ region likely changes the accessibility of the C_ϵ gene to enzymes that mediate switch recombination, although this "accessibility model" cannot explain all cases of class switching. Furthermore, the necessity of RNA splicing also implies that some of the enzymes involved in RNA splicing or processing may be involved in DNA recombination (40).

Class switching joins immunoglobulin switch regions by looping out and excision of intervening DNA (Fig. 3). However, the mechanisms of DNA cleavage, switch region synapsis, and DNA repair after cleavage are not well defined. One of the DNA repair process enzymes that is absolutely required for class switching is DNA-dependent protein kinase (DNA-PK)-Ku complex. This enzyme is involved in nonhomologous end joining following double-strand breaks. Gene disruption of any of the subunits of this enzyme inhibits class switching and VDJ recombination (45,53). DNA-PK-Ku also binds to SWAP-70, a molecule that is up-regulated upon B-cell activation and is specifically required for class switching to IgE (53). The execution of switching also requires the synthesis of new proteins. Muramatsu et al. have identified one of these proteins as activation-induced cytidine deaminase (AID) (54). AID is expressed in activated splenic B cells and in the germinal centers of lymph nodes, and is involved in deletional switch recombination as well as somatic hypermutation. Mice deficient for AID have a major defect in isotype switching, with elevated IgM levels and low or absent IgA, IgE, and IgG. Conversely, overexpression of AID in B cells leads to spontaneous class switching in the absence of cytokine or CD40L stimulation (55). The precise role of AID in the process of deletional switch recombination, requiring double-strand DNA break and repair, is unclear due to the fact that it belongs to a family of RNA-editing enzymes. Recently, it was shown that AID is necessary for the proper localization of the Nijmegen breakage syndrome protein (Nbs1) and phosphorylated H2A histone family member X (γ-H2AX, also known as γ-H2afx), at the C_H region undergoing class switching. Both of these proteins facilitate DNA double-strand break repair, and H2AX knockout mice have deficient class switching (56).

One method to study recent class switching to a particular heavy-chain class is the detection of transcripts of looped-out DNA, in which the I_H promoter is still active. The circular DNA contains a DNA segment between S_μ and a target S region including its I promoter (e.g., I_α), which is driven by specific cytokine stimulation before class switching. The specific I promoter is still active in looped-out circular DNA and directs production of I-C_μ transcripts termed "circle transcripts." A comparison of kinetics between circle transcripts by reverse-transcriptase polymerase chain reaction (RT-PCR) and circular DNA showed more rapid disappearance of circle transcripts. Thus, circle transcripts may serve as a hallmark for active and recent class switching in vitro and in vivo (57). Using this method, it was recently demonstrated that murine B cells undergo class switching to IgA within the lamina propria of the gut (58). This method has not yet been used to detect IgE class switching within sites of allergic inflammation.

B. Induction of IgE Synthesis by CD4⁺ T Cells

B cells require two distinct signals to undergo isotype switching (47,59). This first signal is cytokine dependent and leads to the activation of transcription at the S site of IgH chain locus, allowing the determination of isotype specificity. The second signal activates the recombination machinery (AID and other enzymes), resulting in DNA switch recombination. The two signals required for switching to the IgE are delivered to B cells by T cells through a complex series of secreted signals and cell–surface interactions (Fig. 4). In naive B cells, antigen-specific IgM on the B-cell surface binds antigens, leading to the internalization of antigen-receptor complexes. The antigen then undergoes an endosomal processing in specialized endosomal vesicles (class II-rich vesicles called CIIV) and is subsequently presented to an antigen-specific T cell in the

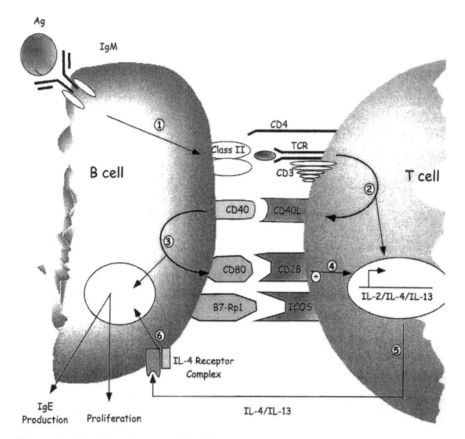

Figure 4 T-cell B-cell cross-talk leading to mutual activation of the cells. **1.** Antigen recognition through the B-cell receptor or through IgE bound to CD23 leads to endocytosis and processing of the antigen in a specialized class II–rich vesicular compartment (CIIV). **2.** Peptides are presented on MHC class II to the T-cell receptor/CD3 complex, leading to up-regulation of CD40L. It is possible that the constitutive expression of B7Rp-1 leads to signaling to ICOS and subsequent CD40L expression by T cells. It is currently unknown if this occurs upstream or downstream of TCR recognition. **3.** CD40 stimulation of B cells leads to up-regulation of CD80/CD86 and to further stimulation of cognate T cells, thus intensifying the interaction between both cell types. **4.** The combined signals of TCR triggering, and ICOS, CD28, and possibly Ox40 stimulation on T cells leads to T-cell differentiation into efficient T-helper cells. **5.** Under particular conditions (ICOS, Ox40), T cells switch to IL-4 and IL-13 production. **6.** IL-4/IL-13 binds to the respective receptors on B cells, effectively contributing together with CD40 stimulation to IgE class switching under conditions of prolonged B-cell stimulation. (Redrawn and modified from Ref. 162.)

form of a peptide associated with MHC class II molecules. Cognate recognition of the antigen/class II complex expressed on B cells by T cells leads to two events: (a) secretion of cytokines such as IL-4 and/or IL-13, and (b) expression of CD40L by T cells. Binding of IL-4 to its receptor on B cells delivers the first signal for isotype switching. The transient expression of CD40L after T-cell activation renders T cells fully competent to induce isotype switching to IgE (60). CD40L engages CD40 that is constitutively expressed on B cells and the CD40L-induced oligomerization of CD40 on B cells delivers the second signal that triggers switch recombination to IgE. However, IL-4 also promotes class switching to IgG and IgA, so that IL-4 cannot be the sole determinant of IgE synthesis. Although the ε and γ1 germline promoters both contain IL-4-responsive elements that bind signal transducer and activator of transcription (STAT)-6, the binding affinity for STAT6 is 10-fold higher in the ε promotor site, explaining a preferential induction of ε germline transcript (61).

Hasbold and Hodgkin have proposed a model in which class switching to a particular class of Ig heavy chain is determined not only by the presence of CD40L and cytokines, but also by the number of cell divisions a B cells undergoes during stimulation, before differentiation into a plasma cell. Thus, it was shown that class switching to IgG occurs after three cell divisions, whereas switching to IgE requires at least five cell divisions. The action of IL-4 and CD40L is merely to accelerate the time that a B cell enters into the first division. In this model, the switching to IgE is a stochastic event of which the chances increase on every successive cell division. This model also explains why switching to IgE requires prolonged stimulation of the B cell (62,63). The fact that certain cell cycle–regulated nuclear proteins, such as myb and PU.1, have binding sites in the I_ε promotor also suggests a link between cell division, germline transcription, and class switching. It is generally accepted that endogenous myb proteins function as cell cycle sensors.

C. IL-4 and IL-13 Are Critical for IgE Class Switching

CD4$^+$ T-helper lymphocytes can be divided into two subsets based on their cytokine production profiles (64). Briefly, Th1 cells preferentially produce IL-2 and IFN-γ and promote delayed-type hypersensitivity responses, whereas Th2 cells produce IL-4, IL-5, IL-6, IL-10, and IL-13, which favor humoral immune responses including isotype switching and the development of allergic diseases. The Th1-derived cytokines inhibit Th2 cytokine production, and Th2 cytokines inhibit Th1 cytokine production. Consistent with this paradigm, whereas IL-4 and IL-13 induce ε germline transcription, IFN-γ suppresses the IL-4 induction of ε germline transcripts (65). The interactions between the cytokines and their receptors delivers the first signal for switching to IgE. IL-4 and IL-13 have been shown to be essential for IgE production. IL-4 and IL-13 are the only cytokines known to induce ε germline transcription and IgE production in vitro when added in recombinant form (66,67). Anti-IL-4 antibodies preferentially inhibit IgE production without affecting IgG, IgM, or IgA synthesis (68). Injection of anti-IL-4 or anti-IL-4 receptor abolishes IgE and IgG_1 production in parasite-infected mice (69). The biological effects of IL-13 overlap those of IL-4, with the exception that IL-13 does not activate human T cells (70). Like IL-4, IL-13 increases MHC class II and CD23 expression on B cells and monocytes, and induces ε germline transcription and isotype switching to IgE and IgG4 (66,67,70). However, IL-13 is less potent that IL-4 in most of these actions. Despite this, cocultures of purified T and B cells from atopic asthmatic donors suggested that IgE synthesis depends more on T-cell-derived IL-13 than IL-4 (71,72).

IL-4 and IL-13 receptors are multimeric and share the IL-4Rα chain. The IL-4 receptor consists of ligand-binding IL-4Rα and the signal-transducing common chain, γc (Fig. 5). The IL-13 receptor is composed of IL-4Rα chain along with an IL-13-binding chain (IL-13Rα1 or IL-13Rα2). The IL-4Rα and γc chains lack known kinase activity and are associated with the Janus family tyrosine kinase JAK1 and JAK3, respectively (73,74). Upon activation, these kinases phosphorylate tyrosine residues in the intracellular domains of the receptor chains which serve as binding sites for STAT6, which is in turn phosphorylated and then dimerizes and translocates to the nucleus (75,76). STAT6 binds to specific DNA sequences in the promoter regions of IL-4-responsive genes, including $C_ε$ (77). Two variants of the IL-4Rα chain gene have been recently identified in association with different atopic disorders, carrying either Val or Ile at position 50 (atopic asthma) and either Gln or Arg at position 551 (hyper-IgE syndrome). The substitution of Ile50 for Val augmented STAT6 activation, proliferation, and transcription activity of $I_ε$ promoter by IL-4, whereas that of 551 Arg for Gln did not change these IL-4 signals (43). The importance of STAT6 in IL-4 signaling is reinforced by the lack of IgE class switching in mice deficient in STAT6 (76).

Although IL-13 activates STAT6 and induces $C_ε$ germline transcript, it does not activate JAK3. Consistent with this, IL-13R signaling is intact in B cells from JAK3-deficient patients (78). There is evidence that the IL13Rα chain associates with JAK2 (79) and with the Janus kinase family member TYK2 (80). Upon ligand binding, heterodimerization of the IL-13R chain results in IL-4Rα chain phosphorylation, docking and phosphorylation of STAT6, followed by STAT6 dimerization and nuclear transcription.

Activation of $C_ε$ gene transcription requires DNA binding transcription factors other than STAT6 (see Fig. 6 for structure of the $C_ε$ promotor region). The promoter region upstream of the $I_ε$ exon also contains binding sites for NF-κB/p50 and for one or more members of the C/EBP family of transcription factors (81). NF-κB/p50-deficient mice have impaired switching to IgE (82) and B cells from mice deficient in the NF-κB inhibitor IkBα have enhanced IgE production (83). C/EBPβ has the potential to transactivate the human, but not the mouse, ε germline promotor. In contrast, AP-1 (fos and jun) transcription factors enhance transcriptional germline activity in synergism with STAT6 in

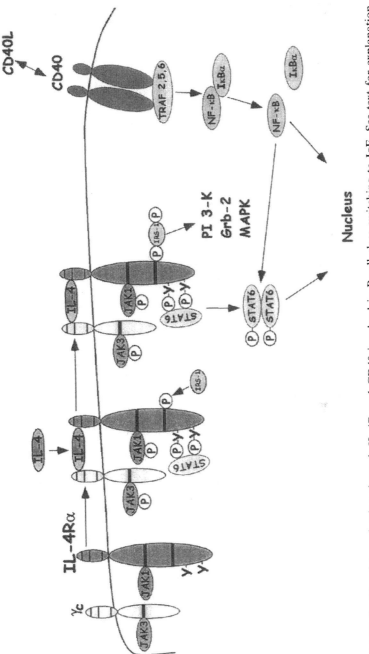

Figure 5 Signal transduction through IL-4R and CD40 involved in B-cell class switching to IgE. See text for explanation. (Redrawn and modified from Ref. 162.)

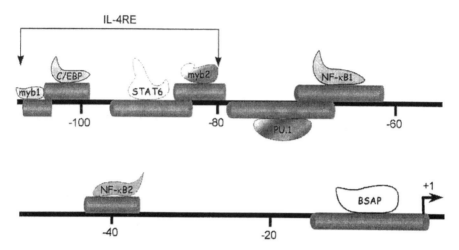

Figure 6 Structure of the human Cε promotor region and transcription factors binding to this region. The IL-4 responsive element is indicated between arrows. There are two binding sites for NF-κB. The STAT6 binding site also binds Bcl-6, but binding of this molecule represses Cε transcription.

the mouse but not in the human (84). One transcription factor that is specifically implied in IgE class switching is BSAP (B-cell-specific activation protein, also known as Pax5). Overexpression of this protein in murine B-cell lines leads to IgE class switching and inhibits class switching to other classes (85). Activation of Cε gene transcription and generation of germline RNA are subject to negative regulation as well. BCL-6, a zinc finger transcription factor expressed in B cells, binds to the same DNA target site as STAT6 and can repress ε germline transcription induced by IL-4 (86). BCL-6-deficient mice have increased IgE isotype switching.

D. Membrane-Associated Molecules Provide a Second Signal for IgE Switching

The CD40–CD40L interaction is critical in the activation of immunoglobulin isotype switching. CD40L is transiently induced on T cells after stimulation of the T-cell receptor by antigen–MHC complexes and ligation of ICOS on T cells by B7-related protein-1 on B cells (14,60). After interaction with CD40L, CD40 aggregation triggers signal transduction through four intracellular proteins, which belong to the family of TNF-receptor associated factors (TRAF1) (Fig. 5). TRAF2, TRAF5, and TRAF6 promote the dissociation of NF-κB from its inhibitor, IκB (87–90). Active NF-κB can then synergize with STAT6 induced by IL-4/IL-13 signaling to activate the Cε gene promoter. CD40L is encoded on the X chromosome, and patients with the X-linked hyper-IgM syndrome are deficient in CD40L expression or have a mutated form of CD40L.

Their B cells are unable to produce IgG, IgA, or IgE (91,92). The activating CD40L signal can also be provided by activated mast cells and DCs expressing CD40L, thus bypassing the need for $CD4^+$ Th cells (93).

E. B-Cell/T-Cell Cross-Talk Contributes to IgE Class Switching

In addition to interaction through MHC/TCR, CD80,86/CD28, CD40/ CD40L, and cytokine secretion, B cells and T cells interact in many more ways to optimize immunoglobulin production. OX40 is a member of the NGFR/TNFR superfamily of receptors expressed on activated T cells, which, upon cross-linking, results in enhanced proliferation and cytokine production (94). Its ligand, OX40L, is expressed on activated B cells and DCs (95). The cross-linking of OX40L in vitro results in the dramatic decrease in B-cell proliferation and in secretion of all Ig isotypes after 5 days of culture (96). OX40-OX40L interaction is critical for the in vivo T-cell-dependent humoral immune response. OX40L expression of DCs induces T cells to up-regulate the expression of CXCR5 and to become responsive to the B-cell follicle–expressed CXCL13 and at the same time induces their differentiation into IL-4 secreting T_{FH} cells (97,98). Blocking this interaction with systemically administered anti-OX40 antibodies caused an inhibition of the specific IgG response to concomitantly administered antigen without affecting IgM response (99). OX40-deficient mice do not produce IgE antibodies and have reduced lung inflammation.

ICOS is a homodimer of 55–60 kD that shares 20% homology with CD28 (13,100). However, unlike CD28, ICOS is not present on naive T cells; instead it is up-regulated after T-cell activation and retained on memory T cells, especially those expressing CXCR5. Activated B cells as well as DCs express the ICOS-ligand B7RP-1, also known as B7-H2 (see Chap. 11). ICOS knockout mice have only few germinal centers, the lymphoid factories where B cells manufacture antibody molecules, and class switching to IgG_1 and IgE is deficient in these mice (14,101,102). Remarkably, GC formation in response to a secondary recall challenge was completely absent in ICOS knockout mice. This can be partly explained by the decrease in production of specific cytokines (such as IL-4 and IL-13) by T cells as well as a lack of CD40L up-regulation by T cells. Indeed, the deficiency in GC formation in ICOS knockout mice could be overcome by exogenous administration of a CD40L stimulus.

F. T-Cell-Independent Second Signals

Two additional stimuli have been described that when present along with IL-4 can induce IgE synthesis in a T-cell-independent manner. The Epstein-Barr virus, in the presence of IL-4, is capable of inducing IgE synthesis by human B cells in vitro (103,104), This may be caused by the Epstein-Barr virus latent infection membrane protein-1, a constitutively active TNFR superfamily member that is similar to CD40 in structure and activation patterns. Studies have demonstrated that TRAF-1, TRAF-2, and TRAF-3 associate with latent infection membrane protein-1 and activate NF-κB (105, 106). The glucocorticoid hydrocortisone, in the presence of IL-4, is also capable of up-regulating total and allergen-specific IgE synthesis by human peripheral blood mononuclear cells from atopic individuals as well as inducing IgE synthesis by sIgE-B cells (107), although the mechanism of this effect is unclear.

III. Regulation of IgE Synthesis

A. Role of CD8 T Cells in Regulation of IgE Synthesis

In non-atopic individuals, short-lived IgE responses can be induced following oral ingestion of food allergens or following immunization of allergens in a Th2-prone adjuvant. Similarly, some rat strains have short-lived IgE responses to inhaled OVA that gradually disappear following exposure (108). This suggests that initial IgE secretion can be suppressed by an active mechanism. Work from Kemeny's lab has identified a crucial role for antigen-specific CD8 cells in the regulation of IgE synthesis (109). Initially it was found that ricin, one of the components of castor bean oil, strongly induces IgE synthesis in rats (110–112). The mechanism behind this observed effect is an in vivo depletion of CD8 T cells, which can be mimicked by depleting CD8 cells using monoclonal Abs. The state of high IgE production could be fully reversed by adoptive transfer of antigen-specific CD8 T cells (113). By cloning experiments it was shown that MHC class I–restricted $CD8^+$ T cells expressing the αβ TCR can inhibit the synthesis of IgE through various mechanisms, of which IFN-γ secretion is an obvious one (111,114). However, the level of IFN-γ secretion by suppressive CD8 T-cell clones and their level of cytotoxicity does not correlate with their ability to suppress IgE synthesis in vivo. Thomas and Kemeny, studying the simultaneous presentation of OVA-antigen to $CD4^+$ and $CD8^+$ OVA-TCR transgenic T cells, recently proposed one additional level of regulation of IgE synthesis (Fig. 7). These authors suggest that antigen-specific $CD8^+$ cells suppress IgE synthesis by their potential to boost IL-12 production in DCs, so that the response of $CD4^+$ T cells is skewed toward Th 1 cytokine (i.e., IFN-γ) synthesis. These Th 1 cells then suppress IgE synthesis. In this model, IFN-γ production by $CD8^+$ T cells was not necessary for IgE suppression, whereas the production by $CD4^+$ T cells clearly was (115,116). Others have shown in the mouse and rat that IgE responses to inhaled antigen are inhibited by $CD8^+$ cells expressing the γδ TCR and producing high levels of IFN-γ. These cells are induced in the draining lymph nodes of the lung and suppress IgE production following adoptive transfer (108,117). IFN-γ directly inhibits the class switching of B cells to IgE and IgG_4 and favors the class switching to IgG_1. Moreover, depletion of IFN-γ-producing cell types also directly increases IgE production through stimulation of Th2 cells producing IL-4 and IL-13 (118). It is not known at present if atopics have a reduced suppressive activity of $CD8^+$ T cells on IgE synthesis.

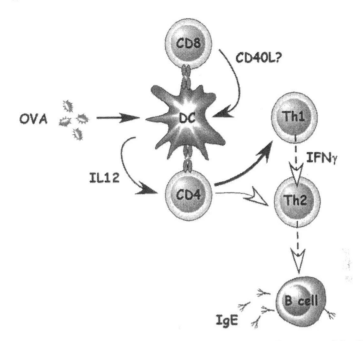

Figure 7 Model of CD8 regulation of IgE responses recently proposed by Kemeny and coworkers. CD8 cells provide an activating signal to DCs to produce IL-12. This leads in turn to Th1 differentiation and IFN-γ secretion by these Th1 cells. At the same time, Th2 differentiation is inhibited, leading to decreased IgE levels.

B. Bacterial Products Influence IgE Synthesis Through Effects on T-Helper-Cell Differentiation

There is an epidemiological link between exposure to bacterial substances and levels of IgE in the general population. Some bacterial antigens, such as those from *Bordetella pertussis*, stimulate IgE synthesis, whereas others, such as mycobacterial antigens, clearly suppress IgE synthesis (119). Therefore, vaccination status of the general population (e.g., with bacillus Calmette-Guérin) can influence the level of IgE production at a population level (120). It is now accepted that this differential regulation of IgE synthesis is due to the type of Th response that is induced by these antigens following recognition by DCs (see Chap. 10). Within the general population, there is a striking polymorphism between levels of soluble lipopolysaccharide (LPS) receptor CD14 and protection against high IgE levels (atopy) in humans (42). LPS is a known inducer of IL-12 production in DCs, and high levels of IL-12 production during encounter of naive T cells with APCs leads to the outgrowth of Th1 cells that suppress IgE synthesis. Increased production of IFN-γ by CD4$^+$ T cells and increased expression of the IFN-γ receptor by B cells is the mechanism behind the suppressive effect of bacterial unmethylated DNA or synthetic CpG oligodesoxynucleotides on IgE production of human B-cell/T-cell cocultures (121). In the same cultures stimulated by CpG motifs, neutralization of IL-12, IFN-α, and IL-10 also led to partial restoration of IgE synthesis, indicating that these cytokines also influence IgE synthesis in response to microbial stimulation.

IV. Local IgE Synthesis

The predominant site of immunoglobulin synthesis is the bone marrow and the B-cell follicles in secondary lymphoid organs. The production of IgA antibodies can, however, occur in peripheral mucosal sites, such as gut lamina propria, with the epithelium delivering some of the cytokines, such as IL-6, and DCs and T cells delivering CD40L, TGF-β, and possibly IL-5 (58). Evidence has also been put forward that IgE class switching and synthesis can occur in peripheral tissues, especially at sites of allergic inflammation. Localized IgE production can occur after contact of primed B lymphocytes with CD40L$^+$ T cells, CD40L$^+$ mast cells, and possibly CD40L$^+$ DCs. Mast cells also produce cytokines such as IL-4 that are necessary for IgE class switching. The class switching occurs locally within the nose and bronchial wall as evidenced by an increased presence of sterile C_ε germline transcripts and I_ε mRNA in nasal and bronchial biopsies of patients with asthma and rhinitis (122–124). The presence of local IgE synthesis relates to asthma *per se* and occurs both in atopic and non-atopic disease, under the regulation of IL-4 (125). In allergic rhinitis patients, C_ε germline transcripts were induced only following allergen challenge to the nose (126). The numbers of airway CD20$^+$ B cells are identical between asthmatic and nonasthmatic individuals (125). The same is true for nasal B cells in allergic rhinitic patients as opposed to healthy controls (126).

One aspect of local IgE synthesis that has not received much attention in human asthma is the induction of organized lympoid tissues in chronically inflamed airways. Date from the OVA-induced asthma model in mice demonstrated the presence of germinal centers in the lung parenchyma. Antigen-driven differentiation of B cells into IgG, IgA, and IgE-secreting plasma cells occurred via induction of an FDC network and germinal centers. These germinal centers would then provide a local source of IgE-secreting plasma cells that contribute to the release of factors mediating inflammatory processes in the lung (127). In mice, OVA-bearing FDCs can induce specific memory T and B cells to produce IgE, which supports the concept that FDC-associated antigen may be involved in the long-term maintenance of specific IgE responses. Despite the fact that the induction of organized lymphoid tissues and the cross-talk between B cells and T cells/mast cells critically depends on chemokine–chemokine receptor interactions, this area has received little attention in the field of asthma and allergy.

V. Role of IgE in Asthma

IgE binds to effector cells through two receptors: the high-affinity FcεRI receptor and the low-affinity FcεRII or CD23 (128) (Fig. 8). These receptors are widely expressed on various cell types (Table 3).

A. Binding to FcεRI

The crystal structure of human FcεRI and its interaction with IgE-Fc has recently been elucidated (129,130). The binding occurs by FcεRIα interaction

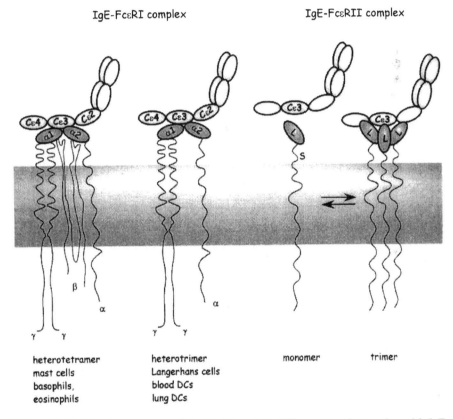

Figure 8 Molecular structure of the FcεRI and FcεRII receptors interacting with IgE through the various constant Cε regions of IgE. The FcεRI has two forms: a tetramer or a trimer lacking the β chain. Binding to IgE occurs via the α2 domain. The FcεRII receptor consists of a type II transmembrane protein that contains an IgE binding lectin (L) domain, a α-helical coiled coil stalk (S) region, a transmembrane domain, and an intracellular domain. Binding to IgE induces oligomerization into a homotrimer through interaction of the stalk regions of the receptor.

Table 3   IgE Receptor Expression

FcεRI
Mast cells
Basophils
Eosinophils
Langerhans cells
Blood monocytes
Blood and lung DCs
FcεRII (CD23)
B cells
Follicular DCs
Alveolar macrophages
Langerhans cells
Bronchial epithelial cells (asthma)
Inducible on blood monocytes by IL-4

through its α_1 and α_2 domains with one IgE molecule through the two Cε3 domains of dimeric IgE-Fc (131). The Cε2 domain of IgE-Fc is necessary to stabilize the interaction and is responsible for the exceptional long half-life of 14 days of the interaction (132). In the immediate hypersensitivity reaction, cross-linking of IgE bound to mast cells through the high-affinity FcεRI receptor by means of polyvalent allergen induces the release of preformed vasoactive mediators, transcription of cytokines, and de novo synthesis of prostaglandins and leukotrienes (see Chap. 5). The signal transduction pathways involved in activation of mast cells through FcεRI have recently been reviewed and will not be discussed here (133). In the airways, the mediators rapidly elicit bronchial mucosal edema, mucus production, and smooth muscle constriction and recruit inflammatory cells resulting in an acute obstruction of airflow (134). In about 50% of atopic asthmatics challenged with a relevant allergen, there is an LPR (late phase response), usually occurring between 3 and 8 h after allergen inhalation. This LPR is associated with an enhanced bronchial hyperresponsiveness (BHR). In some animal models, IgE antibodies can transfer both acute and LPR sensitivity to allergen challenge (135). Interference with mast cell activation or inhibition of the mast cell mediators blocks the onset of both acute and late-phase asthmatic responses (136). Most murine models of asthma developed over the past 5 years have focused on two critical features of the disease, eosinophilic infiltration of the bronchial mucosa and BHR, the enhanced tendency toward airflow obstruction in response to pharmacological stimuli. The data from a large number of studies suggest that IgE can contribute to some aspects of asthmatic pathophysiology but that it is not by itself sufficient to give rise to the characteristic allergic inflammation and BHR seen after allergen exposure. Mast cell activation through FcεRI could certainly provide a critical initiating event in the elicitation of allergic airway symptoms by IgE. In W/W^v

(mast cell–deficient) mice, a role for mast cells in driving eosinophil influx after allergen exposure has been reported. Thus, it seems that under some conditions, IgE-FcεRI-mediated mast cell activation and consequent release of mediators drives both the recruitment of inflammatory cells and the onset of BHR.

The classical FcεRI as expressed on mast cells, basophils, and eosinophils is a heterotetrameric receptor composed of one IgE-binding α chain, one membrane-spanning β chain, and two disulfide-linked γ chains (137) (Fig. 8). Recently, the expression of FcεRI on human professional APCs, such as monocytes, Langerhans cells of the skin, blood DCs, and lung DCs, has received a lot of attention. In these cells, the FcεRI is composed of an $\alpha 2\gamma$ trimer that lacks FcεRIβ (128,138,139). Remarkably, the FcεRI on APCs has not been described in mice. When the receptor is occupied by IgE and cross-linked using specific allergen, the allergen is targeted to an endosomal MHC class II–rich compartment that is specialized for antigen processing, effectively reducing the threshold for allergen recognition (140). When an allergen is targeted to FcεRI through binding with allergen-specific IgE, the dose of allergen can be reduced 1- to 100-fold to obtain a similar degree of T-cell stimulation in allergen-specific T cells. Therefore, an important function of FcεRI expression on Langerhans cells and DCs is to lower the threshold for allergen recognition. This mechanism is particularly involved in the atopy patch test to aeroallergens in atopic dermatitis patients. Only those patients who express IgE for aeroallergen on their LCs demonstrate a delayed reaction to epicutaneously applied allergens.

The expression level of FcεRI is higher on lung DCs from atopic asthmatics than from healthy controls. The total expression of surface FcεRI on blood DCs from healthy and asthmatic subjects was not significantly different. However, in vivo, DCs from atopic asthmatic subjects had higher levels of receptor occupancy by IgE and bound exogenous IgE in vitro more efficiently than DCs from healthy subjects. Therefore, the local environment of the inflamed lung could be important for up-regulating the surface expression of the receptor (141). The intracellular pool of FcεRIα is not different between non-atopics and atopics but its surface expression is much higher on DCs from atopics. In atopics, surface expression of FcεRIα on DCs is regulated by IL-4 and is highly related to the level of IgE in the blood (142).

B. Binding to FcεRII (CD23)

In addition to associating with mast cells, basophils, and APCs through FcεRI, IgE interacts with a number of other cell types by means of the low-affinity IgE receptor (FcεRII or CD23) (Table 3). The extracellular lectin domain of CD23 mediates binding to the Cε3 domain of IgE-Fc. The receptor has different conformations, the trimeric conformation binding IgE with the highest affinity (Fig. 8). Binding of IgE to CD23 induces trimer formation via interaction of the α-helical coiled coil of the extracellular stalk region of CD23. Several investigators have now demonstrated that the binding of allergen with specific IgE facilitates allergen uptake by CD23-bearing cells for processing and presentation to T cells (143,144). Mice immunized with IgE–Ag complexes produce significantly more Ag-specific Abs than mice immunized with Ag alone (145). The enhancement is mediated via the low-affinity receptor for IgE, as shown by its complete absence in mice pretreated with mAbs specific for CD23 and in CD23-deficient mice (146). One of the suggested modes of action of CD23 is to increase the ability of B cells to present Ag bound to IgE to T cells, as demonstrated to take place in vitro and in vivo. Another possibility is that FDCs capture the IgE–Ag complexes and present these directly to B cells.

CD23 is cleaved from the surface of B cells and FDCs by metalloproteases, leading to shedding of soluble CD23 (sCD23). There is some evidence that sCD23 fragments may enhance IgE production, both by direct interaction with B cells (through CD21) and by binding to IgE, thereby blocking its interaction with membrane-bound CD23 (see below). IgE serves as a positive regulator of its receptors, FcεRI and CD23. IgE bound to CD23 protects the receptor from cleavage by metalloproteases, with consequent reduced shedding of sCD23 into the medium (147). Therefore, IgE inhibits its own production by negative feedback.

CD23 has a dual role in allergic responses. In addition to enhancing allergen presentation to T cells and increasing IgE synthesis (sCD23), human and animal studies have shown that ligation of membrane-bound CD23 on B cells can suppress IgE production (148). Also, conditions that give elevated CD23 expression on FDCs (e.g., immunization with antigen in complete Freund's adjuvant or CD23 Tg animals), give a negative signal(s) to B cells and thus inhibit differentiation into IgE Ab-producing cells. FDCs expressing high levels of CD23 inhibit IgE production by sIgE positive B cells in vitro and in vivo (149).

As a consequence, the role of CD23 in atopy and asthma is not clear-cut. Cell-bound CD23 is elevated in atopic individuals and rises with flares of disease (150). Conversely, successful induction of remission of allergy by means of immunotherapy is accompanied by a fall in CD23 levels (151). Endogenous metalloproteases, as well as some allergens, are capable of cleaving CD23, leading to enhanced levels of sCD23. Inhibition of proteolytic activity of Der p1 blocks its ability to induce IgE responses in vivo (152, 153).

C. Treatment with Anti-IgE Antibodies

Recently, humanized monoclonal antibodies (such as omalizumab or E25) directed against the receptor binding domain of IgE have been introduced for the treatment of asthma. These molecules inhibit the effector functions of IgE (Fig. 9). Binding of IgE to anti-IgE and reduction in serum levels of IgE prevents IgE binding to its receptor on mast cells and basophils, thus

binding of IgE
to anti-IgE Ab

Inhibition of effector
functions of IgE

Physiological result

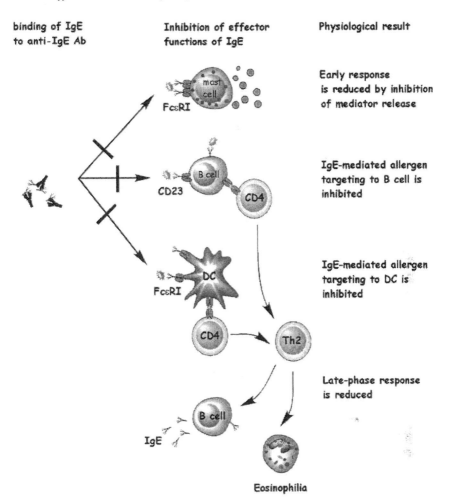

Early response
is reduced by inhibition
of mediator release

IgE-mediated allergen
targeting to B cell is
inhibited

IgE-mediated allergen
targeting to DC is
inhibited

Late-phase response
is reduced

Eosinophilia

Figure 9 Inhibition of IgE effector functions by anti-IgE treatment. See text for explanation.

inhibiting the activation of mast cells and release of mediators during the early response. In addition to this effect, one needs also to envisage that blocking IgE might lead to a reduction of IgE-mediated allergen presentation by B cells (CD23) or DCs (FcεRI) (154). It was indeed shown in murine models that a nonanaphylactogenic anti-IgE antibody has the potential to inhibit the differentiation of allergen-specific Th2 cells during the late-phase response to allergen (144,155). In this way, anti-IgE treatment would increase the threshold for allergen recognition by the immune system. Not surprisingly, anti-IgE has the potential in clinical studies to attenuate both the early-phase response and the late-phase response to allergens (156). Treatment also leads to reduction in plasma levels of IgE and to reduced expression of FcεRI on mast cells, illustrating the positive feedback that IgE levels have on FcεRI expression. In real-life treatment situations, anti-IgE administration to asthmatics leads to improved quality-of-life scores, reduced rescue medication use, reduced corticosteroid use while maintaining asthma control, and increased peak expiratory flow rate (157–159). Although the precise role of these drugs in the current treatment plan of asthma remains to be fully determined, particular patients (those who remain symptomatic despite inhaled and systemic steroids) will benefit from treatment with this new class of drugs (160,161).

VI. Conclusion and Prospects for the Near Future

IgE synthesis is a tightly controlled process involving the interaction of DCs, T cells, and B cells. These interactions occur in the secondary lymphoid organs but also locally within inflamed tissues. In the future, the role of local IgE synthesis in non-atopic asthma as well as the factors controlling this process will be intensively studied. Also, the precise role of DCs and mast cells in the process of B-cell activation and IgE synthesis will have to be determined more precisely. The molecular mechanisms underlying IgE class switching are gradually being unraveled, and studying these mechanisms in atopic and non-atopic individuals should prove to be useful. Finally detailed knowledge of the structure–function relationship of IgE binding to its receptors should allow the design of small-molecule antagonists that have the potential to block the interaction.

References

1. MacLennan IC, Gulbranson-Judge A, Toellner KM, Casamayor-Palleja M, Chan E, Sze DM, Luther SA, Orbea HA. The changing preference of T and B cells for partners as T-dependent antibody responses develop. Immunol Rev 1997; 156:53–66.
2. Toellner KM, Luther SA, Sze DM, Choy RK, Taylor DR, MacLennan IC, Acha-Orbea H. T helper 1 (Th1) and Th2 characteristics start to develop during T cell priming and are associated with an immediate ability to induce immunoglobulin class switching. J Exp Med 1998; 187:1193–1204.
3. Cyster JG. Chemokines and cell migration in secondary lymphoid organs. Science 1999; 286:2098–2102.
4. Forster R, Mattis AE, Kremmer E, Wolf E, Brem G, Lipp M. A putative chemo kine receptor, BLR1, directs B cell migration to defined lymphoid organs and specific anatomic compartments of the spleen. Cell 1996; 87:1037–1047.
5. Ansel KM, Ngo VN, Hyman PL, Luther SA, Forster R, Sedgwick JD, Browning JL, Lipp M, Cyster JG. A chemokine-driven positive feedback loop organizes lymphoid follicles. Nature 2000; 406:309–314.

6. Forster R, Schubel A, Breitfeld D, Kremmer E, Renner-Muller I, Wolf E, Lipp M. CCR7 coordinates the primary immune response by establishing functional microenvironments in secondary lymphoid organs. Cell 1999; 99:23–33.

7. Gunn MD, Kyuwa S, Tam C, Kakiuchi T, Matsuzawa A, Williams LT, Nakano H. Mice lacking expression of secondary lymphoid organ chemokine have defects in lymphocyte homing and dendritic cell localization. J Exp Med 1999; 189:451–460.

8. Ronchese F, Hausmann B. B lymphocytes in vivo fail to prime naive T cells but can stimulate antigen-experienced T lymphocytes. J Exp Med 1993; 177:679–690.

9. Ansel KM, McHeyzer-Williams LJ, Ngo VN, McHeyzer-Williams MG, Cyster JG. In vivo-activated CD4 T cells upregulate CXC chemokine receptor 5 and reprogram their response to lymphoid chemokines. J Exp Med 1999; 190:1123–1134.

10. Schaerli P, Willimann K, Lang AB, Lipp M, Loetscher P, Moser B. CXC chemokine receptor 5 expression defines follicular homing T cells with B cell helper function. J Exp Med 2000; 192:1553–1562.

11. Breitfeld D, Ohl L, Kremmer E, Ellwart J, Sallusto F, Lipp M, Forster R. Follicular B helper T cells express CXC chemokine receptor 5, localize to B cell follicles, and support immunoglobulin production. J Exp Med 2000; 192:1545–1552.

12. Yoshinaga SK, Whoriskey JS, Khare SD, Sarmiento U, Guo J, Horan T, Shih G, Zhang M, Coccia MA, Kohno T, Tafuri-Bladt A, Brankow D, Campbell P, Chang D, Chiu L, Dai T, Duncan G, Elliott GS, Hui A, McCabe SM, Scully S, Shahinian A, Shaklee CL, Van G, Mak TW, et al. T-cell co-stimulation through B7RP-1 and ICOS. Nature 1999; 402:827–832.

13. Coyle AJ, Lehar S, Lloyd C, Tian J, Delaney T, Manning S, Nguyen T, Burwell T, Schneider H, Gonzalo JA, Gosselin M, Owen LR, Rudd CE, Gutierrez-Ramos JC. The CD28-related molecule ICOS is required for effective T-cell-dependent immune responses. Immunity 2000; 13:95–105.

14. McAdam AJ, Greenwald RJ, Levin MA, Chernova T, Malenkovich N, Ling V, Freeman GJ, Sharpe AH. ICOS is critical for CD40-mediated antibody class switching. Nature 2001; 409:102–105.

15. Kim CH, Rott LS, Clark-Lewis I, Campbell DJ, Wu L, Butcher EC. Subspecialization of CXCR5+ T cells: B helper activity is focused in a germinal center-localized subset of CXCR5+ T cells. J Exp Med 2001; 193:1373–1381.

16. van Rooijen N. Direct intrafollicular differentiation of memory B cells into plasma cells. Immunol Today 1990; 11:154–157.

17. Liu YJ, Zhang J, Lane PJ, Chan EY, MacLennan IC. Sites of specific B cell activation in primary and secondary responses to T cell-dependent and T cell-independent antigens. Eur J Immunol 1991; 21:2951–2962.

18. Garcia De Vinuesa C, Gulbranson-Judge A, Khan M, O'Leary P, Cascalho M, Wabl M, Klaus GG, Owen MJ, MacLennan IC. Dendritic cells associated with plasmablast survival. Eur J Immunol 1999; 29:3712–3721.

19. Kosco MH, Burton GF, Kapasi ZF, Szakal AK, Tew JG. Antibody-forming cell induction during an early phase of germinal centre development and its delay with ageing. Immunology 1989; 68:312–318.

20. Benner R, Hijmans W, Haaijman JJ. The bone marrow: the major source of serum immunoglobulins, but still a neglected site of antibody formation. Clin Exp Immunol 1981; 46:1–8.

21. Smith KG, Hewitson TD, Nossal GJ, Tarlinton DM. The phenotype and fate of the antibody-forming cells of the splenic foci. Eur J Immunol 1996; 26:444–448.
22. Hargreaves DC, Hyman PL, Lu TT, Ngo VN, Bidgol A, Suzuki G, Zou YR, Littman DR, Cyster JG. A coordinated change in chemokine responsiveness guides plasma cell movements. J Exp Med 2001; 194:45–56.
23. Gordon J, Pound JD. Fortifying B cells with CD154: an engaging tale of many hues. Immunology 2000; 100:269–280.
24. Wykes M, Pombo A, Jenkins C, MacPherson GG. Dendritic cells interact directly with naive B lymphocytes to transfer antigen and initiate class switching in a primary T-dependent response. J Immunol 1998; 161:1313–1319.
25. Jenkins MK, Khoruts A, Ingulli E, Mueller DL, McSorley SJ, Reinhardt RL, Itano A, Pape KA. In vivo activation of antigen-specific CD4 T cells. Annu Rev Immunol 2001; 19:23–45.
26. Kushnir N, Liu LM, MacPherson GG. Dendritic cells and resting B cells form clusters in vitro and in vivo: T cell independence, partial LFA-1 dependence, and regulation by cross-linking surface molecules. J Immunol 1998; 160:1774–1781.
27. Wykes M, MacPherson G. Dendritic cell-B-cell interaction: dendritic cells provide B cells with CD40-independent proliferation signals and CD40-dependent survival signals. Immunology 2000; 100:1–3.
28. Garcia De Vinuesa C, MacLennan IC, Holman M, Klaus GG. Anti-CD40 antibody enhances responses to polysaccharide without mimicking T cell help. Eur J Immunol 1999; 29:3216–3224.
29. Grouard G, Durand I, Filgueira L, Banchereau J, Liu YJ. Dendritic cells capable of stimulating T cells in germinal centres. Nature 1996; 384:364–367.
30. Dubois B, Barthelemy C, Durand I, Liu YJ, Caux C, Briere F. Toward a role of dendritic cells in the germinal center reaction: triggering of B cell proliferation and isotype switching. J Immunol 1999; 162:3428–3436.
31. Berney C, Herren S, Power CA, Gordon S, Martinez-Pomares L, Kosco-Vilbois MH. A member of the dendritic cells family that enters B cell follicles and stimulates primary antibody responses identified by a mannose receptor fusion protein. J Exp Med 1999; 190:851–860.
32. Kopf M, Herren S, Wiles MV, Pepys MB, Kosco-Vilbois MH. Interleukin 6 influences germinal center development and antibody production via a contribution of C3 complement component. J Exp Med 1998; 188:1895–1906.
33. Vissers JL, Hartgers FC, Lindhout E, Figdor CG, Adema GJ. BLC (CXCL13) is expressed by different dendritic cell subsets in vitro and in vivo. Eur J Immunol 2001; 31:1544–1549.
34. Fayette J, Dubois B, Vandenabeele S, Bridon JM, Vanbervliet B, Durand I, Banchereau J, Caux C, Briere F. Human dendritic cells skew isotype switching of CD40-activated naive B cells towards IgA1 and IgA2. J Exp Med 1997; 185:1909–1918.
35. Dubois B, Vanbervliet B, Fayette J, Massacrier C, Van Kooten C, Briere F, Banchereau J, Caux C. Dendritic cells enhance growth and differentiation of CD40-activated B lymphocytes. J Exp Med 1997; 185:941–951.
36. Pinchuk LM, Klaus SJ, Magaletti DM, Pinchuk GV, Norsen JP, Clark EA. Functional CD40 ligand expressed by human blood dendritic cells is up-regulated by CD40 litigation. J Immunol 1996; 157:4363–4370.

37. Stumbles PA, Thomas JA, Pimm CL, Lee PT, Venaille TJ, Proksch S, Holt PG. Resting respiratory tract dendritic cells preferentially stimulate T helper cell type 2 (Th2) responses and require obligatory cytokine signals for induction of Th1 immunity. J Exp Med 1998; 188:2019–2031.

38. Hammad H, Duez C, Fahy O, Tsicopoulos A, Andre C, Wallaert B, Lebecque S, Tonnel AB, Pestel J. Human dendritic cells in the severe combined immunodeficiency mouse model: their potentiating role in the allergic reaction. Lab Invest 2000; 80:605–614.

39. Lambrecht BN, Salomon B, Klatzmann D, Pauwels RA. Dendritic cells are required for the development of chronic eosinophilic airway inflammation in response to inhaled antigen in sensitized mice. J Immunol 1998; 160:4090–4097.

40. Vercelli D. Immunoglobulin E and its regulators. Curr Opin Allergy Clin Immunol 2001; 1:61–65.

41. Ruiz RG, Richards D, Kemeny DM, Price JF. Neonatal IgE: a poor screen for atopic disease. Clin Exp Allergy 1991; 21:467–472.

42. Baldini M, Lohman IC, Halonen M, Erickson RP, Holt PG, Martinez FD. A polymorphism in the 5′ flanking region of the CD14 gene is associated with circulating soluble CD14 levels and with total serum immunoglobulin E. Am J Respir Cell Mol Biol 1999; 20:976–983.

43. Mitsuyasu H, Yanagihara Y, Mao XQ, Gao PS, Arinobu Y, Ihara K, Takabayashi A, Hara T, Enomoto T, Sasaki S, Kawai M, Hamasaki N, Shirakawa T, Hopkin JM, Izuhara K. Cutting edge: dominant effect of Ile50Val variant of the human IL-4 receptor alpha-chain in IgE synthesis. J Immunol 1999; 162:1227–1231.

44. Oettgen HC, Geha RS. IgE regulation and roles in asthma pathogenesis. J Allergy Clin Immunol 2001; 107:429–440.

45. Gould HJ, Beavil RL, Vercelli D. IgE isotype determination: epsilon-germline gene transcription, DNA recombination and B-cell differentiation. Br Med Bull 2000; 56:908–924.

46. Luby TM, Schrader CE, Stavnezer J, Selsing E. The mu switch region tandem repeats are important, but not required, for antibody class switch recombination. J Exp Med 2001; 193:159–168.

47. Vercelli D, Jabara HH, Arai K, Geha RS. Induction of human IgE synthesis requires interleukin 4 and T/B cell interactions involving the T cell receptor/CD3 complex and MHC class II antigens. J Exp Med 1989; 169:1295–1307.

48. Oettgen HC. Regulation of the IgE isotype switch: new insights on cytokine signals and the functions of epsilon germline transcripts. Curr Opin Immunol 2000; 12:618–623.

49. Gauchat JF, Lebman DA, Coffman RL, Gascan H, de Vries JE. Structure and expression of germline epsilon transcripts in human B cells induced by interleukin 4 to switch to IgE production. J Exp Med 1990; 172:463–473.

50. Jung S, Rajewsky K, Radbruch A. Shutdown of class switch recombination by deletion of a switch region control element. Science 1993; 259:984–987.

51. Bottaro A, Lansford R, Xu L, Zhang J, Rothman P, Alt FW. S region transcription per se promotes basal IgE class switch recombination but additional factors regulate the efficiency of the process. Embo J 1994; 13:665–674.

52. Lorenz M, Jung S, Radbruch A. Switch transcripts in immunoglobulin class switching. Science 1995; 267:1825–1828.

53. Borggrefe S, Keshavarzi S, Gross B, Wabl M, Jessberger R. Impaired IgE response in SWAP-70-deficient mice. Eur J Immunol 2001; 31:2467–2475.
54. Muramatsu M, Sankaranand VS, Anant S, Sugai M, Kinoshita K, Davidson NO, Honjo T. Specific expression of activation-induced cytidine deaminase (AID), a novel member of the RNA-editing deaminase family in germinal center B cells. J Biol Chem 1999; 274:18470–18476.
55. Muramatsu M, Kinoshita K, Fagarasan S, Yamada S, Shinkai Y, Honjo T. Class switch recombination and hypermutation require activation-induced cytidine deaminase (AID), a potential RNA editing enzyme. Cell 2000; 102:553–563.
56. Petersen S, Casellas R, Reina-San-Martin B, Chen HT, Difilippantonio MJ, Wilson PC, Hanitsch L, Celeste A, Muramatsu M, Pilch DR, Redon C, Ried T, Bonner WM, Honjo T, Nussenzweig MC, Nussenzweig A. AID is required to initiate Nbsl/gamma-H2AX focus formation and mutations at sites of class switching. Nature 2001; 414:660–665.
57. Kinoshita K, Harigai M, Fagarasan S, Muramatsu M, Honjo T. A hallmark of active class switch recombination: Transcripts directed by I promoters on looped-out circular DNAs. Proc Natl Acad Sci USA 2001; 98:12620–12623.
58. Fagarasan S, Kinoshita K, Muramatsu M, Ikuta K, Honjo T. In situ class switching and differentiation to IgA-producing cells in the gut lamina propria. Nature 2001; 413:639–643.
59. Vercelli D, Jabara HH, Lauener RP, Geha RS. IL-4 inhibits the synthesis of IFN-gamma and induces the synthesis of IgE in human mixed lymphocyte cultures. J Immunol 1990; 144:570–573.
60. Grewal IS, Flavell RA. A central role of CD40 ligand in the regulation of CD4+ T-cell responses. Immunol Today 1996; 17:410–414.
61. Mao CS, Stavnezer J. Differential regulation of mouse germline Ig gamma 1 and epsilon promoters by IL-4 and CD40. J Immunol 2001; 167:1522–1534.
62. Hodgkin PD, Lee JH, Lyons AB. B cell differentiation and isotype switching is related to division cycle number. J Exp Med 1996; 184:277–281.
63. Hasbold J, Lyons AB, Kehry MR, Hodgkin PD. Cell division number regulates IgG1 and IgE switching of B cells following stimulation by CD40 ligand and IL-4. Eur J Immunol 1998; 28:1040–1051.
64. Abbas AK, Murphy KM, Sher A. Functional diversity of helper T lymphocytes. Nature 1996; 383:787–793.
65. Xu L, Rothman P. IFN-gamma represses epsilon germline transcription and subsequently down-regulates switch recombination to epsilon. Int Immunol 1994; 6:515–521.
66. Defrance T, Carayon P, Billian G, Guillemot JC, Minty A, Caput D, Ferrara P. Interleukin 13 is a B cell stimulating factor. J Exp Med 1994; 179:135–143.
67. Punnonen J, Aversa G, Cocks BG, McKenzie AN, Menon S, Zurawski G, de Waal Malefyt R, de Vries JE. Interleukin 13 induces interleukin 4-independent IgG4 and IgE synthesis and CD23 expression by human B cells. Proc Natl Acad Sci USA 1993; 90:3730–3734.
68. DeKruyff RH, Turner T, Abrams JS, Palladino MA Jr, Umetsu DT. Induction of human IgE synthesis by CD4+ T cell clones. Requirement for interleukin 4 and low molecular weight B cell growth factor. J Exp Med 1989; 170:1477–1493.

69. Finkelman FD, Urban JF Jr, Beckmann MP, Schooley KA, Holmes JM, Katona IM. Regulation of murine in vivo IgG and IgE responses by a monoclonal anti-IL-4 receptor antibody. Int Immunol 1991; 3:599–607.

70. McKenzie AN, Culpepper JA, de Waal Malefyt R, Briere F, Punnonen J, Aversa G, Sato A, Dang W, Cocks BG, Menon S, et al. Interleukin 13, a T-cell-derived cytokine that regulates human monocyte and B-cell function. Proc Natl Acad Sci USA 1993; 90:3735–3739.

71. Van der Pouw Kraan TC, Van der Zee JS, Boeije LC, De Groot ER, Stapel SO, Aarden LA. The role of IL-13 in IgE synthesis by allergic asthma patients. Clin Exp Immunol 1998; 111:129–135.

72. Levy F, Kristofic C, Heusser C, Brinkmann V. Role of IL-13 in CD4 T cell–dependent IgE production in atopy. Int Arch Allergy Immunol 1997; 112:49–58.

73. Witthuhn BA, Silvennoinen O, Miura O, Lai KS, Cwik C, Liu ET, Ihle JN. Involvement of the Jak-3 Janus kinase in signalling by interleukins 2 and 4 in lymphoid and myeloid cells. Nature 1994; 370:153–157.

74. Rolling C, Treton D, Beckmann P, Galanaud P, Richard Y. JAK3 associates with the human interleukin 4 receptor and is tyrosine phosphorylated following receptor triggering. Oncogene 1995; 10:1757–1761.

75. Schindler C, Kashleva H, Pernis A, Pine R, Rothman P. STF-IL-4: a novel IL-4-induced signal transducing factor. Embo J 1994; 13:1350–1356.

76. Shimoda K, van Deursen J, Sangster MY, Sarawar SR, Carson RT, Tripp RA, Chu C, Quelle FW, Nosaka T, Vignali DA, Doherty PC, Grosveld G, Paul WE, Ihle JN. Lack of IL-4-induced Th2 response and IgE class switching in mice with disrupted Stat6 gene. Nature 1996; 380:630–633.

77. Schindler U, Wu P, Rothe M, Brasseur M, McKnight SL. Components of a Stat recognition code: evidence for two layers of molecular selectivity. Immunity 1995; 2:689–697.

78. Izuhara K, Heike T, Otsuka T, Yamaoka K, Mayumi M, Imamura T, Niho Y, Harada N. Signal transduction pathway of interleukin-4 and interleukin-13 in human B cells derived from X-linked severe combined immunodeficiency patients. J Biol Chem 1996; 271:619–622.

79. Palmer-Crocker RL, Hughes CC, Pober JS. IL-4 and IL-13 activate the JAK2 tyrosine kinase and Stat6 in cultured human vascular endothelial cells through a common pathway that does not involve the gamma c chain. J Clin Invest 1996; 98:604–609.

80. Welham MJ, Learmonth L, Bone H, Schrader JW. Interleukin-13 signal transduction in lymphohemopoietic cells. Similarities and differences in signal transduction with interleukin-4 and insulin. J Biol Chem 1995; 270:12286–12296.

81. Delphin S, Stavnezer J. Characterization of an interleukin 4 (IL-4) responsive region in the immunoglobulin heavy chain germline epsilon promoter: regulation by NF- IL-4, a C/EBP family member and NF-kappa B/p50. J Exp Med 1995; 181:181–192.

82. Snapper CM, Zelazowski P, Rosas FR, Kehry MR, Tian M, Baltimore D, Sha WC. B cells from p50/NF-kappa B knockout mice have selective defects in proliferation, differentiation, germ-line CH transcription, and Ig class switching. J Immunol 1996; 156:183–191.

83. Chen CL, Singh N, Yull FE, Strayhorn D, Van Kaer L, Kerr LD. Lymphocytes lacking I kappa B-alpha develop normally, but have selective defects in proliferation and function. J Immunol 2000; 165:5418–5427.

84. Shen CH, Stavnezer J. Activation of the mouse Ig germline epsilon promoter by IL-4 is dependent on AP-1 transcription factors. J Immunol 2001; 166:411–423.

85. Qiu G, Stavnezer J. Overexpression of BSAP/Pax-5 inhibits switching to IgA and enhances switching to IgE in the I.29 mu B cell line. J Immunol 1998; 161:2906–2918.

86. Harris MB, Chang CC, Berton MT, Danial NN, Zhang J, Kuehner D, Ye BH, Kvatyuk M, Pandolfi PP, Cattoretti G, Dalla-Favera R, Rothman PB. Transcriptional repression of Stat6-dependent interleukin-4-induced genes by BCL-6: specific regulation of iepsilon transcription and immunoglobulin E switching. Mol Cell Biol 1999; 19:7264–7275.

87. Ishida T, Mizushima S, Azuma S, Kobayashi N, Tojo T, Suzuki K, Aizawa S, Watanabe T, Mosialos G, Kieff E, Yamamoto T, Inoue J. Identification of TRAF6, a novel tumor necrosis factor receptor–associated factor protein that mediates signaling from an amino-terminal domain of the CD40 cytoplasmic region. J Biol Chem 1996; 271:28745–28748.

88. Ishida TK, Tojo T, Aoki T, Kobayashi N, Ohishi T, Watanabe T, Yamamoto T, Inoue J. TRAF5, a novel tumor necrosis factor receptor–associated factor family protein, mediates CD40 signaling. Proc Natl Acad Sci USA 1996; 93:9437–9442.

89. Nakano H, Oshima H, Chung W, Williams-Abbott L, Ware CF, Yagita H, Okumura K. TRAF5, an activator of NF-kappaB and putative signal transducer for the lymphotoxin-beta receptor. J Biol Chem 1996; 271:14661–14664.

90. Rothe M, Sarma V, Dixit VM, Goeddel DV. TRAF2-mediated activation of NF-kappa B by TNF receptor 2 and CD40. Science 1995; 269:1424–1427.

91. Allen RC, Armitage RJ, Conley ME, Rosenblatt H, Jenkins NA, Copeland NG, Bedell MA, Edelhoff S, Disteche CM, Simoneaux DK, et al. CD40 ligand gene defects responsible for X-linked hyper-IgM syndrome. Science 1993; 259:990–993.

92. Aruffo A, Farrington M, Hollenbaugh D, Li X, Milatovich A, Nonoyama S, Bajorath J, Grosmaire LS, Stenkamp R, Neubauer M, et al. The CD40 ligand, gp39, is defective in activated T cells from patients with X-linked hyper-IgM syndrome. Cell 1993; 72:291–300.

93. Kikuchi T, Worgall S, Singh R, Moore MA, Crystal RG. Dendritic cells genetically modified to express CD40 ligand and pulsed with antigen can initiate antigen-specific humoral immunity independent of CD4$^+$ T cells. Nat Med 2000; 6:1154–1159.

94. Baum PR, Gayle RB, 3rd, Ramsdell F, Srinivasan S, Sorensen RA, Watson ML, Seldin MF, Baker E, Sutherland GR, Clifford KN, et al. Molecular characterization of murine and human OX40/OX40 ligand systems: identification of a human OX40 ligand as the HTLV-1-regulated protein gp34. Embo J 1994; 13:3992–4001.

95. Ohshima Y, Tanaka Y, Tozawa H, Takahashi Y, Maliszewski C, Delespesse G. Expression and function of OX40 ligand on human dendritic cells. J Immunol 1997; 159:3838–3848.

96. Stuber E, Neurath M, Calderhead D, Fell HP, Strober W. Cross-linking of OX40 ligand, a member of the TNF/NGF cytokine family, induces proliferation and differentiation in murine splenic B cells. Immunity 1995; 2:507–521.

97. Flynn S, Toellner KM, Raykundalia C, Goodall M, Lane P. CD4 T cell cytokine differentiation: the B cell activation molecule, OX40 ligand, instructs CD4 T cells to express interleukin 4 and upregulates expression of the chemokine receptor, Blr-1. J Exp Med 1998; 188:297–304.

98. Walker LS, Gulbranson-Judge A, Flynn S, Brocker T, Raykundalia C, Goodall M, Forster R, Lipp M, Lane P. Compromised OX40 function in CD28-deficient mice is linked with failure to develop CXC chemokine receptor 5–positive CD4 cells and germinal centers. J Exp Med 1999; 190:1115–1122.

99. Stuber E, Strober W. The T cell-B cell interaction via OX40-OX40L is necessary for the T cell-dependent humoral immune response. J Exp Med 1996; 183:979–989.

100. Hutloff A, Dittrich AM, Beier KC, Eljaschewitsch B, Kraft R, Anagnostopoulos I, Kroczek RA. ICOS is an inducible T-cell co-stimulator structurally and functionally related to CD28. Nature 1999; 397:263–266.

101. Dong C, Juedes AE, Temann UA, Shresta S, Allison JP, Ruddle NH, Flavell RA. ICOS co-stimulatory receptor is essential for T-cell activation and function. Nature 2001; 409:97–101.

102. Tafuri A, Shahinian A, Bladt F, Yoshinaga SK, Jordana M, Wakeham A, Boucher LM, Bouchard D, Chan VS, Duncan G, Odermatt B, Ho A, Itie A, Horan T, Whoriskey JS, Pawson T, Penninger JM, Ohashi PS, Mak TW. ICOS is essential for effective T-helper-cell responses. Nature 2001; 409:105–109.

103. Thyphronitis G, Tsokos GC, June CH, Levine AD, Finkelman FD. IgE secretion by Epstein-Barr virus-infected purified human B lymphocytes is stimulated by interleukin 4 and suppressed by interferon gamma. Proc Natl Acad Sci USA 1989; 86:5580–5584.

104. Jabara HH, Schneider LC, Shapira SK, Alfieri C, Moody CT, Kieff E, Geha RS, Vercelli D. Induction of germ-line and mature C epsilon transcripts in human B cells stimulated with rIL-4 and EBV. J Immunol 1990; 145:3468–3473.

105. Kaye KM, Izumi KM, Kieff E. Epstein-Barr virus latent membrane protein 1 is essential for B-lymphocyte growth transformation. Proc Natl Acad Sci USA 1993; 90:9150–9154.

106. Devergne O, Hatzivassiliou E, Izumi KM, Kaye KM, Kleijnen MF, Kieff E, Mosialos G. Association of TRAF1, TRAF2, and TRAF3 with an Epstein-Barr virus LMP1 domain important for B-lymphocyte transformation: role in NF-kappaB activation. Mol Cell Biol 1996; 16:7098–7108.

107. Jabara HH, Ahern DJ, Vercelli D, Geha RS. Hydrocortisone and IL-4 induce IgE isotype switching in human B cells. J Immunol 1991; 147:1557–1560.

108. McMenamin C, McKersey M, Kuhnlein P, Hunig T, Holt PG. Gamma delta T cells down-regulate primary IgE responses in rats to inhaled soluble protein antigens. J Immunol 1995; 154:4390–4394.

109. Kemeny DM. CD8+ T cells in atopic disease. Curr Opin Immunol 1998; 10: 628–633.

110. Thorpe SC, Murdoch RD, Kemeny DM. The effect of the castor bean toxin, ricin, on rat IgE and IgG responses. Immunology 1989; 68:307–311.

111. Diaz-Sanchez D, Noble A, Staynov DZ, Lee TH, Kemeny DM. Elimination of IgE regulatory rat CD8+ T cells in vivo differentially modulates interleukin-4 and interferon-gamma but not interleukin-2 production by splenic T cells. Immunology 1993; 78:513–519.

112. Underwood SL, Kemeny DM, Lee TH, Raeburn D, Karlsson JA. IgE production, antigen-induced airway inflammation and airway hyperreactivity in the brown Norway rat: the effects of ricin. Immunology 1995; 85:256–261.

113. Holmes BJ, MacAry PA, Noble A, Kemeny DM. Antigen-specific CD8[+] T cells inhibit IgE responses and interleukin-4 production by CD4[+] T cells. Eur J Immunol 1997; 27:2657–2665.

114. MacAry PA, Holmes BJ, Kemeny DM. Ovalbumin-specific, MHC class I-restricted, alpha beta-positive, Tc1 and Tc0 CD8[+] T cell clones mediate the in vivo inhibition of rat IgE. J Immunol 1998; 160:580–587.

115. Thomas MJ, Noble A, Sawicka E, Askenase PW, Kemeny DM. CD8 T cells inhibit IgE via dendritic cell IL-12 induction that promotes Th1 T cell counterregulation. J Immunol 2002; 168:216–223.

116. Vukmanovic-Stejic M, Thomas MJ, Noble A, Kemeny DM. Specificity, restriction and effector mechanisms of immunoregulatory CD8 T cells. Immunology 2001; 102:115–122.

117. McMenamin C, Pimm C, McKersey M, Holt PG. Regulation of IgE responses to inhaled antigen in mice by antigen-specific gamma delta T cells. Science 1994; 265:1869–1871.

118. Noble A, Staynov DZ, Diaz-Sanchez D, Lee TH, Kemeny DM. Elimination of IgE regulatory rat CD8[+] T cells in vivo increases the co-ordinate expression of Th2 cytokines IL-4, IL-5 and IL-10. Immunology 1993; 80:326–329.

119. Pauwels RA, Van Der Straeten ME, Platteau B, Bazin H. The non-specific enhancement of allergy. I. In vivo effects of *Bordetella pertussis* vaccine on IgE synthesis. Allergy 1983; 38:239–246.

120. Shirakawa T, Enomoto T, Shimazu S, Hopkin JM. The inverse association between tuberculin responses and atopic disorder [see comments]. Science 1997; 275:77–79.

121. Horner AA, Widhopf GF, Burger JA, Takabayashi K, Cinman N, Ronaghy BA, Spiegelberg HL, Raz E. Immunostimulatory DNA inhibits IL4-dependent IgE synthesis by human B cells. J Allergy Clin Immunol 2001; 108:417–423.

122. Cameron L, Hamid Q, Wright E, Nakamura Y, Christodoulopoulos P, Muro S, Frenkiel S, Lavigne F, Durham S, Gould H. Local synthesis of epsilon germline gene transcripts, IL-4, and IL-13 in allergic nasal mucosa after ex vivo allergen exposure. J Allergy Clin Immunol 2000; 106:46–52.

123. Cameron LA, Durham SR, Jacobson MR, Masuyama K, Juliusson S, Gould HJ, Lowhagen O, Minshall EM, Hamid QA. Expression of IL-4, C epsilon RNA, and I epsilon RNA in the nasal mucosa of patients with seasonal rhinitis: effect of topical corticosteroids. J Allergy Clin Immunol 1998; 101:330–336.

124. Smurthwaite L, Walker SN, Wilson DR, Birch DS, Merrett TG, Durham SR, Gould HJ. Persistent IgE synthesis in the nasal mucosa of hay fever patients. Eur J Immunol 2001; 31:3422–3431.

125. Ying S, Humbert M, Meng Q, Pfister R, Menz G, Gould HJ, Kay AB, Durham SR. Local expression of epsilon germline gene transcripts and RNA for the epsilon

heavy chain of IgE in the bronchial mucosa in atopic and nonatopic asthma. J Allergy Clin Immunol 2001; 107:686–692.

126. Durham SR, Gould HJ, Thienes CP, Jacobson MR, Masuyama K, Rak S, Lowhagen O, Schotman E, Cameron L, Hamid QA. Expression of epsilon germ-line gene transcripts and mRNA for the epsilon heavy chain of IgE in nasal B cells and the effects of topical corticosteroid. Eur J Immunol 1997; 27:2899–2906.

127. Chvatchko Y, Kosco-Vilbois MH, Herren S, Lefort J, Bonnefoy JY. Germinal center formation and local immunoglobulin E (IgE) production in the lung after an airway antigenic challenge. J Exp Med 1996; 184:2353–2360.

128. Novak N, Kraft S, Bieber T. IgE receptors. Curr Opin Immunol 2001; 13:721–726.

129. Garman SC, Kinet JP, Jardetzky TS. Crystal structure of the human high-affinity IgE receptor. Cell 1998; 95:951–961.

130. Garman SC, Sechi S, Kinet JP, Jardetzky TS. The analysis of the human high affinity IgE receptor Fc epsilon Ri alpha from multiple crystal forms. J Mol Biol 2001; 311:1049–1062.

131. Wurzburg BA, Garman SC, Jardetzky TS. Structure of the human IgE-Fc C epsilon 3-C epsilon 4 reveals conformational flexibility in the antibody effector domains. Immunity 2000; 13:375–385.

132. McDonnell JM, Calvert R, Beavil RL, Beavil AJ, Henry AJ, Sutton BJ, Gould HJ, Cowburn D. The structure of the IgE C epsilon 2 domain and its role in stabilizing the complex with its high-affinity receptor FcepsilonRIalpha. Nat Struct Biol 2001; 8:437–441.

133. Nadler MJ, Matthews SA, Turner H, Kinet JP. Signal transduction by the high-affinity immunoglobulin E receptor Fc epsilon RI: coupling form to function. Adv Immunol 2000; 76:325–355.

134. Howarth PH, Durham SR, Kay AB, Holgate ST. The relationship between mast cell-mediator release and bronchial reactivity in allergic asthma. J Allergy Clin Immunol 1987; 80:703–711.

135. Shampain MP, Behrens BL, Larsen GL, Henson PM. An animal model of late pulmonary responses to *Alternaria* challenge. Am Rev Respir Dis 1982; 126: 493–498.

136. Cockcroft DW, Murdock KY. Comparative effects of inhaled salbutamol, sodium cromoglycate, and beclomethasone dipropionate on allergen-induced early asthmatic responses, late asthmatic responses, and increased bronchial responsiveness to histamine. J Allergy Clin Immunol 1987; 79:734–740.

137. Sutton BJ, Gould HJ. The human IgE network. Nature 1993; 366:421–428.

138. Maurer D, Fiebiger S, Ebner C, Reininger B, Fischer GF, Wichlas S, Jouvin MH, Schmitt-Egenolf M, Kraft D, Kinet JP, Stingl G. Peripheral blood dendritic cells express FcεRI as a complex composed of FcεRIα- and FcεRIγ-chains and can use their receptor for IgE-mediated allergen presentation. J Immunol 1996; 157: 607–616.

139. Tunon de Lara JM, Redington AE, Bradding P, Church MK, Hartley JA, Semper AE, Holgate ST. Dendritic cells in normal and asthmatic airways: expression of the alfa subunit of the high affinity immunoglobulin E receptor. Clin Exp Allergy 1996; 26:648–655.

140. Maurer D, Fiebiger E, Reininger B, Ebner C, Petzelbauer P, Shi GP, Chapman HA, Stingl G. Fc epsilon receptor I on dendritic cells delivers IgE-bound

multivalent antigens into a cathepsin S–dependent pathway of MHC class II presentation. J Immunol 1998; 161:2731–2739.

141. Holloway JA, Holgate ST, Semper AE. Expression of the high-affinity IgE receptor on peripheral blood dendritic cells: differential binding of IgE in atopic asthma. J Allergy Clin Immunol 2001; 107:1009–1018.

142. Geiger E, Magerstaedt R, Wessendorf JH, Kraft S, Hanau D, Bieber T. IL-4 induces the intracellular expression of the alpha chain of the high-affinity receptor for IgE in in vitro-generated dendritic cells. J Allergy Clin Immunol 2000; 105: 150–156.

143. van der Heijden FL, Joost van Neerven RJ, van Katwijk M, Bos JD, Kapsenberg ML. Serum-IgE-facilitated allergen presentation in atopic disease. J Immunol 1993; 150:3643–3650.

144. Coyle AJ, Wagner K, Bertrand C, Tsuyuki S, Bews J, Heusser C. Central role of immunoglobulin (Ig) E in the induction of lung eosinophil infiltration and T helper 2 cell cytokine production: inhibition by a non-anaphylactogenic anti-IgE antibody. J Exp Med 1996; 183:1303–1310.

145. Kehry MR, Yamashita LC. Low-affinity IgE receptor (CD23) function on mouse B cells: role in IgE-dependent antigen focusing. Proc Natl Acad Sci USA 1989; 86:7556–7560.

146. Fujiwara H, Kikutani H, Suematsu S, Naka T, Yoshida K, Tanaka T, Suemura M, Matsumoto N, Kojima S, et al. The absence of IgE antibody-mediated augmentation of immune responses in CD23-deficient mice. Proc Natl Acad Sci USA 1994; 91:6835–6839.

147. Lee WT, Rao M, Conrad DH. The murine lymphocyte receptor for IgE. IV. The mechanism of ligand-specific receptor upregulation on B cells. J Immunol 1987; 139:1191–1198.

148. Yu P, Kosco-Vilbois M, Richards M, Kohler G, Lamers MC. Negative feedback regulation of IgE synthesis by murine CD23. Nature 1994; 369:753–756.

149. Payet-Jamroz M, Helm SL, Wu J, Kilmon M, Fakher M, Basalp A, Tew JG, Szakal AK, Noben-Trauth N, Conrad DH. Suppression of IgE responses in CD23-transgenic animals is due to expression of CD23 on nonlymphoid cells. J Immunol 2001; 166:4863–4869.

150. Muller KM, Rocken M, Joel D, Bonnefoy JY, Saurat JH, Hauser C. Mononuclear cell-bound CD23 is elevated in both atopic dermatitis and psoriasis. J Dermatol Sci 1991; 2:125–133.

151. Jung CM, Prinz JC, Rieber EP, Ring J. A reduction in allergen-induced Fc epsilon R2/CD23 expression on peripheral B cells correlates with successful hyposensitization in grass pollinosis. J Allergy Clin Immunol 1995; 95:77–87.

152. Gough L, Schulz O, Sewell HF, Shakib F. The cysteine protease activity of the major dust mite allergen Der p 1 selectively enhances the immunoglobulin E antibody response. J Exp Med 1999; 190:1897–1902.

153. Mayer RJ, Bolognese BJ, Al-Mahdi N, Cook RM, Flamberg PL, Hansbury MJ, Khandekar S, Appelbaum E, Faller A, Marshall LA. Inhibition of CD23 processing correlates with inhibition of IL-4-stimulated IgE production in human PBL and hu-PBL-reconstituted SCID mice. Clin Exp Allergy 2000; 30:719–727.

154. van Neerven RJ, van Roomen CP, Thomas WR, de Boer M, Knol EF, Davis FM. Humanized anti-IgE mAb Hu-901 prevents the activation of allergen-specific T cells. Int Arch Allergy Immunol 2001; 124:400–402.

155. Tumas DB, Chan B, Werther W, Wrin T, Vennari J, Desjardin N, Shields RL, Jardieu P. Anti-IgE efficacy in murine asthma models is dependent on the method of allergen sensitization. J Allergy Clin Immunol 2001; 107:1025–1033.

156. Fahy JV, Fleming HE, Wong HH, Liu JT, Su JQ, Reimann J, Fick RB, Jr., Boushey HA. The effect of an anti-IgE monoclonal antibody on the early- and late-phase responses to allergen inhalation in asthmatic subjects. Am J Respir Crit Care Med 1997; 155:1828–1834.

157. Milgrom H, Fick RB, Jr., Su JQ, Reimann JD, Bush RK, Watrous ML, Metzger WJ. Treatment of allergic asthma with monoclonal anti-IgE antibody. rhuMAb-E25 Study Group. N Engl J Med 1999; 341:1966–1973.

158. Salvi SS, Babu KS. Treatment of allergic asthma with monoclonal anti-IgE antibody. N Engl J Med 2000; 342:1292–1293.

159. Soler M, Matz J, Townley R, Buhl R, O'Brien J, Fox H, Thirlwell J, Gupta N, Della Cioppa G. The anti-IgE antibody omalizumab reduces exacerbations and steroid requirement in allergic asthmatics. Eur Respir J 2001; 18:254–261.

160. MacGlashan D, Jr. Anti-IgE antibody therapy. Clin Allergy Immunol 2002; 16:519–532.

161. Busse WW. Anti-immunoglobulin E (omalizumab) therapy in allergic asthma. Am J Respir Crit Care Med 2001; 164:S12–17.

162. Bacharier LB, Geha RS. Molecular mechanisms of IgE regulation. J Allergy Clin Immunol 2000; 105:S547–558.

5

Immune Functions of Mast Cells and Basophils

SARBJIT S. SAINI

Johns Hopkins University School of Medicine
Baltimore, Maryland, U.S.A.

I. Introduction

For several decades mast cells and basophils have been recognized as important effector cells in the pathogenesis of asthma. Elevated numbers of airway mast cells (1) and their activation products have been clearly documented in the airways of asthmatic patients. Likewise, the accumulation of basophils in the lungs of patients with fatal asthma (2) and in the late-phase airway responses of experimental allergen challenge (3–5) has linked this cell type and its mediators to the process of airway inflammation. In this chapter we will review the functions of both of these leukocytes, with an emphasis on their contribution to asthma pathogenesis. Given the complexity of the airway inflammatory response in asthma and the involvement of several immunological pathways and cell types, our discussion of cell-specific functions in vivo will rely on evidence from human studies as well as established animal and in vitro models.

Both mast cells and basophils secrete a range of biologically active mediators, including agents stored in granules as well as newly generated lipid metabolites and cytokines, in response to stimuli such as environmental allergens. Bronchoprovocation tests with relevant allergens of the airways of atopic asthmatic subjects and sensitized animals is a standardized tool to study elements of the asthmatic response in terms of immune cells as well as mediators. In these models of asthma, it is generally accepted that the acute airway response is dependent on allergen binding to specific IgE antibodies bound to lung mast cells. In this early phase, activated mast cells rapidly release spasmogenic and vasoactive mediators that can act on local blood vessels and smooth muscles, leading to airway edema, bronchoconstriction, and symptoms of wheezing. Levels of mast cell mediators have been positively correlated to increasing airway obstruction and bronchial hyperreactivity in asthma patients (6–8). The experimental late-phase airway response, which occurs 4 to 12 h after allergen challenge in 50% of subjects, is characterized by a recurrence in clinical symptoms, mediator release, and leukocyte infiltration of the lung (9). It is during the late-phase airway response that basophils, along with eosinophils and lymphocytes, are recruited to the lung and are activated to release their inflammatory products. A greater understanding of leukocyte recruitment process has resulted from the recognition of chemokines and the expression of their specific receptors on leukocyte subsets (10). Several features of the late-phase airway response are also observed in chronic asthma and have allowed insight into the mechanisms of airway inflammation and the development of airway reactivity.

It is becoming increasingly clear that cytokines released by mast cells and basophils hours after allergen activation may have several immunoregulatory actions that promote a T-helper 2 (Th2)–biased immune response. Evidence for these novel actions by these cells in regulating airway immune responses along with traditional effector functions in asthma will also be presented. It should be noted that a subset of adult and a minority of pediatric asthmatics lack demonstrable allergen sensitization based on standard skin prick testing. Nevertheless, these "intrinsic" asthmatics share several pathological features with the allergen-provoked "extrinsic" asthmatics, including evidence for localized IgE class switching (11) and similar cytokine patterns in tissue biopsies (12–14). Therefore, the focus of the discussions will be allergic-based asthma pathogenesis.

II. Origin and Distribution of Mast Cells and Basophils

Mast cells and basophils share many cellular features such as cytoplasmic granules, which contain acidic molecules that take up basic dyes and stain metachromatically. Both cell types also possess high-affinity IgE receptors (FcεRI) on their surface filled with IgE antibodies that permit interaction with a wide variety of environmental allergens. In addition, they also bear CD40 ligand on their surface and are capable of stimulating B cells to synthesize IgE (15). Mast cells and basophils also both arise from hematopoietic, pluripotent $CD34^+$ stem cells present in the bone marrow but follow divergent maturation paths (16,17). Committed mast cell precursors migrate from the bone marrow to the connective tissues of mucosal and epithelial surfaces of the body to complete their maturation (18,19). These committed precursor cells have been rarely demonstrated in the bloodstream of individuals with mast cell hyperplasia (20). They mature and take up residence in close proximity to blood vessels, lymphatics, and nerves in epithelial surfaces that are at the interface with the external environment. In the lung, large numbers of mast cells are present in the mucosa, submucosa, and alveolar walls (21). This unique anatomical position in the airways allows mast cells the opportunity to sample and respond to external stimuli such as allergen. Mast cells and their precursors also express c-kit (CD117), a tyrosine kinase–linked receptor that binds the growth factor, stem cell factor (SCF). SCF is not only an essential factor for mast cell maturation and survival, but can prime mast cells for IgE-mediated responses (22) and at higher concentrations lead to direct mast cell activation (23), possibly in an autocrine fashion (24). Various activating mutations of c-kit have been identified in subjects who have an excessive number of mast cells or mastocytosis (25,26). The local tissue environment (i.e., fibroblasts and epithelial cells) can provide SCF as well as other factors that may contribute to the heterogeneity noted among populations of mast cells (27) (Table 1). Mature tissue mast cells differ in relation to granule content, with tryptase-bearing cells found mainly in the lung and intestinal mucosa, and chymase- and tryptase-containing cells located in the skin, lymph nodes, and intestinal submucosa. In addition, mast cells vary in granule proteoglycan composition (heparin versus chondroitin sulfate), granule ultrastructure [scroll-like granules or latticework architecture (28)], and functional responses to drugs and stimuli (21). Tissue mast cells appear to be long-lived cells as recently shown by long-term in vitro cultures of human airway mast cells (29). It has also been suggested that tissue-derived mast cells may retain proliferative capacity, as recently observed in studies with skin-derived mast cells (30).

In contrast to mast cells, blood basophils fully mature from $CD34^+$ precursors in the bone marrow under the influence of interleukin-3 (IL-3)(31) and reside in the circulation as nondividing cells. The presence of high levels of the IL-3 receptor α chain on the surface of basophils readily distinguishes them from mast cells. Basophils migrate to tissue sites in response to inflammatory stimuli such as those generated during the late-phase response to allergen challenge of the nose (32), lung (33), or skin (34,35). They possess a wide array of surface adhesion molecules including β_1 integrins like VLA-4, β_2 integrins, ICAMs, as well as numerous chemokine receptors like CCR3, to facilitate their migration and recruitment from the circulation to specific tissue sites (10,36–38). Until recently, identification of basophils in tissues was compromised by lack of a unique marker to separate them from tissue-resident mast cells. In allergen challenge studies, a biological response was assigned to basophils or mast cells based on the pattern of mediators that were detected in the tissue environment or by morphological features. Mediators observed in the allergen-induced early phase, such as histamine, tryptase, and postaglandin D_2 (PGD_2), were most consistent with mast cell activation whereas late-phase airway peaks in histamine without PGD_2 release were attributed to the arrival and activation of basophils (33). In tissue biopsies, mast-cell-specific markers such as tryptase were used given the minimal presence of this protease in basophils (39,40); however, recently this has become controversial (41). The recent development of basophil-specific antibodies, BB1 (42) and 2D7 (43), have confirmed the accumulation of basophils in the late-phase responses of allergen-challenged

Table 1 Selected Mast Cell and Basophil Mediators Released by IgE Activation

Mediator	Cell	Actions
Preformed		
Histamine	MC, B	Vasodilatation, increased vascular permeability, smooth muscle contraction, bronchospasm, mucus secretion, P-selectin induction, fibroblast proliferation
Proteoglycans		
Heparin	MC	Anticoagulant, storage matrix, immunomodulator properties
Chondroitin sulfate	MC, B	Storage matrix
Neutral proteases		
Tryptase	MC$_T$, MC$_{CT}$, B*	Generate C3a, bradykinin, degrades neuropeptides such as VIP, induces epithelial IL-8 and ICAM expression
Chymase	MC$_{CT}$, B*	Bronchial mucus secretion
Carboxypeptidase A	MC$_{CT}$	Undefined
Preformed cytokines		
TNF-α, IL-16	MC	See below
Newly formed		
Arachidonic acid metabolites		
LTB$_4$	MC	Neutrophil chemotaxis

Mediator	Source	Function
LTC$_4$, D$_4$, E$_4$	MC, B	Bronchoconstiction, mucus secretion, vascular permeability, eosinophil chemotaxis and survival, airway hyperresponsiveness
PGD$_2$	MC	Bronchoconstriction, mucus secretion, edema, vasodilatation, neutrophil chemotaxis
Cytokines		
IL-6	MC	Increased IgE synthesis
IL-8	MC, B	Chemotaxis of neutrophils, lymphocytes, and primed eosinophils
IL-4	B, MC	Activation of endothelium adhesion molecules, IgE production, induction of Th2 phenotype, increased FcεRI expression
IL-13	B, MC	Activation of endothelium adhesion molecules, IgE production, mucus secretion
IL-16	MC	Lymphocyte chemotaxis
GM-CSF, IL-5	MC	Eosinophil, growth, activation, survival
TNF-α	MC	Activation of endothelium adhesion molecules, monocyte and neutrophil chemotaxis, mucus secretion, stimulation of leukocyte functions
Chemokines		
IL-8, ENA-78	MC	Neutrophil and eosinophil chemotaxis
MCP-1	MC	Monocyte and T-cell chemotaxis
MIP-1α	MC‡, B	Macrophage differentiation, neutrophil chemotaxis, and cytotoxicity

MC$_{CT}$, Chymase tryptase mast cell, found in skin, blood vessels, intestinal submucosa; MC$_T$, mucosal mast cell, typically found in lung, nasal cavity, intestinal mucosa; B*, extremely low levels of this mediator has been found in basophils (<1% of mast cells); MC‡HMC-1, a human mast cell leukemia cell line produces MIP-1β, RANTES (172).
See also Ref. 173 and 174.

sites such as lung (3,4,44), skin (44,45), nose (46), and eyes (47). In the past, basophils were considered to be a circulating form of mast cell, but the current concensus is that they are closer in lineage to eosinophils (48,49). However, a few recent studies have again suggested that the mast cells and the basophils of atopic subjects can share several biochemical features, such as tryptase (41) and a common lineage marker (50).

Seasonal allergen exposure is known to increase the numbers of circulating basophils (51) and the numbers of mucosal mast cells in nasal epithelium (52) and the conjunctiva of the eye (53). Application of topical steroids can blunt the increase in nasal mast cells that is observed during an allergen season (54). Similar studies of seasonal fluxes in the numbers of lung mast cells are lacking.

III. IgE Receptor Expression and Cellular Activation

Cross-linking of high-affinity IgE receptors by allergen activates the release of all mediator classes by both mast cells and basophils and allows the expression of effector functions commonly associated with these cells. The FcεRI complex is composed of an IgE-binding α chain and a β chain, as well as a β and two γ chains that are involved in signal transduction (55). The FcεRI β chain amplifies downstream signaling pathways (56), and increased FcεRI β expression is linked to enhanced levels of FcεRI surface expression on basophils (57). Bridging of as few as 1% of the total surface FcεRI receptors by allergen is sufficient to activate these cells and mobilize a host response (58). The number of basophil surface FcεRI receptors can range from 5000 to nearly 1 million per cell and is closely linked to serum IgE levels (59,60). Whereas FcεRI receptor expression in rodents is limited to mast cells and basophils, in humans FcεRI is also present at low levels on other leukocytes such as monocytes and dendritic cells (55). The FcεRI on monocytes and dendritic cells is thought to function in antigen presentation (61,62) and also differs from mast cells and basophils in that it is trimeric ($\alpha\gamma_2$) rather than tetrameric ($\alpha\beta\gamma_2$) in structure. The broad expression of FcεRI in humans exemplifies the difficulties in interpretation of allergen-triggered airway studies and their immunological consequences. Likewise, one complexity of murine asthma models is the expression of FcγRIII receptors on mast cells that can be triggered by IgG and activate mediator pathways typical of IgE-triggered reactions (63).

Accumulating evidence from human and mice studies has led to the conclusion that FcεRI is regulated by IgE levels and IL-4 (60,64–68). IgE-deficient mice have roughly four- to fivefold lower levels of FcεRI on their mast cells and basophils, which can be corrected by exogenous administration of IgE (68,69). Furthermore, IgE-dependent enhancement of FcεRI on murine mast cells and human umbilical cord blood–derived mast cells has enhanced sensitivity of these cells to allergen for activation and increased mediator production

(68,70,71). Thus, increased IgE levels can feedback on murine mast cells and enhance their functional responses as well as FcεRI expression. Human experiments with a therapeutic anti-IgE antibody have also supported that IgE-dependent FcεRI regulation occurs on human basophils (72,73); however, effects of FcεRI enhancement on mediator responses and sensitivity to allergen have been somewhat mixed (74). Thus, IgE-dependent modulation of FcεRI in humans is an amplification loop whereby the magnitude and sensitivity of mast cells and basophils can be altered (Fig. 1). As will be discussed, therapies targeting IgE have diminished FcεRI levels on these cell types and led to reduced allergen-related functional responses (75).

IV. Mast Cell and Basophil Mediator Release

Allergen cross-linking of IgE bound to the surface of mast cells and basophils leads to cellular activation and the release of inflammatory products within minutes. These mediators are typically classified according to their pattern of release and include those that are preformed in granules and released by exocytosis, those that are rapidly synthesized from membrane lipids, and,

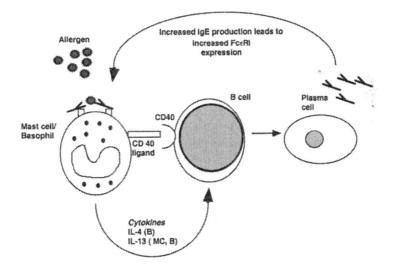

Figure 1 **Proposed pathways of mast cell/basophil promotion of B-cell IgE synthesis**. Allergen activation of mast cells or basophils stimulates the release if IL-4 (basophils) and IL-13 (basophils and mast cells) along with increased surface expression of CD40 ligand. The exposure of B cells to these cytokines along with engagement of CD40 provides the necessary signals for B-cell switching to IgE production. The synthesized IgE released from plasma cells can promote the levels of FcεRI on mast cells and basophils in a feedback loop.

lastly, cytokines that are synthesized and released over several hours. The nature of each mediator, its cellular source and main actions are summarized in Table 1.

Besides allergens there are also numerous biological stimuli that can activate or potentiate mediator release from mast cells and basophils, including histamine-releasing factors (76), products of complement activation such as C3a and C5a (77), nerve-related peptides (tachykinins, nerve growth factor, calcitonin gene-related peptide) (78–80), ATP, IL-3 (81,82), adenosine, SCF (83), and chemokines for basophil histamine release (37,84). Several of the cytokine and chemokine priming factors have been identified in vivo at the sites of late-phase reactions (85,86).

FCεRI receptor aggregation leads to the stimulation of several intracellular signaling events and features calcium influx into the cell. The bridging of adjacent surface-bound IgE molecules by allergen leads to the activation of a receptor-associated src family kinase, Lyn, which phosphorylates the FcεRI β and γ subunits and initiates the signaling cascade. The tyrosine kinase Syk is rapidly recruited to the activated receptor complex, and this is followed by a series of intermediate molecules and secondary messengers that ultimately lead to the end points of granule secretion, lipid metabolite generation and synthesis of cytokines [see recent review by Oliver (87)]. Novel counterregulatory pathways involving phosphatases such as SHIP-1 and SHIP-2 that turnoff the allergen-triggered mediator responses are under active study (88,89). There is wide variation noted in the extent of histamine release from basophils of different individuals, a phenomenon that has been termed "releasability" (90). Factors that determine the sensitivity of basophils or mast cells to allergen activation or the magnitude of their mediator response are also under study as potential therapeutic targets. Thus far only IL-4 and IgE have been linked to the magnitude of mast cell mediator response by effecting FcεRI expression. Among human subjects, a nonreleasing basophil phenotype has been identified and is linked to the selective deficiency of the Syk kinase needed for FcεRI signal transduction (91,92).

V. Specific Mediators of Mast Cells and Basophils

A. Histamine

Preformed histamine is stored in the granules of both mast cells and basophils and is released within 30 min of FcεRI aggregation. Histamine is produced from histidine by histidine decarboxylase and is packaged with chondroitin sulfate or heparin in the granule matrix. Degradation of histamine occurs rapidly in vivo by two pathways, either by deamination by histaminases or methylation by N-methyltransferase. Histamine binding to H_1 receptors is linked to contraction of the airway smooth muscle and increased vascular permeability, whereas H_2 receptor activation leads to increased airway mucus secretion (93).

B. Neutral Proteases and Proteoglycans

Mast cell secretory granules can vary in microscopic appearance as well as in the content of neutral serine proteases. These granules also contain negatively charged proteoglycans, such as chondroitin sulfate or heparin, that influence the activity of the protease by limiting their inactivation as well slowing their rate of diffusion to the local tissue site (94). Neutral proteases are the most abundant proteins in mast cell granules and are represented by tryptase, chymase, and carboxypeptidase A. The proposed functions for these proteases include tissue remodeling by activation of matrix metalloproteases, activation of protease-activated receptors, increased mucus secretion, and, lastly, leukocyte recruitment (95–97).

The serine protease tryptase accounts for up to 20% of all protein produced by the mast cells, and lung mast cells are thought to contain an average of 11 pg/cell. In both animals and humans, tryptase acts as a fibroblast growth factor (98) and has recently been also shown to interact with and activate thrombin as well as the protease-activated receptor-2 (PAR-2) (99). The activation of PAR-2 receptors on airway epithelial cells leads to the release of eotaxin and granulocyte-macrophage colony-stimulating factor (GM-CSF), which recruit eosinophils and increase their survival (100). Given their predominant origin from mast cells, two forms of tryptase in human mast cells have gained utility as biological markers (101). α-Tryptase is constitutively released into the serum at low levels and therefore serves as an indirect measure of the total-body mast cell number (102). Significant elevations in serum α-tryptase are seen in disorders with mast cell hyperplasia, such as mastocytosis (103). In contrast, β-tryptase is released acutely by mast cell activation by allergen or other pathways that involve degranulation and has been proposed as a clinical marker of anaphylaxis (104,105).

The other major mast cell protease is chymase, which is prominent in skin and submucosal-based mast cells and is typically found with carboxypeptidase in the secretory granules. Chymase has been described to stimulate bronchial mucus secretion in animals and possibly is involved in tissue remodeling. Roles for other proteases, such as sulfatases and exoglycosidases, are not well defined in humans.

C. Lipid Mediators

The arachidonic acid derivatives include members of the leukotriene and prostaglandin families generated de novo through the lipoxygenase and cyclooxygenase pathways. Arachidonic acid released from membrane phospholipids by phospholipase A_2 is processed by 5-lipoxygenase (5-LO) to leukotriene A_4. LTA_4 is then converted to dihydroleukotriene $B_4(LTB_4)$ by LTA_4 hydrolase or to the cysteinyl leukotriene C_4 by LTC_4 synthase. LTC_4 is sequentially converted to LTD_4 and LTE_4 by enzymatic cleavage of glutamine and glycine, respectively. The prominent lipoxygenase product of mast cells and basophils with respect to airway reactivity is LTC_4 and its resulting intermediates along with limited LTB_4 production in mast cells. The levels of LTs in bronchoalveolar fluids significantly increase following local challenge with a relevant allergen in atopic asthmatics (106). The cysteinyl LTs (LTC_4, LTD_4, LTE_4) can cause bronchoconstriction with up to a 1000-fold greater potency than histamine by binding to specific receptors on smooth muscle cells (107). Cysteinyl LTs and LTB_4 are also chemotactic for eosinophils and neutrophils, respectively. The effects of the cysteinyl LTs are mediated by two members of the G-protein-coupled receptors, CysLT1 and CysLT2, which have recently been cloned in humans (108,109) and are localized on a variety of cells such as airway smooth muscle (110). Pharmacological antagonists of the CysLT1 receptor as well as an inhibitor of the 5-LO enzyme have been shown to eliminate about 80% of the early-phase bronchoconstrictor response and 50% of the late-phase airway response induced by allergen challenge and ameliorate asthma symptoms (21).

The prostaglandins are also generated from arachidonic acid by cyclooxygenase (COX). COX-1 is constitutively expressed in a wide variety of cell types, whereas COX-2 is highly inducible in mast cells by proinflammatory factors. During the early phase of an allergic reaction, mast cells release prostaglandin D_2 (PGD_2), which causes bronchoconstriction, with up to a 30-fold greater potency than histamine. The importance of PGD_2 as a mediator in asthma has been established by its direct measurement in the bronchoalveolar lavage (BAL) fluid of asthmatics (111) as well as after airway antigen challenge (112). Disruption of the classic PGD_2 receptor, DP, in a mouse model has allowed insight into the importance of this mast cell mediator in allergic inflammation (113). DP receptor–deficient animals have decreased pulmonary inflammation after aerosol allergen challenge, including reductions in T cell numbers, Th2 cytokines, eosinophil infiltration, and airway hyperreactivity. PGD_2 has also been recently described as a chemoattractant for T cells, basophils, and eosinophils via a recently cloned receptor CRTH2 in humans (114).

D. Cytokines

Many recent studies have focused on the identification of cytokines produced by mast cells and basophils, although their exact in vivo role remains unclear. IgE-dependent activation of cultured human mast cells and tissue-derived mast cells has led to the detection of a large number of cytokines, including interleukins 3, 4, 5, 6, 8, 10, 13, 16, as well as GM-CSF, TNF-α, VPF/VEGF, SCF, basic fibroblast growth factor (115,116). As with preformed mediators, cytokine production from mast cells also appears to be heterogeneous (117). In contrast, activated basophils can synthesize and release significant amounts of IL-4 and IL-13 for several hours after receptors activation (118–122). The relative importance of either cell's cytokine products is under review based on the demonstration of in vivo production, quantitative measures, patterns of release, and comparisons to other known sources of these products. In particular, the production of IL-4 and IL-13 from mast cells and basophils has highlighted the potential of these cells to amplify Th2 immune responses. Two independent groups have provided evidence that basophils are recruited to airways after in vivo allergen challenge and produce significant levels of IL-4 protein (3,5). One of these studies employed the basophil-specific antibody 2D7 in airway biopsies before and after allergen challenge and identified a 10-fold rise in basophils in atopic asthmatics, with no change seen in non-atopic healthy controls. Furthermore, a significant fraction of these basophils expressed IL-4 mRNA and protein (3). Twenty percent of IL-4 mRNA–positive cells were basophils, which compares favorably to earlier studies that attributed more than 70% of the IL-4 mRNA to T cells (123). However, no IL-4 protein could be attributed to T cells in the earlier study, but in the basophil study 41% of total IL-4 protein detected was colocalized to basophils. A different study of peripheral blood mononuclear cells cultured after allergen activation also came to the conclusion that the main IL-4 producing cells were basophils (124). A side-by-side comparison of circulating basophils to circulating T cells obtained from allergic asthmatics for IL-4 production after allergen activation showed that 10–20% of basophils were activated by allergen for IL-4 and IL-13 production and accounted for four times as many IL-4 producing cells than similarly activated T cells (125).

Studies of human nasal and lung mast cells have shown the release of IL-4 and IL-13 and secretion of these cytokines after allergen activation (116,126–128). In addition, the release of TNF-α by mast cells can have multiple proinflammatory effects, including the activation of cellular recruitment via enhanced adhesion molecule and chemokine expression on several cell types as well as enhanced airway hyperresponsiveness (129). A small, preformed pool of TNF-α exists in mast cell populations such as dermal mast cells and can activate ICAM-1 expression on endothelium (130,131). IL-5, a cytokine critical to eosinophil activation and survival, has been localized to mast cells in airway biopsies as well as released from activated human lung mast cells (117,132,133).

There is also evidence that cultured mast cells and mast cell lines release a broad array of chemokines, such as MIP1α (70), MIP1β, RANTES, ENA-78 (134), MCP-1, MCP-3, MCP-4, and IL-8, that can recruit a variety of leukocyte species (135).

VI. Cellular Interactions of Mast Cells and Basophils

Several lines of evidence support a role for mast cells and basophils in regulating the functions of leukocytes involved in allergic inflammation. Most of this evidence rests on the cytokines induced after allergen activation of these cells and their diverse roles in asthma pathogenesis. Among the possible scenarios of in vivo effects of IL-4 and IL-13 cytokines are the induction of IgE production from B cells (15,136), promotion of Th2 lymphocyte development (137), and the specific recruitment of leukocytes via the induction of VCAM on endothelial cells (138,139).

For years an association between levels of IgE and the presence of asthma has been known (140). The present understanding of B-cell isotype switching to IgE synthesis is that two signals are necessary. The first is either IL-4 or IL-13, and the second is the ligation of CD40 on the B-cell surface by CD40 ligand (136). In the last decade, it was first reported that purified mast cells with exogenous IL-4 could induce B cells to synthesize IgE (15) (Fig. 1). Likewise, peripheral blood basophils as well as umbilical cord blood–derived basophils were shown to be fully capable of inducing B-cell IgE synthesis without the addition of exogenous cytokines (15,141). A more recent study demonstrated that allergen activation of nasal mast cells in vitro in the presence of B cells was sufficient to stimulate IgE synthesis. Furthermore, this IgE production was blocked by including anti-IL-4 or anti-IL-13 antibodies (128). Likewise, basophils recruited to the airways after allergen exposure could also provide the IL-4 for such isotype switching (3,5). Taken together, the evidence also supports that mast cells and basophils upon activation can express the CD40 ligand necessary for completion of B-cell immunoglobulin switch to IgE (15) and that CD40 ligand is induced on mast cells from subjects with allergic rhinitis and basophils from subjects with allergic asthma (125,128). Several recent studies have provided data that germline switching for IgE synthesis occurs at the tissue level and therefore favors the involvement of tissue-based mast cells or recruited basophils (11,142). Therefore, a novel immunological function for mast cells and basophils is to behave as surrogate Th2 cells under inflammatory states such as allergen exposure. In the peripheral blood compartment, it appears that the vast majority of basophils retain the capacity to secrete large amounts of IL-4 or IL-13 after allergen stimulation (125).

T cells and eosinphils are also key participants in the overall asthmatic inflammatory response and are also specifically recruited to the asthmatic airways (143,144). Efforts at defining interactions between mast cells, basophils, and these cell species are underway. One focus of investigations has been the source of IL-4 that can promote the development of naive T (Th0) cells into Th2 cells (145). The possible cellular candidates for this early IL-4 burst are mast cells, basophils, or a subset of natural killer T cells and remains a topic of debate (146,147).

The release of localized IL-4 and IL-13 can also act to influence endothelial functions by enchancing their expression of VCAM (138,139), a surface adhesion molecule that recruits cells bearing its counterligand VLA-4 such as eosinophils and basophils (38). Furthermore, the induction of local tissue chemokine expression, such as eotaxin, may further assist the arrival of eosinophils to the airway in asthma (86,100).

Whether mast cells and basophils participate in the tissue remodeling observed in asthma has not been formally established. Some of the key pathological determinants of asthma seen on airway pathological specimens or transtracheal biopsies include the presence of fibrosis, collagen deposition, smooth muscle hypertrophy, and mucus gland hyperplasia (148). Elegant studies in mice have clearly established a role for IL-13 in creating airway hyperresponsiveness as well as mucus gland hypertrophy (149,150). IL-13 has also been detected in the environment of local airway allergen challenge in human subjects (151). However, the clear demonstration of the sources of IL-13 or its role in human asthma awaits further investigations.

Mast cell release of the cytokine TNF-α can broadly boost immune responses from chemokine secretion from the epithelium, endothelium adhesion molecule expression like that of ICAM-1(130), and as well as enhance the arrival of leukocytes. More than a decade ago, the use of anti-TNF antibodies was shown to inhibit the passive cutaneous anaphylaxis reaction by 50% (152). Likewise, TNF-α released from lung explants supported the recruitment of eosinophils and neutrophils (153). The rapid release of TNF-α from mast cells has also gained important in host defense against bacterial pathogens as demonstrated by studies of bacterial sepsis in mast cell–deficient animals (154,155). The early TNF-α release from mast cells in these mice was key to the arrival of neutrophils and a reduction in mortality. Thus, TNF-α released from mast cells can clearly focus the resulting immune response from either allergic or infectious challenge.

VII. Animal Models of Allergic Airways Disease

Studies in mast-cell-deficient mice (Kit^W/Kit^{W-v}) with defects in c-kit have established a role for mast cells in mounting acute allergic responses such as in the PCA reaction in the skin (152), lung (156), gut (115), as well as cardiopulmonary changes in passive systemic anaphylaxis models (157). More recent work has concerned the role of mast cells in innate immunity (158,159). However, several murine studies have also raised questions regarding the pivotal need for mast cells and IgE in generating the expected allergen-induced airway response. Experiments with mast cell- (160), B-cell- (161), and IgE-deficient (162) animals have all shown appropriate late-phase airway responses, including the recruitment of eosinophils. Among the explanations for these findings have been the route used for allergen sensitization, the high doses of allergen used for challenges versus the low doses encountered in vivo, as well as inherent difficulties of defining human asthma phenotypes via murine models (163). An example of this latter point is the ability to cause allergen-mediated responses in mice via alternative pathway such as IgG which may not exist in the human system (63). Furthermore, the application of the therapeutic anti-IgE antibody failed to show efficacy in one of two murine asthma models that differed in methods of allergen sensitization which conflicts with the experience of this therapy in human asthma clinical trials (164).

VIII. Lessons from Therapeutic Studies: Anti-IgE

The earliest studies of the use of a monoclonal antibody to reduce IgE levels in allergic asthmatics showed significant protection from early- and late-phase airway responses to allergen challenge of the lungs (165,166). In a separate trial, it was established that in vivo IgE reductions by anti-IgE reducted $Fc\varepsilon RI$ expression on basophils, which led to significant suppression of allergen-related mediator release by basophils (72). A similar reduction in mast cell functional responses assessed by titration of allergen skin test responses was also noted (167). Interestingly, a rapid return to cellular function and $Fc\varepsilon RI$ expression on basophils occurred with the discontinuation of anti-IgE infusions (73). A prediction of these early trials was that the therapeutic effects were largely linked to the magnitude of serum IgE reduction (168). By implication, the therapeutic impact was also linked to levels of $Fc\varepsilon RI$ expression and function of basophils and also likely of mast cells. The completed phase III trials of anti-IgE in asthma with effective IgE reduction have shown reductions in asthma exacerbations and the ability to taper inhaled and oral steroids (169–171). Taken together, the results of anti-IgE therapy can be viewed as in vivo evidence for the role of IgE in asthma and its functional link to the activation of mast cells and basophils in chronic asthma.

IX. Conclusions

As has been noted, there is significant redundancy in inflammation networks seen in allergic airway responses. However, in the context of asthma, the role of allergens in mediating early bronchospastic and delayed responses appears to depend on activation of mast cells and their potent mediators. It is now apparent that the sensitivity and magnitude of mast cells in acute airway responses can be amplified by elevations in serum IgE levels in a positive-feedback loop. In turn, increased IgE levels further arm these cells for subsequent allergen exposures. Levels of IgE are also linked to the presence of asthma and causally related to the expression of $Fc\varepsilon RI$ on both mast cells and basophils. The importance of this amplification loop of IgE upon $Fc\varepsilon RI$ levels in the context of asthma has been highlighted by the results of human studies using anti-IgE. In addition, the expression of IL-4, IL-13, and CD40 ligand by these cells after allergen activation, both in vitro and in vivo, has raised the possibility that mast cells and basophils can themselves enhance IgE levels by inducing B cells to produce IgE at the local tissues. Another consequence of their cytokine release may by the promotion of T-cell development along a Th2 pathway, which again favors asthma progression. Besides providing potent and rapid-acting mediators, mast cells and basophils may now be viewed as providing sustained support of the allergic airway responses by also promoting recruitment of other leukocytes (e.g., eosinophils) to the airway. The diverse distribution of mast cells and basophils recalls their sentinel roles in responding to allergens in the airway environment and focusing the nature of the resulting immune airway response. In the case of the mast cells, undiscovered functions for their mast cell proteases and novel functions for PGD_2 may further expand their roles in vivo.

Acknowledgment

This work was funded in part by NIH grant AI01564.

References

1. Koshino T, Arai Y, Miyamoto Y, et al. Airway basophil and mast cell density in patients with bronchial asthma: relationship to bronchial hyperresponsiveness. J Asthma 1996; 33:89–95.
2. Koshino T, Teshima S, Fukushima N, et al. Identification of basophils by immunohistochemistry in the airways of post-mortem cases of fatal asthma. Clin Exp Allergy 1993; 23:919–925.
3. Nouri-Aria KT, Irani AM, Jacobson MR, et al. Basophil recruitment and IL-4 production during human allergen–induced late asthma. J Allergy Clin Immunol 2001; 108:205–211.
4. Gauvreau GM, Lee JM, Watson RM, Irani AM, Schwartz LB, O'Byrne PM. Increased numbers of both airway basophils and mast cells in sputum after allergen inhalation challenge of atopic asthmatics. Am J Respir Crit Care Med 2000; 161:1473–1478.
5. Schroeder JT, Lichtenstein LM, Roche EM, Xiao H, Liu MC. IL-4 production by human basophils found in the lung following segmental allergen challenge. J Allergy Clin Immunol 2001; 107:265–271.
6. Jarjour NN, Calhoun WJ, Schwartz LB, Busse WW. Elevated bronchoalveolar lavage fluid histamine levels in allergic asthmatics are associated with increased airway obstruction. Am Rev Respir Dis 1991; 144:83–87.
7. Broide DH, Gleich GJ, Cuomo AJ, et al. Evidence of ongoing mast cell and eosinophil degranulation in symptomatic asthma airway. J Allergy Clin Immunol 1991; 88:637–648.
8. Casale TB, Wood D, Richerson HB, Zehr B, Zavala D, Hunninghake GW. Direct evidence of a role for mast cells in the pathogenesis of antigen-induced broncho-constriction. J Clin Invest 1987; 80:1507–1511.
9. Pradalier A. Late-phase reaction in asthma: basic mechanisms. Int Arch Allergy Immunol 1993; 101:322–325.
10. Rothenberg ME, Zimmermann N, Mishra A, et al. Chemokines and chemokine receptors: their role in allergic airway disease. J Clin Immunol 1999; 19:250–265.

11. Ying S, Humbert M, Meng Q, et al. Local expression of epsilon germline gene transcripts and RNA for the epsilon heavy chain of IgE in the bronchial mucosa in atopic and nonatopic asthma. J Allergy Clin Immunol 2001; 107:686–692.

12. Humbert M, Durham SR, Ying S, et al. IL-4 and IL-5 mRNA and protein in bronchial biopsies from patients with atopic and nonatopic asthma: evidence against "intrinsic" asthma being a distinct immunopathologic entity. Am J Respir Crit Care Med 1996; 154:1497–1504.

13. Humbert M, Menz G, Ying S, et al. The immunopathology of extrinsic (atopic) and intrinsic (non-atopic) asthma: more similarities than differences. Immunol Today 1999; 20:528–533.

14. Menz G, Ying S, Durham SR, et al. Molecular concepts of IgE-initiated inflammation in atopic and nonatopic asthma. Allergy 1998; 53(45):15–21.

15. Gauchat JF, Henchoz S, Mazzei G, et al. Induction of human IgE synthesis in B cells by mast cells and basophils. Nature. 1993; 365:340–343.

16. Kirshenbaum AS, Kessler SW, Goff JP, Metcalfe DD. Demonstration of the origin of human mast cells from CD34+ bone marrow progenitor cells. J Immunol 1991; 146:1410–1415.

17. Kirshenbaum AS, Goff JP, Kessler SW, Mican JM, Zsebo KM, Metcalfe DD. Effect of IL-3 and stem cell factor on the appearance of human basophils and mast cells from CD34+ pluripotent progenitor cells. J Immunol 1992; 148:772–777.

18. Kirshenbaum AS, Goff JP, Semere T, Foster B, Scott LM, Metcalfe DD. Demonstration that human mast cells arise from a progenitor cell population that is CD34(+), c-kit(+), and expresses aminopeptidase N (CD13). Blood 1999; 94:2333–2342.

19. Kirshenbaum A. Regulation of mast cell number and function. Hematol Oncol Clin North Am 2000; 14:497–516.

20. Rottem M, Okada T, Goff JP, Metcalfe DD. Mast cells cultured from the peripheral blood of normal donors and patients with mastocytosis originate from a CD34+/Fc epsilon RI-cell population. Blood 1994; 84:2489–2496.

21. Schwartz L, Huff T. Biology of mast cells and basophils. In: Middleton E, Reed CE, Ellis EF, N.F. Adkinson J, Yunginger JW, Busse W, eds. Allergy Principles and Practice, 5th ed. Vol. 1. St. Louis: Mosby, 1998; 261–276.

22. Baghestanian M, Hofbauer R, Kiener HP, et al. The c-kit ligand stem cell factor and anti-IgE promote expression of monocyte chemoattractant protein-1 in human lung mast cells. Blood 1997; 90:4438–4449.

23. Costa JJ, Demetri GD, Harrist TJ, et al. Recombinant human stem cell factor (kit ligand) promotes human mast cell and melanocyte hyperplasia and functional activation in vivo. J Exp Med 1996; 183:2681–2686.

24. Zhang S, Anderson DF, Bradding P, et al. Human mast cells express stem cell factor. J Pathol 1998; 186:59–66.

25. Nagata H, Worobec AS, Oh CK, et al. Identification of a point mutation in the catalytic domain of the protooncogene c-kit in peripheral blood mononuclear cells of patients who have mastocytosis with an associated hematologic disorder. Proc Natl Acad Sci USA 1995; 92:10560–10564.

26. Boissan M, Feger F, Guillosson JJ, Arock M. c-Kit and c-kit mutations in mastocytosis and other hematological diseases. J Leukoc Biol 2000; 67:135–148.

27. Irani AM, Schwartz LB. Human mast cell heterogeneity. Allergy Proc 1994; 15:303–308.
28. Weidner N, Austen KF. Evidence for morphologic diversity of human mast cells. An ultrastructural study of mast cells from multiple body sites. Lab Invest 1990; 63:63–72.
29. Schulman ES, Mohanty JG. Long-tem cultivation of human lung mast cells. J Allergy Clin Immunol 2001; 107:S288.
30. Kambe N, Kambe M, Kochan JP, Schwartz LB. Human skin–derived mast cells can proliferate while retaining their characteristic functional and protease phenotypes. Blood 2001; 97:2045–2052.
31. Brandt J, Srour EF, van Besien K, Briddell RA, Hoffman R. Cytokine-dependent long-term culture of highly enriched precursors of hematopoietic progenitor cells from human bone marrow. J Clin Invest 1990; 86:932–941.
32. Bascom R, Wachs M, Naclerio RM, Pipkorn U, Galli SJ, Lichtenstein LM. Basophil influx occurs after nasal antigen challenge: effects to topical corticosteroid pretreatment. J Allergy Clin Immunol 1988; 81:580–589.
33. Liu MC, Hubbard WC, Proud D, et al. Immediate and late inflammatory responses to ragweed antigen challenge of the peripheral airways in allergic asthmatics. Cellular, mediator, and permeability changes. Am Rev Respir Dis 1991; 144:51–58.
34. Charlesworth EN, Hood AF, Soter NA, Kagey-Sobotka A, Norman PS, Lichtenstein LM. Cutaneous late-phase response to allergen. Mediator release and inflammatory cell infiltration. J Clin Invest 1989; 83:1519–1526.
35. Atkins PC, Schwartz LB, Adkinson NF, von Allmen C, Valenzano M, Zweiman B. In vivo antigen-induced cutaneous mediator release: simultaneous comparisons of histamine, tryptase, and prostaglandin D2 release and the effect of oral corticosteroid administration. J Allergy Clin Immunol 1990; 86:360–370.
36. Saini S, Matusumoto K, Bochner B. Phenotypic and functional characteristics of adhesion molecules on human basophils. In: Bochner BS, ed. Adhesion Molecules in Allergic diseases. New York: Marcel Dekker, 1997.
37. Uguccioni M, Mackay CR, Ochensberger B, et al. High expression of the chemokine receptor CCR3 in human blood basophils. Role in activation by eotaxin, MCP-4, and other chemokines. J Clin Invest 1997; 100:1137–1143.
38. Bochner BS, Schleimer RP. Mast cells, basophils, and eosinophils: distinct but overlapping pathways for recruitment. Immunol Rev 2001; 179:5–15.
39. Xia HZ, Kepley CL, Sakai K, Chelliah J, Irani AM, Schwartz LB. Quantitation of tryptase, chymase, Fc epsilon RI alpha, and Fc epsilon RI gamma mRNAs in human mast cells and basophils by competitive reverse transcription–polymerase chain reaction. J Immunol 1995; 154:5472–5480.
40. Castells MC, Irani AM, Schwartz LB. Evaluation of human peripheral blood leukocytes for mast cell tryptase. J Immunol 1987; 138:2184–2189.
41. Li L, Li Y, Reddel SW, et al. Identification of basophilic cells that express mast cell granule proteases in the peripheral blood of asthma, allergy, and drug-reactive patients. J Immunol 1998; 161:5079–5086.
42. McEuen AR, Buckley MG, Compton SJ, Walls AF. Development and characterization of a monoclonal antibody specific for human basophils and the

identification of a unique secretory product of basophil activation. Lab Invest 1999; 79:27–38.

43. Kepley CL, Craig SS, Schwartz LB. Identification and partial characterization of a unique marker for human basophils. J Immunol 1995; 154:6548–6555.

44. Macfarlane AJ, Kon OM, Smith SJ, et al. Basophils, eosinophils, and mast cells in atopic and nonatopic asthma and in late-phase allergic reactions in the lung and skin. J Allergy Clin Immunol 2000; 105:99–107.

45. Irani AM, Huang C, Xia HZ, et al. Immunohistochemical detection of human basophils in late-phase skin reactions. J Allergy Clin Immunol 1998; 101:354–362.

46. KleinJan A, McEuen AR, Dijkstra MD, Buckley MG, Walls AF, Fokkens WJ. Basophil and eosinophil accumulation and mast cell degranulation in the nasal mucosa of patients with hay fever after local allergen provocation. J Allergy Clin Immunol 2000; 106:677–686.

47. Bacon AS, Ahluwalia P, Irani AM, et al. Tear and conjunctival changes during the allergen-induced early- and late-phase responses. J Allergy Clin Immunol 2000; 106:948–954.

48. Denburg JA, Woolley M, Leber B, Linden M, O'Byrne P. Basophil and eosinophil differentiation in allergic reactions. J Allergy Clin Immunol 1994; 94:1135–1141.

49. Denburg JA, Telizyn S, Messner H, et al. Heterogeneity of human peripheral blood eosinophil-type colonies: evidence for a common basophil-eosinophil progenitor. Blood 1985; 66:312–318.

50. Buhring HJ, Simmons PJ, Pudney M, et al. The monoclonal antibody 97A6 defines a novel surface antigen expressed on human basophils and their multipotent and unipotent progenitors. Blood 1999; 94:2343–2356.

51. Kimura I, Tanizaki Y, Saito K, Takahashi K, Ueda N, Sato S. Appearance of basophils in the sputum of patients with bronchial asthma. Clin Allergy 1975; 5:95–98.

52. Bentley AM, Jacobson MR, Cumberworth V, et al. Immunohistology of the nasal mucosa in seasonal allergic rhinitis: increases in activated eosinophils and epithelial mast cells. J Allergy Clin Immunol 1992; 89:877–883.

53. Anderson DF, MacLeod JD, Baddeley SM, et al. Seasonal allergic conjunctivitis is accompanied by increased mast cell numbers in the absence of leucocyte infiltration. Clin Exp Allergy 1997; 27:1060–1066.

54. Holm AF, Godthelp T, Fokkens WJ, et al. Long-term effects of corticosteroid nasal spray on nasal inflammatory cells in patients with perennial allergic rhinitis. Clin Exp Allergy 1999; 29:1356–1366.

55. Kinet JP. The high-affinity IgE receptor (FcεRI): from physiology to pathology. Annu Rev Immunol 1999; 17:931–972.

56. Lin S, Cicala C, Scharenberg AM, Kinet JP. The FcεRIβ subunit functions as an amplifier of FcεRIγ-mediated cell activation signals. Cell 1996; 85:985–995.

57. Saini SS, Richardson JJ, Wofsy C, Lavens-Phillips S, Bochner BS, Macglashan DW Jr. Expression and modulation of Fc epsilon RI alpha and Fc epsilon RI beta in human blood basophils. J Allergy Clin Immunol 2001; 107:832–841.

58. MacGlashan DW Jr, Lichtenstein LM. Studies of antigen binding on human basophils. I. Antigen binding and functional consequences. J Immunol 1983; 130:2330–2336.

59. Malveaux FJ, Conroy MC, Adkinson NF Jr, Lichtenstein LM. IgE receptors on human basophils: relationship to serum IgE concentration. J Clin Invest 1978; 62:176–181.

60. Saini SS, Klion AD, Holland SM, Hamilton RG, Bochner BS, MacGlashan DW, Jr. The relationship between serum IgE and surface FcεR on human leukocytes in various diseases: correlation of expression with FcεRI on basophils but not on monocytes or eosinophils. J Allergy Clin Immunol 2000; 103:514–520.

61. Maurer D, Ebner C, Reininger B, et al. The high affinity IgE receptor (Fc epsilon RI) mediates IgE-dependent allergen presentation. J Immunol 1995; 154:6285–6290.

62. Maurer D, Fiebiger S, Ebner C, et al. Peripheral blood dendritic cells express FCεRI as a complex composed of FcεRI alpha- and FcεRI gamma-chains and can use this receptor for IgE-mediated allergen presentation. J Immunol 1996; 157:607–616.

63. Miyajima I, Dombrowicz D, Martin TR, Ravetch JV, Kinet JP, Galli SJ. Systemic anaphylaxis in the mouse can be mediated largely through IgG1 and Fc gamma-RIII. Assessment of the cardiopulmonary changes, mast cell degranulation, and death associated with active or IgE- or IgG1-dependent passive anaphylaxis. J Clin Invest 1997; 99:907–914.

64. Xia HZ, Du Z, Craig S, et al. Effect of recombinant human IL-4 on tryptase, chymase, and Fc epsilon receptor type I expression in recombinant human stem cell factor–dependent fetal liver-derived human mast cells. J Immunol 1997; 159:2911–2921.

65. MacGlashan D Jr, Lichtenstein LM, McKenzie-White J, et al. Upregulation of FcεRI on human basophils by IgE antibody is mediated by interaction of IgE with FcεRI. J Allergy Clin Immunol 1999; 104:492–498.

66. MacGlashan D Jr, Xia HZ, Schwartz LB, Gong J. IgE-regulated loss, not IgE-regulated synthesis, controls expression of Fcvar epsilon RI in human basophils. J Leukoc Biol 2001; 70:207–218.

67. MacGlashan D Jr, McKenzie-White J, Chichester K, et al. In vitro regulation of FcεRIα expression on human basophils by IgE antibody. Blood 1998; 91:1633–1643.

68. Yamaguchi M, Lantz CS, Oettgen HC, et al. IgE enhances mouse mast cell Fc(epsilon)RI expression in vitro and in vivo: evidence for a novel amplification mechanism in IgE-dependent reactions. J Exp Med 1997; 185:663–672.

69. Lantz CS, Yamaguchi M, Oettgen HC, et al. IgE regulates mouse basophil Fc epsilon RI expression in vivo. J Immunol 1997; 158:2517–2521.

70. Yano K, Yamaguchi M, de Mora F, et al. Production of Macrophage inflammatory protein-1alpha by human mast cells: increased anti-IgE-dependent secretion after IgE-dependent enhancement of mast cell IgE-binding ability. Lab Invest 1997; 77:185–193.

71. Yamaguchi M, Sayama K, Yano K, et al. IgE enhances Fc epsilon receptor I expression and IgE-dependent release of histamine and lipid mediators from human umbilical cord blood–derived mast cells: synergistic effect of IL-4 and IgE on human mast cell Fc epsilon receptor I expression and mediator release. J Immunol 1999; 162:5455–5465.

72. MacGlashan DW Jr, Bochner BS, Adelman DC, et al. Down-regulation of FcεRI expression on human basophils during in vivo treatment of atopic patients with anti-IgE antibody. J Immunol 1997; 158:1438–1445.

73. Saini SS, MacGlashan DW Jr, Sterbinsky SA, et al. Down-regulation of human basophil IgE FcεRIα surface densities and mediator release by anti-IgE infusions is reversible in vitro and in vivo. J Immunol 1999; 162:5624–5630.

74. MacGlashan D Jr, Schroeder JT. Functional consequences of FcepsilonRIalpha up-regulation by IgE in human basophils. J Leukoc Biol 2000; 68:479–486.

75. Macglashan DW Jr, Schroeder JT, Lichtenstein LM, Saini SS, Bochner BS. Mediator release from basophils and mast cells and its relationship to FcεRI expression and IgE suppressing therapies. In: Jardieu PM, Fick RB, Jr, eds. Anti-IgE and Allergic Diseases. New York: Marcel Dekker, 2002.

76. MacDonald SM. Human recombinant histamine-releasing factor. Int Arch Allergy Immunol 1997; 113:187–189.

77. Galli SJ. New concepts about the mast cell. N Engl J Med 1993; 328:257–265.

78. Bonini S, Lambiase A, Levi-Schaffer F, Aloe L. Nerve growth factor: an important molecule in allergic inflammation and tissue remodeling. Int Arch Allergy Immunol 1999; 118:159–162.

79. Burgi B, Otten UH, Ochensberger B, et al. Basophil priming by neurotrophic factors. Activation through the trk receptor. J Immunol 1996; 157:5582–5588.

80. Heaney LG, Cross LJ, Stanford CF, Ennis M. Substance P induces histamine release from human pulmonary mast cells. Clin Exp Allergy 1995; 25:179–186.

81. MacDonald SM, Schleimer RP, Kagey-Sobotka A, Gillis S, Lichtenstein LM. Recombinant IL-3 induces histamine release from human basophils. J Immunol 1989; 142:3527–3532.

82. Bischoff SC, De Weck AL, Dahinden CA. Interleukin-3 and granulocyte/macrophase colony-stimulating factor render basophils responsive to low concentrations of complement component C3a. Proc Natl Acad Sci USA 1990; 87:6813.

83. Hogaboam C, Kunkel SL, Strieter RM, et al. Novel role of transmembrane SCF for mast cell activation and eotaxin production in mast cell–fibroblast interactions. J Immunol 1998; 160:6166–6171.

84. Dahinden CA, Geiser T, Brunner T, et al. Monocyte chemotactic protein 3 is a most effective basophil- and eosinophil-activating chemokine. J Exp Med 1994; 179:751–756.

85. Kay AB, Ying S, Varney V, et al. Messenger RNA expression of the cytokine gene cluster, interleukin 3 (IL-3), IL-4, IL-5, and granulocyte/macrophage colony-stimulating factor, in allergen-induced late-phase cutaneous reactions in atopic subjects. J Exp Med 1991; 173:775–778.

86. Ying S, Robinson DS, Meng Q, et al. C-C chemokines in allergen-induced late-phase cutaneous responses in atopic subjects: association of eotaxin with early 6-hour eosinophils, and of eotaxin-2 and monocyte chemoattractant protein-4 with the later 24-hour tissue eosinophilia, and relationship to basophils and other C-C chemokines (monocyte chemoattractant protein-3 and RANTES). J Immunol 1999; 163:3976–3984.

87. Oliver JM, Kepley CL, Ortega E, Wilson BS. Immunologically mediated signaling in basophils and mast cells: finding therapeutic targets for allergic diseases in the

human Fcvar epsilon R1 signaling pathway. Immunopharmacology 2000; 48: 269–81.

88. Krystal G, Damen JE, Helgason CD, et al. SHIPs ahoy. Int J Biochem Cell Biol 1999; 31:1007–1010.

89. Huber M, Helgason CD, Damen JE, Liu L, Humphries RK, Krystal G. The src homology 2–containing inositol phosphatase (SHIP) is the gatekeeper of mast cell degranulation. Proc Natl Acad Sci USA 1998; 95:11330–11335.

90. MacGlashan DW Jr. Releasability of human basophils: cellular sensitivity and maximal histamine release are independent variables. J Allergy Clin Immunol 1993; 91:605–615.

91. Kepley CL, Youssef L, Andrews RP, Wilson BS, Oliver JM. Syk deficiency in nonreleaser basophils. J Allergy Clin Immunol 1999; 104:279–284.

92. Lavens-Phillip S, MacGlashan D. The tyrosine kinases, p53 lyn, p72 syk are differentially expressed at the protein level, not the mRNA level in non-releasing human basophils. Am J Cell Respir Mol Med 2000; 23:566–571.

93. White MV. The role of histamine in allergic diseases. J Allergy Clin Immunol 1990; 86:599–605.

94. Humphries DE, Wong GW, Friend DS, et al. Heparin is essential for the storage of specific granule proteases in mast cells. Nature 1999; 400:769–772.

95. Huang C, Sali A, Stevens RL. Regulation and function of mast cell proteases in inflammation. J Clin Immunol 1998; 18:169–183.

96. Huang C, De Sanctis GT, O'Brien PJ, et al. Evaluation of the substrate specificity of human mast cell tryptase beta I and demonstration of its importance in bacterial infections of the lung. J Biol Chem 2001; 276:26276–26284.

97. He S, Walls AF. Human mast cell chymase induces the accumulation of neutrophils, eosinophils and other inflammatory cells in vivo. Br J Pharmacol 1998; 125:1491–1500.

98. Cairns JA, Walls AF. Mast cell tryptase stimulates the synthesis of type I collagen in human lung fibroblasts. J Clin Invest 1997; 99:1313–1321.

99. Macfarlane SR, Seatter MJ, Kanke T, Hunter GD, Plevin R. Proteinase-activated receptors. Pharmacol Rev 2001; 53:245–282.

100. Vliagoftis H, Befus AD, Hollenberg MD, Moqbel R. Airway epithelial cells release eosinophil survival–promoting factors (GM-CSF) after stimulation of proteinase-activated receptor 2. J Allergy Clin Immunol 2001; 107:679–685.

101. Miller JS, Moxley G, Schwartz LB. Cloning and characterization of a second complementary DNA for human tryptase. J Clin Invest 1990; 86:864–870.

102. Schwartz LB, Sakai K, Bradford TR, et al. The alpha form of human tryptase is the predominant type present in blood at baseline in normal subjects and is elevated in those with systemic mastocytosis. J Clin Invest 1995; 96:2702–2710.

103. Schwartz LB, Irani AM. Serum tryptase and the laboratory diagnosis of systemic mastocytosis. Hematol Oncol Clin North Am 2000; 14:641–657.

104. Schwartz LB, Metcalfe DD, Miller JS, Earl H, Sullivan T. Tryptase levels as an indicator of mast-cell activation in systemic anaphylaxis and mastocytosis. N Engl J Med 1987; 316:1622–1626.

105. Lin RY, Schwartz LB, Curry A, et al. Histamine and tryptase levels in patients with acute allergic reactions: an emergency department–based study. J Allergy Clin Immunol 2000; 106:65–71.

106. Wenzel SE, Wescott JY, Larsen GL. Bronchoalveolar lavage fluid mediator levels 5 minutes after allergen challenge in atopic subjects with asthma: relationship to the development of late asthmatic responses. J Allergy Clin Immunol 1991; 87: 540–548.

107. Griffin M, Weiss JW, Leitch AG, et al. Effects of leukotriene D on the airways in asthma. N Engl J Med 1983; 308:436–439.

108. Lynch KR, O'Neill GP, Liu Q, et al. Characterization of the human cysteinyl leukotriene CysLT1 receptor. Nature 1999; 399:789–793.

109. Heise CE, O'Dowd BF, Figueroa DJ, et al. Characterization of the human cysteinyl leukotriene 2 receptor. J Biol Chem 2000; 275:30531–30536.

110. Figueroa DJ, Breyer RM, Defoe SK, et al. Expression of the cysteinyl leukotriene 1 receptor in normal human lung and peripheral blood leukocytes. Am J Respir Crit Care Med 2001; 163:226–233.

111. Liu MC, Bleecker ER, Lichtenstein LM, et al. Evidence for elevated levels of histamine, prostaglandin D_2, and other bronchoconstricting substances in the airways of mild asthmatic subjects. Am Rev Respir Dis 1990; 142:126–132.

112. Murray JJ, Tonnel AB, Brash AR, et al. Release of prostaglandin D_2 into human airways during acute antigen challenge. N Engl J Med 1986; 315:800–804.

113. Matsuoka T, Hirata M, Tanaka H, et al. Prostaglandin D2 as a mediator of allergic asthma. Science 2000; 287:2013–2017.

114. Hirai H, Tanaka K, Yoshie O, et al. Prostaglandin D2 selectively induces chemotaxis in T helper type 2 cells, eosinophils, and basophils via seven-transmembrane receptor CRTH2. J Exp Med 2001; 193:255–261.

115. Williams CM, Galli SJ. The diverse potential effector and immunoregulatory roles of mast cells in allergic disease. J Allergy Clin Immunol 2000; 105:847–859.

116. Jaffe JS, Raible DG, Post TJ, et al. Human lung mast cell activation leads to IL-13 mRNA expression and protein release. Am J Respir Cell Mol Biol 1996; 15:473–481.

117. Bradding P, Okayama Y, Howarth PH, Church MK, Holgate ST. Heterogeneity of human mast cells based on cytokine content. J Immunol 1995; 155:297–307.

118. Arock M, Merle-Béral H, Dugas B, et al. IL-4 release by human leukemic and activated normal basophils. J Immunol 1993; 151:1441–1447.

119. Brunner T, Heusser C, Dahinden C. Human peripheral blood basophils primed by interleukin 3 produce IL-4 in response to immunoglobulin E receptor stimulation. J Exp Med 1993; 177:605–612.

120. MacGlashan D, White JM, Huang SK, Ono SJ, Schroeder JT, Lichtenstein LM. Secretion of IL-4 from human basophils—the relationship between IL-4 mRNA and protein in resting and stimulated basophils. J Immunol 1994; 152:3006–3016.

121. Li H, Sim TC, Alam R. IL-13 released by and localized in human basophils. J Immunol 1996; 156:4833–4838.

122. Schroeder JT, MacGlashan DW Jr, Lichtenstein LM. Human basophils: mediator release and cytokine production. Adv Immunol 2001; 77:93–122.

123. Ying S, Humbert M, Barkans J, et al. Expression of IL-4 and IL-5 mRNA and protein product by CD4+ and CD8+ T cells, eosinophils, and mast cells in bronchial biopsies obtained from atopic and nonatopic (intrinsic) asthmatics. J Immunol 1997; 158:3539–3544.

124. Kasaian MT, Clay MJ, Happ MP, Garman RD, Hirani S, Luqman M. IL-4 production by allergen-stimulated primary cultures: identification of basophils as the major IL-4-producing cell type. Int Immunol 1996; 8:1287–1297.

125. Devouassoux G, Foster B, Scott LM, Metcalfe DD, Prussin C. Frequency and characterization of antigen-specific IL-4- and IL-13-producing basophils and T cells in peripheral blood of healthy and asthmatic subjects. J Allergy Clin Immunol 1999; 104:811–819.

126. Kobayashi H, Okayama Y, Ishizuka T, Pawankar R, Ra C, Mori M. Production of IL-13 by human lung mast cells in response of Fc epsilon receptor cross-linkage [see comments]. Clin Exp Allergy 1998; 28:1219–1227.

127. Toru H, Pawankar R, Ra C, Yata J, Nakahata T. Human mast cells produce IL-13 by high-affinity IgE receptor cross-linking: enhanced IL-13 production by IL-4-primed human mast cells. J Allergy Clin Immunol 1998; 102:491–502.

128. Pawankar R, Okuda M, Yssel H, Okumura K, Ra C. Nasal mast cells in perennial allergic rhinitics exhibit increased expression of the Fc eipsilonRI, CD40L, IL-4, and IL-13, and can induce IgE synthesis in B cells. J Clin Invest 1997; 99:1492–1499.

129. Thomas PS. Tumour necrosis factor-alpha: the role of this multifunctional cytokine in asthma. Immunol Cell Biol 2001; 79:132–140.

130. Walsh LJ, Trinchieri G, Waldorf HA, Whitaker D, Murphy GF. Human dermal mast cells contain and release tumor necrosis factor α, which induces endothelial leukocyte adhesion mmolecule 1. Proc Natl Acad Sci USA 1991; 88:4220–4224.

131. Bradding P, Roberts JA, Britten KM, et al. Interleukin-4, -5, and -6 and tumor necrosis factor-alpha in normal and asthmatic airways: evidence for the human mast cell as a source of these cytokines. Am J Respir Cell Mol Biol 1994; 10:471–480.

132. Ying S, Durham SR, Barkans J, et al. T cells are the principal source of interleukin-5 mRNA in allergen-induced rhintis. Am J Respir Cell Mol Biol 1993; 9:356–360.

133. Jaffe JS, Glaum MC, Raible DG, et al. Human lung mast cell IL-5 gene and protein expression: temporal analysis of upregulation following IgE-mediated activation. Am J Respir Cell Mol Biol 1995; 13:665–675.

134. Lukacs NW, Hogaboam CM, Kunkel SL, et al. Mast cells produce ENA-78, which can function as a potent neutrophil chemoattractant during allergic airway inflammation. J Leukoc Biol 1998; 63:746–751.

135. Nickel R, Beck LA, Stellato C, Scheleimer RP. Chemokines and allergic disease. J Allergy Clin Immunol 1999; 104:723–742.

136. Bacharier LB, Geha RS. Molecular mechanisms of IgE regulation. J Allergy Clin Immunol 2000; 105:S547–S558.

137. Mosmann TR, Coffman RL. TH1 and TH2 cells: different patterns of lymphokine secretion lead to different functional properties. Annu Rev Immunol 1989; 7:145–173.

138. Bochner BS, Klunk DA, Sterbinsky SA, Coffman RL, Schleimer RP. Interleukin-13 selectively induces vascular cell adhesion molecule-1 (VCAM-1) expression in human endothelial cells. J Immunol 1995; 154:799–803.

139. Schleimer RP, Sterbinsky SA, Kaiser J, et al. Interleukin-4 induces adherence of human eosinophils and basophils but not neutrophils to endothelium: association with expression of VCAM-1. J Immunol 1992; 148:1086–1092.

140. Oettgen HC, Geha RS. IgE regulation and roles in asthma pathogenesis. J Allergy Clin Immunol 2001; 107:429–440.

141. Yanagihara Y, Kajiwara K, Basaki Y, et al. Cultured basophils but not cultured mast cells induce human IgE synthesis in B cells after immunologic stimulation. Clin Exp Immunol 1998; 111:136–143.

142. Cameron L, Hamid Q, Wright E, et al. Local synthesis of epsilon germline gene transcripts, IL-4, and IL-13 in allergic nasal mucosa after ex vivo allergen exposure. J Allergy Clin Immunol 2000; 106:46–52.

143. Robinson DS, Hamid Q, Ying S, et al. Predominant T_{H2}-like bronchoalveolar T-lymphocyte population in atopic asthma. N Eng J Med 1992; 326:298–304.

144. Bentley AM, Menz G, Storz C, et al. Identification of T-lymphocytes, macrophages, and activated eosinophils in the bronchial mucosa in intrinsic asthma—relationship to symptoms and bronchial responsiveness. Am Rev Respir Dis 1992; 146:500–506.

145. Romagnani S. Human T_{H1} and T_{H2} subsets: doubt no more. Immunol Today 1991; 12:256–259.

146. Coffman RL, von der Weid T. Multiple pathways for the initiation of T helper 2 (Th2) responses. J Exp Med 1997; 185:373–375.

147. Hass H, Falcone FH, Holland MJ, et al. Early interleukin-4: its role in the switch towards a Th2 response and IgE-mediated allergy. Int Arch Allergy Immunol 1999; 119:86–94.

148. Jeffrey PK. Morphology of the airway wall in asthma and in chronic obstructive pulmonary disease. Am Rev Respir Dis 1991; 143:1152–1158.

149. Grunig G, Warnock M, Wakil AE, et al. Requirement for IL-13 independently of IL-4 in experimental asthma [see comments]. Science 1998; 282:2261–2263.

150. Wills-Karp M, Luyimbazi J, Xu X, et al. Interleukin-13: central mediator of allergic asthma. Science 1998; 282:2258–2261.

151. Kroegel C, Julius P, Matthys H, Virchow JC Jr, Luttmann W. Endobronchial secretion of interleukin-13 following local allergen challenge in atopic asthma: relationship to interleukin-4 and eosinophil counts. Eur Respir J 1996; 9:899–904.

152. Wershil BK, Wang ZS, Gordon JR, Galli SJ. Recruitment of neutrophils during IgE-dependent cutaneous late phase reactions in the mouse is mast cell-dependent—partial inhibition of the reaction with antiserum against tumor necrosis factor-α. J Clin Invest 1991; 87:446–453.

153. Casale TB, Costa JJ, Galli SJ. TNF alpha is important in human lung allergic reactions. Am J Respir Cell Mol Biol 1996; 15:35–44.

154. Echtenacher B, Mannel DN, Hultner L. Critical protective role of mast cells in a model of acute septic peritonitis. Nature 1996; 381:75–77.

155. Malaviya R, Ikeda T, Ross E, Abraham SN. Mast cell modulation of neutrophil influx and bacterial clearance at sites of infection through TNF-alpha. Nature 1996; 381:77–80.

156. Martin TR, Takeishi T, Katz HR, Austen KF, Drazen JM, Galli SJ. Mast cell activation enhances airway responsiveness to methacholine in the mouse. J Clin Invest 1993; 91:1176–1182.

157. Takeishi T, Martin TR, Katona IM, Finkelman FD, Galli SJ. Differences in the expression of the cardiopulmonary alterations associated with anti-immunoglobulin E–induced or active anaphylaxis in mast cell–deficient and normal mice.

Mast cells are not required for the cardiopulmonary changes associated with certain fatal anaphylactic responses. J Clin Invest 1991; 88:598–608.

158. Abraham SN, Arock M. Mast cells and basophils in innate immunity. Semin Immunol 1998; 10:373–381.

159. Galli SJ, Wershil BK. The two faces of the mast cell. Nature 1996; 381:21–22.

160. Takeda K, Hamelmann E, Joetham A, et al. Development of eosinophilic airway inflammation and airway hyperresponsiveness in mast cell–deficient mice. J Exp Med 1997; 186:449–454.

161. MacLean JA, Sauty A, Luster AD, Drazen JM, De Sanctis GT. Antigen-induced airway hyperresponsiveness, pulmonary eosinophilia, and chemokine expression in B cell–deficient mice. Am J Respir Cell Mol Biol 1999; 20:379–387.

162. Mehlhop PD, van de Rijn M, Goldberg AB, et al. Allergen-induced bronchial hyperreactivity and eosinophilic inflammation occur in the absence of IgE in a mouse model of asthma. Proc Natl Acad Sci USA 1997; 94:1344–1349.

163. Galli SJ. Complexity and redundancy in the pathogenesis of asthma: reassessing the roles of mast cells and T cells. J Exp Med 1997: 186:343–347.

164. Tumas DB, Chan B, Werther W, et al. Anti-IgE efficacy in murine asthma models is dependent on the method of allergen sensitization. J Allergy Clin Immunol 2001; 107:1025–1033.

165. Fahy JV, Fleming HE, Wong HH, et al. The effect of an anti-IgE monoclonal antibody on the early- and late-phase responses to allergen inhalation in asthmatic subjects. Am J Respir Crit Care Med 1997; 155:1828–1834.

166. Boulet LP, Chapman KR, Cote J, et al. Inhibitory effects of anti-IgE antibody E25 on allergen-induced early asthmatic response. Am J Respir Crit Care Med 1997; 155:1835–1840.

167. Togias A, Corren J, Shapiro G, et al. Anti-IgE infusions reduces skin test reactivity. J Allergy Clin Immunol 1998; 101:S171.

168. Casale TB, Bernstein IL, Busse WW, et al. Use of an anti-IgE humanized monoclonal antibody in ragweed-induced allergic rhinitis. J Allergy Clin Immunol 1997; 100:110–121.

169. Busse W, Corren J, Lanier BQ, et al. Omalizumab, anti-IgE recombinant humanized monoclonal antibody, for the treatment of severe allergic asthma. J Allergy Clin Immunol 2001; 108:184–190.

170. Boushey HA Jr. Experiences with monoclonal antibody therapy for allergic asthma. J Allergy Clin Immunol 2001; 108:77S–83S.

171. Milgrom H, Fick RB Jr, Su JQ, et al. Treatment of allergic asthma with monoclonal anti-IgE antibody. rhuMAb-E25 Study Group. N Engl J Med 1999; 341:1966–1973.

172. Selvan RS, Butterfield JH, Krangel MS. Expression of multiple chemokine genes by a human mast cell leukemia. J Biol Chem 1994; 269:13893–13898.

173. Compton SJ, Cairns JA, Holgate ST, Walls AF. The role of mast cell tryptase in regulating endothelial cell proliferation, cytokine release, and adhesion molecule expression: tryptase induces expression of mRNA for IL-1 beta and IL-8 and stimulates the selective release of IL-8 from human umbilical vein endothelial cells. J Immunol 1998; 161:1939–1946.

174. Moller A, Henz BM, Grutzkau A, et al. Comparative cytokine gene expression: regulation and release by human mast cells. Immunology 1998; 93:289–295.

6

Immune Functions of Human Eosinophils

PAUL J. COFFER and
LEO KOENDERMAN

University Medical Center
Utrecht, The Netherlands

PATRICIA M. R. e SILVA and
MARCO A. MARTINS

Oswaldo Cruz Foundation
Rio de Janeiro, Brazil

I. Introduction

For more than 100 years, eosinophils have been readily recognized by microscopic examination of blood, bone marrow, and other tissues due to their property of staining strongly with eosin dye (1–3). Maturated and differentiated in the bone marrow, eosinophils are released at a low rate into the blood circulation, and their levels are only 1–2% of the total peripheral leukocytes in healthy subjects (2). Traditionally viewed as killer-effector cells in helminth parasitic infections and as proinflammatory cells in allergic diseases, eosinophils are known to be attracted from the peripheral blood circulation toward the inflamed tissues, where they can modulate the inflammatory process by releasing a range of toxic basic proteins, lipid mediators, cytokines, and superoxide anions (1). It is noteworthy, however, that under physiological conditions 95% of the total eosinophil population are found marginated in submucosal region of the respiratory, gastrointestinal, and genitourinary tracts (2). A recent study has demonstrated a causative relationship between eosinophil recruitment and class 1–restricted T-cell selection in the thymus, indicating an immunomodulatory role for eosinophils under nonpathological conditions (4).

Studies on the mechanisms associated with tissue eosinophil homing in normal immunological homeostasis have emphasised the importance of the β-chemokine eotaxin—an eosinophil-specific CCR3 ligand—which was first described as a crucial and selective eosinophil chemotactic protein in an animal model of asthma (5). A close correlation between eotaxin mRNA expression and constitutive eosinophil numbers has been shown to occur in distinct tissues, including segments of the gastrointestinal tract, thymus, and lymph nodes in health states (6,7). This gives support to the interpretation that eotaxin might promote eosinophil homing to these tissues. Furthermore, eotaxin-null mice have demonstrated a selective reduction in both gastro-intestinal and circulating eosinophil levels with normal eosinophil counts in the bone marrow, indicating that alternative factors are implicated in the regulation of eosinophil growth in hematopoietic compartments (6). It has also been demonstrated that eotaxin-evoked eosinophil accumulation in vivo is up-regulated by the coadministration of interleukin-5 (IL-5) (8). Several Th2-derived cytokines, including IL-3, granulocyte-macrophage colony-stimulating factor (GM-CSF), and IL-5 have been shown to stimulate maturation, survival, and priming of eosinophils (9). Of these cytokines, IL-5 is the most selective to the eosinophil population (10). It strongly stimulates the release of these cells from the bone marrow into the blood circulation and facilitates the eosinophil recruitment process triggered by local generated chemoattractants such as eotaxin (8).

While trying to assess the fundamental signals underlying eosinophil homing to the gastrointestinal tract, Mishra et al. (6) observed that 19-day-old embryos and germ-free mice exhibited eosinophil levels in the lamina propria at levels comparable to those present in control colonized adult mice. This investigation clearly demonstrated eosinophil trafficking into the gastro-intestinal tract occurring during embryonic development and entirely independent of a pathogenic challenge. Furthermore, IL-5 transgenic mice in an eotaxin-null background have a marked reduction in the level of their gut eosinophils, as compared with IL-5 transgenic mice that have the wild-type eotaxin gene. This demonstrates that the eosinophil homing to the gut under normal physiological conditions is mainly dependent on eotaxin rather than on IL-5 (6). Thus, these findings highlight the existence of an eotaxin-dependent mechanism for preferential localization of eosinophils within submucosal sites under healthy conditions and add support to the interpretation that these cells may have a pivotal role in innate mucosal immune response.

II. Eosinophil Differentiation

A. Regulation of Eosinophil Levels

It has long been known that elevated numbers of eosinophils are associated with asthma and helminth infections, and levels are increased in animal tissues after acute anaphylaxis. However, the molecular mechanisms by which the levels of eosinophils can be specifically and rapidly modulated remain somewhat elusive. It is a combination of an increase in eosinophil production and a sustained survival in the tissues and peripheral blood that are defining factors in this phenomenon. Here we will discuss the current understanding of the molecular mechanisms regulating these processes.

B. Eosinophil Differentiation In Vitro and In Vivo

Eosinophils develop and mature in the bone marrow from IL-5-responsive $CD34^+$-expressing eosinophil/basophil colony-forming units (Eo/B-CFUs) (see also Fig. 2A). The development and differentiation of eosinophils is promoted by three cytokines: GM-CSF, IL-3, and IL-5. IL-3 tends to primarily stimulate basophil differentiation, whereas the presence of IL-5 will generally force differentiation toward the eosinophil lineage (11). In the presence of GM-CSF differentiation is of mixed eosinophil-basophil lineages. IL-5 also acts to release a pool of already developed eosinophils from the marrow into the circulation. While the bone marrow provides the major source of Eo/B-CFUs, these cells have also been found in the peripheral blood and can also be differentiated toward mature eosinophils in vitro (12). Higher numbers of both circulating Eo/B-CFUs and $CD34^+$ progenitors are found in the blood of atopic subjects compared with normals (13). It has also been demonstrated that allergen challenge can cause an increase in Eo/B-CFUs in the bone marrow of subjects (14). These progenitor cells specifically up-regulate the IL-5 receptor α chain (15). This up-regulation of receptor expression is itself most likely triggered by allergen-mediated increases in IL-5 levels.

While eosinophil differentiation is thought to occur predominantly in the bone marrow, recent reports have identified increased levels of $CD34^+$ progenitor cells within the peripheral blood and lungs of atopic individuals compared with normals (13,16). Furthermore, elevated numbers of cells producing IL-5 have been observed in the nasal mucosa of individuals with allergic rhinitis following allergen challenge (17). These studies present the possibility that a population of eosinophils may actually differentiate in situ. Indeed, a recent study provided evidence for possible local eosinophil differentiation within allergic nasal mucosa (18).

Initial studies analyzing eosinophil production in vitro identified an eosinophil colony-stimulating activity in mouse spleen–conditioned media (19). This was later more clearly defined as eosinophil differentiation factor and termed IL-5 (11). There is now good evidence that IL-5 is the major, and probably the only, cytokine involved *specifically* in the production of eosinophils. Certainly, IL-5 is responsible for the large increase in cell production observed in specific eosinophilia observed in helminth infections and allergic diseases. For example, the treatment of helminth-infected mice with anti-IL-5 antibodies abrogates the development of eosinophilia (20). Null mutant IL-5Rα (-/-) mice are unable to respond to *Angiostrongylus cantonensis* challenge with an effective increase in eosinophil levels (21). Furthermore, transgenic mice constitutively expressing IL-5 develop eosinophilia specifically despite being healthy otherwise (22). These data underscore the critical nature of IL-5 as a cytokine controlling eosinophil maturation in vivo.

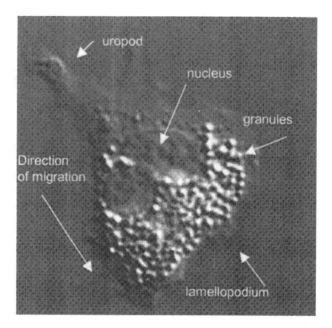

Figure 1   Moving eosinophil on an albumin-coated surface.

C. Molecular Mechanisms Regulating Eosinophil Differentiation

Granulopoiesis is a complex process by which primitive blood progenitors mature into fully differentiated, functionally active granulocytes (see also Fig. 2B). Transcription factors are master regulatory switches of differentiation, including development of specific hematopoietic lineages. Recent studies have started to unravel the intricate and essential roles played by various transcription factor families in myeloid differentiation (23). Such transcription factors can act both positively and negatively to regulate the expression of a wide range of genes critical for granulocyte maturation. These include cytokines, growth factors, other transcription factors and molecules important for function of mature cells. In a recent analysis to define the genes expressed during eosinophil differentiation of umbilical cord blood CD34$^+$ progenitors, a cDNA library was prepared from cells treated with IL-5 (24). Sequencing of this library revealed that many of the most abundant genes were those encoding for granule proteins. The most abundant mRNA was that major basic protein (MBP), which constituted more than 8% of the total transcripts.

In addition to the regulation of expression of transcription factors controlling granulopoiesis, the activity of these molecules can also be regulated by cytokines adding a further level of complexity to the system. The transcription factors C/EBP, PU.1, CBF, and c-Myb have emerged as key regulators of gene

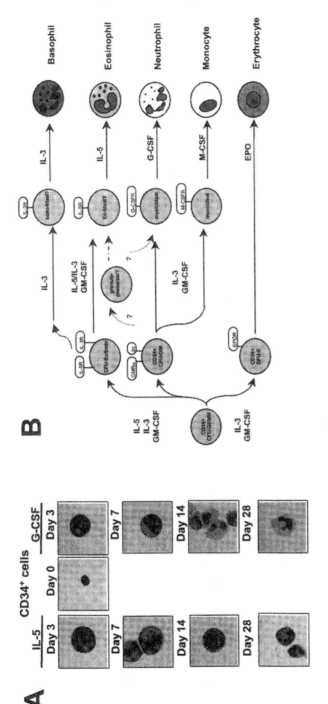

Eosinophils   Neutrophils

Figure 2 (A) In vitro differentiation of eosinophils and neutrophils. CD34[+] stem cells were isolated from cord blood and allowed to differentiate in the presence of G-CSF (neutrophils) and IL-5 (eosinophils). (B) Control of differentiation of myeloid cells by key cytokines.

expression during early granulopoiesis. Target genes up-regulated through action of these proteins include myeloperoxidase (MPO), neutrophil elastase, G-CSF receptor, GM-CSF receptor, and lysozyme. In the hematopoietic system, C/EBPα is expressed selectively in myeloid but not lymphoid or erythroid cells. Mice with a targeted disruption of the C/EBPα or C/EBPε genes demonstrate a selective block in the development of eosinophils (25,26). Peripheral blood and bone marrow smears show only myeloblastic cells of the myeloid lineage. These data suggest a critical role for members of the C/EBP transcription factor family in eosinophil maturation. The most elegant studies addressing this hypothesis have been performed by Graf and coworkers (27–29). This group has focused on the differentiation of transformed avian multipotent hematopoietic progenitors (MEPs). These studies have revealed that forced expression of either the α or β isoforms of C/EBP in MEPs induced eosinophil differentiation. Conversely, dominant-negative versions of C/EBP inhibited myeloid differentiation. C/EBP-induced eosinophil differentiation could be separated into two distinct events: lineage commitment and maturation. Using a powerful system to induce and transiently activate C/EBPs, it was found that short periods of C/EBPβ activation led to the formation of immature, nongranulated eosinophils, whereas sustained activation produced mature eosinophils. Recent data have added another level of complexity to this system. The transcriptional cofactor FOG (Friend of GATA) was found to antagonize eosinophil lineage commitment of MEPs (29). Multipotent cells were found to express high levels of FOG mRNA which were rapidly down-regulated upon C/EBP-mediated commitment to the eosinophil lineage. Expression of FOG in avian eosinophils led to a loss of eosinophil markers and the acquisition of a multipotent, immature phenotype. Indeed FOG was found to repress activation of the eosinophil-specific MBP promoter (30). These results suggest that FOG is a repressor of eosinophil maturation and that C/EBP-mediated down-regulation is an essential step in commitment of hematopoietic progenitors to the eosinophil lineage.

Previously high levels of protein kinase C (PKC) activity were found to specifically induce eosinophil lineage commitment in MEPs (31) and C/EBPβ is induced under these conditions (29). Taken together, these data suggest a molecular model whereby extracellular signals may regulate C/EBP transcription factors leading to eosinophil differentiation through both the direct activation of eosinophil-specific genes and the removal of FOG, a promoter of multipotency and repressor of eosinophil gene expression.

D. Eosinophil Survival and Regulation of Apoptosis

Eosinophils, like many hematopoietic lineages, have a default program of cell death. In the absence of survival factors these cells undergo a controlled process of active cell destruction termed *apoptosis* (32,33). In contrast to necrotic death, apoptosis is characterized by defined changes such as chromosomal condensation, DNA laddering, cell shrinkage, and expression of adhesion molecules at the cell surface that facilitate detection and engulfment by phagocytic cells in vivo. Aged apoptotic eosinophils exhibit increased red autofluorescence and are recognized and ingested as intact cells by macrophages, often before they manifest signs of the morphological changes associated with apoptosis (34). Since the life span of eosinophils is normally as short as 4 days, prolonged survival at sites where they have migrated is essential for them to exert their function (35). The fact that eosinophils undergo a default program of apoptosis is, however, critical to the resolution of inflammatory reactions. Once eosinophils have entered the tissues there is no mechanism by which they can leave when their contribution to the inflammatory reaction is complete. Thus, their removal is contingent on controlled cell death and phagocytosis by macrophages. In allergic inflammation, activated eosinophils are known to accumulate at the site of inflammation at least in part because of their prolonged survival (35,36). This can occur through exposure to several cytokines including, IL-3, IL-5, and GM-CSF (37). Importantly, activated T cells, which produce eosinophil survival cytokines, have been found at sites of allergic inflammation with eosinophilia in bronchial asthma and atopic dermatitis.

Corticosteroids are potent anti-inflammatory drugs that can act by directly inducing apoptosis as well as repressing the secretion of survival factors (38). The acceleration of apoptosis induced by steroids is overcome by increasing amounts of cytokines ruling out a direct toxic effect and suggesting that they are directly antagonistic to each other (38). Interestingly, peripheral blood eosinophils isolated from asthmatic patients have delayed apoptosis (39). This delay may be partly explained by production of GM-CSF, which is inhibited by the use of inhaled glucocorticoids. Transforming growth factor-β (TGF-β) is a pleiotropic cytokine that has a number of inhibitory effects on proinflammatory cells. TGF-β induces apoptosis in eosinophils cultured with IL-5, IL-3, or GM-CSF (40). TGF-β is expressed in chronically inflamed airways where it may modulate the inflammatory response.

The molecular mechanisms underlying the ability of cytokines to inhibit eosinophil apoptosis remain to be clearly defined. However, recent studies have started to unravel the mechanisms by which survival factors inhibit apoptosis. Addition of actinomycin D or cycloheximide to eosinophils inhibits the anti-apoptotic effect of cytokines, suggesting that RNA and protein synthesis are important for this phenomenon (33,37). Intracellular signal transduction pathways important for the inhibition of eosinophil apoptosis by cytokines include several protein kinases such as JAK2, Lyn, Raf-1, and the lipid kinase phosphatidylinositol 3-kinase (PI3K) (41–43). The precise mechanisms by which these signaling molecules impinge on the default pathway of apoptosis remains to be clearly defined in eosinophils. However, recent studies have suggested an important role for proteins of the Bcl-2 family.

Members of the Bcl-2 family of proteins are important regulators of apoptosis in many systems (44). There are both anti-apoptotic and pro-apoptotic

Bcl-2 family members, and the first member, Bcl-2, was identified due to its dysregulation in B-cell lymphomas bearing the t(14;18) translocation resulting in constitutive Bcl-2 expression. Many more Bcl-2 members have been identified based on homology in conserved regions called BH domains. Anti-apoptotic Bcl-2 family members have been found to inhibit apoptosis by preventing the release of cytochrome *c* from the mitochondria, a process that appears to be critical for inducing the apoptotic program after cytokine withdrawal (45). The release cytochrome *c* triggers the activation of intracellular proteases, termed caspases, which then proceed to degrade the cell in a controlled manner. Pro-apoptotic Bcl-2 family members induce this process; thus, their expression and/or activity must be kept in check for cell survival.

Simon and coworkers have examined the expression of various Bcl-2 family members in eosinophils (46). Freshly isolated eosinophils were found to express significant amounts of Bcl-2 family members Bcl-xl and Bax. Spontaneous eosinophil apoptosis was found to correlate with a decrease in Bcl-xl mRNA and protein levels. In contrast, stimulation of cells with GM-CSF or IL-5 resulted in up-regulation of Bcl-xl. Using an antisense approach, specific inhibition of Bcl-xl was further found to partially block cytokine-mediated rescue of eosinophil apoptosis. In a similar study, a patient with hyper-eosinophilia was found to have enhanced levels of Bcl-2, which is normally not expressed in eosinophils (47). This was associated with delayed death of peripheral blood eosinophils in vitro, suggesting that Bcl-2 acted as an apoptosis repressor in this system. Thus, the up-regulation of anti-apoptotic members of the Bcl-2 family appears to have critical role in maintaining eosinophil survival.

Recently, a role for PI3K in the regulation of apoptosis in eosinophils has been demonstrated (43). Pharmacological inhibition of PI3K results in antagonism of IL-5-induced eosinophil survival. Interestingly, this correlates with the up-regulation of the cell cycle inhibitor $p27^{KIP1}$ (48). It appears that IL-5 represses the expression of p27 in a PI3K-dependent manner. Whereas high p27 levels are normally associated with an inhibition of cellular proliferation, eosinophils are terminally differentiated, nondividing cells. What is the function of this protein in eosinophils? In cytokine-dependent cell lines, ectopic expression of p27 results in induction of the apoptotic program through an as yet unresolved mechanism. Thus, in human eosinophils p27 levels may play a critical role in the regulation of cell survival. The regulation of p27 levels is controlled by members of the Forkhead family of transcription factors: AFX, FKHR, and FKHR-L1 (49). FKHR-L1 has also been demonstrated to up-regulate the expression of Bim, a pro-apoptotic Bcl-2 family member (48). We recently demonstrated that FKHR-L1 is regulated in eosinophils in a PI3K manner (PJC and LK, unpublished data). In eosinophils isolated from hyper-eosinophilic patients, we have observed increased survival correlating with inhibition of FKHR-L1. Thus, inhibition of FKHR-L1 by PI3K is likely to be a critical mechanism by which IL-5 rescues eosinophils from the default program of apoptosis.

One molecule that has been shown to induce apoptosis in a variety of cell types is Fas (APO-1/CD95), a transmembrane member of the tumor necrosis factor (TNF) superfamily (50). Cross-linking of Fas on receptor-bearing cells with its ligand, FasL, is sufficient to induce apoptosis. Eosinophils have been shown to express low levels of Fas, and cross-linking leads to induction of apoptosis (51,52). Increasing the concentration of IL-5 does not rescue cells from Fas-induced apoptosis, indicating that Fas ligation triggers apoptosis through a mechanism independent of the effects of IL-5. Interestingly, Fas expression is regulated in human eosinophils. Incubation of cells with interferon-γ or TNF-α alone or together causes an increase in Fas expression, which is reversed by addition of survival cytokines (53). Eosinophils isolated by bronchoalveolar lavage (BAL) of sensitized mice following allergen challenge express Fas and are sensitive to Fas-induced killing (54). It remains to be determined whether the Fas/FasL system is important for the regulation of eosinophil survival in the resolution of an inflammatory response. Importantly, there is at least one counterregulatory mechanism preventing Fas-induced eosinophil apoptosis. A recent study reported that nitric oxide, which is released in increased amounts during chronic inflammatory responses, can inhibit CD95-induced signals in eosinophils (55). This may help to protect eosinophils by providing an additional survival signal.

III. Eosinophil Priming

A. The Concept of Priming

Because the eosinophil is one of the most cytotoxic cells in the human body, its mobilization and activation is under tight control of cytokines and chemokines (for review, see 56, 57). Eosinophils leave the bone marrow with a so-called nonprimed phenotype that is refractory to activation. Upon interaction with cytokines and/or chemokines these cells change their phenotype and become prone for activation by physiologically relevant activators (58–60). This whole process is generally referred to as "priming." Typically a priming agent does not provoke a cytotoxic response by itself but enhances this response upon activation of heterologous stimulus. Virtually all eosinophil responses are under the control of this cytokine/chemokine-induced priming mechanism (56) (Fig. 3). The process acts as a safety lock preventing specific activation of this highly cytotoxic cell.

B. Multistep Paradigm of Eosinophil Priming

Cytokine and chemokine-induced priming is not a one-hit event, but is better characterized by a gradual increase in extent and/or type of priming phenotype. Eosinophil responses can be arbitrarily divided into adhesion, cytotoxic, and proinflammatory responses. It turns out that these different groups of responses are regulated very differently by priming cytokines and/or chemokines.

1. Adhesion-associated responses are very sensitive to priming by cytokines such as GM-CSF, IL-3, and IL-5. Eosinophil chemotaxis in both Boyden chamber assays (61) and transmigration assays through endothelial cell layers (62,63) are modulated by pre-incubation of eosinophils with these cytokines. These cytokines greatly facilitate the movement of these cells in both assays. This facilitation is characterized by a marked increase in responsiveness toward, for example, platelet-activating factor (PAF) (61) and RANTES (64). In addition, this priming reaction is essential for the cells to be responsive to chemokines such as IL-8. Interestingly, when eosinophils adhere to physiological substrates a more pronounced priming phenotype is induced (65, and see below).

2. Cytoxic responses such as degranulation and activation of the respiratory burst are very sensitive to priming in vitro by the same cytokines involved in priming of adhesion-associated responses. Apart from these cytokines, chemotaxins are also potent priming agents. Especially lipids such as inflammatory cell–derived PAF and leukotriene B_4 (LTB$_4$) and bacterial products such as lipopolysaccharide (LPS) are very active (56). These semiphysiological agonists are not the only ones to cause priming; compounds that increase the intracellular free Ca^{2+} concentration [Ca^{2+}-ionophores] (66), activate PKC (67), or disrupt the cytoskeleton (68) can also induce the priming phenotype. The cytotoxic responses of eosinophils induced by opsonized targets are especially sensitive to priming by the aforementioned compounds.

3. Proinflammatory responses such as the release of cytokines/chemokines and/or bioactive lipids are also sensitive to priming (69,70). This implies that eosinophils participate in a clear feed-forward mechanism that can accelerate the inflammatory response.

C. Priming In Vivo

Priming of eosinophils occurs in the peripheral blood of allergic (asthmatic) individuals. In particular, priming of adhesion-associated responses of eosinophils has been found to be elevated upon isolation from these patient groups. This in vivo priming response has the following characteristics: Eosinophils from allergic patients exhibit a marked increase in sensitivity for activation with PAF (58), which is very similar to experiments performed with normal eosinophils primed in vitro with IL-3, IL-5, or GM-CSF (58,61).

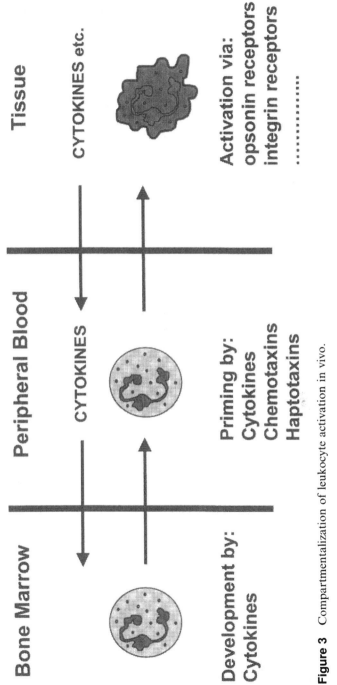

Figure 3 Compartmentalization of leukocyte activation *in vivo*.

In addition, chemotaxis of eosinophils from allergic asthmatics is induced by IL-8 in marked contrast to cells from normal control donors (59,71). This cannot be explained by increased expression of CXCR1 or CXCR2 because both IL-8 receptors are not expressed by eosinophils from both sources. There is some evidence that a small subpopulation of eosinophils isolated from allergic patients express these receptors at very low levels (72). In addition to chemotaxis, transendothelial migration is also primed in allergic asthma. Ebisawa et al. (63) and Moser et al. (62) have presented convincing evidence that this response is sensitive for priming by cytokines in vitro and that in vivo primed cells exhibit a marked increase in this transendothelial migration response. Interestingly, in vivo primed eosinophils migrate spontaneously through IL-4 activated endothelial cells in the absence of a stimulus (60).

The situation is less clear when cytotoxic responses are evaluated in the context of in vivo priming (73). We could show in the late 1980s that activation of the NADPH-oxidase induced by chemotaxins is up-regulated in patients with allergic asthma. However, luminol-enhanced chemiluminescence is a highly sensitive but not very quantitative measure of oxidase responses. It proved somewhat difficult to show a clear in vivo primed respiratory burst response (74,75). Similar observations were made evaluating the degranulation response of human eosinophils. The differences between in vivo priming of adhesion responses and cytotoxic responses are yet unresolved. However, several points may be taken into account. First of all, priming of cytotoxic responses in the peripheral blood does not seem to be very advantageous because of the danger of systemic activation of this cytotoxic cell type. It might be that (1) the mix of cytokines only allows adhesion to be primed; (2) priming of adhesion-associated responses are irreversible whereas the priming of cytotoxic responses is transient (see below); or (3) fully primed eosinophils will attach to the tissues and disappear as "suspended" cells from the peripheral blood. At present it remains unresolved which of these hypotheses explains the apparent lack of appreciable priming of cytotoxic responses in the peripheral blood. It also remains unresolved which cytokine(s) mediate(s) the in vivo primed phenotype. The most appealing hypothesis is that different sets of cytokines can mediate priming in vivo and that complex cross-talk determines the extent and type of priming response (for underlying mechanisms, see below).

D. Mechanisms of Priming

Despite the very clear priming phenotype induced by cytokines, surprisingly little is known about the underlying mechanisms. In recent years, several studies have provided the first insight into the complex intracellular mechanisms mediating the priming response:

1. *Receptor expression.* Priming of eosinophils is accompanied by a change in expression of several relevant receptors. Best studied are

Macl (CD11b/CD18) whose expression is clearly induced upon interaction in vitro with cytokines/chemokines (76), whereas L-selectin is down-regulated (77). However, an increased expression of Mac-1 *per se* is not sufficient for enhanced functionality (78). The expression of several other receptors is increased upon interaction with cytokines/chemokines: e.g., ICAM-1 (79), CD69 (80), CXC4R (81), and FcαR (CD89) (82).

2. *Inside-out control of receptor function.* This phenomenon has been studied in eosinophils in the context of cytokine induced inside-out control of adhesion and immunoglobulin receptors (83,84). It turns out that the functionality of both receptor families is under the control of intracellular signals. This results in the observation that these receptors can only bind and signal after appropriate preactivation or priming by a cytokine, chemokine, or growth factor. Despite this broadly recognized phenomenon surprisingly little is known about the molecular mechanisms by which this is regulated in primary eosinophils. We recently designed experiments to study the mechanisms underlying the inside-out control of the human IgA receptor (FcαRI, CD89) (85). The functionality of this receptor is under complex control by several signal transduction pathways. The best characterized is the phosphatidylinositol 3-kinase (PI3K)–mediated modulation of receptor functionality. Normal eosinophils express FcαRI as a nonfunctional receptor on the cell surface (86). Upon interaction with chemokines or cytokines a rapid up-regulation of receptor functionality is induced without an apparent increase of receptor expression. Inhibition with specific inhibitors blocking the function of PI3K prevents this cytokine-induced increase in receptor function (86). In a cell line model used to study this cytokine-mediated control of FcαRI the crucial role of PI3K was confirmed by expressing dominant-negative and constitutive active forms of the PI3K (85). Exploring this model in more detail we were able to demonstrate that FcαRI mutants lacking a critical serine residue at position 263 were fully functional and did not require cytokine priming (87). These findings are consistent with a model in which eosinophils actively down-regulate the function of FcαRI in the absence of cytokines. Upon activation with cytokines, such as IL-4, IL-5, and/or GM-CSF, this negative signal is antagonized by a mechanism involving PI3K and Ser263 in the C terminus of FcαRI. It is possible that the main β_2-integrin on eosinophils Mac-1 (α_m/β_2, CD11b/CD18) is under similar control (88).

3. *Modulation of signaling pathways.* A complex mechanism of cytokine-induced priming concerns the finding that some cytokines can activate certain effector molecules only in the context of already activated signaling pathways. This form of cross-talk is difficult to

study, but two clear examples have recently been published (89,90). Bates et al. (89) have shown that certain stimuli, such as IL-8, can only activate certain signaling pathways provided the cells are first primed with IL-5 in vitro. The authors could also show that extravasated cells in the lung that were primed in vivo responded to IL-8 in the context of ERK1/ERK2 activation. A similar finding was found evaluating the effect of TNF on human eosinophils. Cells isolated from the blood of normal individuals did not respond to TNF with an increase of FcαRI function despite a clear expression of TNFRI and TNFRII (90), whereas cells isolated from symptomatic allergic asthmatics increase the affinity-state FcαRI upon interaction with TNF. Further analysis revealed that eosinophils from allergic asthmatics contain a constitutively activated PI3K-based signaling pathway allowing the cells to be responsive to TNF.

E. Priming as a Therapeutic Target

It is clear from the issues described above that cytokine-induced priming is an important mechanism in controlling the function of eosinophils in vivo. Antagonism of eosinophil priming is an important target for future specific therapy of eosinophil-mediated diseases. Effective antagonism of priming of these cells will not cure the disease but might prevent the tissue damage seen in chronic inflammatory lesions. However, a clear dilemma is present in the design of such an approach. Single cytokine antagonists are not likely to be successful because several combinations of cytokines will steer eosinophil priming in different disease phenotypes. In addition, antagonism of priming by inhibition of intracellular signaling pathways will be difficult because it is very likely that no priming specific signaling molecules exist. Rather unique combinations of general signaling pathways localized at an activated cytokine receptor complex will lead to specific priming responses (57). Therefore, a few critical questions have to be resolved before a novel therapeutic priming antagonism can be developed: (1) Which combinations of cytokines cause the priming response *in vivo*? (2) Can a therapeutic agent be targeted specifically to the eosinophil, a cytokine-receptor, or both? (3) Which minimal combination of signaling molecules is essential to mediate the priming response? If these issues can be adequately addressed, antagonism of priming of inflammatory cells will be a very interesting therapeutic target in the future.

IV. Eosinophil Activation

Eosinophils are activated by different stimuli and this process is intimately related to cytokine/chemokine induced priming. Here we will focus on activation of adhesion processes, cytotoxic responses, and production of cytokines.

A. Adhesion Processes

The extravasation response of eosinophils from the peripheral blood into the tissues is a tightly regulated process. Under conditions of shear as are found *in vivo*, two families of adhesion molecules are dominant in the regulation of adhering to and moving through the endothelial cell layer. Selectins mediate rolling adhesion slowing the eosinophils down, and integrins mediate firm arrest and transendothelial movement. The selectin family consists of three members: E(endothelial)-selectin, P(platelet)-selectin, and L(leukocyte)-selectin. E- and P-selectin are expressed on activated endothelial cells and L-selectin is constitutively expressed by leukocytes [for a review, see Diamond et al. (91)]. Inflammatory cells express ligands for all three selectins and endothelial cells express ligands for L-selectin (91). Eosinophils can roll on a surface expressing P-selectin (92) or E-selectin (93). The interaction between selectin and their ligands does not require cellular activation and even occurs at 4°C (94). Rolling by itself (physiological cross-linking of selectin ligands) does not induce/activate the cells to stop rolling and firmly attach to the surface.

These last phenomena are mediated by integrins, which are heterodimers consisting of α chains non-covalently linked to β chains. Many of these integrins have in common that they need cellular activation in order to be functional. On eosinophils two integrins are dominant in mediating the transition of rolling cells to firmly attached cells guided by the presence of an activating chemotaxin (chemokine): α_m/β_2 (Mac-1, CD11b/CD18) and α_4/β_1 (VLA-4, CD49e/CD29). On isolated eosinophils VLA-4 seems to be present in a partly functional configuration (93), while Mac-1 is not a functional adhesion molecule for activated endothelial cells under flow conditions in the absence of stimulus (93). Upon interaction with most activating chemotaxins/chemokines the cells immediately activate their integrins in a process generally referred to as "inside-out control" and the cells stop rolling, firmly attach, and migrate through the endothelial cell layer. Interestingly not all activating chemotaxins induce the same adhesion phenotype. Recently, we (95) have shown that IL-8 can activate both VLA-4 and Mac-1, resulting in the transition from rolling to firm attachment. However, in marked contrast to stimuli such as eotaxin, this firm attachment is transient. It is not yet clear which signaling molecules are involved in mediating transient and prolonged arrest of eosinophils to endothelial surfaces. When experiments are performed on surfaces coated with isolated proteins it could be shown that eotaxin-2 causes detachment of cells from surfaces coated with ICAM-1 and VCAM-1 (96). These findings indicate that adhesion is the result of a cycle of adhesion and deadhesion mediated by several processes that can be controlled independently: (1) expression level of different adhesion molecules and/or different chemokines, (2) inside-out control of adhesion molecules, and (3) activation of deadhesion.

B. Activation of Cytotoxicity

Eosinophils contain two main cytotoxic mechanisms: a membrane bound NADPH oxidase producing cytotoxic oxygen intermediates, and cytotoxic proteins stored in granules that are released upon activation (97,98). These cytotoxic mechanisms are shown to be synergistic in the killing of helminths *in vitro* (99). Interestingly, eosinophils are well equipped to extracellularly kill these macroparasites, which are many times their own size. Not much is known about the intracellular signaling pathways underlying these responses, and it is difficult to distinguish mechanisms involved in priming and actual activation of cytotoxicity.

The best semiphysiological activators that can induce cytotoxicity-associated responses are surfaces covered with immunoglobulins and/or complement fragments. Several groups have shown that surfaces covered with IgG (100), IgA (101), opsonized zymosan particles (covered with both immunoglobulins and complement), and opsonized microorganisms (102) are excellent activators for degranulation and activation of the respiratory burst provided that the cells are first primed by addition of cytokines (102) or paracrine-produced PAF (103). The requirement of these preactivating substances seems to be particularly necessary to induce a high-affinity state of the opsonin receptors, which facilitates the interaction between cell and surface. It is not only this affinity/avidity that changes but also signal transduction processes shift upon priming of eosinophils (102). A complicating factor is the finding that Mac-1 seems to be important in several of these assays even in the absence of a recognized ligand on the studied surface. It has been proposed that optimal activation of leukocytes only occurs when a proper adhesiosome (with Mac-1 present) is formed (104).

C. Production of Proinflammatory Mediators

Apart from being important effector cells in different acute and chronic inflammatory illnesses, eosinophils can act as proinflammatory cells. These cells have the capability of producing large amounts of cytokines and chemokines, such as IL-4, IL-5, GM-CSF, IFN-γ, TNF, RANTES, IL-8, IL-10, and platelet-derived growth factor (PDGF), and TFG-β (105,106). In addition, several bioactive lipids are formed such as leukotrienes and PAF (107). All of these mediators are involved in different steps of the human inflammatory response and can act in an autocrine and paracrine fashion on eosinophils or activate other inflammatory cells or bystander cells in the vicinity of these eosinophils. Relevant processes are, for example, rescue of eosinophil apoptosis, increased killing of microorganisms by different phagocytes, increased chemotaxis of newly recruited leukocytes, increased expression of adhesion molecules, and proliferation of fibroblasts. However, some inflammatory responses can also be inhibited by cytokines such as TGF-β and IL-10. In contrast to the lymphocyte compartment, many cytokines, chemokines, and growth factors are preformed in granules. This can enable eosinophils to liberate these inflammatory mediators instantly upon activation of the appropriate stimulus, which can accelerate pro- or anti-inflammatory mechanisms that are characterized by eosinophil involvement.

V. Eosinophils in Disease

A. Eosinophils in Parasitic Disease

Eosinophils are strongly associated with infection caused by macroparasites, specially helminths, and may play a role in protective immunity and/or in the pathogenesis of these diseases (2,3). Besides their marked involvement in helminthiasis, eosinophils can also appear associated in variable magnitudes with other microendoparasites, including *Toxoplasma gondii*, *Trypanosoma cruzi* (108), *Plasmodium falciparum* (109), and *Pneumocystis carinii* (110), as well as with ectoparasites, including head lice, scabies, and ticks (3).

Infection with helminths, including trematodes, cestodes, and nematodes, is the commonest cause of peripheral blood eosinophilia in humans and animals (3,111). In addition to the increase in the number of circulating eosinophils, a massive eosinophil infiltration and degranulation can be observed either at the site of parasite invasion or migration, or in local tissue fluids. For instance, *Angionstrongylus cantonensis*–induced eosinophilic meningitis is accompanied by intense eosinophilic response in the cerebrospinal fluid (112,113). Likewise, following the migratory phase of several lungworms it is possible to observe substantial eosinophil accumulation both in the lung tissue and in the bronchoalveolar effluent (114). Other anatomical sites frequently associated with marked eosinophilic response following parasite infection include intestinal mucosa, liver, skin, bladder, and pleural cavity (111). In all of these cases, local and systemic eosinophilia is frequently related to the extension of tissue damage, worm burden, and products generated from live (including larvae and eggs), dying, and dead organisms (3,115). Blood and tissue eosinophilia following parasite infection are also dependent on host factors that regulate eosinophilopoiesis within the bone marrow, the adherence of the eosinophil to vascular endothelia, and maintenance of eosinophil viability at extramedullar sites (111).

In a series of classical studies performed in the early 1970s it became clear that parasite-evoked eosinophilia involves the activation of T lymphocytes (116,117). It was shown, for instance, that the eosinophilic inflammatory response to the nematode *Trichinella spiralis* was prevented by antilymphocyte serum treatment, chronic thoracic duct draining, or neonatal thymectomy in rats. Moreover, eosinophilia was restored when lymphocytes obtained from *T. spiralis*–infected animals were used in the reconstitution procedure (116,117). Similar abrogation of eosinophilia was obtained following infection with *Ascaris suum* (118) or *Schistosoma mansoni* in athymic mice (119).

It is now well established that immune responses to protein antigens are indeed strongly influenced by the nature of the helper T-lymphocyte (Th) subsets participating in the response. Helminthic parasites are highly antigenic multicellular organisms that typically promote a Th2-type response, marked by an IL-5-driven eosinophilia, associated with an IL-4- and IL-13-mediated increase in IgE levels. Augmented levels of antiparasite IgE and eosinophilia have been associated with increased resistance to helminth infections (111). On the other hand, Th1-type cytokines (IFN-γ, IL-2), typically produced during immune responses to intracellular pathogens, inhibit protective immunity to gut parasites (120). However, it is noteworthy that Th1 cytokines are able to enhance the clearance of tissue-dwelling parasites, such as schistosoma (121).

The concept that the major "beneficial" role of eosinophils is to participate in host defense against helminth parasites is mainly based on observations that eosinophils can kill some species of parasites and/or impair larval migration and development (122,123). In vitro studies have demonstrated that eosinophils in the presence of different antibody isotypes, including subclasses of IgE, IgG, and IgA, are able to adhere closely to worms from distinct species, including *S. mansoni*, *T. spiralis*, and *Nippostrongylus brasiliensis*, and to release their cationic granule content on the surface of the target organism. The interaction between eosinophils and parasites is dependent on sensitization of the target by parasite-specific antibodies, in a reaction known as antibody-dependent cellular cytotoxicity (ADCC). Opsonization with complement components, including C3b, selectins, and Lewis X-related structures, has also been implicated in the eosinophil–parasite adhesion mechanism (124).

Evaluation of the parasite-induced eosinophil exocytotic process revealed that the granules are released either individually or sequentially to a restricted space defined by the site of contact with the opsonized larvae (125). As attested by phase contrast and electron microscopy, the massive granule discharge induces the formation of vacuoles in the syncytial tegument and damage of the tegumental membrane, leading to parasite death (126–128). A similar pattern of damage has been shown to occur when *S. mansoni* (129), *T. spiralis* (130), and *T. cruzi* (131) were exposed to isolated major basic protein, which represents a large proportion of protein in eosinophil granules. Other eosinophil granule proteins, such as eosinophil peroxidase, eosinophil cationic protein, and eosinophil-derived protein, are also highly toxic for a number of parasites (132,133).

Histological examination of the reaction at the site of parasite death in experimental animal models revealed that distinct parasites, including *S. mansoni* (134), *Schistosoma japonicum* (135), *Trichostrongylus colubriforms* (136,137), and *Strongyloides ratti* (138) were clearly damaged and surrounded by a massive infiltration of eosinophils, which were seen attached to and degranulating onto the surface of the parasite. In a particular case of baboon infected with *S. mansoni* followed by challenge with cercaria, eosinophils were observed invading the schistosomulum interior (134). An alternative mechanism implicated in the process of parasite killing is the generation of toxic oxygen metabolites by eosinophils. Oxygen radical production by granulomatous inflammatory cells in close contact with the eggs were observed in the liver of mice infected with *S. mansoni* (139). Studies by Pincus et al. indicated that although oxidative reactions are not essential for the killing, they can clearly enhance the toxic effect of eosinophil cationic proteins (140).

The major problem of such in vivo experiments is in identifying whether an eosinophil-rich infiltrate around the dead parasite is due to either the eosinophil killing of parasite or to dead parasite killed by some other mechanism eliciting an eosinophil response. *S. mansoni* cercariae mechanically transformed into schistosomula were injected, either dead or alive, into the tail vein of Balb/c mice that were previously infected with *S. mansoni*. Histological examination of the lungs within 24 h revealed that eosinophilic inflammatory reaction around schistosomula occurred only in the groups injected with dead schistosomula (141). Furthermore, a sudden increase in the circulating eosinophil numbers and intense eosinophil infiltrate toward tissue focus of dead parasites have been observed after chemotherapy in filariasis (142), onchocerciasis (115), and schistosomiasis in humans (143), indicating that the parasite-related eosinophil accumulation may be secondary to and not necessarily the cause of the parasite death.

Mast cells and IgE play an important role in immunity against intestinal helminth infections (144–146). The major known functions of IgE are mediated by its high-affinity receptor FcεRI, which appears expressed on mast cells and basophils as $\alpha\beta\gamma_2$ tetramer. No consensus is present about the expression of a functional FcεRI receptor on eosinophils from humans (147,148) while the receptor is absent on murine eosinophils (149). The association of IgE responses and eosinophilia that is observed in helminth infections can have at least two consequences. IgE can act as ligand for eosinophil-mediated ADCC reactions (150) and/or it can mediate mast cell degranulation at the site of the invading parasite leading to the release of mediators capable of inducing plasma leakage and eosinophil recruitment and activation (151). Evidence that mast cells play a role in host protection against *T. spiralis* (152), *S. ratti* (153), and *Hyminolepis nana* (154) have been reported in mast cell–deficient mice. In contrast, the course of the infection by *N. brasiliensis* remained unchanged in the absence of mast cells (155).

B. Outcomes of Helminth Infection in IL-5-Deficient and IL-5-Transgenic Mice

In a broad number of diseases, including parasitosis and allergy, eosinophilia in the bone marrow, blood circulation, and targeted tissue is largely associated with IL-5, a cytokine critically required for maturation, bone marrow mobilization, and activation of eosinophils (10). Coffman et al. (20) first reported that a monoclonal antibody to IL-5 completely suppressed the blood eosinophilia and the infiltration of eosinophils in the lungs of mice parasitized with *N. brasiliensis* but had no effect on the concomitant increased levels of serum IgE. The dissociation between both phenomena was also observed after treatment with a monoclonal antibody to IL-4 which inhibited the up-regulation of IgE but not the eosinophilia. The data are consistent with the interpretation that IL-5 is indeed a pivotal cytokine in the induction of eosinophilia following helminth infection, and that IgE and eosinophil production are distinctly regulated by IL-4 and IL-5 (20).

Antiserum raised against eosinophils were previously used to illustrate the requirement for eosinophils in the resistance to both *S. mansoni* and *T. spiralis* (156,157), and these early findings were considered important evidence for the putative helminthotoxic role of eosinophils. Nevertheless, more recent studies have indicated that the eosinophil depletion, via either antibody-mediated neutralization of IL-5 or IL-5 gene deletion (IL-5 knockout), has a different impact in different helminth parasites (Table 1). Selective abrogation of the eosinophilia failed to modify the pattern of worm burden and other pathological outcomes of the infection caused by the cestode *Mesocestoides corti* (158), the trematodes *S. mansoni* (159) and *Fasciola hepatica* (160), and by the nematodes *Trichinella spiralis* (161) and *Toxocara canis* (160). In contrast, the immunity was lost when IL-5 and eosinophil levels were depleted in animals infected with the nematodes *A. cantonensis* (162,163), *Strongyloides venezuelensis* (164), *S. ratti* (165), *Onchocerca volvulus* (166), *Onchocerca lienalis* (167), and *Litomosoides sigmodontis* (168).

The immune resistance to a range of helminth parasite species has been also assessed in IL-5 transgenic mice with lifelong constitutive eosinophilia. The findings, similar to those from IL-5-deficient mice, appeared quite heterogeneous (Table 2). For the three parasite species *N. brasiliensis* (169–171), *Angiostrongylus cantonensis* (163), and *L. sigmodontis* (172), the primary infection in IL-5 transgenic mice resulted in increased resistance as compared to non-transgenic littermates. For these species, the findings were not compatible with those obtained in IL-5-deficient mice, as expected, reinforcing the view that IL-5 and eosinophils have a critical role in host defense to certain parasites. Le Goff et al. (168) reported that IL-5 is essential for vaccine-mediated immunity but not innate resistance to *L. sigmodontis*. These data contrast studies with *S. ratti* in mice, where IL-5 is important in the primary but not in the protective response against a challenge infection (165). According to Le Goff et al. (168), the findings are not surprising since each parasite has evolved independently and developed distinct survival strategies that may or may not involve the avoidance of eosinophil-mediated killing. In addition, the location and migration patterns of the parasite certainly influence their susceptibility to innate or adaptive immune mechanisms. However, it is noteworthy, that in cases of infections by *A. cantonensis* and *N. brasiliensis* in IL-5 transgenic mice, the enhanced resistance occurred in the absence of a preexisting specific immunity, strongly suggesting that eosinophils can play an effective role in host innate protection (170). Further evidence supporting that interpretation was provided by Daly et al. (169), while addressing the migratory kinetics of *N. brasiliensis* larvae through the skin in primary infection of IL-5 transgenic mice. By monitoring the retention of larvae injected in preformed subcutaneous air pouches, the authors found that 75–95% of the injected larvae in IL-5 transgenic mice were retained in the pouches for at least 24 h, whereas less than 20% of the organisms could be recovered from the air pouch 2 h postinjection in non-transgenic mice. In addition, in pouch fluids recovered from IL-5 transgenic mice, eosinophil peroxidase activity was elevated 10- to 25-fold above the levels noted in uninfected conditions. The rapid entrapment and killing of *N. brasiliensis* larvae at the site of inoculation in IL-5 transgenic mice strongly suggest that eosinophils may confer some degree of immediate and nonspecific resistance in primary infection with certain parasites (169).

On the other hand, for a number of parasite species, including *T. canis* (170), *T. spiralis* (123,173), *S. mansoni* (123,174), and *Mesocestoides corti* (175), there were no differences in the worm burdens or pathology when the infection occurred in IL-5 transgenic mice, confirming data obtained in IL-5-deficient mice. Collectively, the findings emphasize that there is an important group of parasite species that is clearly refractory to either depletion or overproduction of eosinophils, suggesting that eosinophilia is a redundant or unimportant phenomenon for immune protection against these parasites in mice. It may be relevant to note that mice are not the natural host of many of the parasites used experimentally (122). It is known that eosinophils from mice do not bind or express receptor for IgE, which has been correlated with the fact that mice eosinophils are indeed less effective in killing certain parasites (123).

But what might be the mechanistic pathway(s) underlying eosinophil-independent protective immunity to parasites? It has been reported that Th1 cytokines IL-12 and IFN-γ clearly enhance protective immunity to the tissue-dwelling parasite *S. mansoni* (121), but delay worm expulsion in case of the infection induced by the gut parasite *N. brasiliensis* (120). Rajan et al. (176) demonstrated that treatment of mice with nitric oxide synthase inhibitor abrogated resistance to infection with the human filarial parasite *Brugia malayi*, raising the possibility that classic Th1-mediated responses, such as nitric oxide release by IFN-γ-activated macrophages, may be of extreme relevance either to act together with or as an alternative route to eosinophils.

VI. Eosinophils in Allergic Diseases

Blood and tissue eosinophilia is a hallmark of chronic allergic disorders, including asthma, dermatitis, rhinitis, and atopic gastroenteritis (2,177–179).

Table 1 Helminth Infections in IL-5-Depleted Mice

Parasite	IL-5 status	Infection	Comparative effect	Ref.
Trematodes				
Schistosoma mansoni	α-IL-5	Immunized with irradiated cercaria	Slight reduction in ganuloma volume; hepatic fibroses unaffected; similar egg elimination	159
Schistosoma japonicum	α-IL-5, α-IL-5R	Primary	Similar egg output	218
Asciola hepatica	IL-5 KO	Primary	Similar establishment and host pathology	160
Cestodes				
Mesocestoides corti	IL-5 KO	Primary	Similar number of worms and host pathology	158
Hymenolepis diminuta	IL-5 KO	Primary	Similar worms failed to develop and persist	160
Nematodes				
Angiostrongylus cantonensis	α-IL-5	Primary	Increased intracranial worms	219
	IL-5RKO	Primary	Increased intracranial worm burden; larger worms	163;162
Toxocara canis	IL-5 KO	Primary	Similar number of tissue larvae; reduced lung pathology	220

Organism	Treatment	Infection	Effect	Ref.
Strongyloides ratti	IL-5-KO	Primary	Increased worm burden; more fecund parasites; increased host pathology	165
	IL-5 KO	Secondary	Similar host protection	165
Strongyloides venezuelensis	α-IL-5	Primary	Similar egg output and worm elimination	164
Trichinella spiralis	α-IL-5	Primary	Slightly delayed of adult worm expulsion; similar number of intestinal adult and muscle larvae	161
	α-IL-5	Secondary	Similar muscle larvae burden	161
	IL-5 KO	Primary	Delayed worm expulsion; less intestinal contractility	221
Onchocerca lienalis	α-IL-5	Primary	Increased parasite killing	167;222
Onchocerca volvulus		Immunized with irradiated L3	Reduced parasite killing	166
Litomosoides sigmodontis	IL-5 KO	Primary	Similar parasite survival	168
	IL-5 KO	Immunized with irradiated larvae	Abrogated parasite recovery after challenge	168
Heligmosomoides polygyrus	IL-5 KO	Primary	Failure of worm development and growth	160

α-IL-5, anti-IL-5 antiserum; α-IL-5R, anti-IL-5 receptor α antiserum; IL-5 KO, IL-5 knockout; IL-5 KOR, IL-5 receptor α knockout.

Table 2 Helminth Infections in IL-5 Transgenic Mice

Parasite	Infection	Comparative effect	Ref.
Trematodes			
Schistosoma mansoni	Primary	Similar recovery of adult worms	174
	Immunized with irradiated cercaria	Similar resistance to challenge infection	174
Cestodes			
Mesocestoides corti	Primary	Similar number of tissue larvae	223
Nematodes			
Nippostrongylus brasiliensis	Primary	Lower numbers of larvae in lungs and adult in intestine	171
	Primary	Smaller and fewer intestinal worms; reduced egg output; females less fecund	123;170
	Secondary	Similar number of intestinal worms	123
	Primary	Increased trapping and immobilization of inoculated larvae	170
Angiostrongylus cantonensis	Primary	Smaller and fewer intracranial worms	163
Toxocara canis	Primary	Similar number of tissue larvae	224
	Primary	Similar number of tissue larvae	170
	Immunized with larval antigen	Similar number of tissue larvae	224
Trichinella spiralis	Primary	Similar number of intestinal adult worms; similar female fecundity	123; 173
	Immunized with larval antigen	Similar number of intestinal adult worms and tissue larvae; similar female fecundity	123
Onchocerca volvulus	Immunized with irradiated L3	Blockage of larvae killing	166
Litomosoides sigmodontis	Primary	Reduced recovery of adult worms	172

A consistent finding in many studies has been that the eosinophilic inflammatory infiltrate increases during an allergen-induced late-phase response.

Allergic asthma is a complex syndrome marked by variable airflow obstruction, bronchial hyperresponsiveness, and chronic airway inflammation (177). The association between eosinophilia and asthma was first raised in autopsy tissue studies, which documented the presence of remarkable eosinophilic inflammatory infiltrates, disintegrated eosinophils, and numerous free eosinophil granules in the bronchial epithelium (180). These early findings were further extended in studies utilizing pulmonary biopsy specimen from symptomatic patients. Especially notable in asthmatics were (a) prominent inflammatory infiltrate in the lamina propria; and (b) eosinophilia in tissue, sputum, and blood. The more recent development of fiberoptic bronchoscopy has been instrumental for a better understanding of the pathological and immunological changes in asthma, since it has allowed bronchial biopsies and BAL fluid to be examined under controlled conditions. These studies demonstrated that particularly eosinophils and T cells are increased in numbers and activation status in asthmatic airways in comparison with controls, even in those with very mild disease (181). Furthermore, they have revealed a close correlation between the number of activated eosinophils and the abnormalities in bronchial reactivity and severity of illness (182,183). Therefore, understanding the mechanisms implicated in the regulation and control of airway eosinophilia has become a central line of interest in asthma research.

The prevalent opinion that eosinophils are implicated in the pathogenesis of asthma is largely based on circumstantial observations that (1) eosinophils contain and can generate substances that are toxic and/or injurious to the bronchial epithelium; (2) increased quantities of these substances are detectable in the targeted site; and (3) reducing eosinophil numbers leads to amelioration of the asthma symptoms (184–186). Eosinophils are believed to cause long-term tissue damage when activated to release their granular content of cationic proteins, including EPO, EDN, MBP, and ECP. The capacity of these highly charged proteins to damage airways epithelium has been demonstrated in vitro and in vivo (187,188). A prerequisite for tissue eosinophil accumulation to occur is the recruitment of such cells into the affected area. Chemoattractants such as a C5a, LTB_4, PAF, and chemokines were identified many years ago as substances capable of activating tissue eosinophil recruitment from the blood to sites of allergic inflammation (189,190). However, most of them have no cell specificity attracting different leukocyte subtypes. Belonging to the CC family of chemokines, eotaxin-1 and eotaxin-2 are potent and selective chemoattractants for eosinophils (5,191,192). They signal via the chemokine receptor CCR3, which is restricted to eosinophils, basophils, and some Th2 lymphocytes (5,192,193). Evidence from an in situ bone marrow perfusion system indicates that eotaxin has potent and selective effect in mobilizing bone marrow eosinophils and their progenitors in the guinea pig via a chemotactic gradient. In addition, a marked synergism was observed by combining eosinophil chemotaxis stimulated by eotaxin and eosinophil chemokinesis evoked by IL-5, showing that chemotaxis and chemokinesis may be critical cooperative phenomena in the acceleration of the leukocyte migration across the vascular endothelium (194).

It is now widely accepted that the eosinophilic inflammatory response in asthma, as well as in other allergic disorders, is associated with a Th2-polarized immune response. This concept is supported by a number of studies showing that the infiltrating cells, following nasal or bronchial allergen provocation of atopic individuals, express mRNA and produce proteins for IL-3, IL-4, IL-5, and GM-CSF, but not IL-2 or IFN-γ (1,184). For the induction of an eosinophilic response, IL-5—a cytokine derived from Th2 cells, NK cells, mast cells, and eosinophils—appears to be the main promoting factor (184). It enhances the proliferation, survival, activation, and recruitment of eosinophils into the focus of the allergic inflammatory response. Important evidence that IL-5 might be harmful in asthma is that its inhalation by asthmatic patients led to increased airway hyperresponsiveness and accumulation of eosinophils in the BAL fluid, bronchial mucosa, and sputum (195). On the other hand, particular attention has also been paid to IL-4 and IL-13, which stimulate commitment of naive T cells to Th2 phenotype, isotype switching in B cells toward IgE synthesis, up-regulation of VCAM-1$^+$ expression on endothelial cells, and eotaxin generation to facilitate eosinophil recruitment (196,197). Inhalation of IL-4 by asthmatic patients also caused increased airway hyperresponsiveness (198). Thus, it is widely believed that allergen-specific Th2-type cells and the cytokines IL-4, IL-5, and IL-13 play a crucial role in triggering and maintaining an asthmatic response by promoting eosinophil recruitment and activation (1,184).

A. Lessons from Animal Models of Asthma

Multiple animal studies have pointed to a central role for Th2 cells and potentially important roles for Th2 type cytokines in asthma pathogenesis. However, there are some conflicting data regarding the relative importance of IL-4 and IL-5 in the mechanisms underlying allergen-evoked airway hyperreactivity (199). An obligatory role for IL-5 in the induction of the asthma phenotype has been proposed based on the demonstration that IL-5 deficiency in genetically modified mice entirely abolished lung eosinophilia, bronchial damage, and hyperreactivity (199). In addition, the asthmatic response in IL-5-null mice could be restored by reconstitution of IL-5 levels with recombinant vaccinia viruses (199). A pivotal role for IL-5 has also been suggested by studies based on the treatment with antibodies against IL-5 in sensitized guinea pig (200,201), rat (202), mice (203), and primates (204). Brusselle et al. (205) have shown that allergen-induced bronchial responsiveness and inflammation appeared markedly attenuated in IL-4-null mice, and Corry et al. (206) reported that IL-4 but not IL-5 is required in a murine model of acute airway hyperreactivity.

In contrast, by studying the asthma phenotype established in IL-4-null mice and CD40-deficient mice, Hogan et al. (207) have provided evidence that aeroallergen-induced eosinophilic inflammation, lung damage, and airways hyperresponsiveness can occur independently of IL-4 and allergen-specific immunoglobulins.

VII. Eosinophil-Mediated Inhibitory Mechanisms in Allergic Inflammation

Much of the research in the immunobiological role of eosinophils has been focused on the multiple proinflammatory actions exhibited by these cells in the context of chronic allergic disorders. Much less attention has been dedicated to the anti-inflammatory properties of eosinophils particularly illustrated by early studies developed in the 1960s and 1990s (188). In fact, eosinophils are not simple killer or proinflammatory cells. They have the ability to release enzymes such as histaminase and arylsulfatase, which are recognized to degrade histamine and sulfidopeptide leukotrienes, respectively (188). Following appropriate stimulation eosinophils can also secrete substances with marked negative immunoregulatory activities, including PGE_2, LXA_4, and TGF-β (1). Studies by Hubscher (208) demonstrated that eosinophils stimulated with allergen- or anti-IgE-secreted PGE_2, which prevented blood leukocyte histamine release in vitro. More recently, it was observed that mice and guinea pigs infected with *Toxocara canis* developed airway eosinophilia in parallel with tracheal hyporeactivity (209). The downward shift in the responsiveness to several contracting agonists coincides with an increased concentration in PGE_2 in the BAL fluid and was prevented by cyclooxygenase blockade. Additional evidence for the anti-inflammatory role of eosinophils comes from observations from our laboratory, in which allergen-induced pleural edema response appeared markedly shortened when the reaction was triggered in spontaneous eosinophilic AM1/TOR rats (210), or in animals undergoing selective local eosinophilia caused by distinct eosinophil chemoattractants (211). This phenomenon, which was clearly reversed by pharmacological or immunological blockade of the eosinophilia, also seemed to be dependent on prostaglandins (210–212). Likewise, accelerated resolution of allergen-induced edema was noted in IgE-passively sensitized rats subjected to prior infection with the nematode *Angiostrongylus costaricensis* or pretreatment with IL-5, both conditions clearly associated with blood eosinophilia. Particularly notable in these models is that the accelerated resolution of allergic edema is (1) coincident with marked eosinophil accumulation in the focus of the lesion; (2) associated with increased levels of PGE_2 and LXA_4 in the pleural effluent; (3) overcome by cyclooxygenase type 2-preferring inhibitors; and (4) mimicked by pretreatment with the PGE_1 analogue misoprostol or LXA_4 analogues 15-methyl-LXA_4 and 15-epi-16-*p*-fluorophenoxy-LXA_4 (213). It is noteworthy that

LXA_4 and aspirin-triggered lipoxin derivatives, though not affecting the onset of the allergen-mediated pleurisy, block the subsequent production of proinflammatory cytokines, including IL-5 and eotaxin, and the eosinophil recruitment (214). The notion that in situ LXA_4 could display beneficial actions on allergic diseases came also from clinical results showing that lipoxins are recovered from airway tissue from patients with asthma (215), and that LXA_4 inhalation by asthmatic subjects reduces LTC_4-evoked airways obstruction (216).

Assuming that eosinophil products, including prostaglandins and LXA_4, may be necessary for self-limitation and/or resolution of the allergic inflammatory process, it is tempting to speculate whether a defect in eosinophil-dependent inhibitory mechanisms might be occurring in asthmatics, resulting in increased or more prolonged inflammation.

VIII. Concluding Remarks

As reviewed here eosinophils are fascinating cells. The general consensus that these cells are proinflammatory and important effector cells in parasitic infections has yet to be proved. A recent study (217) denies an important role of eosinophils in human allergic asthma, but these studies are short term, with a limited number of patients, and do not consider the possibility that only particular forms of allergic asthma will benefit from a single anti-eosinophil strategy. It is clear from a range of rare eosinophilic conditions that extravasation and activation of these cells can result in life-threatening clinical conditions. In addition, eosinophils have been shown to be able to process and present antigen to T cells. Therefore, new research will help to identify the precise role of eosinophils in normal and pathological immune reactions.

References

1. Giembycz MA, Lindsay MA. Pharmacology of the eosinophil. Pharmacol Rev 1999; 51:213–340.
2. Spry CJ. Smith H, Cook RM, editors. The Natural History of Eosinophils. London: Academic Press, 1993:1–19.
3. Spry CJ. Spry CJ, editor. Eosinophils: a comprehensive review and guide to the scientific and medical literature. Oxford: Oxford University Press, 1988:1–21.
4. Throsby M, Herbelin A, Pleau JM, Dardenne M. CD11c+ eosinophils in the murine thymus: developmental regulation and recruitment upon MHC class I–restricted thymocyte deletion. J Immunol 2000; 165:1965–1975.
5. Jose PJ, Adcock IM, D.A., Berkman N, Wells TN, Williams TJ, et al. Eotaxin: cloning of an eosinophil chemoattractant cytokine and increased mRNA expression in allergen-challenged guinea-pig lungs. Biochem Biophys Res Commun 1994; 205:788–794.

6. Mishra A, Hogan SP, Lee JJ, Foster PS, Rothenberg ME. Fundamental signals that regulate eosinophil homing to the gastrointestinal tract. J Clin Invest 1999; 103:1719–1727.

7. Rothenberg ME, Luster AD, Lilly CM, Drazen JM, Leder P. Constitutive and allergen-induced expression of eotaxin mRNA in the guinea pig lung. J Exp Med 1995; 181:1211–1216.

8. Collins PD, Marleau S, D.A., Jose PJ, Williams TJ. Cooperation between interleukin-5 and the chemokine eotaxin to induce eosinophil accumulation in vivo. J Exp Med 1995; 182:1169–1174.

9. Tai PC, Sun L, Spry CJ. Effects of IL-5, granulocyte/macrophage colony-stimulating factor (GM-CSF) and IL-3 on the survival of human blood eosinophils in vitro. Clin Exp Immunol 1991; 85:312–316.

10. Sanderson CJ. Pharmacological implications of interleukin-5 in the control of eosinophilia. Adv Pharmacol 1992; 23:163–177.

11. Sanderson CJ, Warren DJ, Strath M. Identification of a lymphokine that stimulates eosinophil differentiation in vitro. Its relationship to interleukin 3, and functional properties of eosinophils produced in cultures. J Exp Med 1985; 162:60–74.

12. Shalit M, Sekhsaria S, Mauhorter S, Mahanti S, Malech HL. Early commitment to the eosinophil lineage by cultured human peripheral blood CD34+cells: messenger RNA analysis. J Allergy Clin Immunol 1996; 98:344–354.

13. Sehmi R, Howie K, Sutherland DR, Schragge W, O'Byrne PM, Denburg JA. Increased levels of CD34+ hemopoietic progenitor cells in atopic subjects. Am J Respir Cell Mol Biol 1996; 15:645–655.

14. Wood LJ, Inman MD, Watson RM, Foley R, Denburg JA, O'Byrne PM. Changes in bone marrow inflammatory cell progenitors after inhaled allergen in asthmatic subjects. Am J Respir Crit Care Med 1998; 157:99–105.

15. Sehmi R, Wood LJ, Watson R, Foley R, Hamid Q, O'Byrne PM, et al. Allergen-induced increases in IL-5 receptor alpha-subunit expression on bone marrow-derived CD34+ cells from asthmatic subjects. A novel marker of progenitor cell commitment towards eosinophilic differentiation. J Clin Invest 1997; 100:2466–2475.

16. Robinson DS, Damia R, Zeibecoglou K, Molet S, North J, Yamada T, et al. CD34(+)/interleukin-5Ralpha messenger RNA+ cells in the bronchial mucosa in asthma: potential airway eosinophil progenitors. Am J Respir Cell Mol Biol 1999; 20:9–13.

17. Durham SR, Ying S, Varney VA, Jacobson MR, Sudderick RM, Mackay IS, et al. Cytokine messenger RNA expression for IL-3, IL-4, IL-5, and granulocyte/macrophage-colony-stimulating factor in the nasal mucosa after local allergen provocation: relationship to tissue eosinophilia. J Immunol 1992; 148:2390–2394.

18. Cameron L, Christodoulopoulos P, Lavigne F, Nakamura Y, Eidelman D, McEuen A, et al. Evidence for local eosinophil differentiation within allergic nasal mucosa: inhibition with soluble IL-5 receptor. J Immunol 2000; 164:1538–1545.

19. Metcalf D, Parker J, Chester HM, Kincade PW. Formation of eosinophilic-like granulocytic colonies by mouse bone marrow cells in vitro. J Cell Physiol 1974; 84:275–289.

20. Coffman RL, Seymour BW, Hudak S, Jackson J, Rennick D. Antibody to inter-leukin-5 inhibits helminth-induced eosinphilia in mice. Science 1989; 245:308–310.
21. Yoshida T, Ikuta K, Sugaya H, Maki K, Takagi M, Kanazawa H, et al. Defective B-1 cell development and impaired immunity against *Angiostrongylus cantonensis* in IL-5R alpha-deficient mice. Immunity 1996; 4:483–494.
22. Dent LA, Strath M, Mellor AL, Sanderson CJ. Eosinophilia in transgenic mice expressing interleukin 5. J Exp Med 1990; 172:1425–1431.
23. Ward AC, Loeb DM, A.A., Touw IP, Friedman AD. Regulation of granulo-poiesis by transcription factors and cytokine signals. Leukemia 2000; 14:973–990.
24. Plager DA, Loegering DA, Weiler DA, Checkel JL, Wagner JM, Clarke NJ, et al. A novel and highly divergent homolog of human eosinophil granule major basic protein. J Biol Chem 1999; 274:14464–14473.
25. Zhang DE, Zhang P, Wang ND, Hetherington CJ, Darlington GJ, Tenen DG. Absence of granulocyte colony-stimulation factor signaling and neutrophil development in CCAAT enhancer binding protein alpha-deficient mice. Proc Natl Acad Sci USA 1997; 94:569–574.
26. Yamanaka R, Barlow C, Lekstrom-Himes J, Castilla LH, Liu PP, Eckhaus M, et al. Impaired granulopoiesis, myelodysplasia, and early lethality in CCAAT/ enhancer binding protein epsilon-deficient mice. Proc Natl Acad Sci USA 1997; 94:13187–13192.
27. Muller C, Kowenz-Leutz E, Grieser-Ade S, Graf T, Leutz A. NF-M (chicken C/EBP beta) induces eosinophilic differentiation and apoptosis in a hematopoietic progenitor cell line. EMBO J 1995; 14:6127–6135.
28. Nerlov C, McNagny KM, Doderlein G, Kowenz-Leutz E, Graf T. Distinct C/EBP functions are required for eosinophil lineage commitment and matura-tion. Genes Dev 1998; 12:2413–2423.
29. Querfurth E, Schuster M, Kulessa H, Crispino JD, Doderlein G, Orkin SH, et al. Antagonism between C/EBPbeta and FOG in eosinophil lineage commitment of multipotent hematopoietic progenitors. Genes Dev 2000; 14:2515–2525.
30. Yamaguchi Y, Nishio H, Kishi K, Ackerman SJ, Suda T. C/EBPbeta and GATA-1 synergistically regulate activity of the eosinophil granule major basic protein promoter: implication for C/EBPbeta activity in eosinophil gene expression. Blood 1999; 94:1429–1439.
31. Rossi F, McNagny M, Smith G, Frampton J, Graf T. Lineage commitment of transformed haematopoietic progenitors is determined by the level of PKC activity. EMBO J 1996; 15:1894–1901.
32. Kerr JF, Wyllie AH, Currie AR. Apoptosis: a basic biological phenomenon with wide-ranging implications in tissue kinetics. Br J Cancer 1972; 26:239–257.
33. Yamaguchi Y, Suda T, Ohta S, Tominaga K, Miura Y, Kasahara T. Analysis of the survival of mature human eosinophils: interleukin-5 prevents apoptosis in mature human eosinophils. Blood 1991; 78:2542–2547.
34. Stern M, Meagher L, Savill J, Haslett C. Apoptosis in human eosinophils. Pro-grammed cell death in the eosinophil leads to phagocytosis by macrophages and is modulated by IL-5. J Immunol 1992; 148:3543–3549.
35. Simon HU, Yousefi S, Schranz C, Schapowal A, Bachert C, Blaser K. Direct demonstration of delayed eosinophil apoptosis as a mechanism causing tissue eosinophilia. J Immunol 1997; 158:3902–3908.

36. Bousquet J, Chanez P, Lacoste JY, Barneon G, Ghavanian N, Enander I, et al. Eosinophilic inflammation in asthma. N Engl J Med 1990; 323:1033–1039.
37. Tai PC, Sun L, Spry CJ. Effects of IL-5, granulocyte/macrophage colony-stimulating factor (GM-CSF) and IL-3 on the survival of human blood eosinophils in vitro. Clin Exp Immunol 1991; 85:312–316.
38. Hallsworth MP, Litchfield TM, Lee TH. Glucocorticoids inhibit granulocyte-macrophage colony-stimulating factor-1 and interleukin-5 enhanced in vitro survival of human eosinophils. Immunology 1992; 75:382–385.
39. Kankaanranta H, Lindsay MA, Giembycz MA, Zhang X, Moilanen E, Barnes PJ. Delayed eosinophil apoptosis in asthma. J Allergy Clin Immunol 2000; 106:77–83.
40. Alam R, Forsythe P, Stafford S, Fukuda Y. Transforming growth factor beta abrogates the effects of hematopoietins on eosinophils and induces their apoptosis. J Exp Med 1994; 179:1041–1045.
41. Simon H, Alam R. Regulation of eosinophil apoptosis: transdution of survival and death signals. Int Arch Allergy Immunol 1999; 118:7–14.
42. Walsh GM. Eosinophil apoptosis: mechanisms and clinical relevance in asthmatic and allergic inflammation. Br J Haematol 2000; 111:61–67.
43. Dijkers PF, Medema RH, Pals C, Banerji L, Thomas NS, Lam EW, et al. Forkhead transcription factor FKHR-L1 modulates cytokine-dependent transcriptional regulation of p27(KIPI). Mol Cell Biol 2000; 20:9138–9148.
44. Chao DT, Korsmeyer SJ. BCL-2 family: regulators of cell death. Annu Rev Immunol 1998; 16:395–419.
45. Yang J, Liu X, Bhalla K, Kim CN, Ibrado AM, Cai J, et al. Prevention of apoptosis by Bcl-2: release of cytochrome c from mitochondria blocked. Science 1997; 275:1129–1132.
46. Dibbert B, Daigle I, Braun D, Schranz C, Weber M, Blaser K, et al. Role for Bcl-xL in delayed eosinophil apoptosis mediated by granulocyte-macrophage colony-stimulating factor and interleukin-5. Blood 1998; 92:778–783.
47. Plotz SG, Dibbert B, Abeck D, Ring J, Simon HU. Bcl-2 expression by eosinophils in a patient with hypereosinophilia. J Allergy Clin Immunol 1998; 102:1037–1040.
48. Dijkers PF, Medema RH, Lammers JW, Koenderman L, Coffer PJ. Expression of the pro-apoptotic Bcl-2 family member Bim is regulated by the forkhead transcription factor FKHR-L1. Curr Biol 2000; 10:1201–1204.
49. Datta SR, Brunet A, Greenberg ME. Cellular survival: a play in three Akts. Genes Dev 1999; 13:2905–2927.
50. Nagata S, Golstein P. The Fas death factor. Science 1995; 267:1449–1456.
51. Matsumoto K, Schlemier RP, Saito H, Iikura Y, Bochner BS. Induction of apoptosis in human eosinophils by anti-Fas antibody treatment in vitro. Blood 1995; 86:1437–1443.
52. Druilhe A, Cai Z, Haile S, Chouaib S, Pretolani M. Fas-mediated apoptosis in cultured human eosinophils. Blood 1996; 87:2822–2830.
53. Luttmann W, Opfer A, Dauer E, Foerster M, Matthys H, Eibel H, et al. Differential regulation of CD95 (Fas/APO-1) expression in human blood eosinophils. Eur J Immunol 1998; 28:2057–2065.
54. Tsuyuki S, Bertrand C, Erard F, Trifilieff A, Tsuyuki J, Wesp M, et al. Activation of the Fas receptor on lung eosinophils leads to apoptosis and the resolution of eosinohilic inflammation of the airways. J Clin Invest 1995; 96:2924–2931.

55. Hebestreit H, Dibbert B, Balatti I, Braun D, Schapowal A, Blaser K, et al. Disruption of fas receptor signaling by nitric oxide in eosinophils. J Exp Med 1998; 187:415–425.

56. Koenderman L, van der BT, Schweizer RC, Warringa RA, Coffer P, Caldenhoven E, et al. Eosinophil priming by cytokines: from cellular signal to in vivo modulation. Eur Respir J Suppl 1996; 22:119s–125s.

57. Koenderman L, Coffer PJ. Controlling allergic inflammation by signaling regulation of eosinophils. Allergy 2001; 56:204–214.

58. Warringa RA, Mengelers HJ, Kuijper PH, Raaijmakers JA, Bruijnzeel PL, Koenderman L. In vivo priming of platelet-activating factor-induced eosinophil chemotaxis in allergic asthmatic individuals. Blood 1992; 79:1836–1841.

59. Sehmi R, Wardlaw AJ, Cromwell O, Kurihara K, Waltmann P, Kay AB. Interleukin-5 selectively enhances the chemotactic response of eosinophils obtained from normal but not eosinophilic subjects. Blood 1992; 79:2952–2959.

60. Moser R, Fehr J, Bruijnzeel PL. IL-4 controls the selective endothelium-driven transmigration of eosinophils from allergic individuals. J Immunol 1992; 149:1432–1438.

61. Warringa RA, Koenderman L, Kok PT, Kreukniet J, Bruijnzeel PL. Modulation and induction of eosinophil chemotaxis by granulocyte-macrophage colony-stimulating factor and interleukin-3. Blood 1991; 77:2694–2700.

62. Moser R, Fehr J, Olgiati L, Bruijnzeel PL. Migration of primed human eosinophils across cytokine-activated endothelial cell monolayers. Blood 1992; 79:2937–2945.

63. Ebisawa M, Liu MC, Yamada T, Kato M, Lichtenstein LM, Bochner BS, et al. Eosinophil transendothelial migration induced by cytokines. II. Potentiation of eosinophil transendothelial migration by eosinophil-active cytokines. J Immunol 1994; 152:4590–4596.

64. Schweizer RC, Welmers BA, Raaijmakers JA, Zanen P, Lammers JW, Koenderman L. RANTES- and interleukin-8-induced responses in normal human eosinophils: effects of priming with interleukin-5. Blood 1994; 83:3697–3704.

65. Dri P, Cramer R, Spessotto P, Romano M, Patriarca P. Eosinophil activation on biologic surfaces. Production of O2- in response to physiologic soluble stimuli is differentially modulated by extracellular matrix components and endothelial cells. J Immunol 1991; 147:613–620.

66. van der BT, Kok PT, Raaijmakers JA, Verhoeven AJ, Kessels RG, Lammers JW, et al. Cytokine priming of the respiratory burst in human eosinophils is Ca^{2+} independent and accompanied by induction of tyrosine kinase activity. J Leukoc Biol 1993; 53: 347–353.

67. Tyagi SR, Tamura M, Burnham DN, Lambeth JD. Phorbol myristate acetate (PMA) augments chemoattractant-induced diglyceride generation in human neutrophils but inhibits phosphoinositide hydrolysis. Implications for the mechanism of PMA priming of the respiratory burst. J Biol Chem 1988; 263: 13191–13198.

68. Daniels RH, Elmore MA, Hill ME, Shimizu Y, Lackie JM, Finnen MJ. Priming of the oxidative burst in human neutrophils by physiological agonists or cytochalasin B results from the recruitment of previously non-responsive cells. Immunology 1994; 82:465–472.

69. Lacy P, Logan MR, Bablitz B, Moqbel R. Fusion protein vesicle-associated membrane protein 2 is implicated in IFN-gamma-induced piecemeal degranulation in human eosinophils from atopic individuals. J Allergy Clin Immunol 2001; 107:671–678.

70. Shindo K, Koide K, Hirai Y, Sumitomo M, Fukumura M. Priming effect of platelet activating factor on leukotriene C4 from stimulated eosinophils of asthmatic patients. Thorax 1996; 51:155–158.

71. Warringa RA, Schweizer RC, Maikoe T, Kuijper PH, Bruijnzeel PL, Koendermann L. Modulation of eosinophil chemotaxis by interleukin-5. Am J Respir Cell Mol Biol 1992; 7:631–636.

72. Shute J. Interleukin-8 is a potent eosinophil chemo-attractant. Clin Exp Allergy 1994; 24:203–206.

73. Koenderman L, Bruijnzeel PL. Increased sensitivity of the chemoattractant-induced chemiluminescence in eosinophils isolated from atopic individuals. Immunology 1989; 67:534–536.

74. Grutter JC, Brinkman L, Aslander MM, van den Bosch JM, Koenderman L, Lammers JW. Asthma therapy modulates priming-associated blood eosinophil responsiveness in allergic asthmatics. Eur Respir J 1999; 14:915–922.

75. Evans DJ, Lindsay MA, O'Connor BJ, Barnes PJ. Priming of circulating human eosinophils following late response to allergen challenge. Eur Respir J 1996; 9:703–708.

76. Tenscher K, Metzner B, Schopf E, Norgauer J, Czech W. Recombinant human eotaxin induces oxygen radical production, Ca(2+)-mobilization, actin reorganization, and CD11b upregulation in human eosinophils via a pertussis toxin-sensitive heterotrimeric guanine nucleotide-binding protein. Blood 1996; 88:3195–3199.

77. Mengelers HJ, Maikoe T, Hooibrink B, Kuypers TW, Kreukniet J, Lammers JW, et al. Down modulation of L-selectin expression on eosinophils recovered from bronchoalveolar lavage fluid after allergen provocation. Clin Exp Allergy 1993; 23:196–204.

78. Vedder NB, Harlan JM. Increased surface expression of CD11b/CD18 (Mac-1) is not required for stimulated neutrophil adherence to cultured endothelium. J clin Invest 1988; 81:676–682.

79. Czech W, Krutmann J, Budnik A, Schopf E, Kapp A. Induction of intercellular adhesion molecule 1 (ICAM-1)expression in normal human eosinophils by inflammatory cytokines. J Invest Dermatol 1993; 100:417–423.

80. Hartnell A, Robinson DS, Kay AB, Wardlaw AJ. CD69 is expressed by human eosinophils activated in vivo in asthma and in vitro by cytokines. Immunology 1993; 80:281–286.

81. Nagase H, Miyamasu M, Yamaguchi M, Fujisawa T, Ohta K, Yamamoto K, et al. Expression of CXCR4 in eosinophils: functional analyses and cytokine-mediated regulation. J Immunol 2000; 164:5935–5943.

82. Monteiro RC, Hostoffer RW, Cooper MD, Bonner JR, Gartland GL, Kubagawa H. Definition of immunoglobulin A receptors on eosinophils and their enhanced expression in allergic individuals. J Clin Invest 1993; 92:1681–1685.

83. Blom M, Tool AT, Kok PT, Koenderman L, Roos D, Verhoeven AJ. Granulocyte-macrophage colony-stimulating factor, interleukin-3 (IL-3), and IL-5

greatly enhance the interaction of human eosinophils with opsonized particles by changing the affinity of complement receptor type 3. Blood 1994; 83:2978–2984.

84. Bracke M, Dubois GR, Bolt K, Bruijnzeel PL, Vaerman JP, Lammers JW, et al. Differential effects of the T helper cell type 2-derived cytokines IL-4 and IL-5 on ligand binding to IgG and IgA receptors expressed by human eosinophils. J Immunol 1997; 159:1459–1465.

85. Bracke M, Nijhuis E, Lammers JW, Coffer PJ, Koenderman L. A critical role for PI 3-kinase in cytokine-induced Fcalpha-receptor activation. Blood 2000; 95:2037–2043.

86. Bracke M, Coffer PJ, Lammers JW, Koenderman L. Analysis of signal transduction pathways regulating cytokine-mediated Fc receptor activation on human eosinophils. J Immunol 1998; 161:6768–6774.

87. Bracke M, Lammers JW, Coffer PJ, Koenderman L. Cytokine-induced inside-out activation of FcalphaR (CD89) is mediated by a single serine residue (S263) in the intracellular domain of the receptor. Blood 2001; 97:3478–3483.

88. Blom M, Tool AT, Roos D, Verhoeven AJ. Priming of human eosinophils by platelet-activating factor enhances the number of cells able to bind and respond to opsonized particles. J Immunol 1992; 149:3672–3677.

89. Bates ME, Green VL, Bertics PJ. ERK1 and ERK2 activation by chemotactic factors in human eosinophils is interleukin 5-dependent and contributes to leukotriene C(4) biosynthesis. J Biol Chem 2000; 275:10968–10975.

90. Bracke M, van de GE, Lammers JW, Coffer PJ, Koenderman L. In vivo priming of FcalphaR functioning on eosinophils of allergic asthmatics. J Leukoc Biol 2000; 68:655–661.

91. Diamond MS, Springer TA. The dynamic regulation of integrin adhesiveness. Curr Biol 1994; 4:506–517.

92. Kitayama J, Fuhlbrigge RC, Puri KD, Springer TA. P-selectin, L-selectin, and alpha 4 integrin have distinct roles in eosinophil tethering and arrest on vascular endothelial cells under physiological flow conditions. J Immunol 1997; 159:3929–3939.

93. Ulfman LH, Kuijper PH, van der Linden JA, Lammers JW, Zwaginga JJ, Koenderman L. Characterization of eosinophil adhesion to TNF-alpha-activated endothelium under flow conditions: alpha 4 integrins mediate initial attachment, and E-selectin mediates rolling. J Immunol 1999; 163:343–350.

94. Knol EF, Tackey F, Tedder TF, Klunk DA, Bickel CA, Sterbinsky SA, et al. Comparison of human eosinophil and neutrophil adhesion to endothelial cells under nonstatic conditions. Role of L-selectin. J Immunol 1994; 153:2161–2167.

95. Ulfman LH, Joosten DP, van der Linden JA, Lammers JW, Zwaginga JJ, Koenderman L. IL-8 induces a transient arrest of rolling eosinophils on human endothelial cells, J Immunol 2001; 166:588–595.

96. Tachimoto H, Burdick MM, Hudson SA, Kikuchi M, Konstantopoulos K, Bochner BS. CCR3-active chemokines promote rapid detachment of eosinophils from VCAM-1 in vitro. J Immunol 2000; 165:2748–2754.

97. Bolscher BG, Koenderman L, Tool AT, Stokman PM, Roos D. NADPH:O2 oxidoreductase of human eosinophils in the cell-free system. FEBS Lett 1990; 268:269–273.

98. Walsh GM. Eosinophil granule proteins and their role in disease. Curr Opin Hematol 2001; 8:28–33.

99. Yazdanbakhsh M, Tai PC, Spry CJ, Gleich GJ, Roos D. Synergism between eosinophil cationic protein and oxygen metabolites in killing of schistosomula of *Schistosoma mansoni*. J Immunol 1987; 138:3443–3447.

100. Kaneko M, Horie S, Kato M, Gleich GJ, Kita H. A crucial role for beta 2 integrin in the activation of eosinophils stimulated by IgG. J Immunol 1995; 155:2631–2641.

101. Kita H, Horie S, Gleich GJ. Extracellular matrix proteins attenuate activation and degranulation of stimulated eosinophils. J Immunol 1996; 156:1174–1181.

102. Koenderman L, Tool AT, Roos D, Verhoeven AJ. Priming of the respiratory burst in human eosinophils is accompanied by changes in signal transduction. J Immunol 1990; 145:3883–3888.

103. Tool AT, Koenderman L, Kok PT, Blom M, Roos D, Verhoeven AJ. Release of platelet-activating factor is important for the respiratory burst induced in human eosinophils by opsonized particles. Blood 1992; 79:2729–2732.

104. van Spriel AB, Leusen JH, van Egmond M, Dijkman HB, Assmann KJ, Mayadas TN, et al. Mac-1 (CD11b/CD18) is essential for Fc receptor–mediated neutrophil cytotoxicity and immunologic synapse formation. Blood 2001; 97:2478–2486.

105. Capron M, Woerly G, Kayaba H, Loiseau S, Roger N, Dombrowicz D. Invited lecture: role of membrane receptors in the release of T helper 1 and 2 cytokines by eosinophils. Int Arch Allergy Immunol 2001; 124:223–226.

106. Levi-Schaffer F, Garbuzenko E, Rubin A, Reich R, Pickholz D, Gillery P, et al. Human eosinophils regulate human lung- and skin-derived fibroblast properties in vitro: a role for transforming growth factor beta (TGF-beta). Proc Natl Acad Sci USA 1999; 96:9660–9665.

107. Henderson WRJ. Eicosanoids and platelet-activating factor in allergic respiratory diseases. Am Rev Respir Dis 1991; 143:S86–S90.

108. Molina HA, Kierszenbaum F. Interaction of human eosinophils or neutrophils with *Trypanosoma cruzi* in vitro causes bystander cardiac cell damage. Immunology 1989; 66:289–295.

109. Waters LS, Taverne J, Tai PC, Spry CJ, Targett GA, Playfair JH. Killing of *Plasmodium falciparum* by eosinophil secretory products. Infect Immun 1987; 55:877–881.

110. Pattison N, Wright T, Herrod HG. Pneumocystis carinii pneumonitis, eosinophilia and hypogammaglobulinemia. Pediatr Infect Dis J 1987; 6:293–294.

111. Butterworth AE, Thorne KJI, Smith H, Cook RM, editors. Immunopharmacology of Eosinophils. London: Academic Press, 1993, pp 119–131.

112. Hua XX, Sugaya H, Yoshimura K. Alteration in density of eosinophils in the cerebrospinal fluid of mice infected with Angiostrongylus cantonensis. Int Parasitol 1990; 20:681–683.

113. Perez O, Lastre M, Capron M, Neyrinck JL, Jouault T, Bazin H, et al. Total and specific IgE in serum and cerebrospinal fluid of rats and guinea pigs infected with *Angiostrongylus cantonensis*. Parasitol Res 1989; 75:476–481.

114. Boon JH, Grondel JL, Hemmer JG, Booms GH. Relationship between cytologic changes in bronchoalveolar lavage fluid and weight gain in calves with gastrointestinal nematodes and lungworms. Vet Parasitol 1987; 24:251–261.

115. Guerra-Caceres JG, Bryceson AD, Quaki K, Spry CJ. Studies on the mechanisms of adverse reactions produced by diethylcarbamazine in patients with onchocerciasis: the Mazotti reaction. Parasite Immunol 1980; 2:121 Abstract.

116. Basten A, Beeson PB. Mechanism of eosinophilia. II. Role of the lymphocyte. J Exp Med 1970; 131:1288–1305.

117. Bastern A, Boyer MH, Beeson PB. Mechanism of eosinophilia. I. Factors affecting the eosinophil response of rats to *Trichinella spiralis*. J Exp Med 1970; 131:1271–1287.

118. Nielsen K, Fogh L, Andersen S. Eosinophil response to migrating *Ascaris suum* larvae in normal and congenitally thymus-less mice. Acta Pathol Microbiol Scand [B] Microbiol Immunol 1974; 82:919–920.

119. Hsu CK, Hsu SH, Whitney RAJ, Hansen CT. Immunopathology of schistosomiasis in athymic mice. Nature 1976; 262:397–399.

120. Urban JFJ, Madden KB, Cheever AW, Trotta PP, Katona IM, Finkelman FD. IFN inhibits inflammatory responses and protective immunity in mice infected with the nematode parasite, *Nippostrongylus brasiliensis*. J Immunol 1993; 151:7086–7094.

121. Abbas AK, Murphy KM, Sher A. Functional diversity of helper T lymphocytes. Nature 1996; 383:787–793.

122. Behm CA, Ovington KS. The role of eosinophils in parasitic helminth infections: insights from genetically modified mice. Parasitol Today 2000; 16:202–209.

123. Dent LA, Daly C, Geddes A, Cormie J, Finlay DA, Bignold L, et al. Immune responses of IL-5 transgenic mice to parasites and aeroallergens. Mem Inst Oswaldo Cruz 1997; 92 Suppl 2:45–54.

124. Nutten S, Papin JP, Woerly G, Dunne DW, MacGregor J, Trottein F, et al. Selectin and Lewis(x) are required as co-receptors in antibody-dependent cell-mediated cytotoxicity of human eosinophils to *Schistosoma mansoni* schistosomula. Eur J Immunol 1999; 29:799–808.

125. Scepek S, Lindau M. Focal exocytosis by eosinophils—compound exocytosis and cumulative fusion. EMBO J 1993; 12:1811–1817.

126. Glauert AM, Butterworth AE. Morphological evidence for the ability of eosinophils to damage antibody-coated schistosomula. Trans R Soc Trop Med Hyg 1977; 71:392–395.

127. McLaren DJ, McKean JR, Olsson I, Venges P, Kay AB. Morphological studies on the killing of schistosomula of Schistosoma mansoni by human eosinophil and neutrophil cationic proteins in vitro. Parasite Immunol 1981; 3:359–373.

128. McLaren DJ, Mackenzie CD, F.J. Ultrastructural observations on the in vitro interaction between rat eosinophils and some parasitic helminths (*Schistosoma mansoni, Trichinella spiralis* and *Nippostrongylus brasiliensis*). Clin Exp Immunol 1977; 30:105–118.

129. Butterworth AE, Wassom DL, Gleich GJ, Loegering DA, David JR. Damage to schistosomula of *Schistosoma mansoni* induced directly by eosinophil major basic protein. J Immunol 1979; 122:221–229.

130. Hamann KJ, Barker RL, Loegering DA, Gleich GJ. Comparative toxicity of purified human eosinophil granule proteins for newborn larvae of *Trichinella spiralis*. J Parasitol 1987; 73:523–529.

131. Kierszenbaum F, Ackerman SJ, Gleich GJ. Destruction of bloodstream forms of *Trypanosoma cruzi* by eosinophil granule major basic protein. Am J Trop Med Hyg 1981; 30:775–779.

132. Jong EC, Klebanoff SJ. Eosinophil-mediated mammalian tumor cell cytotoxicity: role of the peroxidase system. J Immunol 1980; 124:1949–1953.

133. McLaren DJ, Peterson CG, Venge P. *Schistosoma mansoni*: further studies of the interaction between schistosomula and granulocyte-derived cationic proteins in vitro. Parasitology 1984; 88 (Pt 3):491–503.

134. Seitz HM, Cottrell BJ, Sturrock RF. A histological study of skin reactions of baboons to *Schistosoma mansoni* schistosomula. Trans R Soc Trop Med Hyg 1987; 81:385–390.

135. Hsu SY, Hsu HF. Recovery of schistosomula in the skin of rhesus monkeys immunized with cercariae of *Schistosoma japonicum* exposed to high dose of x-irradiation. J Parasitol 1975; 61:1108–1109.

136. Dawkins HJ, Windon RG, Eagleson GK. Eosinophil responses in sheep selected for high and low responsiveness of *Trichostrongylus colubriformis*. Int J Parasitol 1989; 19:199–205.

137. Douch PG, Harrison GB, Elliott DC, Buchanan LL, Greer KS. Relationship of gastrointestinal histology and mucus antiparasite activity with the development of resistance to trichostrongyle infections in sheep. Vet Parasitol 1986; 20:315–331.

138. Moqbel R, McLaren DJ. Strongyloides ratti: structural and functional characteristics of normal and immune-damaged worms. Exp Parasitol 1980; 49:139–152.

139. Abdallahi OM, Hanna S, De Reggi M, Gharib B. Visualization of oxygen radical production in mouse liver in response to infection with *Schistosoma mansoni*. Liver 1999; 19:495–500.

140. Pincus SH, Butterworth AE, David JR, Robbins M, Vadas MA. Antibody-dependent eosinophil-mediated damage to schistosomula of *Schistosoma mansoni*: lack of requirement for oxidative metabolism. J Immunol 1981; 126:1794–1799.

141. Andrade ZA, M.G. [Role of eosinophils in the destruction of schistosomula of *Schistosoma mansoni* in vivo (preliminary report)]. Mem Inst Oswaldo Cruz 1984; 79:371–373.

142. Neva FA, Ottesen EA. Tropical (filarial) eosinophilia. N Engl J Med 1978; 298:1129–1131.

143. Butterworth AE, Capron M, Cordingley JS, Dalton PR, Dunne DW, Kariuki HC, et al. Immunity after treatment of human schistosomiasis mansoni. II. Identification of resistant individuals, and analysis of their immune responses. Trans R Soc Trop Med Hyg 1985; 79:393–408.

144. Bell SJ, Metzger WJ, Welch CA, Gilmour MI. A role for Th2 T-memory cells in early airway obstruction. Cell Immunol 1996; 170:185–194.

145. Maizels RM, Holland MJ. Parasite immunology: pathways for expelling intestinal helminths. Curr Biol 1998; 8:R711–R714.

146. Urban JFJ, Madden KB, Svetic A, Cheever A, Trotta PP, Gause WC, et al. The importance of Th2 cytokines in protective immunity to nematodes. Immunol Rev 1992; 127:205–220.

147. Dombrowicz D, Quatannens B, Papin JP, Capron A, Capron M. Expression of a functional Fc epsilon RI on rat eosinophils and macrophages. J Immunol 2000; 165:1266–1271.

148. Kita H, Kaneko M, Bartemes KR, Weiler DA, Schimming AW, Reed CE, et al. Does IgE bind to and activate eosinophils from patients with allergy? J Immunol 1999; 162:6901–6911.

149. de Andres B, Rakasz E, Hagen M, McCormik ML, Mueller AL, Elliot D, et al. Lack of Fc-epsilon receptors on murine eosinophils: implications for the functional significance of elevated IgE and eosinophils in parasitic infections. Blood 1997; 89:3826–3836.

150. Gounni AS, Lamkhioued B, Ochiai K, Tanaka Y, Delaporte E, Carpon A, et al. High-affinity IgE receptor on eosinophils is involved in defence against parasites. Nature 1994; 367:183–186.

151. Larsh JEJ. Trichinella spiralis: phospholipase in sensitized mice after challenge. Exp Parasitol 1975; 37:233–238.

152. Alizadeh H, Murrell KD. The intestinal mast cell response to *Trichinella spiralis* infection in mast cell–deficient w/wv mice. J Parasitol 1984; 70:767–773.

153. Nawa Y, Kiyota M, Korenaga M, Kotani M. Defective protective capacity of W/Wv mice against *Strongyloides ratti* infection and its reconstitution with bone marrow cells. Parasite Immunol 1985; 7:429–438.

154. Watanabe N, Nawa Y, Okamoto K, Kobayashi A. Expulsion of *Hymenolepis nana* from mice with congenital deficiencies of IgE production of mast cell development. Parasite Immunol 1994; 16:137–144.

155. Uber CL, Roth RL, Levy DA. Expulsion of *Nippostrongylus brasiliensis* by mice deficient in mast cells. Nature 1980; 287:226–228.

156. Grove DI, Mahmoud AA, Warren KS. Eosinophils and resistance to *Trichinella spiralis*. J Exp Med 1977; 145:755–759.

157. Mahmoud AA, Warren KS, Graham RCJ. Antieosinophil serum and the kinetics of eosinophilia in schistosomiasis mansoni. J Exp Med 1975; 142:560–574.

158. Kopf M, Brombacher F, Hodgkin PD, Ramsay AJ, Milbourne EA, Dai WJ, et al. IL-5 deficient mice have a developmental defect in CD5+B-1 cells and lack eosinophilia but have normal antibody and cytotoxic T cell responses. Immunity 1996; 4:15–24.

159. Sher A, Coffman RL, Hieny S, Cheever AW. Ablation of eosinophil and IgE responses with anti-IL-5 or anti-IL-4 antibodies fails to affect immunity against *Schistosoma mansoni* in the mouse. J Immunol 1990; 145:3911–3916.

160. Ovington KS, Behm CA. The enigmatic eosinophil: investigation of the biological role of eosinophils in parasitic helminth infection. Mem Inst Oswaldo Cruz 1997; 92 Suppl 2:93–104.

161. Herndon FJ, Kayes SG. Depletion of eosinophils by anti-IL-5 monoclonal antibody treatment of mice infected with *Trichinella spiralis* does not alter parasite burden or immunologic resistance to reinfection. J Immunol 1992; 149:3642–3647.

162. Sugaya H, Aoki M, Yoshida T, Takatsu K, Yoshimura K. Eosinophilia and intracranial worm recovery in interleukin-5 transgenic and interleukin-5 receptor

alpha chain-knockout mice infected with *Angiostrongylus cantonensis*. Parasitol Res 1997; 83:583–590.

163. Yoshida M, Masuryama K, Ogata N, Samejima Y, Eura M, Ishikawa T. Local production of interleukin-5 by T lymphocytes is associated with recruitment of eosinophils in patients with eosinophilic granuloma of the soft tissue. Int Arch Allergy Immunol 1996; 111:133–141.

164. Korenaga M, Hitoshi Y, Yamaguchi N, Sato Y, Takatsu K, Tada I. The role of interleukin-5 in protective immunity to *Strongyloides venezuelensis* infection in mice. Immunology 1991; 72:502–507.

165. Ovington KS, McKie K, Matthaei KI, Young IG, Behm CA. Regulation of primary *Strongyloides ratti* infections in mice: a role for interleukin-5. Immunology 1998; 95:488–493.

166. Lange AM, Yutanawiboonchai W, Scott P, Abraham D. IL-4- and IL-5-dependent protective immunity to *Onchocerca volvulus* infective larvae in BALB/cBYJ mice. J Immunol 1994; 153:205–211.

167. Folkard SG, Hogarth PJ, Taylor MJ, Bianco AE. Eosinophils are the major effector cells of immunity to microfilariae in a mouse model of onchocerciasis. Parasitology 1996; 112 (Pt 3):323–329.

168. Le Goff L, Martin C, Oswald IP, Vuong PN, Petit G, Ungeheuer MN, et al. Parasitology and immunology of mice vaccinated with irradiated *Litomosoides sigmodontis* larvae. Parasitology 2000; 120 (Pt 3):271–280.

169. Daly CM, Mayrhofer G, Dent LA. Trapping and immobilization of *Nippostrongylus brasiliensis* larvae at the site of inoculation in primary infections of interleukin-5 transgenic mice. Infect Immun 1999; 67:5315–5323.

170. Dent LA, Daly CM, Mayrhofer G, Zimmerman T, Hallett A, Bignold LP, et al. Interleukin-5 transgenic mice show enhanced resistance to primary infections with *Nippostrongylus brasiliensis* but not primary infections with *Toxocara canis*. Infect Immun 1999; 67:989–993.

171. Shin EH, Osada Y, Chai JY, Matsumoto N, Takatsu K, Kojima S. Protective roles of eosinophils in *Nippostrongylus brasiliensis* infection. Int Arch Allergy Immunol 1997; 114 Suppl 1:45–50.

172. Martin C, Al-Qaoud KM, Ungeheuer MN, Paehle K, Vuong PN, Bain O, et al. IL-5 is essential for vaccine-induced protection and for resolution of primary infection in murine filariasis. Med Microbiol Immunol (Berl) 2000; 189:67–74.

173. Hokibara S, Takamoto M, Tominaga A, Takatsu S, Sugane K. Marked eosinophilia in interleukin-5 transgenic mice fails to prevent *Trichinella spiralis* infection. J Parasitol 1997; 83:1186–1189.

174. Freeman GLJ, Tominaga A, Takatsu K, Secor WE, Colley DG. Elevated innate peripheral blood eosinophilia fails to augment irradiated cercarial vaccine-induced resistance to *Schistosoma mansoni* in IL-5 transgenic mice. J Parasitol 1995; 81:1010–1011.

175. Strath M, Dent L, Sanderson C. Infection of IL5 transgenic mice with *Mesocestoides corti* induces very high levels of IL5 but depressed production of eosinophils. Exp Hematol 1992; 20:229–234.

176. Rajan TV, Paciorkowski N. Role of B lymphocytes in host protection against the human filarial parasite, *Brugia malayi*. Curr Top Microbiol Immunol 2000; 252:179–187.

177. Busse WW, Lemanske RFJ. Asthma. N Engl J Med 2001; 344:350–362.

178. De Monchy JG, Kauffman HF, Venge P, Koeter GH, Jansen HM, Sluiter HJ, et al. Bronchoalveolar eosinophilia during allergen-induced late asthmatic reactions. Am Rev Respir Dis 1985; 131:373–376.

179. Kay AB. Allergy and allergic diseases. First of two parts. N Engl J Med 2001; 344:30–37.

180. Huber HL, Koessler KK. The pathology of bronchial asthma. Arch Intern Med 1922; 30:689–697.

181. Laitinen LA, Laitinen A, Haahtela T. Airway mucosal inflammation even in patients with newly diagnosed asthma. Am Rev Respir Dis 1993; 147:697–704.

182. Bousquet J, Chanez P, Lacoste JY, Barneon G, Ghavanian N, Enander I, et al. Eosinophilic inflammation in asthma. N Engl J Med 1990; 323:1033–1039.

183. Walker C, Bauer W, Braun RK, Menz G, Braun P, Schwarz F, et al. Activated T cells and cytokines in bronchoalveolar lavages from patients with various lung diseases associated with eosinophilia. Am J Respir Crit Care Med 1994; 150:1038–1048.

184. Holt PG, Macaubas C, Stumbles PA, Sly PD. The role of allergy in the development of asthma. Nature 1999; 402:B12–B17.

185. Gleich GJ. Mechanisms of eosinophil-associated inflammation. J Allergy Clin Immunol 2000; 105:651–663.

186. Cookson W. The alliance of genes and environment in asthma and allergy. Nature 1999; 402:B5.

187. Noguchi H, Kephart GM, Colby TV, Gleich GJ. Tissue eosinophilia and eosinophil degranulation in syndromes associated with fibrosis. Am J Pathol 1992; 140:521–528.

188. Weller PF, Goetzl EJ. The regulatory and effector roles of eosinophils. Adv Immunol 1979; 27:339–371.

189. Silva PM, Martins MA, Lima MC, Alves AC, Diaz BL, Cordeiro RS. Pharmacological modulation of the late eosinophilia induced by antigen in actively sensitized rats. Int Arch Allergy Immunol 1992; 98:355–360.

190. Silva PM, Martins MA, H.C., Cordeiro RS, Vargaftig BB. Generation of an eosinophilotactic activity in the pleural cavity of platelet-activating factor–injected rats. J Pharmacol Exp Ther 1991; 257:1039–1044.

191. Forssman U, Uguccioni M, Loetscher P, Dahinden CA, Langen H, Thelen M, et al. Eotaxin-2, a novel CC chemokine that is selective for the chemokine receptor CCR3, and acts like eotaxin on human eosinophil and basophil leukocytes. J Exp Med 1997; 185:2171–2176.

192. Jose PJ, D.A., Collins PD, Walsh DT, Moqbel R, Totty NF, et al. Eotaxin: a potent eosinophil chemoattractant cytokine detected in a guinea pig model of allergic airways inflammation. J Exp Med 1994; 179:881–887.

193. Rothenberg ME, Zimmermann N, Mishra A, Brandt E, Birkenberger LA, Hogan SP, et al. Chemokines and chemokine receptors: their role in allergic airway disease. J Clin Immunol 1999; 19:250–265.

194. Palframan RT, Collins PD, Williams TJ, Rankin SM. Eotaxin induces a rapid release of eosinophils and their progenitors from the bone marrow. Blood 1998; 91:2240–2248.

195. Shi H, Qin S, Huang G, Chen Y, Xiao C, Xu H, et al. Infiltration of eosinophils into the asthmatic airways caused by interleukin 5. Am J Respir Cell Mol Biol 1997; 16:220–224.

196. Larbi KY, Allen AR, Tam FW, Haskard DO, Lobb RR, Silva PM, et al. VCAM-1 has a tissue-specific role in mediating interleukin-4-induced eosinophil accumulation in rat models: evidence for a dissociation between endothelial-cell VCAM-1 expression and a functional role in eosinophil migration. Blood 2000; 96:3601–3609.

197. Li L, Xia Y, Nguyen A, Lai YH, Feng L, Mosmann TR, et al. Effects of Th2 cytokines on chemokine expression in the lung: IL-13 potently induces eotaxin expression by airway epithelial cells. J Immunol 1999; 162:2477–2487.

198. Shi HZ, Deng JM, Xu H, Nong ZX, Xiao CQ, Liu ZM, et al. Effects of inhaled interleukin-4 on airway hyperreactivity in asthmatics. Am J Respir Crit Care Med 1998; 157:1818–1821.

199. Foster PS, Hogan SP, Ramsay AJ, Matthaei KI, Young IG. Interleukin 5 deficiency abolishes eosinophilia, airways hyperreactivity, and lung damage in a mouse asthma model. J Exp Med 1996; 183:195–201.

200. Chand N, Harrison JE, Rooney S, Pillar J, Jakubicki R, Nolan K, et al. Anti-IL-5 monoclonal antibody inhibits allergic late phase bronchial eosinophilia in guinea pigs: a therapeutic approach. Eur J Pharmacol 1992; 211:121–123.

201. Mauser PJ, Pitman A, Witt A, Fernandez X, Zurcher J, Kung T, et al. Inhibitory effect of the TRFK-5 anti-IL-5 antibody in a guinea pig model of asthma. Am Rev Respir Dis 1993; 148:1623–1627.

202. Yagi T, Sato A, Hayakawa H, Ide K. Failure of aged rats to accumulate eosinophils in allergic inflammation of the airway. J Allergy Clin Immunol 1997; 99:38–47.

203. Egan RW, Athwahl D, Chou CC, Chapman RW, Emtage S, Jenh CH, et al. Pulmonary biology of anti-interleukin 5 antibodies. Mem Inst Oswaldo Cruz 1997; 92 Suppl 2:69–73.

204. Mauser PJ, Pitman AM, Fernandez X, Foran SK, Adams GK3, Kreutner W, et al. Effects of an antibody to interleukin-5 in a monkey model of asthma. Am J Respir Crit Care Med 1995; 152:467–472.

205. Brusselle G, Kips J, Joos G, Bluthmann H, Pauwels R. Allergen-induced airway inflammation and bronchial responsiveness in wild-type and interleukin-4-deficient mice. Am J Respir Cell Mol Biol 1995; 12:254–259.

206. Corry DB, Folkesson HG, Warnock ML, Erle DJ, Matthay MA, J.P., et al. Interleukin 4, but not interleukin 5 or eosinophils, is required in a murine model of acute airway hyperreactivity. J Exp Med 1996; 183:109–117.

207. Hogan SP, Foster PS. Cellular and molecular mechanisms involved in the regulation of eosinophil trafficking in vivo. Med Res Rev 1996; 16:407–432.

208. Hubscher T. Role of the eosinophil in the allergic reactions. II. Release of prostaglandins from human eosinophilic leukocytes. J Immunol 1975; 114:1389–1393.

209. Buijs J, Egbers MW, Nijkamp FP. *Toxocara canis*-induced airway eosinophilia and tracheal hyporeactivity in guinea pigs and mice. Eur J Pharmacol 1995; 293:207–215.

210. Bandeira-Melo C, Cordeiro RS, Silva PM, Martins MA. Modulatory role of eosinophils in allergic inflammation: new evidence for a rather outdated concept. Mem Inst Oswaldo Cruz 1997; 92 Suppl 2:37–43.

211. Bandeira-Melo C, Silva PM, Cordeiro RS, Martins MA. Pleural fluid eosinophils suppress local IgE-mediated protein exudation in rats. J Leukoc Biol 1995; 58:395–402.

212. Bandeira-Melo C, Singh Y, Cordeiro RS, Silva PM, Martins MA. Involvement of prostaglandins in the down-regulation of allergic plasma leakage observed in rats undergoing pleural eosinophilia. Br J Pharmacol 1996; 118:2192–2198.

213. Bandeira-Melo C, Bozza PT, Diaz BL, Cordeiro RS, Jose PJ, Martins MA, et al. Cutting edge: lipoxin (LX) A4 and aspirin-triggered 15-epi-LXA4 block allergen-induced eosinophil trafficking. J Immunol 2000; 164:2267–2271.

214. Bandeira-Melo C, Serra MF, Diaz BL, Cordeiro RS, Silva PM, Lenzi HL, et al. Cyclooxygenase-2-derived prostaglandin E2 and lipoxin A4 accelerate resolution of allergic edema in *Angiostrongylus costaricensis*–infected rats: relationship with concurrent eosinophilia. J Immunol 2000; 164:1029–1036.

215. Lee TH, Crea AE, Gant V, Spur BW, Marron BE, Nicolaou KC, et al. Identification of lipoxin A4 and its relationship to the sulfidopeptide leukotrienes C4, D4, and E4 in the bronchoalveolar lavage fluids obtained from patients with selected pulmonary diseases. Am Rev Respir Dis 1990; 141:1453–1458.

216. Christie PE, Hawksworth R, Spur BW, Lee TH. Effect of indomethacin on leukotriene 4-induced histamine hyperresponsiveness in asthmatic subjects. Am Rev Respir Dis 1992; 146:1506–1510.

217. Leckie MJ, ten Brinke A, Khan J, Diamant Z, O'Connor BJ, Walls CM, et al. Effects of an interleukin-5 blocking monoclonal antibody on eosinophils, airway hyperresponsiveness, and the late asthmatic response. Lancet 2000; 356:2144–2148.

218. Cheever AW, Xu YH, Sher A, Macedonia JG. Analysis of egg granuloma formation in Schistosoma japonicum-infected mice treated with antibodies to interleukin-5 and gamma interferon. Infect Immun 1991; 59:4071–4074.

219. Sasaki O, Sugaya H, Ishida K, Yoshimura K. Ablation of eosinophils with anti-IL-5 antibody enhances the survival of intracranial worms of *Angiostrongylus cantonensis* in the mouse. Parasite Immunol 1993; 15:349–354.

220. Takamoto M, Ovington KS, Behm CA, Sugane K, Young IG, Matthaei KI. Eosinophilia, parasite burden and lung damage in *Toxocara canis* infection in C57Bl/6 mice genetically deficient in IL-5. Immunology 1997; 90:511–517.

221. Vallance BA, Blennerhassett PA, Deng Y, Matthaei KI, Young IG, Collins SM. IL-5 contributes to worm expulsion and muscle hypercontractility in a primary *T. spiralis* infection. Am J Physiol 1999; 277:G400–G408.

222. Hogarth PJ, Taylor MJ, Bianco AE. IL-5-dependent immunity to microfilariae is independent of IL-4 in a mouse model of onchocerciasis. J Immunol 1998; 160:5436–5440.

223. Dent LA, Strath M, Mellor AL, Sanderson CJ. Eosinophilia in transgenic mice expressing interleukin 5. J Exp Med 1990; 172:1425–1431.

224. Sugane K, Kusama Y, Takamoto M, Tominaga A, Takatsu K. Eosinophilia, IL-5 level and recovery of larvae in IL-5 transgenic mice infected with *Toxocara canis*. J Helminthol 1996; 70:153–158.

7

Immune Functions of Airway Epithelium

SUNDEEP S. SALVI and STEPHEN T. HOLGATE

University of Southampton
Southampton, England

I. Introduction

On a daily basis, epithelial cells that line the mucosal surface of the human airways are exposed to around 10,000 liters of air, which consists of a complex mixture of gases, particulates, dust, bacteria, viruses, allergens, and other toxic substances. In addition to providing a tight physical barrier, thereby preventing the entry of harmful substances, airway epithelial cells play an integral role in the airway defense mechanisms via their mucociliary action and secretion of a wide array of mediators. Recently, substantial evidence has emerged indicating that airway epithelial cells also serve as an important part of the local immune system. They have the capacity to act as phagocytic as well as antigen-presenting cells and produce and release a wide range of biologically active compounds, including lipid mediators, peptides, reactive oxygen species, growth factors, cytokines, and chemokines, which have an important role not only in normal physiological processes but also in the initiation and progression of various airway inflammatory disorders. Airway epithelial cells are also believed to have a crucial role in airway remodeling by secreting various growth factors that drive smooth muscle, vascular, and neuronal proliferation and deposition of matrix including collagen. This chapter describes our current understanding of the immune functions of the airway epithelium and its role in the pathogenesis of asthma.

II. Phagocytic Function of Airway Epithelial Cells

Airway epithelial cells possess phagocytic functions as demonstrated by phagocytosis of different particulate substances (1), surfactant (2), iron oxide aerosols (3), carbon particles (4), nickel dust (5), asbestos chrysotile fibers (6,7),

189

and titanium dioxide (8,9). More recently, airway epithelial cells have been shown to actively phagocytose diesel particles (10) as well as ultrafine particles in vitro (8), an effect mediated by extension of pseudopods and actin assembly.

It has been recently demonstrated that human small airway epithelial cells are capable of recognizing and ingesting apoptotic eosinophils, an effect that is enhanced by stimulation with the proinflammatory cytokines inter-leukin-1α (IL-1α) and tumor necrosis factor-α (TNF-α) (11). The membrane receptors involved in epithelial cell recognition of apoptotic eosinophils appear similar to those reported for human macrophages. These observations suggest that airway epithelial cells might be active participants in the removal of apop-totic eosinophils and may therefore have an important role in the resolution of eosinophilic inflammation in the asthmatic lung.

III. Epithelial Cells as Antigen-Presenting Cells

Being the primary interface for inhaled antigenic material, the respiratory epi-thelium has a key part in the interaction between the lung and the external environment. Experimental studies have suggested that epithelial cells can act as nonprofessional antigen-presenting cells when appropriate conditions are provided (12). All levels of the airway epithelial cells express functional major histocompatibility complex (MHC) class I and class II antigens (12–14). The levels of expression of these molecules are low at baseline but can be rapidly induced by a number of inflammatory stimuli, including cytokines (15,16), allergens (17), and heat-shock proteins (18). Interferon-γ (IFN-γ) has been shown to up-regulate the expression of MHC class II molecules (19), while IFN-β increases the expression of MHC class I molecules on airway epithelial cells (20), thereby increasing the ability of epithelial cells to present intact protein antigens to specifically sensitized T cells. Following viral infections, airway epithelial cells up-regulate the expression of costimulatory molecules B7-1 (CD80) and B7-2 (CD86) on the cell surface (21) and thereby enhance antigen presentation to T cells. Type II alveolar epithelial cells have also been shown to express the costimulatory sign molecules (HLA-DR, CD54, CD58, CD80, and CD86) and are able to deliver costimulatory signals for T cells, an effect that is under the inhibitory control of endogenously released transforming growth factor-β (TGF-β) (22).

IV. Antimicrobial Activity of Airway Epithelial Cells

The respiratory epithelium helps maintain an effective antimicrobial environ-ment to prevent colonization by microorganisms from inspired air. In addition to the barrier function, secretion of mucus and the mucociliary escalator, epi-thelial cells also respond to the presence of microbes by the induction of two complementary parts of an innate immune response. The first response is the increased production of antimicrobial agents, and the second is the induction of a signal network to recruit phagocytic cells to contain the infection.

Airway epithelial cells produce β-defensins, a class of homologous antibiotic peptides that keep the mucosal surfaces free from infection (23). Tracheal antimicrobial peptide (TAP), a 38-amino-acid peptide with broad-spectrum antimicrobial activity, was the first described β-defensin (24). The *TAP* gene has been shown to be expressed in the ciliated airway epithelial cells (25) at baseline, and its expression level are dramatically increased following experimentally induced bacterial infection (26). In vitro incubation of bovine tracheal epithelial cells with heat-killed bacteria or bacterial lipopolysaccharide (LPS) has also been shown to markedly increase TAP mRNA levels (27). This response is mediated by CD14, a well-characterized mammalian coreceptor for LPS. Although initially characterized as a cell surface marker for cells of the monocyte/macrophage lineages, CD14 is also expressed by epithelial cells (28), and likely provides these cells with the capacity to detect and respond to bacteria at their luminal surface. Airway epithelial cells, therefore, have the cellular machinery to autonomously detect bacteria and respond by mounting a direct antimicrobial action (28). Inflammatory mediators released by epithelial cells further induce the expression of antimicrobial agents. The result is effective prevention of microbial colonization (23).

Bronchial epithelial cells also provide components of the complement system, which act as opsonins allowing efficient phagocytosis by macrophages (29). C-reactive protein, an acute-phase reactant protein that activates complement and enhances opsonophagocytosis, has recently been demonstrated to be produced by human airway epithelial cells in amounts sufficient for anti-microbial effects (30). Lysozyme (31) and lactoferrin (32) produced by epithelial cells also have direct antibacterial activities. Surfactant protein A produced by airway epithelial cells acts as an opsonin, allowing for efficient phagocytosis (33). Recently, airway epithelial cells have been shown to produce IL-12p40, a protein that was originally known to be produced only by immune cells. It has potent antiviral properties and is thought to play an important role in airway mucosal immune defenses (34).

In addition to generating mediators subserving innate immune responses, epithelial cells induce a signal network that can recruit phagocytic cells to the site of infection. Infection of airway epithelial cells (A549) in vitro has been shown to activate multiple protein kinase C (PKC) isoforms, which lead to activation of MAP kinase and synthesis of cytokines, chemokines, and other inflammatory mediators (35,36) aimed at recruiting and activating phagocytic cells.

A. Role of Airway Epithelial Cells in Mucosal IgA Synthesis

Immunoglobulin A (IgA), the major immunoglobulin of the healthy respiratory tract, is probably the most important immunoglobulin for mucosal lung

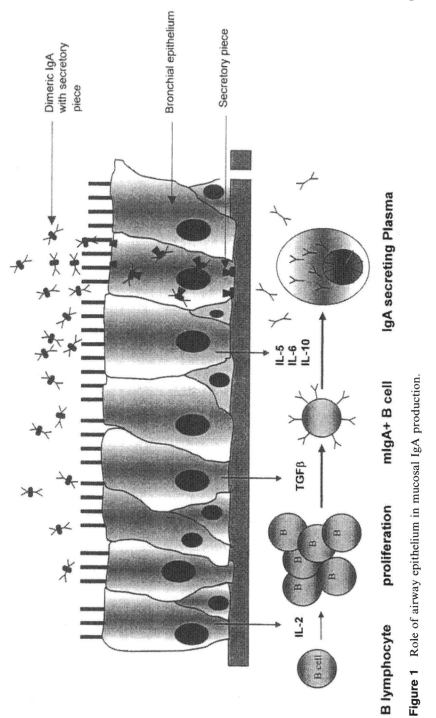

Figure 1   Role of airway epithelium in mucosal IgA production.

defense (Fig. 1). IgA present in the airway secretions binds via its carbohydrate moieties to lectin-like bacterial adhesins, thereby blocking their epithelial colonization, and provides an immune exclusion barrier against microbes, toxins, and other antigens. IgA also promotes phagocytosis by binding to Fcα receptors expressed on the surface of phagocytic cells and activates the alternative pathway of the complement system. In addition, it synergizes with non-specific antimicrobial substances in the airway secretions, and excretes antigens from subepithelial compartments across the epithelium into luminal secretions, thereby ridding the body of locally formed immune complexes and decreasing their access to the systemic circulation (37,38). Almost all of the IgA in the airway mucosa is produced locally, and it has been suggested that airway epithelial cells play an important role in airway mucosal IgA synthesis (39). Airway epithelial cells constitutively produce IL-2, TGF-β, IL-5, IL-6, and IL-10—factors that are essential for B-cell clonal proliferation (IL-2), IgA isotype switch (TGF-β), and differentiation into IgA-secreting plasma cells (IL-5, IL-6, IL-10) (39). In addition, the epithelial cells produce a glycoprotein, called secretory component, which not only confers increased stability to secretory(S)-IgA but is also quantitatively the most important receptor of the mucosal immune system because it is responsible for the external transport of locally produced polymeric IgA and IgM (40).

V. Epithelial Cells as Cellular Sources of Mediator Generation

A. Airway Epithelial Cells as Cellular Sources of Cytokines, Chemokines, and Growth Factors

Cytokines are extracellular signaling proteins, usually less than 80 kDa in size, that are involved in cell-to-cell interactions through specific receptors on the surface of target cells. They usually have an effect on closely adjacent cells and therefore function in a predominantly paracrine fashion, although they may also act in an endocrine or autocrine manner. They act on target cells to cause a wide array of cellular functions including activation, proliferation, chemotaxis, immunomodulation, release of other cytokines or mediators, growth and cell differentiation, and apoptosis (41). Airway epithelial cells have been shown to be a cellular source of a wide array of cytokines in the airways that are responsible for normal physiological processes as well as various pathological states (Fig. 2; Table 1).

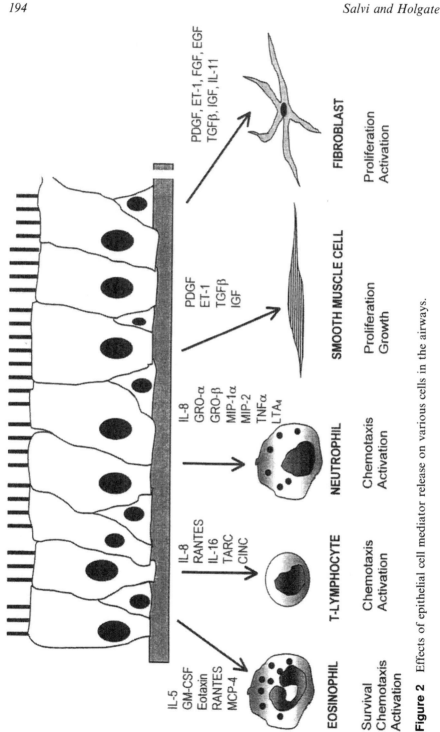

Figure 2   Effects of epithelial cell mediator release on various cells in the airways.

Table 1 Inflammatory Mediators Released by Airway Epithelial Cells

Cytokines	IL-1α, IL-1β, IL-2, IL-3, IL-5, IL-6, IL-7, IL-10, IL-11, IL-12, IL-13, IL-16, IL-18, TNF-α
Colony-stimulating factors	G-CSF, GM-CSF, M-CSF, CSF-1
Growth factors	TGF-α, TGF-β, SCF, bFGF, IGF-1, IGF-2, EGF, ET-1, amphiregulin, β-cellulin, neuregulins
Chemokines	RANTES, MCP-1, MCP-3, MCP-4, MIP-1α, MIP-2, eotaxin, Gro-α, Gro-β, Gro-γ, IP-10, Mig, I-TAC, IL-8, IL-16, TARC, CINC
Lipid mediators	15-HETE, PGE_2, $PGF_{2\alpha}$, PAF
Peptide mediators	ET-1, vasopressin, substance P, CGRP, β-defensin
Other mediators	CC16, complement factor C3, C5a, phosphodiesterase enzymes
Adhesion molecules	ICAM-1, VCAM-1, $\alpha_2\beta_6$, $\alpha_v\beta_6$
Reactive oxygen species	OH^-, O_2^-, H_2O_2
Nitric oxide	NO

Epithelial Cell–Derived Cytokines

1. **Pleiotropic cytokines**
   IL-1α (42)
   IL-1β (42)
   IL-2 (43)
   IL-3 (42)
   IL-5 (44)
   IL-6 (45)
   IL-7 (42)
   IL-10 (46)
   IL-11 (47)
   IL-12 (34)
   IL-13 (mRNA) (48)
   IL-16 (49)
   IL-18 (50)
   TNF-α (51)
2. **Colony-stimulating factors**
   G-CSF (42)
   GM-CSF (42)
   M-CSF (52)
   CSF-1 (53)
3. **Growth factors**
   TGF-α (54)
   TGF-β (55)
   Stem cell factor (SCF) (56)

       Basic fibroblast growth factor (bFGF) (57)
       Insulin-like growth factor (IGF) (58)
4. **Chemoattractant cytokines C-C**
       RANTES (59)
       Monocyte chemotactic protein-1 (60)
       Monocyte chemotactic protein-3 (61)
       Monocyte chemoattractant protein-4 (62)
       Macrophage inflammatory protein-1α (63)
       Macrophage inflammatory protein-2 (64)
       Eotaxin (65)
       Eotaxin-1 (61)
       Eotaxin-2 (61)
5. **C-X-C**
       IL-8
       Growth-related oncogene-α (60)
       Growth-related oncogene-β (60)
       Growth-related oncogene-γ (60)
       Interferon-induced protein of 10 kDa (IP-10) (66)
       Monokine induced by IFN-γ (Mig) (66)
       IFN-inducible T-cell α chemoattractant (I-TAC) (66)
6. **Lymphocyte chemoattractant factor**
       IL-16 (67)
       Thymus- and activation-regulated chemokine (TARC) (68)
       Cytokine-induced neutrophil chemoattractant-2 (CINC-2) (69)

B. Epithelial Cells as Sources of Lipid Mediators

The impressive capacity of lung cells to release arachidonic acid from membrane phospholipid stores via the actions of phospholipases, both constitutively and in response to a variety of biological or mechanical stimuli, has been recognized for more than three decades (70). Once released, the free arachidonic acid is available for oxidation along one of three major metabolic pathways: (1) the lipoxygenase pathway, which produces the leukotrienes, midchain hydroxyeicosatetraenoic acids (HETEs), and lipoxins; (2) the cyclo-oxygenase pathway, which produces the prostaglandins; and (3) the cytochrome P-450 mono-oxygenase pathway, which produces midchain and ω-terminal HETEs and *cis*-epoxyeicosatrienoic acids (EETs) (71,72).

    Animal and human studies have shown that epithelial cells contain abundant stores of fatty acid substrates, produced via phospholipase activity, and produce high levels of lipoxygenase and cyclo-oxygenase activity. Human airway epithelial cells have the ability to convert arachidonic acid to a range of lipid mediators involved in immune responses as well as local physiological responses (73). The 15-lipoxygenase pathway present in epithelial cells predominates and converts arachidonic acid to 15-HETE and a broad range of biologically active hydroperoxy, epoxyhydroxy, keto, and dihydroxy acids (74–77). Human airway epithelial cells also express 5-lipoxygenase, 12-lipoxygenase, LTA_4 hydrolase, and 5-lipoxygenase activating protein (FLAP) (78–80), and may, therefore, have an important role in metabolizing arachidonic acid through the lipoxygenase pathway.

Prostanoids have a crucial role as endogenous mediators participating in inflammation and immune responses. Cyclo-oxygenase (COX), the enzyme responsible for converting arachidonic acid to prostanoids, exists in two iso-forms: COX-1 and COX-2. Human bronchial epithelial cells express both COX-1 and COX-2 isoenzymes under basal conditions, and the expression of COX-2 is further enhanced by TNF-α, IL-1β, and bradykinin (81). There is a considerable predominance of COX-1 in epithelial cells, and basal levels of COX-2 are higher than in human airway smooth muscle cells and fibroblasts (81). Prostaglandin E_2 (PGE_2) and $PGF_{2\alpha}$ are the major COX products made by epithelial cells (82). PGE_2 has a $3',5'$-cyclic AMP-dependent bronchodilator and anti-inflammatory role, and increases synthesis and release of IL-6 (83), whereas $PGF_{2\alpha}$ is pro-inflammatory prostanoid. Production of COX metabolites by airway epithelial cells is believed to play an important part in the regulation of immune responses (84). Although the lipoxygenase pathway often predominates in epithelial cells, the preferred route of metabolism depends on the available arachidonic acid concentrations because maximal cyclo-oxygenase activity occurs at lower sub-strate concentrations than for lipoxygenases.

Airway epithelial cells also express cytochrome P-450 monoxygenase enzymes with the capacity to metabolize arachidonic acid into a series of regiospecific and stereospecific fatty acid oxides and alcohols that affect pul-monary vascular and bronchial smooth muscle tone as well as epithelial ion transport (85).

Moreover, human bronchial epithelial cells also synthesize and release platelet-activating factor (PAF) (86), a potent proinflammatory mediator that increases vascular permeability and helps in the recruitment of neutrophils and eosinophils. Human airway epithelial cells have a functional receptor for PAF (87), stimulation of which activates the cyclo-oxygenase and lipoxygenase pathway to generate prostanoids and 15-HETE (88,89).

C. Epithelial Cells as Sources of Peptide Mediators

Airway epithelial cells are a source of various peptide mediators, including endothelins (ET), vasopressin, substance P, calcitonin gene–related peptide (CGRP), and β-defensins (90). Among these the endothelin family has been best characterized (91). Epithelial cells produce low levels of ET-1 at baseline. However, stimulation with allergens (92), thrombin, LPS, phorbol ester and phorbol 12-myristate-13-acetate (PMA) (93), and infection with respiratory syncytial viruses (94) have been shown to enhance ET-1 synthesis and release. Endothelins are potent bronchoconstrictors, stimulate mucus production, mediate smooth muscle proliferation, and serve as an autocrine regulatory factor capable of stimulating release of lipid mediators from the epithelium (82).

D. Epithelial Cells as Sources of Other Mediators

Clara cell protein (CC16) is one of the most abundant respiratory tract–derived proteins (5–10% of the total proteins recovered from bronchial lavage fluid). It is constitutively secreted by nonciliated airway epithelial cells, mainly bronchiolar Clara cells and probably by other nonciliated columnar epithelial cells as demonstrated by in situ hybridization. Putative roles for CC16 include an anti-inflammatory effect mediated by the inhibition of phospholipase A_2 and detoxification of xenobiotics (95).

Airway epithelial cells are also an important source of growth factors that can mediate airway fibrosis during the progression of diseases such as asthma and chronic obstructive pulmonary disease (COPD). Insulin-like growth factor-2 (IGF-2), epidermal growth factor (EGF), heparin-binding epidermal-like growth factor (HB-EGF), and fibroblast growth factor-2 (FGF-2), which promote fibroblast proliferation and growth, have been shown to be produced and released by human airway epithelial cells (96,97). TGF-β_1 released by epithelial cells following damage is believed to induce collagen synthesis and contribute to subepithelial fibrosis.

Human airway epithelial cells express group X and group V secretory phospholipases A_2, enzymes that contribute to inflammatory injury in human lung by mechanisms including eicosanoid production and hydrolytic damage to surfactant phospholipids (98). Airway epithelial cells have also been shown to express GPI (glycosylphosphatidylinositol)–linked proteins of the RT6 superfamily (ART1, ART3, and ART4), which contribute to airway inflammatory responses (99).

When stimulated with IL-1β and TNF-α, human bronchial epithelial cells have been shown to produce the complement factor C3 (100). In addition, epithelial cells constitutively express receptors for C5a (C5aR, CD88), stimulation of which increases IL-8 synthesis (101). Airway epithelial cells express CD40, a member of the TNF-α family, which includes the TNF receptor, nerve growth factor (N6F), and Fas. Engagement of epithelial CD40 induces a significant increase in the expression of chemokines RANTES, MCP-1, IL-8, and the intracellular adhesion molecule ICAM-1 (102). Epithelial cells have recently been shown to express protease activated receptor (PAR)-1, PAR-2, and PAR-4 receptors, ligands for tryptase (103). However, their functional role remains to be determined. Expression of high- as well as low-affinity IgE receptor (CD23) has been described in bronchial epithelial cells of asthmatic patients, but not of healthy controls (104,105). Stimulation of bronchial epithelial cells of asthmatics with IgE has been shown to be associated with increased release of ET-1, suggesting that bronchial epithelial cells of asthmatic subjects may be directly activated with IgE-dependent mechanisms.

Cultured human bronchial epithelial cells express glucocorticoid receptors (106), suggesting that airway epithelial cells may be an actual target for inhaled glucocorticoid therapy. Moreover, columnar and basal epithelial cells of intact human lung tissue express cell surface Fas (CD95) and FasL (CD95L) (107). Ligation of Fas receptor can lead to induction of apoptosis. Expression of these molecules by airway epithelial cells may play an important role in the regulation of airway inflammation (108) by reducing the generation of inflammatory mediators.

Phosphodiesterases are enzymes that degrade intracellular levels of cAMP (*i*cAMP) and cGMP. Among the seven different isotypes of phosphodiesterase enzymes identified so far, human airway epithelial cells have been shown to express PDE-1, PDE-4 (alternatively spliced variants: 4A5, 4C1, 4D1, 4D2, 4D3), PDE-5, and PDE-7 isoenzymes (109). PDE-4 appears to be the major cAMP-degrading pathway, whereas PDE-1 and PDE-5 are responsible for the metabolism of cGMP. Increased levels of *i*cAMP are generally associated with anti-inflammatory properties; hence, degradation of cAMP by these phosphodiesterase enzymes could play an important proinflammatory role.

Expression of Adhesion Molecules by Epithelial Cells

Epithelial cells lining the airways express cell surface adhesion molecule receptors (110). These are glycoproteins that mediate the contact between two cells or between the cell and the components of the extracellular matrix (ECM). Intercellular ICAM-1 is constitutively expressed by bronchial and type I alveolar epithelial cells and during inflammation ICAM-1 has been reported to be induced in type 2 alveolar epithelial cells (111,112). Constitutive expression of ICAM-1 on bronchial and alveolar epithelial cells may contribute to the transmigration of macrophages, neutrophils, and lymphocytes from the submucosa into the airway lining fluid, but may also be involved in the retention of inflammatory cells at the site of inflammation, thereby promoting cytokine cellular host defense mechanisms that result in damage to the airway epithelium. Overexpression of ICAM-1 in airway epithelial cells may cause activation of alveolar macrophages, neutrophils, and eosinophils and thereby further amplify the inflammatory responses.

Human bronchial epithelial cells express molecules of the integrin family, mainly $\alpha_2\beta_6$, and $\alpha_v\beta_6$ integrins (113–115). The epithelial expression of these adhesion molecules is increased after epithelial injury and inflammation (116). Studies using transgenic mice indicate that $\alpha_v\beta_6$ may be involved in the downregulation of airway inflammation (116).

E. Epithelial Cells as Sources of Reactive Oxygen Species

Reactive oxygen species (ROS) have traditionally been believed to be produced by macrophages, eosinophils, and neutrophils. Epithelial cells are also an important cellular source of ROS. Bovine tracheal and bronchial epithelial cells have been shown to release hydrogen peroxide at baseline as well as after stimulation with PAF and TNF-α (117). Although the amount generated is small in comparison with that derived from macrophages, when taken as a whole, the epithelial cells lining the entire respiratory tract could be a significant source of reactive oxygen molecules. Ozone exposure has been shown to generate hydroxyl radicals from guinea pig airway epithelial cells (118). Reactive oxygen species have been shown to alter the expression and activation of oxidant-regulated transcription factors, such as NFκB and AP-1, many of which are involved in regulating the expression of proinflammatory cytokines and adhesion molecules (119,120).

Nitric oxide is a highly reactive compound with multiple roles in immune effector mechanisms. It is produced from L-arginine by a small group of specific nitric oxide synthase (NOS) enzymes. The inducible form of NOS has been localized to airway epithelium (121,122). Release of nitric oxide from airway epithelium occurs following exposure to various cytokines, endotoxins (123,124), and viral infections (125,126). Nitric oxide regulates mucus secretion as well as ciliary activity in airway epithelial cells, and also plays an important role in modulating immune responses, both as a proinflammatory and an anti-inflammatory agent (127,128).

F. Epithelial Cells as Sources of Antioxidants

The airway epithelium is constantly exposed to an oxidant-rich environment. Airway epithelial cells have been shown to possess both intracellular and extracellular antioxidant activities. The major intracellular antioxidant systems present in the airway epithelial cells are the glutathione redox cycle, superoxide dismutase, and catalase (129). Superoxide dismutase reduces the superoxide radical to H_2O_2 and catalase reduces H_2O_2 to water. The glutathione redox system maintains a high ratio of reduced glutathione to oxidized glutathione, which reduces intracellular hydroperoxides, lipid peroxides, as well as products of lipoxygenase-catalyzed reactions. Exposure of epithelial cells to oxidant stress leads to up-regulation of intracellular antioxidant mechanisms (129).

The extracellular epithelial lining fluid is rich in antioxidant activities. Although much of the antioxidant activity is derived from the serum, epithelial cells also release substances with specific antioxidant activities. Prominent among these are lactoferrin, transferrin, ferritin, glutathione, vitamin A, vitamin C, vitamin E, uric acid, and albumin. Human airway epithelial cells are also a cellular source for extracellular glutathione peroxidase, a critical first-line antioxidant defense on the airway epithelium surface (130). Recent data suggest a role for surfactant apoprotein-A (SP-A), produced by epithelial cells as an antioxidant in the lower respiratory tract (131). At physiologically relevant concentrations, SP-A has been found to inhibit superoxide production by alveolar macrophages stimulated by PMA or zymosan-activated serum.

VI. Epithelial Cells as Regulators of Airway Inflammation

Airway epithelial cells represent the first structural airway cell exposed to environmental factors in the inspired air. In the past two decades, the classical view that the epithelium is merely a physical barrier between the lung and the environment has been rapidly replaced by a more complex description in which epithelial cells act as central modulators of the inflammatory cascade.

In addition to performing nonspecific phagocytic functions, epithelial cells also have the potential to act as antigen-presenting cells. They express functional MHC class I and II molecules at all levels in the airways, and these molecules can be further rapidly up-regulated by a number of inflammatory stimuli, including cytokines, allergens, and heat-shock proteins. In addition, they also express several costimulatory molecules on activation and thereby enhance antigen presentation and activation of specifically sensitized T cells. IL-2 production by airway epithelial cells may further stimulate local T-cell proliferation and activation.

A. Role of Epithelial Cells in the Recruitment of Inflammatory Cells

Recruitment of inflammatory cells into the airways is dependent upon the presence of chemoattractants. Epithelial cells can synthesize and release a wide range of such chemoattractants, including arachidonic acid metabolites (15-HETE—neutrophils; LTB_4—neutrophils), chemokines (IL-8—neutrophils, basophils, lymphocytes; GRO-α—neutrophils; GRO-γ—neutrophils; MCP-1—monocytes, eosinophils, basophils; eotaxin—eosinophils, RANTES—T cells, monocytes, eosinophils, basophils; MIP-1—monocytes, lymphocytes, basophils; MIP-2—neutrophils; MCP-4—eosinophils; IL-16—T cells and eosinophils; IL-5—eosinophils; CINC—leukocytes). More recently, airway epithelial cells have been shown to be a cellular source of thymus- and activation- regulated chemokine (TARC), a Th2-specific CC chemokine, and may therefore play an important role in the specific recruitment of Th2 cells into the airways. Production of these chemoattractants by airway epithelial cells may therefore have an important function in the recruitment of inflammatory cells into the airways.

B. Expression of Adhesion Molecules by Epithelial Cells

Airway epithelial cells interact with other cells by direct contact mediated via surface membrane-bound molecules. Bronchial and alveolar type 1 airway epithelial cells express the adhesion molecule ICAM-1 at baseline. This likely helps in the transmigration of leukocytes from the blood into the airway-lining surface. Following stimulation with allergens, viruses, and cytokines, the expression of ICAM-1 on epithelial cells is further up-regulated, and this is believed to play an important role in the recruitment, localization, and activation of various leukocytes, including neutrophils, eosinophils, and lymphocytes. Epithelial expression of integrins $\alpha_v\beta_6$ has been also shown to help regulate inflammatory responses. More recently, human alveolar airway epithelial cells have been shown to express vascular cell adhesion molecule-1 (VCAM-1) following viral infection (132). VCAM-1 is an adhesion molecule that is specifically involved in the recruitment and activation of eosinophils.

C. Synthesis and Release of Pleiotropic Cytokines

Epithelial cells release various maturation and cell survival enhancing factors that may further promote inflammatory processes. Studies with conditioned medium from cultures of human bronchial epithelial cells have been shown to markedly enhance the survival of neutrophils, macrophages, and eosinophils (52,133,134). Release of growth factors from epithelial cells has also been shown to induce monocytic (135) and mast cell (136) differentiation. IL-5, RANTES, granulocyte-macrophage colony-stimulating factor (GM-CSF), and eotaxin synthesized and released by airway epithelial cells are believed to contribute to eosinophil growth, survival, and activation in the airway mucosa. IL-8 released by epithelial cells is not only a potent chemoattractant for neutrophils and lymphocytes; it also activates neutrophils and basophils to release various proinflammatory mediators. TNF-α release by airway epithelial cells contributes to epithelial, leukocyte, and endothelial expression of adhesion molecules, generation of ROS, and activation of leukocytes and macrophages. IL-1α and IL-1β possess proinflammatory as well as anti-inflammatory activities. GM-CSF released by epithelial cells can induce the expression of adhesion molecules on epithelial cells and can further prime granulocytes to release increased amounts of mediators of stimulation (137). GM-CSF is also an important cytokine for the differentiation and function of dendritic cells (138), and increased local production of GM-CSF has been shown to be responsible for the accumulation and differentiation of dendritic cells in patients with diffuse panbronchiolitis (139).

Surfactant synthesized by airway epithelial cells also can modulate inflammatory cell activity. Studies with whole surfactant have demonstrated inhibition of lymphocyte activities, including natural killer cells activity, proliferation, and immunoglobulin synthesis (140–142). The lymphocyte suppressor activities of surfactant have been isolated to the lipid fraction of the surfactant (141). In contrast, SP-A has macrophage-enhancing effects (143). It enhances macrophage migration (144), opsonophagocytosis (145), and intracellular killing of *Staphylococcus aureus* (146).

Experimental evidence therefore suggests that airway epithelial cells interact with inflammatory cells via a number of mechanisms. Airway epithelial cells recruit inflammatory cells to the airways via the release of chemoattractants, to direct inflammatory cell migration across the epithelium via the expression of cell surface molecules, and to regulate inflammatory cell activity via the release of chemokines, growth factors, and cytokines. Each of these steps amplifies the inflammatory response, establishing the importance of airway epithelial cells for the modulation of airway inflammatory diseases (90).

VII. Anti-Inflammatory Role of Airway Epithelium

Besides the potential of human airway epithelial cells to recruit and activate leukocytes or parenchymal cells, airway epithelial cells may also down-regulate inflammatory responses (Table 2). This occurs via the release of anti-inflammatory mediators, the release of soluble receptors, and the inactivation of pro-inflammatory mediators.

Airway epithelial cells release IL-1α and IL-1β, which are both pro-inflammatory mediators. They act through stimulation of IL-1 receptors present on the plasma membrane. The extracellular portions of both receptors may be shed from the plasma membrane and act as IL-1 inhibitors (147). It has been shown that human bronchial epithelial cells are able to produce and release the extracellular portions of the IL-1 receptor, which may counteract the pro-inflammatory effects of IL-1α and IL-1β (148,149). Airway epithelial cells have also been shown to release the IL-6 receptor and the p55-soluble TNF-α receptor, which may down-regulate the effects of IL-6 and TNF-α, respectively (150,151).

Active TGF-β secreted by airway epithelial cells has many anti-inflammatory properties, including inhibition of IL-2-dependent proliferation of T lymphocytes, inhibition of cytokine production by macrophages, and inhibition of IL-4-induced IL-8 release by human bronchial epithelial cells (152,153). PGE$_2$ and IL-6 produced by bronchial epithelial cells have both pro- and anti-inflammatory properties. PGE$_2$, however, is a potent anti-inflammatory mediator (154) and can both reduce the production of neutrophil chemoattractants by macrophages and inhibit fibroblast matrix production (155), whereas IL-6 has been shown to reduce inflammatory reactions in several models of in vivo pulmonary inflammation (152). IL-10, which is produced

Table 2 Anti-Inflammatory Mediators Released by Airway Epithelial Cells

Cytokines	Soluble IL-1 receptor, soluble IL-6 receptor, soluble TNF-α receptor, IL-6, IL-10, TGF-β
Lipid mediators	PGE$_2$
Other mediators	Nitric oxide, histamine *N*-methyltransferase
Antioxidants	Glutathione, superoxide dismutase, catalase, lactoferrin, transferrin, ferritin, surfactant protein A

constitutively by airway epithelial cells (46), is a potent regulatory cytokine that decreases inflammatory responses and T-cell activation (156,157).

Epithelial cells express the inducible form of NOS and produce nitric oxide from L-arginine. The levels of nitric oxide are greatly increased during airway inflammatory responses, and this is implicated in both proinflammatory and anti-inflammatory processes in the lung. Nitric oxide has been shown to decrease inflammatory cytokine production, including that of IL-1β, TNF-α, and MIP-1α. In vitro studies with alveolar macrophages have demonstrated that nitric oxide suppresses NFκB activation by LPS in a dose-dependent manner (158). Nitric oxide has also been shown to decrease cytokine-induced endothelial cell activation and expression of adhesion molecules and pro-inflammatory cytokines (159).

Airway epithelial cells also express several enzymes that can degrade and thereby often inactivate a variety of mediators, including neuropeptides, hisa-mine, bradykinin, and cytokines. Epithelial cells express histamine N-methyl-transferase and thus are capable of modulating histamine effects (160–162).

VIII.   Role of Epithelial Cells in Asthma Pathogenesis

With the understanding that epithelial cells play an important role in regulating inflammatory and repair processes in the airways, emphasis has now shifted to airway epithelium as one of the major cell types implicated in asthma patho-genesis. The bronchial epithelium in asthma is structurally disturbed, with separation of columnar cells from their basal attachments (163,164), and there are more CD44$^+$ and EGFR$^+$ epithelial cells (165,166), reflecting increased repair activity. The shedding of epithelial cells from basal cells is believed to be due to release of eosinophil granule proteins, TNF-α, proteases, and oxygen free radicals by several cell types (167,168).

Several studies have identified an association between epithelial damage and the degree of bronchial hyperresponsiveness (163,169). This association may be caused by several mechanisms: (1) epithelial damage results in loss of the permeability barrier enabling noxious agents or allergens to directly penetrate the airway wall and reach the submucosa; (2) loss of ciliated cells results in impaired transport of mucus; (3) epithelial damage may expose nonmyelinated afferent nerve endings, and as a consequence these nerves may be more easily stimulated by inflammatory mediators or inhaled particles; (4) the epithelium secretes factors that suppress airway contraction (PGE$_2$, PGI$_2$, nitric oxide, and a putative epithelial-derived relaxing factor). Loss of these factors may con-tribute to bronchial hyperresponsiveness; (5) bronchial epithelial cells contain neutral endopeptidase, which is involved in the metabolism of a variety of pep-tides with contractile effects on smooth muscles; and (6) epithelial damage may trigger the production and release of mediators such as PGF$_{2α}$, 13-hydro-xylinoleic acid, and ET-1, which can affect airway responsiveness.

Epithelial damage caused by allergens, pollutants, and mediators released by inflammatory cells results in an altered phenotype, with the epithelium becoming a significant source of autacoid mediators, cytokines, chemokines, and growth factors with the potential to promote inflammation, fibroblast, and smooth muscle proliferation and matrix deposition (170). Epithelial cells obtained from asthmatic airways seem to be in an activated state as shown by the increased expression of membrane markers such as ICAM-1 or human leukocyte antigen-DR (HLA-DR) (14) and increased spontaneous release of inflammatory mediators (171). Primary cultures of asthmatic epithelial cells established from mucosal biopsy specimens demonstrate higher basal production of IL-8, GM-CSF, MCP-1, and RANTES and increased sensitivity to air pollutants such as diesel particles, ozone, and nitrogen dioxide (17,172,173), suggesting an intrinsic difference in the set point for the expression of certain cytokines in asthmatic epithelial cells.

In asthma the "stressed" epithelial phenotype is reflected in functional changes, with this structure becoming an important source of autacoid mediators, chemokines, and growth factors. These include oxidative arachidonic acid metabolites (PGE_2, 15-HETE, 12,15-diHETE, and 8,15-diHETE), lipoxins, nitric oxide, ET-1, fibronectin, ROS, IL-8, GRO-α, MCP-1, RANTES, eotaxin, TNF-α, IL-1β, IL-5, IL-6, oncostatin-M, IL-11, IL-10, IL-16, IL-18, GM-CSF, bFGF, TGF-β_1, TGF-β_2, IGF, PDGF, stem cell factor, IL-5, and IL-13 (17,50,67,174,175).

More recently, bronchial epithelial cells have been shown to be a source of TARC protein, a ligand for CCR4, expressed predominantly on Th2 cells (68), comparable with that reported by monocytes on a single-cell basis (176). In vitro secretion of TARC by bronchial epithelial cells strongly suggests the in vivo elaboration of a Th2-specific chemokine from the bronchial epithelium could potentially contribute to the accumulation of Th2 cells in the airways.

In asthma, epithelial cells obtained by bronchial brushings were shown to release a greater amount of 15-HETE spontaneously or after stimulation (171). 15-HETE is a biological mediator with the potential of influencing the inflammatory response. It is capable of stimulating the chemotaxis of inflammatory cells, including the release of mucus glycoprotein from human airways in culture, influencing 5-lipoxygenase activity in leukocytes and enhancing the early bronchoconstrictor response to inhaled allergen in atopic asthmatic subjects. Eosinophils coincubated with bronchial epithelial cells for 1hr have been shown to produce significantly higher quantities of leukotriene C4 (LTC4) in response to PAF (177).

Epithelial cells of asthmatics bear the FcϵRI and FcϵRII receptors (104), suggesting that they can be directly activated by anti-IgE and allergens. Addition of crude *Dermatophagoides pteronysinus* in the presence of 1.5 mM dithiothreitol (activator of cysteine protease) on epithelial cells induces a progressive increase in bioelectric conductance, an index of epithelial permeability (178).

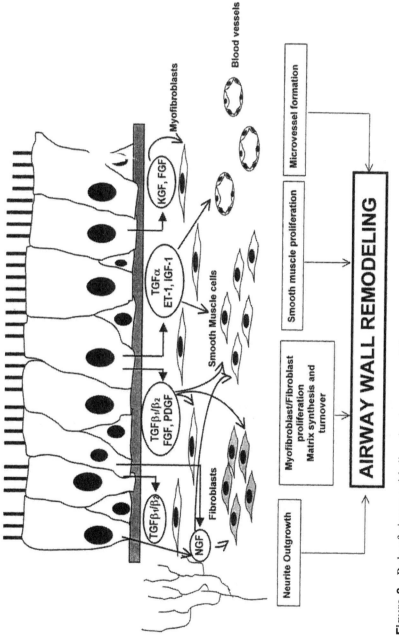

Figure 3   Role of airway epithelium in airway remodeling.

Epithelial cells of asthmatics show increased expression of ICAM-1 compared with normals (179), and blockade of ICAM-1 has been shown to attenuate asthmatic responses (110). A CD18/ICAM-1-dependent pathway mediates eosinophil adhesion to human bronchial epithelial cells (180).

IX. Role of Epithelial Cells in Airway Remodeling

Although inflammation is important in asthma pathogenesis, it is not sufficient to explain the chronic nature of the disease and its progression. Remodeling or restructuring of the airway wall is believed to account for the chronicity of the disease and the incomplete therapeutic efficacy of corticosteroids with persistence of bronchial hyperresponsiveness (181). Bronchial biopsy study in children aged 1–11 years has shown increased epithelial subbasement membrane collagen thickening as early as 4 years before asthma was clinically expressed (182). It has been suggested that the disordered epithelium observed in asthmatic airways can provide a basis for airway remodeling in asthma (170) (Fig. 3). Injury to human airway epithelial cells grown on a collagen gel seeded with human myofibroblasts in vitro results in enhanced proliferation of the mesenchymal cells due to the combined effects of bFGF, IGF, PDGF, TGF-β, and ET-1 (58) and increased collagen gene expression.

Among the growth factor receptors, the EGFR serves a central role as a primary regulator of epithelial function (183). A pivotal role of the EGFR is in controlling the behavior of the bronchial epithelium. Unlike the normal bronchial epithelium, where EGFR expression is only observed in areas of structural damage (184), the epithelium in asthmatic airways shows a striking disease-related overexpression of the EGFR both in damaged and morphologically intact epithelium, the extent of which correlates with subbasement membrane collagen thickness (165). Contrasting with normal epithelium, EGFR immunostaining in asthma occurs throughout the epithelial layer, which is indicative of widespread functional changes. It is possible that EGFR expression occurs as an early response to damage and that high levels of EGFR is a reporter of damage, and that the extent of epithelial injury is more widespread than previously appreciated (174).

The extensive deposition of interstitial collagens and other matrix proteins in the lamina reticularis in asthma in vivo is strong evidence that the epithelial-mesenchymal trophic unit is reactivated in asthma. This results in alteration of the set point for communication between the two compartments, leading to a subsequent increase in mesenchymal volume. Such a hypothesis is consistent with the increased amount of TGF-β detected in asthmatic airways (185), the low degree of epithelial proliferation in areas of epithelial damage (186), and the concomitant decrease in MMP/TIMP ratio in asthmatic airways, especially in severe disease (187). Abnormal interactions between epithelial cells and mesenchymal cells may therefore contribute to the development of collagen thickening seen in the subbasement membrane.

References

1. Greenberg SD, Gyorkey F, Jenkins DE, Gyorkey P. Phagocytosis and the granular pneumonocyte. Am Rev Respir Dis 1972;105(2):302–303.
2. Corrin B. Phagocytic potential of pulmonary alveolar epithelium with particular reference to surfactant metabolism. Thorax 1969;24:110–115.
3. Sorokin SP, Brain JD. Pathways of clearance in mouse lungs exposed to iron oxide aerosols. Anat Rec 1975;181(3):581–625.
4. Adamson IY, Bowden DH. Adaptive responses of the pulmonary macrophagic system to carbon. II. Morphologic studies. Lab Invest 1978;38(4):430–438.
5. Johansson A, Camner P, Robertson B. Effects of long-term nickel dust exposure on rabbit alveolar epithelium. Environ Res 1981;25(2):391–403.
6. Suzuki Y. Interaction of asbestos with alveolar cells. Environ Health Persp 1974;9:241–252.
7. Pinkerton KE, Pratt PC, Brody AR, Crapo JD. Fiber localization and its relationship to lung reaction in rats after chronic inhalation of chrysotile asbestos. Am J Pathol 1984;117(3):484–498.
8. Stearns RC, Paulauskis JD, Godleski JJ. Endocytosis of ultrafine particles by A549 cells. Am J Respir Cell Mol Biol 2001;24(2):108–115.
9. Churg A, Stevens B, Wright JL. Comparison of the uptake of fine and ultrafine TiO2 in a tracheal explant system. Am J Physiol 1998;274(1 Pt 1):L81–86.
10. Boland S, Baeza-Squiban A, Fournier T, Houcine O, Gendron MC, Chevrier M et al. Diesel exhaust particles are taken up by human airway epithelial cells in vitro and alter cytokine production. Am J Physiol 1999;276(4 Pt 1): L604–613.
11. Walsh GM, Sexton DW, Blaylock MG, Convery CM. Resting and cytokine-stimulated human small airway epithelial cells recognize and engulf apoptotic eosinophils. Blood 1999;94(8):2827–2835.
12. Mezzetti M, Soloperto M, Fasoli A, Mattoli S. Human bronchial epithelial cells modulate CD3 and mitogen-induced DNA synthesis in T cells but function poorly as antigen-presenting cells compared to pulmonary macrophages. J Allergy Clin Immunol 1991;87(5):930–938.
13. Vignola AM, Chanez P, Campbell AM, Bousquet J, Michel FB, Godard P. Functional and phenotypic characteristics of bronchial epithelial cells obtained by brushing from asthmatic and normal subjects. Allergy 1993;48(17):32–38; discussion 48–49.
14. Vignola AM, Campbell AM, Chanez P, Bousquet J, Paul-Lacoste P, Michel FB et al. HLA-DR and ICAM-1 expression on bronchial epithelial cells in asthma and chronic bronchitis. Am Rev Respir Dis 1993;148(3):689–694.
15. Ibrahim L, Dominguez M, Yacoub M. Primary human adult lung epithelial cells in vitro: response to interferon-gamma and cytomegalovirus. Immunology 1993;79(1):119–124.
16. Cunningham AC, Zhang JG, Moy JV, Ali S, Kirby JA. A comparison of the antigen-presenting capabilities of class II MHC- expressing human lung epithelial and endothelial cells. Immunology 1997;91(3):458–463.

17. Thompson PJ. Unique role of allergens and the epithelium in asthma. Clin Exp Allergy 1998;28 (suppl 5):110–116; discussion 117–118.

18. Bertorelli G, Bocchino V, Zhuo X, Chetta A, Del Donno M, Foresi A et al. Heat shock protein 70 upregulation is related to HLA-DR expression in bronchial asthma. Effects of inhaled glucocorticoids. Clin Exp Allergy 1998;28(5):551–560.

19. Suda T, Sato A, Sugiura W, Chida K. Induction of MHC class II antigens on rat bronchial epithelial cells by interferon-gamma and its effect on antigen presentation. Lung 1995;173(2):127–137.

20. Jamaluddin M, Wang S, Garofalo RP, Elliott T, Casola A, Baron S et al. IFN-beta mediates coordinate expression of antigen-processing genes in RSV-infected pulmonary epithelial cells. Am J Physiol Lung Cell Mol Physiol 2001;280(2):L248–L257.

21. Papi A, Stanciu LA, Papadopoulos NG, Teran LM, Holgate ST, Johnston SL. Rhinovirus infection induces major histocompatibility complex class I and costimulatory molecule upregulation on respiratory epithelial cells. J Infect Dis 2000;181(5):1780–1784.

22. Zissel G, Ernst M, Rabe K, Papadopoulos T, Magnussen H, Schlaak M et al. Human alveolar epithelial cells type II are capable of regulating T-cell activity. J Invest Med 2000;48(1):66–75.

23. Diamond G, Legarda D, Ryan LK. The innate immune response of the respiratory epithelium. Immunol Rev 2000;173:27–38.

24. Diamond G, Zasloff M, Eck H, Brasseur M, Maloy WL, Bevins CL. Tracheal antimicrobial peptide, a cysteine-rich peptide from mammalian tracheal mucosa: peptide isolation and cloning of a cDNA. Proc Natl Acad Sci USA 1991;88(9):3952–3956.

25. Diamond G, Jones DE, Bevins CL. Airway epithelial cells are the site of expression of a mammalian antimicrobial peptide gene. Proc Natl Acad Sci USA 1993;90(10):4596–4600.

26. Stolzenberg ED, Anderson GM, Ackermann MR, Whitlock RH, Zasloff M. Epithelial antibiotic induced in states of disease. Proc Natl Acad Sci USA 1997;94(16):8686–8690.

27. Diamond G, Russell JP, Bevins CL. Inducible expression of an antibiotic peptide gene in lipopolysaccharide-challenged tracheal epithelial cells. Proc Natl Acad Sci USA 1996;93(10):5156–5160.

28. Diamond G, Kaiser V, Rhodes J, Russell JP, Bevins CL. Transcriptional regulation of beta-defensin gene expression in tracheal epithelial cells. Infect Immun 2000;68(1):113–119.

29. Rothman BL, Merrow M, Bamba M, Kennedy T, Kreutzer DL. Biosynthesis of the third and fifth complement components by isolated human lung cells. Am Rev Respir Dis 1989;139(1):212–220.

30. Gould JM, Weiser JN. Expression of C-reactive protein in the human respiratory tract. Infect Immun 2001;69(3):1747–1754.

31. Ellison RT, Giehl TJ. Killing of gram-negative bacteria by lactoferrin and lysozyme. J Clin Invest 1991;88(4):1080–1091.

32. Arnold RR, Cole MF, McGhee JR. A bactericidal effect for human lactoferrin. Science 1977;197(4300):263–265.

33. Tenner AJ, Robinson SL, Borchelt J, Wright JR. Human pulmonary surfactant protein (SP-A), a protein structurally homologous to C1q, can enhance FcR- and CR1-mediated phagocytosis. J Biol Chem 1989;264(23):13923–13928.

34. Walter MJ, Kajiwara N, Karanja P, Castro M, Holtzman MJ. Interleukin 12 p40 production by barrier epithelial cells during airway inflammation. J Exp Med 2001;193(3):339–352.

35. Monick MM, Staber JM, Thomas KW, Hunninghake GW. Respiratory syncytial virus infection results in activation of multiple protein kinase C isoforms leading to activation of mitogen-activated protein kinase. J Immunol 2001;166(4):2681–2687.

36. Arnold R, Humbert B, Werchau H, Gallati H, Konig W. Interleukin-8, interleukin-6, and soluble tumour necrosis factor receptor type I release from a human pulmonary epithelial cell line (A549) exposed to respiratory syncytial virus. Immunology 1994;82(1):126–133.

37. Lamm ME. Interaction of antigens and antibodies at mucosal surfaces. Annu Rev Microbiol 1997;51:311–340.

38. Fujioka H, Emancipator SN, Aikawa M, Huang DS, Blatnik F, Karban T et al. Immunocytochemical colocalization of specific immunoglobulin A with sendai virus protein in infected polarized epithelium. J Exp Med 1998;188(7):1223–1229.

39. Salvi S, Holgate ST. Could the airway epithelium play an important role in mucosal immunoglobulin A production? Clin Exp Allergy 1999;29(12):1597–1605.

40. Brandtzaeg P, Berstad AE, Farstad IN, Haraldsen G, Helgeland L, Jahnsen FL et al. Mucosal immunity–a major adaptive defence mechanism. Behring Inst Mitt 1997(98):1–23.

41. Chung KF, Barnes PJ. Cytokines in asthma. Thorax 1999;54(9):825–857.

42. Stadnyk AW. Cytokine production by epithelial cells. FASEB J 1994;8(13):1041–1047.

43. Aoki Y, Qiu D, Uyei A, Kao PN. Human airway epithelial cells express interleukin-2 in vitro. Am J Physiol 1997;272(2 Pt 1):L276–286.

44. Salvi S, Semper A, Blomberg A, Holloway J, Jaffar Z, Papi A et al. Interleukin-5 production by human airway epithelial cells. Am J Respir Cell Mol Biol 1999;20(5):984–991.

45. Takizawa H, Ohtoshi T, Ohta K, Hirohata S, Yamaguchi M, Suzuki N et al. Interleukin 6/B cell stimulatory factor-II is expressed and released by normal and transformed human bronchial epithelial cells. Biochem Biophys Res Commun 1992;187(2):596–602.

46. Bonfield TL, Konstan MW, Burfeind P, Panuska JR, Hilliard JB, Berger M. Normal bronchial epithelial cells constitutively produce the anti-inflammatory cytokine interleukin-10, which is downregulated in cystic fibrosis. Am J Respir Cell Mol Biol 1995;13(3):257–261.

47. Minshall E, Chakir J, Laviolette M, Molet S, Zhu Z, Olivenstein R et al. IL-11 expression is increased in severe asthma: association with epithelial cells and eosinophils. J Allergy Clin Immunol 2000;105(2 Pt 1):232–238.

48. Salvi SS, Papadopoulos N, Frew AJ, Holgate ST. Rhinovirus infection upregulates IL-13 mRNA expression in human airway epithelial cells. Immunology 1999;98(1):164 (Abstract).

49. Arima M, Plitt J, Stellato C, Bickel C, Motojima S, Makino S et al. Expression of interleukin-16 by human epithelial cells. Inhibition by dexamethasone. Am J Respir Cell Mol Biol 1999;21(6):684–692.

50. Cameron LA, Taha RA, Tsicopoulos A, Kurimoto M, Olivenstein R, Wallaert B et al. Airway epithelium expresses interleukin-18. Eur Respir J 1999;14(3):553–559.

51. Devalia JL, Campbell AM, Sapsford RJ, Rusznak C, Quint D, Godard P et al. Effect of nitrogen dioxide on synthesis of inflammatory cytokines expressed by human bronchial epithelial cells in vitro. Am J Respir Cell Mol Biol 1993;9(3):271–278.

52. Xing Z, Ohtoshi T, Ralph P, Gauldie J, Jordana M. Human upper airway structural cell-derived cytokines support human peripheral blood monocyte survival: a potential mechanism for monocyte/macrophage accumulation in the tissue. Am J Respir Cell Mol Biol 1992;6(2):212–218.

53. Bedard M, McClure CD, Schiller NL, Francoeur C, Cantin A, Denis M. Release of interleukin-8, interleukin-6, and colony-stimulating factors by upper airway epithelial cells: implications for cystic fibrosis. Am J Respir Cell Mol Biol 1993;9(4):455–462.

54. Strandjord TP, Clark JG, Hodson WA, Schmidt RA, Madtes DK. Expression of transforming growth factor-alpha in mid-gestation human fetal lung. Am J Respir Cell Mol Biol 1993;8(3):266–272.

55. Sacco O, Romberger D, Rizzino A, Beckmann JD, Rennard SI, Spurzem JR. Spontaneous production of transforming growth factor-beta 2 by primary cultures of bronchial epithelial cells. Effects on cell behavior in vitro. J Clin Invest 1992;90(4):1379–1385.

56. Wen LP, Fahrni JA, Matsui S, Rosen GD. Airway epithelial cells produce stem cell factor. Biochim Biophys Acta 1996;1314(3):183–186.

57. Han RN, Liu J, Tanswell AK, Post M. Expression of basic fibroblast growth factor and receptor: immunolocalization studies in developing rat fetal lung. Pediatr Res 1992;31(5):435–440.

58. Zhang S, Smartt H, Holgate ST, Roche WR. Growth factors secreted by bronchial epithelial cells control myofibroblast proliferation: an in vitro coculture model of airway remodeling in asthma. Lab Invest 1999;79(4):395–405.

59. Stellato C, Beck LA, Gorgone GA, Proud D, Schall TJ, Ono SJ et al. Expression of the chemokine RANTES by a human bronchial epithelial cell line. Modulation by cytokines and glucocorticoids. J Immunol 1995;155(1):410–418.

60. Becker S, Quay J, Koren HS, Haskill JS. Constitutive and stimulated MCP-1, GRO alpha, beta, and gamma expression in human airway epithelium and bronchoalveolar macrophages. Am J Physiol 1994;266(3 Pt 1):L278–286.

61. Ying S, Meng Q, Zeibecoglou K, Robinson DS, Macfarlane A, Humbert M et al. Eosinophil chemotactic chemokines (eotaxin, eotaxin-2, RANTES, monocyte chemoattractant protein-3 (MCP-3), and MCP-4), and C-C chemokine receptor 3 expression in bronchial biopsies from atopic and nonatopic (Intrinsic) asthmatics. J Immunol 1999;163(11):6321–6329.

62. Stellato C, Collins P, Ponath PD, Soler D, Newman W, La Rosa G et al. Production of the novel C-C chemokine MCP-4 by airway cells and comparison of its biological activity to other C-C chemokines. J Clin Invest 1997;99(5):926–936.

63. Olszewska-Pazdrak B, Casola A, Saito T, Alam R, Crowe SE, Mei F et al. Cell-specific expression of RANTES, MCP-1, and MIP-1alpha by lower airway epithelial cells and eosinophils infected with respiratory syncytial virus. J Virol 1998;72(6):4756–4764.

64. Haeberle HA, Kuziel WA, Dieterich HJ, Casola A, Gatalica Z, Garofalo RP. Inducible expression of inflammatory chemokines in respiratory syncytial virus-infected mice: role of MIP-1alpha in lung pathology. J Virol 2001;75(2):878–890.

65. Lilly CM, Nakamura H, Kesselman H, Nagler-Anderson C, Asano K, Garcia-Zepeda EA et al. Expression of eotaxin by human lung epithelial cells: induction by cytokines and inhibition by glucocorticoids. J Clin Invest 1997;99(7): 1767–1773.

66. Sauty A, Dziejman M, Taha RA, Iarossi AS, Neote K, Garcia-Zepeda EA et al. The T cell-specific CXC chemokines IP-10, Mig, and I-TAC are expressed by activated human bronchial epithelial cells. J Immunol 1999;162(6):3549–3558.

67. Laberge S, Ernst P, Ghaffar O, Cruikshank WW, Kornfeld H, Center DM et al. Increased expression of interleukin-16 in bronchial mucosa of subjects with atopic asthma. Am J Respir Cell Mol Biol 1997;17(2):193–202.

68. Sekiya T, Miyamasu M, Imanishi M, Yamada H, Nakajima T, Yamaguchi M et al. Inducible expression of a Th2-type CC chemokine thymus- and activation-regulated chemokine by human bronchial epithelial cells. J Immunol 2000;165(4):2205–2213.

69. Amano H, Oishi K, Sonoda F, Senba M, Wada A, Nakagawa H et al. Role of cytokine-induced neutrophil chemoattractant-2 (CINC-2) alpha in a rat model of chronic bronchopulmonary infections with Pseudomonas aeruginosa. Cytokine 2000;12(11):1662–1668.

70. Hyman AL, Mathe AA, Lippton HL, Kadowitz PJ. Prostaglandins and the lung. Med Clin North Am 1981;65(4):789–808.

71. Holtzman MJ. Arachidonic acid metabolism. Implications of biological chemistry for lung function and disease. Am Rev Respir Dis 1991;143(1):188–203.

72. McGiff JC. Cytochrome P-450 metabolism of arachidonic acid. Annu Rev Pharmacol Toxicol 1991;31:339–369.

73. Holtzman MJ. Arachidonic acid metabolism in airway epithelial cells. Annu Rev Physiol 1992;54:303–329.

74. Nadel JA, Conrad DJ, Ueki IF, Schuster A, Sigal E. Immunocytochemical localization of arachidonate 15-lipoxygenase in erythrocytes, leukocytes, and airway cells. J Clin Invest 1991;87(4):1139–1145.

75. Adler KB, Akley NJ, Glasgow WC. Platelet-activating factor provokes release of mucin-like glycoproteins from guinea pig respiratory epithelial cells via a lipoxygenase-dependent mechanism. Am J Respir Cell Mol Biol 1992;6(5):550–556.

76. Sigal E, Dicharry S, Highland E, Finkbeiner WE. Cloning of human airway 15-lipoxygenase: identity to the reticulocyte enzyme and expression in epithelium. Am J Physiol 1992;262(4 Pt 1):L392–398.

77. Bradding P, Redington AE, Djukanovic R, Conrad DJ, Holgate ST. 15-Lipoxygenase immunoreactivity in normal and in asthmatic airways. Am J Respir Crit Care Med 1995;151(4):1201–1204.

78. Dixon RA, Jones RE, Diehl RE, Bennett CD, Kargman S, Rouzer CA. Cloning of the cDNA for human 5-lipoxygenase. Proc Natl Acad Sci USA 1988;85(2):416–420.
79. Hansbrough JR, Takahashi Y, Ueda N, Yamamoto S, Holtzman MJ. Identification of a novel arachidonate 12-lipoxygenase in bovine tracheal epithelial cells distinct from leukocyte and platelet forms of the enzyme. J Biol Chem 1990;265(3):1771–1776.
80. James AJ, Lackie PM, Sampson AP. The expression of leukotriene pathway enzymes in human bronchial epithelial cells. Eur Respir J 1999; 14(suppl 30):365s.
81. Petkova DK, Pang L, Range SP, Holland E, Knox AJ. Immunocytochemical localization of cyclo-oxygenase isoforms in cultured human airway structural cells. Clin Exp Allergy 1999;29(7):965–972.
82. Polito AJ, Proud D. Epithelia cells as regulators of airway inflammation. J Allergy Clin Immunol 1998;102(5):714–718.
83. Tavakoli S, Cowan MJ, Benfield T, Logun C, Shelhamer JH. Prostaglandin E(2)-induced interleukin-6 release by a human airway epithelial cell line. Am J Physiol Lung Cell Mol Physiol 2001;280(1):L127–133.
84. Watkins DN, Peroni DJ, Lenzo JC, Knight DA, Garlepp MJ, Thompson PJ. Expression and localization of COX-2 in human airways and cultured airway epithelial cells. Eur Respir J 1999;13(5):999–1007.
85. Jacobs ER, Zeldin DC. The lung HETEs (and EETs) up. Am J Physiol 2001;280(1):H1–H10.
86. Holtzman MJ, Ferdman B, Bohrer A, Turk J. Synthesis of the 1-o-hexadecyl molecular species of platelet-activating factor by airway epithelial and vascular endothelial cells. Biochem Biophys Res Commun 1991;177(1):357–364.
87. Kang JX, Man SF, Hirsh AJ, Clandinin MT. Characterization of platelet-activating factor binding to human airway epithelial cells: modulation by fatty acids and ion-channel blockers. Biochem J 1994;303(Pt 3):795–802.
88. Wu T, Rieves RD, Logun C, Shelhamer JH. Platelet-activating factor stimulates eicosanoid production in cultured feline tracheal epithelial cells. Lung 1995;173(2):89–103.
89. Lai CK, Holgate ST. Stimulation of human airway epithelial cells by platelet activating factor (PAF) and arachidonic acid produces 15-hydroxyeicosatetraenoic acid (15-HETE) capable of contracting bronchial smooth muscle. Pulm Pharmacol 1992;5(1):75–76.
90. Thompson AB, Robbins RA, Romberger DJ, Sisson JH, Spurzem JR, Teschler H et al. Immunological functions of the pulmonary epithelium. Eur Respir J 1995;8(1):127–149.
91. Aubert JD, Leuenberger P, Juillerat-Jeanneret L. Endothelin-1 expression in airway epithelial cells. Eur Respir J 1999;13(1):225–226.
92. Salmon M, Liu YC, Mak JC, Rousell J, Huang TJ, Hisada T et al. Contribution of upregulated airway endothelin-1 expression to airway smooth muscle and epithelial cell DNA synthesis after repeated allergen exposure of sensitized brown-norway rats. Am J Respir Cell Mol Biol 2000;23(5):618–625.
93. Hay DW, Van Scott MR, Muccitelli RM. Characterization of endothelin release from guinea-pig tracheal epithelium: influence of proinflammatory mediators including major basic protein. Pulm Pharmacol Ther 1997;10(4):189–198.

94. Samransamruajkit R, Gollapudi S, Kim CH, Gupta S, Nussbaum E. Modulation of endothelin-1 expression in pulmonary epithelial cell line (A549) after exposure to RSV. Int J Mol Med 2000;6(1):101–105.

95. Bernard A, Marchandise FX, Depelchin S, Lauwerys R, Sibille Y. Clara cell protein in serum and bronchoalveolar lavage. Eur Respir J 1992;5(10): 1231–1238.

96. Cambrey AD, Kwon OJ, Gray AJ, Harrison NK, Yacoub M, Barnes PJ et al. Insulin-like growth factor I is a major fibroblast mitogen produced by primary cultures of human airway epithelial cells. Clin Sci (Colch) 1995;89(6):611–617.

97. Zhang L, Rice AB, Adler K, Sannes P, Martin L, Gladwell W et al. Vanadium stimulates human bronchial epithelial cells to produce heparin-binding epidermal growth factor-like growth factor. A mitogen for lung fibroblasts. Am J Respir Cell Mol Biol 2001;24(2):123–131.

98. Seeds MC, Jones KA, Duncan Hite R, Willingham MC, Borgerink HM, Woodruff RD et al. Cell-specific expression of group X and group V secretory phospholipases A(2) in human lung airway epithelial cells. Am J Respir Cell Mol Biol 2000;23(1): 37–44.

99. Balducci E, Horiba K, Usuki J, Park M, Ferrans VJ, Moss J. Selective expression of RT6 superfamily in human bronchial epithelial cells. Am J Respir Cell Mol Biol 1999;21(3):337–346.

100. Varsano S, Kaminsky M, Kaiser M, Rashkovsky L. Generation of complement C3 and expression of cell membrane complement inhibitory proteins by human bronchial epithelium cell line. Thorax 2000;55(5):364–369.

101. Floreani AA, Heires AJ, Welniak LA, Miller-Lindholm A, Clark-Pierce L, Rennard SI et al. Expression of receptors for C5a anaphylatoxin (CD88) on human bronchial epithelial cells: enhancement of C5a-mediated release of IL-8 upon exposure to cigarette smoke. J Immunol 1998;160(10):5073–5081.

102. Propst SM, Denson R, Rothstein E, Estell K, Schwiebert LM. Proinflammatory and Th2-derived cytokines modulate CD40-mediated expression of inflammatory mediators in airway epithelia: implications for the role of epithelial CD40 in airway inflammation. J Immunol 2000;165(4):2214–2221.

103. Chow JM, Moffatt JD, Cocks TM. Effect of protease-activated receptor (PAR)-1, -2 and -4-activating peptides, thrombin and trypsin in rat isolated airways. Br J Pharmacol 2000;131(8):1584–1591.

104. Campbell AM, Vachier I, Chanez P, Vignola AM, Lebel B, Kochan J et al. Expression of the high-affinity receptor for IgE on bronchial epithelial cells of asthmatics. Am J Respir Cell Mol Biol 1998;19(1):92–97.

105. Campbell AM, Vignola AM, Chanez P, Godard P, Bousquet J. Low-affinity receptor for IgE on human bronchial epithelial cells in asthma. Immunology 1994;82(4):506–508.

106. Verheggen MM, Adriaansen-Soeting PW, Berrevoets CA, van Hal PT, Brinkmann AO, Hoogsteden HC et al. Glucocorticoid receptor expression in human bronchial epithelial cells: effects of smoking and COPD. Mediators Inflamm 1998;7(4): 275–281.

107. Hamann KJ, Dorscheid DR, Ko FD, Conforti AE, Sperling AI, Rabe KF et al. Expression of Fas (CD95) and FasL (CD95L) in human airway epithelium. Am J Respir Cell Mol Biol 1998;19(4):537–542.

108. Gochuico BR, Miranda KM, Hessel EM, De Bie JJ, Van Oosterhout AJ, Cruikshank WW et al. Airway epithelial Fas ligand expression: potential role in modulating bronchial inflammation. Am J Physiol 1998;274(3 Pt 1): L444–449.

109. Fuhrmann M, Jahn HU, Seybold J, Neurohr C, Barnes PJ, Hippenstiel S et al. Identification and function of cyclic nucleotide phosphodiesterase isoenzymes in airway epithelial cells. Am J Respir Cell Mol Biol 1999;20(2):292–302.

110. Wegner CD, Gundel RH, Reilly P, Haynes N, Letts LG, Rothlein R. Intercellular adhesion molecule-1 (ICAM-1) in the pathogenesis of asthma. Science 1990;247(4941):456–459.

111. Bloemen PG, Van den Tweel MC, Henricks PA, Engels F, Van de Velde MJ, Blomjous FJ et al. Stimulation of both human bronchial epithelium and neutrophils is needed for maximal interactive adhesion. Am J Physiol 1996;270(1 Pt 1):L80–87.

112. Christensen PJ, Kim S, Simon RH, Toews GB, Paine R. Differentiation-related expression of ICAM-1 by rat alveolar epithelial cells. Am J Respir Cell Mol Biol 1993;8(1):9–15.

113. Mette SA, Pilewski J, Buck CA, Albelda SM. Distribution of integrin cell adhesion receptors on normal bronchial epithelial cells and lung cancer cells in vitro and in vivo. Am J Respir Cell Mol Biol 1993;8(5):562–572.

114. Pilewski JM, Latoche JD, Arcasoy SM, Albelda SM. Expression of integrin cell adhesion receptors during human airway epithelial repair in vivo. Am J Physiol 1997;273(1 Pt 1):L256–263.

115. Sheppard D. Epithelial integrins. Bioessays 1996;18(8):655–660.

116. Huang XZ, Wu JF, Cass D, Erle DJ, Corry D, Young SG et al. Inactivation of the integrin beta 6 subunit gene reveals a role of epithelial integrins in regulating inflammation in the lung and skin. J Cell Biol 1996;133(4):921–928.

117. Rochelle LG, Fischer BM, Adler KB. Concurrent production of reactive oxygen and nitrogen species by airway epithelial cells in vitro. Free Radic Biol Med 1998;24(5):863–868.

118. Chen LC, Qu Q. Formation of intracellular free radicals in guinea pig airway epithelium during in vitro exposure to ozone. Toxicol Appl Pharmacol 1997;143(1):96–101.

119. Remacle J, Raes M, Toussaint O, Renard P, Rao G. Low levels of reactive oxygen species as modulators of cell function. Mutat Res 1995;316(3):103–122.

120. Martin LD, Krunkosky TM, Voynow JA, Adler KB. The role of reactive oxygen and nitrogen species in airway epithelial gene expression. Environ Health Persp 1998;106 Suppl 5:1197–1203.

121. Robbins RA, Barnes PJ, Springall DR, Warren JB, Kwon OJ, Buttery LD et al. Expression of inducible nitric oxide in human lung epithelial cells. Biochem Biophys Res Commun 1994;203(1):209–218.

122. Kobzik L, Bredt DS, Lowenstein CJ, Drazen J, Gaston B, Sugarbaker D et al. Nitric oxide synthase in human and rat lung: immunocytochemical and histochemical localization. Am J Respir Cell Mol Biol 1993;9(4):371–377.

123. Robbins RA, Springall DR, Warren JB, Kwon OJ, Buttery LD, Wilson AJ et al. Inducible nitric oxide synthase is increased in murine lung epithelial cells by cytokine stimulation. Biochem Biophys Res Commun 1994;198(3):835–843.

124. Gutierrez HH, Pitt BR, Schwarz M, Watkins SC, Lowenstein C, Caniggia I et al. Pulmonary alveolar epithelial inducible NO synthase gene expression: regulation by inflammatory mediators. Am J Physiol 1995;268(3 Pt 1):L501–508.

125. Kao YJ, Piedra PA, Larsen GL, Colasurdo GN. Induction and regulation of nitric oxide synthase in airway epithelial cells by respiratory syncytial virus. Am J Respir Crit Care Med 2001;163(2):532–539.

126. Sanders SP, Siekierski ES, Richards SM, Porter JD, Imani F, Proud D. Rhinovirus infection induces expression of type 2 nitric oxide synthase in human respiratory epithelial cells in vitro and in vivo. J Allergy Clin Immunol 2001;107(2):235–243.

127. Sanders SP, Siekierski ES, Porter JD, Richards SM, Proud D. Nitric oxide inhibits rhinovirus-induced cytokine production and viral replication in a human respiratory epithelial cell line. J Virol 1998;72(2):934–942.

128. Gaston B, Drazen JM, Loscalzo J, Stamler JS. The biology of nitrogen oxides in the airways. Am J Respir Crit Care Med 1994;149(2 Pt 1):538–551.

129. Heffner JE, Repine JE. Pulmonary strategies of antioxidant defense. Am Rev Respir Dis 1989;140(2):531–554.

130. Comhair SA, Bhathena PR, Farver C, Thunnissen FB, Erzurum SC. Extracellular glutathione peroxidase induction in asthmatic lungs: evidence for redox regulation of expression in human airway epithelial cells. FASEB J 2001;15(1):70–78.

131. Katsura H, Kawada H, Konno K. Rat surfactant apoprotein A (SP-A) exhibits antioxidant effects on alveolar macrophages. Am J Respir Cell Mol Biol 1993;9(5):520–525.

132. Papi A, Johnston SL. Respiratory epithelial cell expression of vascular cell adhesion molecule–1 and its up-regulation by rhinovirus infection via NF-kappaB and GATA transcription factors. J Biol Chem 1999;274(42):30041–30051.

133. Cox G, Gauldie J, Jordana M. Bronchial epithelial cell–derived cytokines (G-CSF and GM-CSF) promote the survival of peripheral blood neutrophils in vitro. Am J Respir Cell Mol Biol 1992;7(5):507–513.

134. Cox G, Ohtoshi T, Vancheri C, Denburg JA, Dolovich J, Gauldie J et al. Promotion of eosinophil survival by human bronchial epithelial cells and its modulation by steroids. Am J Respir Cell Mol Biol 1991;4(6):525–531.

135. Ohtoshi T, Vancheri C, Cox G, Gauldie J, Dolovich J, Denburg JA et al. Monocyte-macrophage differentiation induced by human upper airway epithelial cells. Am J Respir Cell Mol Biol 1991;4(3):255–263.

136. Ohtoshi T, Tsuda T, Vancheri C, Abrams JS, Gauldie J, Dolovich J et al. Human upper airway epithelial cell–derived granulocyte-macrophage colony-stimulating factor induces histamine-containing cell differentiation of human progenitor cells. Int Arch Allergy Appl Immunol 1991;95(4):376–384.

137. Soloperto M, Mattoso VL, Fasoli A, Mattoli S. A bronchial epithelial cell–derived factor in asthma that promotes eosinophil activation and survival as GM-CSF. Am J Physiol 1991;260(6 Pt 1):L530–538.

138. Markowicz S, Engleman EG. Granulocyte-macrophage colony-stimulating factor promotes differentiation and survival of human peripheral blood dendritic cells in vitro. J Clin Invest 1990;85(3):955–961.

139. Todate A, Chida K, Suda T, Imokawa S, Sato J, Ide K et al. Increased numbers of dendritic cells in the bronchiolar tissues of diffuse panbronchiolitis. Am J Respir Crit Care Med 2000;162(1):148–153.
140. Baughman RP, Strohofer S. Lung derived surface active material (SAM) inhibits natural killer cell tumor cytotoxicity. J Clin Lab Immunol 1989;28(2):51–54.
141. Catanzaro A, Richman P, Batcher S, Hallman M. Immunomodulation by pulmonary surfactant. J Lab Clin Med 1988;112(6):727–734.
142. Wilsher ML, Parker DJ, Haslam PL. Immunosuppression by pulmonary surfactant: mechanisms of action. Thorax 1990;45(1):3–8.
143. van Iwaarden F, Welmers B, Verhoef J, Haagsman HP, van Golde LM. Pulmonary surfactant protein A enhances the host-defense mechanism of rat alveolar macrophages. Am J Respir Cell Mol Biol 1990;2(1):91–98.
144. Schwartz LW, Christman CA. Alveolar macrophage migration. Influence of lung lining material and acute lung insult. Am Rev Respir Dis 1979;120(2):429–439.
145. van Iwaarden JF, van Strijp JA, Ebskamp MJ, Welmers AC, Verhoef J, van Golde LM. Surfactant protein A is opsonin in phagocytosis of herpes simplex virus type 1 by rat alveolar macrophages. Am J Physiol 1991;261(2 Pt 1):L204–209.
146. Juers JA, Rogers RM, McCurdy JB, Cook WW. Enhancement of bactericidal capacity of alveolar macrophages by human alveolar lining material. J Clin Invest 1976;58(2):271–275.
147. Symons JA, Eastgate JA, Duff GW. Purification and characterization of a novel soluble receptor for interleukin 1. J Exp Med 1991;174(5):1251–1254.
148. Sousa AR, Lane SJ, Nakhosteen JA, Lee TH, Poston RN. Expression of interleukin-1 beta (IL-1beta) and interleukin-1 receptor antagonist (IL-1ra) on asthmatic bronchial epithelium. Am J Respir Crit Care Med 1996;154(4 Pt 1):1061–1066.
149. Levine SJ, Wu T, Shelhamer JH. Extracellular release of the type I intracellular IL-1 receptor antagonist from human airway epithelial cells: differential effects of IL-4, IL-13, IFN-gamma, and corticosteroids. J Immunol 1997;158(12):5949–5957.
150. Takizawa H, Ohtoshi T, Yamashita N, Oka T, Ito K. Interleukin 6-receptor expression on human bronchial epithelial cells: regulation by IL-1 and IL-6. Am J Physiol 1996;270(3 Pt 1):L346–352.
151. Levine SJ, Logun C, Chopra DP, Rhim JS, Shelhamer JH. Protein kinase C, interleukin-1 beta, and corticosteroids regulate shedding of the type I, 55 kDa TNF receptor from human airway epithelial cells. Am J Respir Cell Mol Biol 1996;14(3):254–261.
152. Ulich TR, Yin S, Guo K, Yi ES, Remick D, del Castillo J. Intratracheal injection of endotoxin and cytokines. II. Interleukin-6 and transforming growth factor beta inhibit acute inflammation. Am J Pathol 1991;138(5):1097–1101.
153. Strober W, Kelsall B, Fuss I, Marth T, Ludviksson B, Ehrhardt R et al. Reciprocal IFN-gamma and TGF-beta responses regulate the occurrence of mucosal inflammation. Immunol Today 1997;18(2):61–64.
154. Gauvreau GM, Watson RM, O'Byrne PM. Protective effects of inhaled PGE2 on allergen-induced airway responses and airway inflammation. Am J Respir Crit Care Med 1999;159(1):31–36.

155. Christman JW, Christman BW, Shepherd VL, Rinaldo JE. Regulation of alveolar macrophage production of chemoattractants by leukotriene B4 and prostaglandin E2. Am J Respir Cell Mol Biol 1991;5(3):297–304.

156. de Vries JE. Immunosuppressive and anti-inflammatory properties of interleukin 10. Ann Med 1995;27(5):537–541.

157. Mosmann TR. Properties and functions of interleukin-10. Adv Immunol 1994;56:1–26.

158. Raychaudhuri B, Dweik R, Connors MJ, Buhrow L, Malur A, Drazba J et al. Nitric oxide blocks nuclear factor-kappaB activation in alveolar macrophages. Am J Respir Cell Mol Biol 1999;21(3):311–316.

159. De Caterina R, Libby P, Peng HB, Thannickal VJ, Rajavashisth TB, Gimbrone MA et al. Nitric oxide decreases cytokine-induced endothelial activation. Nitric oxide selectively reduces endothelial expression of adhesion molecules and proinflammatory cytokines. J Clin Invest 1995;96(1):60–68.

160. Lindstrom EG, Andersson RG, Granerus G, Grundstrom N. Is the airway epithelium responsible for histamine metabolism in the trachea of guinea pigs? Agents Actions 1991;33(1–2):170–172.

161. Okayama M, Yamauchi K, Sekizawa K, Okayama H, Sasaki H, Inamura N et al. Localization of histamine N-methyltransferase messenger RNA in human nasal mucosa. J Allergy Clin Immunol 1995;95(1 Pt 1):96–102.

162. Yamauchi K. [Regulation of gene expression of L-histidine decarboxylase and histamine N-methyl-transferase, and its relevance to the pathogenesis of bronchial asthma]. Nippon Rinsho 1996;54(2):377–388.

163. Laitinen LA, Heino M, Laitinen A, Kava T, Haahtela T. Damage of the airway epithelium and bronchial reactivity in patients with asthma. Am Rev Respir Dis 1985;131(4):599–606.

164. Montefort S, Roberts JA, Beasley R, Holgate ST, Roche WR. The site of disruption of the bronchial epithelium in asthmatic and non-asthmatic subjects. Thorax 1992;47(7):499–503.

165. Puddicombe SM, Polosa R, Richter A, Krishna MT, Howarth PH, Holgate ST et al. Involvement of the epidermal growth factor receptor in epithelial repair in asthma. FASEB J 2000;14(10):1362–1374.

166. Lackie PM, Baker JE, Gunthert U, Holgate ST. Expression of CD44 isoforms is increased in the airway epithelium of asthmatic subjects. Am J Respir Cell Mol Biol 1997;16(1):14–22.

167. Robinson BW, Venaille T, Blum R, Mendis AH. Eosinophils and major basic protein damage but do not detach human amniotic epithelial cells. Exp Lung Res 1992;18(5):583–593.

168. Mendis AH, Venaille TJ, Robinson BW. Study of human epithelial cell detachment and damage: effects of proteases and oxidants. Immunol Cell Biol 1990;68(Pt 2):95–105.

169. Ohashi Y, Motojima S, Fukuda T, Makino S. Airway hyperresponsiveness, increased intracellular spaces of bronchial epithelium, and increased infiltration of eosinophils and lymphocytes in bronchial mucosa in asthma. Am Rev Respir Dis 1992;145(6):1469–1476.

170. Holgate ST, Lackie P, Wilson S, Roche W, Davies D. Bronchial epithelium as a key regulator of airway allergen sensitization and remodeling in asthma. Am J Respir Crit Care Med 2000;162(3 Pt 2):S113–117.

171. Campbell AM, Chanez P, Vignola AM, Bousquet J, Couret I, Michel FB et al. Functional characteristics of bronchial epithelium obtained by brushing from asthmatic and normal subjects. Am Rev Respir Dis 1993;147(3):529–534.

172. Devalia JL, Bayram H, Abdelaziz MM, Sapsford RJ, Davies RJ. Differences between cytokine release from bronchial epithelial cells of asthmatic patients and non-asthmatic subjects: effect of exposure to diesel exhaust particles. Int Arch Allergy Immunol 1999;118(2–4):437–439.

173. Bayram H, Devalia JL, Khair OA, Abdelaziz MM, Sapsford RJ, Sagai M et al. Comparison of ciliary activity and inflammatory mediator release from bronchial epithelial cells of nonatopic nonasthmatic subjects and atopic asthmatic patients and the effect of diesel exhaust particles in vitro. J Allergy Clin Immunol 1998;102(5):771–782.

174. Holgate ST, Davies DE, Lackie PM, Wilson SJ, Puddicombe SM, Lordan JL. Epithelial-mesenchymal interactions in the pathogenesis of asthma. J Allergy Clin Immunol 2000;105(2 Pt 1):193–204.

175. Shim JJ, Dabbagh K, Ueki IF, Dao-Pick T, Burgel PR, Takeyama K et al. IL-13 induces mucin production by stimulating epidermal growth factor receptors and by activating neutrophils. Am J Physiol Lung Cell Mol Physiol 2001;280(1):L134–140.

176. Imai T, Nagira M, Takagi S, Kakizaki M, Nishimura M, Wang J et al. Selective recruitment of CCR4-bearing Th2 cells toward antigen-presenting cells by the CC chemokines thymus and activation-regulated chemokine and macrophage-derived chemokine. Int Immunol 1999;11(1):81–88.

177. Dent G, Ruhlmann E, Bodtke K, Magnussen H, Rabe KF. Up-regulation of human eosinophil leukotriene C4 generation through contact with bronchial epithelial cells. Inflamm Res 2000;49(5):236–239.

178. Roche N, Chinet TC, Belouchi NE, Julie C, Huchon GJ. Dermatophagoides pteronyssinus and bioelectric properties of airway epithelium: role of cysteine proteases. Eur Respir J 2000;16(2):309–315.

179. Bentley AM, Durham SR, Robinson DS, Menz G, Storz C, Cromwell O et al. Expression of endothelial and leukocyte adhesion molecules interacellular adhesion molecule-1, E-selectin, and vascular cell adhesion molecule-1 in the bronchial mucosa in steady-state and allergen-induced asthma. J Allergy Clin Immunol 1993;92(6):857–868.

180. Burke-Gaffney A, Hellewell PG. A CD18/ICAM-1-dependent pathway mediates eosinophil adhesion to human bronchial epithelial cells. Am J Respir Cell Mol Biol 1998;19(3):408–418.

181. Lange P, Parner J, Vestbo J, Schnohr P, Jensen G. A 15-year follow-up study of ventilatory function in adults with asthma. N Engl J Med 1998;339(17):1194–1200.

182. Warner JO, Marguet C, Rao R, Roche WR, Pohunek P. Inflammatory mechanisms in childhood asthma. Clin Exp Allergy 1998;28 (suppl 5):71–75; discussion 90–91.

183. Hackel PO, Zwick E, Prenzel N, Ullrich A. Epidermal growth factor receptors: critical mediators of multiple receptor pathways. Curr Opin Cell Biol 1999;11(2):184–189.

184. Davies DE, Polosa R, Puddicombe SM, Richter A, Holgate ST. The epidermal growth factor receptor and its ligand family: their potential role in repair and remodelling in asthma. Allergy 1999;54(8):771–783.

185. Redington AE, Madden J, Frew AJ, Djukanovic R, Roche WR, Holgate ST et al. Transforming growth factor-beta 1 in asthma. Measurement in bronchoalveolar lavage fluid. Am J Respir Crit Care Med 1997;156(2 Pt 1):642–647.

186. Demoly P, Simony-Lafontaine J, Chanez P, Pujol JL, Lequeux N, Michel FB et al. Cell proliferation in the bronchial mucosa of asthmatics and chronic bronchitics. Am J Respir Crit Care Med 1994;150(1):214–217.

187. Mautino G, Henriquet C, Jaffuel D, Bousquet J, Capony F. Tissue inhibitor of metalloproteinase-1 levels in bronchoalveolar lavage fluid from asthmatic subjects. Am J Respir Crit Care Med 1999;160(1):324–330.

8

Tolerance to Inhaled Antigen

ELIZABETH R. JARMAN
JONATHAN R. LAMB

University of Edinburgh Medical School
Edinburgh, Scotland

GERARD F. HOYNE

Australian National University
Canberra, Australia

I. Asthma: An Inflammatory Response of the Airways to Inhaled Antigen

Asthma is a clinical syndrome caused by chronic bronchial inflammation, reversible airway obstruction, and airway hyperresponsiveness (AHR). A number of factors, such as allergens, irritants, or infections, which induce or exacerbate inflammation of the airways, may play a role in initiating asthma. Allergic or extrinsic asthma is an inflammatory-mediated disease characterized by infiltration of the airways by T lymphocytes, mast cells, and eosinophils in response to inhalation of ubiquitous aeroallergens (1). Analysis of bronchoscopic biopsies and bronchoalveolar lavage (BAL) samples taken from allergic asthmatics revealed that CD4$^+$ T cells expressing an activated memory Th2 phenotype are the predominant lymphocyte population. These cells expressed elevated levels of mRNA for the cytokines interleukin-4 (IL-4), IL-5, IL-13, and granulocyte-macrophage colony-stimulating factor (GM-CSF), indicating that have play a role in initiating and sustaining allergic inflammation (2,3). The reason only a proportion of atopic individuals develop asthma in response to inhalation of allergens is not fully understood. The mucosal surfaces of the airways are continually exposed to substances from the environment, and the immune system has evolved mechanisms to distinguish between pathogenic and innocuous substances. In most individuals, soluble proteins delivered to the nasal mucosa do not invoke an immune response but induce a state of nonresponsiveness, or tolerance, to the antigen. There has been considerable interest in understanding the mechanisms involved in the induction and maintenance of mucosal tolerance to inhaled antigen and in exploiting this as a therapeutic approach for preventing pathogenic responses to inhaled allergens (4).

II. Disruption of Immunoregulation and Homeostasis Leads to Induction of Airway Inflammation

Under conditions that result in antigen sensitization, the cytokine milieu in the airways provides a microenvironment that favors development of Th2-dependent humoral and inflammatory responses. Stumbles et al. demonstrated that dendritic cells (DCs) isolated from the airways, when pulsed with antigen and adoptively transferred into naive animals, induce Th2 responses. These cells also expressed mRNA for the immunoregulatory cytokine IL-10, suggesting that in vivo they may induce tolerance (5). Therefore, factors that disrupt the state of homeostasis and cause inflammation of the lower airways act as a trigger for the subsequent development of asthma in genetically predisposed individuals. Allergic asthma often develops during infancy, when the immune system displays a strong bias toward Th2 immunity (6,7). Respiratory viral infections, by inducing the release of inflammatory mediators such as IL-1β tumor necrosis factor-α (TNF-α), IL-8, and IL-6 have been shown to predispose individuals to the development of asthma. Respiratory syncytial virus infection of epithelial cells leads to enhanced absorption of aeroallergens across the airway wall and subsequent allergen sensitization. IL-1β, IL-6, and TNF-α stimulate the maturation of DCs and their migration to draining lymph nodes where they prime T-cell responses. In addition, the induction and up-regulation in expression of adhesion molecules such as ICAM-1 on nasal and bronchial epithelial cells promotes the adhesion of activated T lymphocytes and inflammatory cells (8).

Some allergens themselves exhibit enzymatic activity, which may contribute to the pathophysiology of airway inflammation (9). For example, Der p1, a major allergen of house dust mite, is a 25-kDa cysteine protease that can disrupt the epithelial architecture of the airways, facilitating entry of allergens from the lumen across the epithelium and into the mucosa, where it is taken up by antigen-presenting cells (APCs). Enzymatic properties of Der p1 may perturb regulatory mechanisms in the bronchial tissues, thus potentiating the development of asthma. Proteolytic cleavage of CD23 on B cells leads to disruption of the negative regulation of IgE production. Cleavage of the IL-2Rα subunit leads to the selective loss in expansion of Th1 cells and a possible shift to Th2 responses (10–12).

III. Mucosal Tissues of the Airways and Nasal Cavity

The mucosal tissues of the airways and nasal cavity are central to the induction and maintenance of tolerance to inhaled antigen (13). The mucosal surfaces are covered by a layer of epithelial cells, whose function is to sample antigen while providing a protective barrier against pathogens and environmental agents. Intraepithelial dendritic cells (IDCs) form an extensive network in the basal layers of the pseudostratified epithelium, which line the nasal cavity and trachea, as well as in the simple bronchiolar epithelium (14). These IDCs are similar both in function and in appearance to Langerhans cells in the skin. They have an immature phenotype, express major histocompatibility complex (MHC) class II in intracellular lysosomal compartments, and their primary function is to take up antigen from the airway lumen. An essential function of DCs is to transport antigen from peripheral tissues to secondary lymphoid tissues where immune responses are initiated. In the presence of the cytokines TNF-α, IL-1β, and IL-6, which are released during inflammation, these DCs are stimulated to up-regulate the chemokine receptor CCR7 and migrate to draining lymph nodes. These cells undergo functional maturation en route (15,16). In the lymph nodes, mature DCs are very potent APCs, capable of priming naive T cells. Mature DCs express high levels of MHC class II and the costimulatory molecules CD80 and CD86. The rapid recruitment of DC precursors to the airways during inflammation suggests that these cells are important in initiating immune responses to pathogens (17,18). IDCs, are not the only potential APCs present in the airways. Follicular DCs expressing a mature phenotype have been identified in the lung parenchyma (19). Following inflammation, epithelial cells lining the nasal cavity and bronchioles up-regulate MHC II, CD40, B7, and intracellular adhesion molecule 1 (ICAM-1), suggesting that epithelial cells have the capacity to present antigen (20).

The state of activation or functional phenotype of the APC population may determine whether T-cell receptor (TCR) ligation results in the induction of immunity or tolerance. DCs in the airways, through their role in sampling antigen from the environment and their ability to prime naive T-cell responses, are critical in determining the outcome of immunity versus tolerance (21,22). IDCs express an immature phenotype. In the resting state or in the absence of infection, the presentation of specific antigen to T cells by immature DCs leads to TCR ligation in the absence of activating signals transmitted through costimulatory molecules. Under these conditions, T cells undergo tolerance and loss of antigen responsiveness. Similarly, CD40 ligation stimulates DC activation, maturation, and the release of cytokines, which enables the DC to maintain sustained T-cell responses (23–26). This failure of IDC to prime T-cell responses in the absence of appropriate stimuli may be important in maintaining a nonresponsive state of environmental antigens and to self antigens derived from tissues during tissue damage and repair (27). Many of the products of known pathogens act as inflammatory mediators, including lipo polysaccharide (LPS), certain bacterial CpG motifs, and viral constituents such as dsRNA, stimulating release of TNF-α and IL-1β, which leads to IDC maturation, up-regulation of MHC class II, CD80, and CD86 expression, and migration to draining lymph nodes. Under these conditions, exposure to antigen results in priming of T-cell responses and a loss of tolerance (28,29).

IV. In Vivo Models of Mucosal Tolerance

The development of experimental models and the application of genetically manipulated mouse strains has facilitated the study of the mechanisms involved in the induction of immunity and tolerance. Studies on animal models of autoimmune disease have demonstrated that the intranasal or oral administration of autoantigen can prevent the subsequent induction or exacerbation of disease, following parenteral challenge with autoantigen in an immunogenic form. Exposure of mucosal surfaces of the nasal or gastrointestinal tract to soluble antigen commonly results in the induction of tolerance or hyporesponsiveness. The mucosa is continually exposed to foreign antigens, and it is likely that mechanisms have evolved to prevent or down-regulate T-cell-mediated responses to nonpathogenic agents and can therefore be exploited to induce tolerance to self antigens. A number of factors influence the type of response that is generated, including the nature of the antigen, antigen dose, length of exposure, and mode of administration, as well as the genetic and immunological status of the host. The response of the innate immune system to infection or the presence of adjuvants will also influence the outcome. It has been demonstrated that whereas intranasal administration of antigen alone results in tolerance, when coadsorbed to a bacterial adjuvant such as *Cholera* toxin, both systemic and mucosal T-cell-mediated responses are generated in the nasal associated lymphoid tissue (30). Oral administration of high doses of antigen results in tolerance induction by clonal deletion. In contrast, low doses of antigen cause induction of regulatory cells, which are responsible for inhibiting T-cell effector function. The cytokine milieu in the mucosal tissues of the gastrointestinal tract are favorable for the development of Th2 responses, associated with production of IL-4, IL-5, and IL-10 or the development of Th3 responses and transforming growth factor-β (TGF-β) production (31,32). However, the increase in production of Th2-like cytokines, such as IL-4, observed following oral administration of antigen is independent of the induction of hyporesponsiveness (33). Similarly, exposure of the mucosal surfaces of the upper airways or the nasal cavity to antigen leads to the induction of a state of nonresponsiveness. A number of groups have demonstrated that the intranasal administration of autoantigens, or peptides covering defined T-cell epitopes of the antigen, prior to parenteral sensitization with the autoantigen in an immunogenic form protected against the development of disease (34–38).

V. A Protective Role of IFN-γ in Preventing Th2-Mediated Inflammatory Responses

Holt and colleagues showed that allergic sensitization of the airways could be prevented by an early immune deviation away from a potentially pathogenic

Th2 response to a protective Th1 response. They demonstrated that the repeated exposure of naive rats to a low concentration of aerosolized antigen resulted in initial production of IL-2, and IL-4, which was rapidly replaced by a sustained production of interferon-γ (IFN-γ) by ovalbumin (OVA)–specific CD8[+] T cells. Furthermore, these rats failed to develop IgE responses when subsequently immunized with OVA in adjuvant. The state of antigen-specific tolerance could be adoptively transferred to naive animals, indicating that regulatory cells had been induced (39). Further studies suggested that these regulator cells were $\gamma\delta^+$ T cells (40). The response in rodents to aerosolized antigen was strain dependent, suggesting that induction of IFN-γ-secreting regulatory cells is genetically determined (41). Similarly, C3H/HeJ mice, which are low IgE responders, could be induced to develop AHR and eosinophilia following blockage of endogenous IL-12, suggesting that the inherent ability of DC to produce IL-12 may influence the development of asthma (42). Furthermore, the observation that infants with a reduced capacity to produce IFN-γ were more likely to develop allergic asthma supports the concept that the disposition to develop asthma is associated with a genetic defect in the production of "protective" Th1 cytokines (43,44). Data obtained from other animal studies are conflicting, suggesting that the role of IFN-γ is not solely protective and under certain circumstances may exacerbate airway inflammation (45–49). A recent study published by Tsitoura et al. demonstrated that the intranasal administration of OVA led to CD4[+] T-cell unresponsiveness and a loss in airway inflammation and AHR induction. However, if IL-12 was coadministered with the OVA, Th1 responses were primed, leading to IFN-γ production, eosinophilia, and airway inflammation (50). Studies by Hamelmann et al. (51) demonstrated a critical role for CD8[+] T cells in the production of IL-5 and the induction of eosinophilia and AHR. They showed that mice depleted of CD8[+] T cells prior to sensitization developed normal levels of specific IgE antibodies but failed to develop airway inflammatory responses (51). Interestingly, Holt and coworkers induced the development of IFN-γ-producing CD8[+] regulatory cells by aerosolized exposure to OVA of naive mice, but not of mice that had an established IgE response. This study suggests that IFN-γ-producing CD8[+] $\gamma\delta$ cells may be part of the regulatory network in the airway mucosa, which prevents the induction of responses to nonpathogenic inhaled antigen but does not possess the capacity to down-regulate established T-cell-mediated responses.

VI. Immunoregulatory Role of $\gamma\delta^+$ T Cells in the Airway Mucosa

There is conflicting evidence for a role of $\gamma\delta$ T cells in regulating airway responsiveness. Seymour et al. found that regulation of Th2-mediated responses and the reduction in specific IgE levels was independent of IFN-γ production and could be mediated in the absence of CD8[+] or $\gamma\delta^+$ T cells (39,40,52).

Their approach was to investigate the effect of aerosolized allergen exposure on the reduction of IgE responses in CD8$^+$ or γδ$^+$T-cell-depleted mice. Since Holt and coworkers investigated the regulatory potential of these cells following adoptive transfer into recipient mice, one could hypothesize that in the absence of either γδ$^+$ or CD8$^+$ T cells, other mechanisms may take over the role of downregulating these responses. It is likely that there is a degree of redundancy in the immunoregulatory mechanisms, which have evolved to control T-cell responses and inflammation.

Other studies have also implicated a role for γδ$^+$ T cells in mucosal tolerance (53). Within the NALT and the bronchial-associated tissue of the respiratory tract, these cells are located between the epithelial layer and the basement membrane. They make a number of cytokines, including IL-2, IFN-γ, and TNF-α as well as IL-4, IL-10, and TGF-β. Production of these latter cytokines may account for some of their immunoregulatory effects. Recently, Lahn et al. demonstrated a role for γδ$^+$ T cells in maintaining normal airway responsiveness. Mice genetically deficient in γδ$^+$ T cells or whose γδ$^+$ T cells had been depleted by antibody treatment developed increased AHR, though, surprisingly, levels of eosinophils present in the BAL and lung tissue were reduced (54). In addition to regulating αβ-mediated T-cell responses, γδ T cells may also have an independent role in controlling the growth of epithelial cells in the respiratory tract and thus may influence tissue repair. This could account for the increased presence of γδ$^+$ T cells in the airways of asthmatic individuals (55).

VII. Induction of Tolerance Following Mucosal Delivery of Antigen: The Role of Immunosuppressive Cytokines TGF-β and IL-10 in Suppressing Inflammatory Responses to Inhaled Antigens

TGF-β is a cytokine that has been shown to inhibit a wide variety of inflammatory responses. TGF-β-deficient mice develop a wasting syndrome, which is characterized by the multiorgan infiltration of inflammatory cells (56,57). A role for TGF-β has been demonstrated in mucosal tolerance. Weiner and coworkers demonstrated that regulatory T cells, induced following oral administration of myelin basic protein, protected mice against subsequent development of autoimmune encephalomyelitis. CD4$^+$ T-cell clones isolated form these mice produced high levels of TGF-β, but also IL-4 and IL-10 (58,59). A role for TGF-β in the regulation of Th2-mediated airway inflammation following the mucosal administration of antigen has also been demonstrated. Wiedermann et al. showed that multiple intranasal administrations of a low dose of recombinant Bet vl (the major allergen of birch pollen), prior to parenteral immunization with rBet vl in adjuvant, and subsequent exposure to aerosolized rBet vl lead to T-cell tolerance. They observed a loss in T-cell-mediated systemic responses, including suppression of Bet vl-specific antibodies of all isotypes. In vitro restimulation with antigen revealed a reduction in production of the cytokines IL-4, IL-5, and, to as lesser extent, IL-10, as well as IFN-γ. However, mice treated with intranasal rBet vl showed a marked increase in levels of TGF-β mRNA (60). TGF-β appears to play an important role in regulating inflammatory responses in the airways. Using the murine DO11.10 OVA-TCR transgenic model, Haneda et al. demonstrated that in mice sensitized to OVA by parenteral immunization, administration of a single low dose of antigen directly into the airways induced eosinophilia. In contrast, a high dose of antigen failed to induce eosinophilia and airway inflammation, leading instead to a loss of functional CD4$^+$ T-cell responses to antigen. This was accompanied by a reduction in IL-4 levels in BAL and following in vitro stimulation of cells with antigen. The inability of CD4$^+$ T cells obtained from these mice to adoptively transfer suppression indicates that regulatory cells were not induced. If, however, a single high dose of OVA was administered to the airways of naive DO11.10 OVA transgenic mice, CD4$^+$ regulatory T cells were generated. Adoptive transfer of CD4$^+$ T cells isolated from the mediastinal lymph nodes of these mice into mice sensitized by parenteral immunization with OVA/alum led to active suppression of T-cell-mediated responses and eosinophilic infiltration of the airways following inhalation of antigen. The regulatory effect was antigen specific and was mediated by the local production of TGF-β because the intratracheal instillation of an anti-TGF-β neutralizing antibody at the time of cell transfer revoked this regulatory effect. In contrast, the systemic, intraperitoneal injection of an equal concentration of anti-TGF-β antibody failed to reverse the suppressive effect of transferred cells. This may be because, in contrast to other cytokines, TGF-β, due to its nature of activation and a short half-life, mediates more localized suppression (61). The role of TGF-β in regulating airway inflammation and AHR was demonstrated by Nakao et al. (62). Transgenic mice were generated that selectively overexpressed Smad 7, an intracellular antagonist of TGF-β signaling, in peripheral T cells. By blocking TGF-β signaling in mature T cells, they demonstrated that TGF-β has a critical role in down-regulating immune-mediated inflammatory responses in the airways to an aerosolized challenge with antigen. The absence of TGF-β signaling led to enhanced airway inflammation and AHR, an increase in eosinophilia, and an increase in both IL-5 and IFN-γ levels in the BAL fluid.

Wraith and coworkers demonstrated that IL-10 is central to protection against development of experimental autoimmune encephalomyelitis in mice intranasally administered a peptide derived from myelin basic protein (63). However, a role for IL-10 in the suppression of Th2-mediated responses following the mucosal delivery of antigens into the airways has not been clearly established. Although IL-10 was originally defined as a Th2 cytokine (64), it is now recognized that IL-10 is principally involved in immunoregulation of both Th1 and Th2 responses (65,66). The loss of tolerance leading to an induction of airway responsiveness following viral infection may be due to the ability of certain viruses to inhibit IL-10 production. This would support the view that IL-10 plays a role in maintaining homeostasis in the airways (67). Recent data from Hawrylowicz and coworkers demonstrated that CD4$^+$ T cells isolated from asthmatic individuals who responded to steroid treatment produced IL-10 when stimulated polyclonally in the presence of IL-4 and dexamethasone, whereas CD4$^+$ T cells obtained from steroid-resistant patients failed to produce IL-10. Murine CD4$^+$ T cells cultured under similar conditions could prevent the induction of experimental autoimmune encephalomyelitis in recipient mice following adoptive transfer. These data suggest that the reduction in severity of asthmatic disease to inhaled allergen following steroid treatment may be due to the induction of IL-10-producing regulatory T cells (68,69). IL-10 has been shown to inhibit DC maturation, leading to the induction of a tolerogenic phenotype (70). The observations from the laboratories of Groux and Powrie confirm that IL-10 is also an important growth factor for CD4$^+$ T-regulatory cells (71,72).

VIII. Mechanisms Underlying Induction of Tolerance to Inhaled Antigen

In an effort to define the requirements for the development of protective immunity following mucosal administration of antigen, Tsitoura et al. investigated the effect on the antigen-reactive CD4$^+$ T-cell population of multiple intranasal administrations of a high dose of antigen prior to parenteral sensitization (73). They demonstrated a reduction in specific IgE, with an increase in specific IgG$_1$ and IgG$_{2a}$ levels in sera. The recall response to antigen was impaired, with a reduction in the Th2 and Th1 cytokines IL-4, IL-5, IL-10, and IFN-γ. Tolerance could be induced in mice treated with anti-CD8 antibody, which suggested that the CD8$^+$ regulatory T cells implicated by McMenamin et al. in the induction of nonresponsiveness to inhaled antigen (39) were not involved in mucosal tolerance. There was no evidence for an active role of regulatory cells in the loss of responsiveness, with no increase in IL-10 or TGF-β levels produced by splenocytes. This was confirmed by treatment of mice with anti-IL-10 or anti-TGF-β antibodies prior to intranasal administration of antigen. The possibility that TGF-β is produced locally was not investigated. These observations contrast with those of Haneda et al. who demonstrated a role for TGF-β and CD4$^+$ regulatory T cells in the induction and transfer of tolerance following the intratracheal instillation directly into the airways of a single high dose of antigen (61). The route of administration as well as the dose of antigen may, therefore, be critical in determining the immune response generated and the nature of immunoregulation.

By using the model established by Jenkins and coworkers (74), which involved transferring OVA-specific TCR transgenic CD4$^+$ T cells. Tsitoura et al. followed the fate of the OVA-reactive T-cell population on the basis of positive staining with a TCR clonotype–specific monoclonal antibody, KJ1.26. Within 48 h after intranasal administration of OVA there was a massive expansion in the draining lymph nodes of CD4$^+$KJ1.26$^+$ cells, expressing an activated phenotype. By day 13, at which point mice would have received OVA parenterally, the majority of the population were deleted, leaving a small residual population, which was functionally impaired and persisted for only a few months. After this time an immune response could be induced on immunization with OVA in adjuvant. This suggests that the presence of antigen is required to maintain tolerance, an observation consistent with the independent findings of Jenkins and Whiticare. Using TCR transgenic models, they demonstrated that peripheral tolerance, induced following the intravenous or mucosal administration of soluble antigen, leads to a rapid but transient activation of the antigen-reactive CD4$^+$ T-cell population, followed by a state of functional inactivation (or anergy) and subsequent deletion with an increase in apoptosis (75,76). The existence of a residual population of functionally impaired cells in both of these studies suggests that these T cells have a role in maintaining tolerance, which is dependent on the presence of antigen. This is plausible when one considers that generally the tolerized population would be self-reactive T cells in the periphery, which would be continually exposed to autoantigen (77).

The activation of naive T cells requires two signals, which are transmitted following the specific engagement of the TCR with MHC peptide complexes, and following the engagement of CD28, expressed on the T cell with its ligands CD80 and CD86, expressed on the APCs (78). Early studies with T-cell clones demonstrated that TCR ligation in the absence of APCs derived costimulatory signals led to functional inactivation and anergy (79). However, in vivo studies suggest that the process is more complex. Depending on the route of antigen administration or the dose of antigen, tolerance may result from immune deviation, active suppression, or deletion. Indeed, both T-cell activation and deletion share a number of common features, including initial up-regulation of the activation markers TCR and CD69, and an increase in functional activities, such as proliferation and cytokine production. The requirement for antigen to maintain tolerance suggests that defective signaling occurs following TCR ligation. Studies on tolerized T-cell clones have shown that TCR ligation results in Ca^{2+} mobilization in the absence of protein kinase signaling (80,81).

Signals transmitted following ligation of CD28 and CD86, which is constitutively expressed on DC, are thought to be important in initiating T-cell responses (82,83), whereas CD80 is required to sustain T-cell signaling. Studies have demonstrated that blocking the CD86/CD28 interaction during antigen challenge leads to a loss in the induction of T-cell responses. The cytolytic T-lymphocyte-associated antigen 4 immunoglobulin (CTLA-4Ig) fusion protein, which competes with CD28 for binding to the B7 isoforms, when administered to the airways of mice prior to allergen challenge led to a loss of T-cell responses and a reduction in production of specific IgE antibodies in airway inflammation and AHR. T-cell-mediated responses could also be inhibited by the administration of anti-CD86, but not anti-CD80 antibodies, indicating that ligation of CD28 by CD86 is critical for priming T-cell responses in vivo (84–86). The induction of peripheral tolerance to soluble antigen administered intravenously can be prevented by blocking the B7-CD28 signaling pathway (87). Signals transmitted following B7-CD28 ligation are also essential for the induction of immunoregulation. Bluestone and coworkers demonstrated that the development of spontaneous diabetes in (NOD) transgenic nonobese diabetius mice was exacerbated in mice deficient in CD28, or in NOD mice that express soluble CTLA-4Ig, which blocks the B7–CD28 interaction (88). This was due to a profound decrease in the number of immunoregulatory CD4$^+$ CD25$^+$ T cells present in CD28-deficient NOD mice (89). Tsitoura et al. demonstrated that the induction of tolerance following the mucosal delivery of OVA into the nasal cavity could be prevented by pretreating mice with anti-CD86 antibodies, but not anti-CD80 antibodies. However, they failed to abrogate tolerance induction by treating mice with anti-CTLA-4 antibodies. Other studies have demonstrated a critical role for signals transmitted through CTLA-4 in the induction of peripheral T-cell tolerance (87). T cells up-regulate CTLA-4 expression following signaling through CD28. CTLA-4 is expressed on activated rather than resting T cells and binds with at least a 10-fold higher affinity to the B7 isoforms, thus competing with CD28 for B7 ligation. Through the transmission of negative signals, CTLA-4 appears to be important for the induction of T-cell tolerance and in maintaining homeostasis (87,90,91). This is supported by the finding that mice deficient in CTLA-4 exhibit fatal lymphoproliferative disorders (92). Signaling through CD45RB induces a shift to expression of the CD45RB low isoform and up-regulation of CTLA-4 expression on T cells, making them more susceptible to negative signaling (93). Whether signals transmitted through CTLA-4 trigger the development of an immunoregulatory phenotype has not been established (94). It has been demonstrated that CD4$^+$ CD25$^+$ regulatory T cells constitutively express CTLA-4 and the immunosuppressive function of these cells in vitro and in vivo is dependent ON CTLA-4 costimulation (95,96). The immunosuppressive cytokines IL-10 and TGF-β have been shown to be involved in immunoregulation. TCR ligation in conjunction CTLA-4 cross-linking leads to a loss of IL-2 gene expression and induction of TGF-β production (97). Signaling involved in the induction of IL-10 production by regulatory CD4$^+$ T cells has not been characterized. However, it is known that ligation of the inducible costimulator (ICOS), expressed on activated T cells or an as-yet-unidentified ligand of B7-H1 on APCs, results in induction of high levels of IL-10 production. Signaling through these molecules may be critical for controlling peripheral T-cell responses (for more information, see Chap. 11) (98–100).

IX. Role of Regulatory Cells and Linked Suppression in the Induction of Peripheral Tolerance

A series of studies by Hoyne et al. demonstrated that tolerance to a whole protein could be induced following the mucosal administration of a single peptide incorporating the immunodominant T-cell epitope of that protein and, furthermore, that the mechanism appeared to involve bystander or linked suppression. For the purpose of these studies they used Der p1, which is a major allergen of the *Dermatophagoides pteronyssinus* species of house dust mite. In earlier studies, Hoyne et al. demonstrated that a state of tolerance resulting in a loss of responses to Der p1 could be induced by oral adminis-tration of peptides containing either major or minor T-cell epitopes (101). They subsequently demonstrated that multiple intranasal administrations of a peptide encoding either a major (p111-139) or minor (p81-102) T-cell epitope of Der p1, but not an irrelevant peptide, could induce a state of tolerance in naive mice, which failed to respond to a subsequent systemic challenge with intact Der p1 administered in an immunogenic form (102). There was no decrease in specific IgE levels in sera, although the production of Der p1-specific antibodies in vitro was suppressed in mice tolerized by intranasal administration of peptide. T cells derived from the draining lymph nodes showed a loss in proliferation and IL-2 production following in vitro stimu-lation, either with the dominant peptide p111-139, the intact Der p1, or pep-tides covering minor epitopes of Der p1. This suggested that in addition to a specific down-regulation of the response to p111-139, there was also a loss of responsiveness to other epitopes within Der p1, which may have arisen as a result of bystander tolerance induction. Furthermore, Hoyne et al. were able to inhibit ongoing responses by the intranasal administration of peptide to mice, that had been previously sensitized to Der p1, suggesting that this may prove to be a potential therapeutic approach (103). Investigation of the mechanisms involved demonstrated a hierarchy in the potency of peptides as tolerogens, which reflected their immunogenicity in vivo. The response to Der p1 was inhibited to a greater extent in mice treated with the major epitope p111-139. This was reflected in the loss in production of the cytokines IL-2 and IFN-γ as well as IL-5 and IL-3, following in vitro rechallenge with Der p1 of cells derived from the spleen or lymph nodes. The induction of tolerance fol-lowing inhalation of peptide was CD8$^+$ T-cell independent. Tolerance was presumably mediated by CD4$^+$ T cells, which exhibited broad immuno-regulatory effects, since mice administered a peptide of Der p1 not only failed to respond to a subsequent challenge with Der p1, but also failed to elicit recall T-cell responses following immunization with an irrelevant protein antigen, OVA (102). The induction of peripheral T-cell tolerance, following intranasal administration of a high dose of peptide, appears to involve a strong but transient activation of CD4$^+$ T cells, which is rapidly followed by progression to a long-term state of nonresponsiveness. The recall responses to peptide, investigated at various time points following inhalation of peptide, revealed an initial hyperactivation of CD4$^+$ T cells that peaked at day 4 and lead to an increase in IL-2, IL-3, and IFN-γ. The response generated was comparable to that obtained in mice immunized with Der p1/CFA and was associated with an increase in cell numbers present in the cervical lymph nodes (LN) (104).

Linked suppression may account for the loss of responsiveness to the intact Der p1 protein, following the mucosal delivery of a single peptide covering a T-cell epitope. Suppression may arise as a result of direct cell–cell contact, or due to the release of suppressive cytokines such as IL-10 and TGF-β (Corsin-Jimenez M, Lamb JR, Hoyne GF, unpublished). There is evidence for both mechanisms operating in linked suppression. Powrie and coworkers identified a phenotypically and functionally distinct population of CD4$^+$ T cells. These CD45RB^{low} T cells were capable of controlling intestinal inflammation and maintaining homeostasis. Cotransfer of CD4$^+$ CD45RB^{low} cells into SCID mice protected against development of inflammatory bowel disease induction by the pathogenic CD4$^+$ CD45RB^{high} population (105). Immune suppression by the CD4$^+$ CD45RB^{low} regulatory T-cell population was dependent on production of TGF-β (106) and IL-10 (65). Two separate laboratories have independently identified a CD25$^+$ CD4$^+$ T-cell population, which is present in the thymus of the neonate and constitutes approximately 5% of the peripheral T-cell population in adults. These cells exhibit an anergic phenotype but on stimulation with antigen potently suppress the proliferative response of CD4$^+$ CD25$^-$ T cells in a cell–cell contact–dependent manner, which is mediated in part by the release of TGF-β and IL-10. The sensitivity of these cells to antigen may be due to their constitutive expression of CTLA-4 (107,108). The immunoregulatory capacity of Tr1 cell lines isolated by Groux et al. following chronic activation of murine CD4$^+$ T cells in the presence of IL-10 could only be partially reversed by the addition of anti-IL-10- and anti-TGF-β-neutralizing antibodies, indicating that cell–cell contact was required for complete suppression (71,109).

Within the lymph nodes, APCs such as DCs, on processing antigen, can simultaneously present a number of different MHC–peptide complexes to T cells of different specificities. Thus, it would be possible for the same APC to present different epitopes derived from the same antigen to a regulatory CD4$^+$ T cell as well as a naive or memory T cell, in this way facilitating linked suppression. Shevach and coworkers demonstrated that antigen-dependent CD4$^+$ CD25$^+$ regulatory T cells mediate suppression via an antigen-nonspecific cognate interaction with APC, suggesting that a similar mechanism may operate in vivo (110). The Notch signaling pathway was first identified for its role in cell–cell signaling during developmental stages, which determined the fate of precursor stem cells (111,112). Peripheral T cells express multiple Notch receptors (1–4) and Notch ligands (Jagged 1, 2 and Delta 1, 3), suggesting that Notch signaling may be involved in determining the state of differentiation of peripheral $CD4^+$ T cells (113). The influence of Notch signaling on the differentiation of hematopoietic precursors is influenced by the presence of different cytokines. Recently, we showed a correlation between the expression of IL-10 during the induction of tolerance and the expression of Notch receptors and ligands on $CD4^+$ T cells. Notch signaling may, therefore, act in concert with inhibitory cytokines, such as TGF-β and IL-10, and may induce the expression of these cytokines, thus acting in conjunction with other immunoregulatory pathways. IL-10 by inhibiting up-regulation of MHC class II and B7 expression induces a tolerogenic phenotype in DC. In addition, IL-10 directly inhibits IL-2 production by T cells. This loss of both antigen presentation and T-cell expansion would result in bystander suppression (70,114,115). Similarly, negative signals transmitted through Notch receptor–ligand interactions could result in an immunoregulatory state, analogous to a state of linked suppression. To investigate whether signaling through the Notch-1 receptor contributes to the differentiation of $CD4^+$ T cells into helper or regulatory cells, Serrate-1 (the ligand for Notch) was overexpressed on APCs. The Serrate-1$^+$ APCs were pulsed with a dominant peptide of Der p1 (p110-131) prior to adoptive transfer into either naive mice or mice immunized with Der p1/CFA. Serrate-1 expression on APCs inhibited priming of both primary and established secondary T-cell responses to Der p1, but not to OVA, an irrelevant antigen. Mice that had received Serrate-1$^+$ APCs showed a loss in the proliferative and cytokine response in the draining lymph nodes to the Der p1 protein and peptides, providing evidence for a role of Notch signaling in linked suppression. Furthermore, the suppression induced by Serrate-1$^+$ APC was long lived, suggesting that it may be analogous to the suppression induced by regulatory cells following mucosal administration of antigen, and as described for $CD4^+$ $CD45RB^{low}$ $CD25^+$ regulatory T cells (116).

X. Conclusions

The airways are continually exposed to inhaled antigen and have therefore evolved mechanisms to distinguish between pathogenic and innocuous substances. In the absence of inflammation, inhalation of soluble antigen leads to the induction of a state of nonresponsiveness or tolerance. Data obtained from various studies suggests that there is a degree of redundancy in the mechanisms involved in the regulation of immune responses to inhaled antigen. A role has been demonstrated for IFN-γ-producing $\gamma\delta^+$ $CD8^+$ T cells in preventing responses to aerosolized antigen. However, the administration of antigen via the nasal mucosa leads to functional inactivation, tolerance, and clonal deletion, although active suppression is also involved. A residual population of anergic, antigen-dependent $CD4^+$ T cells appears to mediate suppression by a mechanisms involving both cell–cell contact and the release of immunoregulatory cytokines IL-10 and TGF-β. The state of activation of APCs and in particular DCs may be influential in the induction of tolerance. This is supported by the recent finding that signaling through the Notch pathway leads to tolerance induction. The identification of a functionally and phenotypically distinct population of CD4$^+$ CD25$^+$ CD45RB^{low} T cells in periphery, which exhibit regulatory functions, raises the question as to whether these cells are also involved in the induction of tolerance to inhaled antigen.

References

1. Hamid QA, Minshall EM. Molecular pathology of allergic disease. I: Lower airway disease. J Allergy Clin Immunol 2000;105:20–36.
2. Robinson DS, Hamid Q, Ying S, Tsicopoulos A, Barkans J, Bentley AM, Corrigan C, Durham SR, Kay AB. Predominant TH2 like branchoalveolar T-lymphocyte population in atopic asthma. N Engl J Med 1992;326:298–304.
3. Del Prete GF, De Carli M, D'Elios MM, Maestrelli P, Ricci M, Fabbri L, Romagniani S. Allergen exposure induces the activation of allergen specific Th2 cells in the airway mucosa of patients with allergic respiratory disorders. Eur J Immunol 1993;23:1445–1449.
4. Lowrey JA, Savage NDL, Palliser D, Corsin-Jimenez M, Forsyth LMG, Hall G, Lindey S, Stewart GA, Tan KAL, Hoyne GF, Lamb JR. Induction of tolerance via the respiratory mucosa. Int Arch Allergy Immunol 1998;116:93–102.
5. Stumbles PA, Thomas JA, Pimm CL, Lee PT, Venaille TJ, Proksch S, Holt PG. Resting respiratory tract dendritic cells preferentially stimulate T helper cell type 2 (Th2) responses and require obligatory cytokine signals for induction of Th1 immunity. J Exp Med 1998;188:2019–2031.
6. Gern JE, Lemanske, Jr RF, Busse. WW. Early life origins of asthma. J Clin Investigation 1999;104:837–843.
7. Prescott SL, Macaubas C, Holt BJ, Smallacombe TB, Loh R, Sly PD, Holt PG. Transplacental priming of the human immune system to environmental allergens: universal skewing of the initial T cell responses towards the Th2 cytokine profile. J Immunol 1998;160:4730–4737.
8. Lukas NW, Tekkanat KK. Role of Chemokines in ashmatic airway inflammation. Immunol Rev 2000;177:21–30.
9. Thomas WR. Mite allergens groups I–VII. A catalogue of enzymes. Clin Exp Allergy 1993;23:350–353.
10. Shultz O, Sewell HF, Shakib F. Proteolytic cleavage of CD25, the subunit of the human T cell interleukin-2 receptor, by Der p1, a major mite allergen with cysteine protease activity. J Exp Med 1998;187:271–275.
11. Shakib F, Schultz O, Sewell H. A mite subversive: cleavage of CD23 and CD25 by Der p1 enhances allergenicity. Immunol Today 1998;19:313–316.
12. King C, Brennan S, Thompson PJ, Stewart GA. Dust mite proteolytic allergens induce cytokine release from cultured airway epithelium. J Immunol 1998;161:3645–3651.
13. Czerkinsky C, Anjuere F, McGhee JR, George-Chandy A, Holmgren J, Kieny M-P, Fujiyashi K, Mestecky JF, Pierrefite-Carle V, Rask C, Sun J-B. Mucosal

immunity and tolerance: relevance to vaccine development. Immunol Rev 1999;170:197–222.

14. Neutra MR, Pringault E, Kraehenbuhl J-P. Antigen sampling across epithelial barriers and induction of mucosal immune responses. Annu Rev Immunol 1996;14:275–300.

15. Cumberbach M, Dearman RJ, Kimber I. Langerhans cells require signals from both tumour necrosis factor-alpha and interleukin-1 beta for migration Immunology 1997;92:388–395.

16. Sallusto F, P. Schaerli P, Loetscher C, Schaniel D, Lenig CR, Mackay S. Qin, Lanzavecchia A. Rapid and coordinated switch in chemokine receptor expression during dendritic cell maturation. Eur J Immunol 1998;28:2760–2769.

17. Holt PG, Schon-Hegrad MA, McMenamin PG. Dendritic cells in the respiratory tract. Int Rev Immunol 1990;6:139–149.

18. Mc William AS, Nelson D, Thomas JA, Holt PG. Rapid dendritic cell recruitment in a hallmark of the acute inflammatory response at mucosal surfaces. J Exp Med 1994;179:1331–1336.

19. Gong JL, McCarthy KM, Telford J, Tamatani T, Miyasaka M, Schneeberger EE. Intraepithelial airway dendritic cells: a distinct subset of pulmonary dendritic cells obtained by microdissection. J Exp Med 1992;175:797–807.

20. Nakajima J, Ono M, Takeda M, Kawauchi M, Furuse A, Takizawa H. Role of costimulatory molecules on airway epithelial cells acting as alloantigen presenting cells. Transplant Proc 1997;29:2297–2300.

21. Lambrecht BN, Salomon B, Klatzmann D, Pauwels RA. Dendritic cells are required for the development of chronic eosinophilic airway inflammation in response to inhaled antigen in sensitized mice. J Immunol 1998;160:4090–4097.

22. Dhodapkar MV, Steinman RM, Sapp M, Desai H, Fossella C, Krasovsky J, Donahoe SM, Dunbar PR, Cerundolo V, Nixon DF, Bhardwaj N. Rapid generation of broad T-cell immunity in humans after a single injection of mature dendritic cells. J Clin Invest. 1999;104:173–180.

23. Graza KM, Chan SM, Suri R, Nguyen LT, Odermatt B, Schoenberger SP, Ohashi PS. Role of antigen-presenting cells in mediating tolerance and autoimmunity. J Exp Med 2000;191:2021–2027.

24. Jonuleit H, Schmitt E, Schuler G, Knop J, Enk AH. Induction of interleukin 10–producing, non-proliferating CD4(+) T cells with regulatory properties by repetitive stimulation with allogeneic immature human dendritic cells. J Exp Med 2000;192:1213–1222.

25. Howland KC, Ausubel LJ, London CA, Abbas AK. The roles of CD28 and CD40 ligand in T cell activation and tolerance. J Immunol 2000;164:4465–4470.

26. Cella M, Sheidegger D, Palnmer-Lehmann K, Lane P, Lanzavecchia A, Alber G. Ligation of CD40 on dendritic cells triggers production of high levels of interleukin-12 and enhances T cell stimulatory capacity. J Exp Med 1996;184:747–752.

27. Steinman RM, Turley S, Mellman I, Inaba K. The induction of tolerance by dendrtic cells that have captured apoptotic cells. J Exp Med 2000;191:411–416.

28. Cella M, Engering A, Pinet V, Pieters J, Lanzavecchia A. Inflammatory stimuli induce accumulation of MHC class II complexes on dendritic cells. Nature 1997;388:782–787.

29. Sparwasser T, Koch E.S, Vabulas R.M, Heeg K, Lipford G.B, Ellwart J.W. Bacterial DNA and immunostimulatory CpG oligonucleotides trigger maturation and activation of murine dendritic cells. Eur J Immunol 1998;28:2045–2054.

30. Pogador A, Staats HF, Itoh Y, Kelsall BL. Intranasal immunization with cytotoxic T-Lymphocyte epitope peptide and muosal adjuvant cholera toxin: selective augmentation of peptide-presenting dendritic cells in nasal mucosa-associated Lymphoid Tissue. Infect Immun 1998;66:5876–5881.

31. Chen Y, Inobe J, Marks R, Gonnella P, Kuchroo VK, Weiner H.L. Peripheral deletion of antigen reactive T cells in oral tolerance. Nature 1995;376:177–180.

32. Weiner H.L. Oral Tolerance for the treatment of autoimmune diseases. Annu Rev Med 1997;48:341–351.

33. Wolvers DA, van der Cammen MJ, Kraal G. Mucosal tolerance is associated with, but independent of up-regulation Th2 responses. Immunology 1997;92:328–333.

34. Dick, AD, Cheng Y, Liversidge J, Forrester J. Intranasal administration of retinal antigens suppresses retinal antigen-induced experimental autoimmune uveoretinititis. Immunology 1994;82:625–631.

35. Ma CG, Zhang GX, Xiao BG, Link J, Olsson T, Link H. Suppression of experimental autoimmune myasthenia gravis by nasal administration of acetylcholine receptor. J Neuroimmunol 1995;58:51–60.

36. Metzler B, Wraith DC. Mucosal tolerance in a murine model of experimental autoimmune encephalomyelitis. Ann NY Acad Sci 1996;778:228–242.

37. Myers LK, Seyer JM, Stuart JM, Kang A.H. Suppression of murine collagen-induced arthritis by nasal administration of collagen. Immunology 1997;90:161–164.

38. Shi, H-D, Li, H, Wang, H, Bai, X, Peter, H van der Meide, Link, H, Ljunggren H-G. Mechanisms of nasal tolerance induction in experimental autoimmune myasthenia gravis: identification of regulatory cells. J Immunol 1999;162:5757–5763.

39. McMenamin C, Holt PG. The natural immune response to inhaled soluble protein antigens involves major histocompatability complex (MHC) class I–restricted CD8+ T cell–mediated but MHC class II–restricted CD4+ T cell–dependent immune deviation resulting in selective suppression of immunoglobulin E production. J Exp Med 1993;178:889–899.

40. McMenamin C, Pimm C, McKersey M, Holt PG. Regulation of IgE responses to inhaled antigen in mice by antigen-specific $\gamma\delta$ T cells. Science 1994;65:1869–1871.

41. Sedgwick JD, Holt PG. Suppression of IgE responses in inbred rats by repeated respiratory tract exposure to antigen: responder phenotype influences isotype specificity of induced tolerance. Eur J Immunol 1984;14:893–897.

42. Keane-Myers M, Wysocka M, Trinchieri G, Wills-Karp M. Resistance to antigen-induced hyperresponsiveness requires endogenous production of interleukin- 12. J Immunol 1998;162:919–926.

43. Martinez FD, Stern DA, Wright AL, Holberg CJ, Taussig LM, Halonen M. Association of interleukin-2 and interferon-gamma production by blood mononuclear cells in infancy with parental allergy skin tests and wit subsequent development of atopy. J Allergy Clin Immunol 1995;96:652–660.

44. Shirakawa T, Enomoto T, Shimazu S, Hopkin JM. The inverse association between tuberculin responses and atopic disorder. Science 1997;275:77–79.
45. Germann T, Guckes S, Bongartz M, Dlugonska H, Schmitt E, Kolbe L, Kolsch E, Podlaski F.J, Gately M.K, Rude E. Administration of IL-12 during ongoing immune responses fails to permanently suppress and can even enhance the synthesis of antigen-specific IgE. Int Immunol 1995;7:1649–1657.
46. Coyle A.J, Tsuyuki C, Bertrand S, Huang M, Aguet S, Alkan S, Anderson GP. Mice lacking the IFN-γ receptor have impaired ability to resolve a lung eosino-philic inflammatory response associated with a prolonged capacity of T cells to exhibit a Th2 cytokine profile. J Immunol 1996;156:2680–2685.
47. Lack G, Renz H, Saloga J, Bradley KL, Loader J, Leung DYM, Larsen G, Gelfand EW. Nebulized IFN-gamma inhibits the development of secondary allergic responses in mice. J Immunol 1996;157:1432–1439.
48. Gavett SH, O'Hearn DJ, Li X, Huang S-H, Finkelman FD, Wills-Karp M. Interleukin 12 inhibits Antigen-induced airway hyperresponsiveness, inflamma-tion, and Th2 cytokine expression in mice. J Exp Med 1995;2:1–10.
49. Cohn L, Homer RJ, Niu N, Bottomly K. T Helper 1 cells and interferon γ reg-ulate allergic airway inflammation and mucus production. J Exp Med 1999;190:1309–1317.
50. Tsitoura DC, Blumenthal RL, Berry G, DeKruyff RH, Umetsu DT. Mechanisms preventing allergen-induced airway hyperreactivity: role of tolerance and immune deviation. J Allergy Clin Immunol 2000;106:239–246.
51. Hamelmann E, Oshiba A, Paluh J, Bradley K, Loader J, Potter TA, Larson GL, Gelfand EW. Requirement for CD8+ T cells in the development of airway hyperresponsiveness in a murine model of airway sensitisation. J Exp Med 1996;183:1719–1729.
52. Seymour BWP, Gershwin LJ, Coffman RL. Aerosol-induced immunoglobulin (Ig) E unresponsiveness to ovalbumin does not require CD8+ or T cell receptor (TCR)-γ/δ+ T cells or interferon (IFN)-γ in a murine model of allergen sensiti-zation. J Exp Med 1998;187:721–731.
53. Hannien A, Harrison LC. γδ T cells as mediators of mucosal tolerance: the autoimmune diabetes model. Immunol Rev 2000;173:109–119.
54. Lahn M, Kanehio A, Takeda K, Joetham A, Schwarze J, Kohler G, O'Brien, Gelfand EW, Born W. Negative regulation of airway responsiveness that is dependent on γδ T cells and independent of αβ T cells. Nat Med 1999;5:1150–1156.
55. Jahnsen FL, Farstad IN, Aanesen JP, Brandtzaeg P. Phenotypic distribution of T cells in human nasal mucosa differs from that in the gut. Am J Respi Cell Mol Biol 1998;18:392–401.
56. Skull MM, Ormsby L, Kier AB, Pawlowski S, Diebold DJ, Yin M, Allen R, Sidman C, Proetzel G, Calvin D, Annuziata N, Doetschman T. Targeted dis-ruption of the mouse transforming growth factor-β1 gene results in multifactoral inflammatory disease. Nature 1992;359:693–699.
57. Christ M, McCartney-Francis NL, Kulkarni AB, Ward JM, Mizel DR, Mackall CL, Gress RE, Hines KL, Tian H, Karlsson S. Immune dysregulation in TGF-beta 1-deficient mice. J Immunol 1994;153:1936–1946.

58. Chen Y, Kuchroo VK, Inobe J, Hafler DA, Weiner HL. Regulatory T cell clones induced by oral tolerance: suppression of autoimmune encephalomyelitis. Science 1994;265:1237–1240.

59. Weiner HL, van Rees EP. Mucosal Tolerance. Immunol Lett 1999;69:3–4.

60. Wiedermann U, Jahn-Schmid B, Bohle B, Repa A, Renz H, Kraft D, Ebner C. Suppression of antigen-specific T and B cell responses by intranasal or oral administration of recombinant Bet v1, the major birch pollen allergen, in a murine model of type I allergy. J Allergy Clin Immunol 1999;103:102–110.

61. Haneda K, Sano K, Tamura G, Shirota H, Ohkawara Y, Sato T, Habu S, Shirato K. Transforming growth factor-β secreted from CD4+ T cells ameliorates antigen-induced eosinophilic inflammation. Am J Respir Cell Mol Biol 1999;21:268–274.

62. Nakao A, Miike S, Hatano M, Okumura K, Tokuhisa T, Ra C, Iwamoto I. Blockade of transforming growth factor β/Smad signaling in T cells by over-expression of Smad7 enhances antigen-induced airway inflammation and airway reactivity. J Exp Med 2000,192:151–158.

63. Burkhart C, Liu GY, Anderton SM, Netzler B, Wraith DC. Peptide-induced T cell regulation of experimental autoimmune encephalomyelitis: a role for IL-10. Int Immunol 1999;11:1625–1634.

64. Mosmann TR, Coffman RL. Th1 and Th2 cells: Different patterns of lymphokine secretion lead to different functional properties. Annu Rev Immunol 1989;7:145–173.

65. Asseman C, Mauze S, Leach MW, Coffman RL, Powrie F. An essential role for interleukin 10 in the function of regulatory T cells that inhibit intestinal inflammation. J Exp Med 1999;190:995–1003.

66. Zuany-Amorin C, Haile S, Leduc D, Dumarey C, Huerre M, Vargaftig BB, Pretolani M. Interleukin-10 inhibits antigen-induced cellular recruitment into the airway of sensitised Mice. J Clin Invest 1995;95:2644–2651.

67. Gentile DA, Patel A, Ollila C, Fireman P, Zeevi A, Doyle WJ, Skoner DP. Diminished IL-10 production in subjects with allergy after infection with influenza A virus. J Allergy Clin Immunol 1999;103:1045–1048.

68. Hawrylowicz C, Richards D, Lee T. Failure of glucocorticoids to induce CD4+ T cells with an IL-10 high cytokine phenotype in patients with steroid resistant asthma. Keystone Symposia Regulation of Immunity and Autoimmunity. 2001;Abs 315.

69. Barrat FJ, Boonstra A, Cua DJ, Richards DF, de Wall Malefyt R, Coffman RL, Savelkoul HF, Hawrylowicz CM, O'Garra A. In vitro generation of regulatory T cells using a combination of immunosuppressive drugs. Keystone Symposia Regulation of Immunity and Autoimmunity. 2001;Abs 406.

70. Steinbrink K, Wolf M, Jonuleit H, Knop J, Enk AH. Induction of tolerance by IL-10 treated dendritic cells. J Immunol 1997;159:4772–4780.

71. Groux H, O'Garra A, Bigler M, Rouleau M, Antonenko S, de Vries JE, Grazia Roncarolo M. A CD4+ T-cell subset inhibits antigen-specific T-cell responses and prevents colitis. Nature 1997;389:737–741.

72. Asseman C, Powrie F. Interleukin 10 is a growth factor for a population of regulatory T cells. Gut 1998;42:157–158.

73. Tsitoura DC, DeKruyff RH, Lamb JR, Umetsu DT. Intranasal exposure to protein antigen induces immunological tolerance mediated by functionally disabled CD4+ T cells. J Immunol 1999;163:2592–2600.

74. Kearney ER, Pape KA, Loh DY, Jenkins MK. Visualization of peptide-specific T cell immunity and peripheral tolerance induction in vivo. Immunity 1994;1:327–229.

75. Pape KA, Merica R, Mondino A, Khoruts A, Jenkins MJ. Direct evidence that functionally impaired CD4+ T cells persist in vivo following induction of peripheral tolerance. J Immunol 1998;160:4719–4729.

76. Benson JM, Campbell KA, Guan Z, Gienapp IE, Stuckman SS, Forsthuber T, Whitacre CC. T-cell activation and receptor downmodulation precede deletion induced by mucosally administered antigen. J Clin Invest 2000;106:1031–1038.

77. Asano M, Toda M, Sakaguchi N, Sakaguchi S. Autoimmune disease as a consequence of developmental abnormality of a T cell subpopulation. J Exp Med 1996;184:387–396.

78. Chambers CA, Allison JP. Co-stimulation in T cell responses. Curr Opin Immunol 1997;9:369–404.

79. Mueller DL, Jenkins MK, Schwartz RH. Clonal expansion versus functional inactivation: a co-stimulatory signalling pathway determines the outcome of T cell antigen receptor occupancy. Annu Rev Immunol 1989;7:445–480.

80. Li W, Whaley CD, Mondino A, Mueller DL. Blocked signal transduction in the ERK and JNK protein kinases in anergic CD4+ T cells. Science 1996;271:1272–1276.

81. Mondino A, Whaley CD, DeSilva DR, Li W, Jenkins MK, Mueller DL. Defective transcription of the IL-2 gene is associated with impaired c-Fos, FosB and JunB in anergic T helper 1 cells. J Immunol 1996;157:2048–2057.

82. Inaba K, Witmer-Pack M, Inaba M, Hathcock KS, Sakuta H, Azuma M, Yagita H, Okumura K, Linsley PS, Ikehara S. The tissue distribution of the B7-2 costimulator in mice: abundant expression on dendritic cells in situ and during maturation in vitro. J Exp Med 1994;180:1849–1860.

83. Lenschow DJ, Walunas TL, Bluestone JA. CD28/B7 system of T cell costimulation. Annu Rev Immunol 1996;14:233–258.

84. Tsuyuki S, Tsuyuki J, Einsle K, Kopf M, Coyle AJ. Costimulation through B7-2 (CD86) is required for the induction of a lung mucosal T helper cell 2 (TH2) immune response and altered airway responsiveness. 1997;185:1671–1679.

85. Keane-Myers AM, Gause WC, Finkelman FD, Xhou D, Wills-Karp M. Development of murine allergic asthma is dependent upon B7-2 costimulation. J Immunol 1998;160:1036–1043.

86. Larche M, Till S, Haselden BM, North J, Barkans J, Corrigan CJ, Kay AB, Robinson DS. Costimulation through CD86 is involved in airway antigen-presenting cell and T cell responses to allergen in atopic asthmatics. J Immunol 1998;161:6375–6382.

87. Perez VL, Van Parijs A, Biuckians X, Zheng XX, Strom TB, Abbas AK. Induction of peripheral T cell tolerance in vivo requires CTLA-4 engagement. Immunity 1997;6:411–417.

88. Lenschow DJ, Herold KC, Rhee L, Patel B, Koons A, Qin H-Y, Fuchs E, Singh B, Thompson CB, Bluestone JA. CD28/B7 Regulation of Th1 and Th2 subsets in the development of autoimmune diabetes. Immunity 1996;5:285–293.

89. Salomon B, Lenschow DJ, Rhee L, Ahourian N, Singh B, Sharpe A, Bluestone J. B7/CD28 Costimulation is essential for the homeostasis of the CD4+CD25+ immunoregulatory T cells that control autoimmune diabetes. Immunity 2000;12:432–440.

90. Linsley PS, Goldstein P. Lymphocyte activation: T-cell regulation by CTLA-4. Curr Biol 1996;6:398–400.

91. Ostrov DA, Shi W, Schwartz J-CD, Almo SC, Nathenson SG. Structure of murine CTLA-4 and its role in modulating T cell responsiveness. Science 2000;290:816–819.

92. Tivol EA, Borriello F, Schweitezer AN, Lynch WP, Bluestone JA, Sharpe AH. Loss of CTLA-4 leads to massive lymphoproliferation and fatal multi-organ tissue destruction, revealing a critical negative role of CTLA-4. Immunity 1995;3:541–547.

93. Fecteau S, Basadonna G, Freitas A, Ariyan C, Sayegh MH, Rothstein DM. CTLA-4 up-regulation plays a role in tolerance mediated by CD45. Nat Immunol 2001;2:58–63.

94. Metz DP, Farber DL, Taylor T, Bottomly K. Differential role of CTLA-4 in regulation of resting memory versus naive CD4 T cell activation. J Immunol 1998;161:5855–5861.

95. Takahashi T, Tagami T, Yamazaki S, Uede T, Shimizu J, Sakaguchi N, Mak TM, Sakaguchi S. Immunologic self-tolerance maintained by CD25+ CD4+ regulatory T cells constitutively expressing cytotoxic T lymphocyte–associated antigen 4. J Exp Med 2000;192:303–309.

96. Read S, Malmstrom V, Powrie F. Cytotoxic T lymphocyte-associated antigen 4 plays an essential role in the function of CD25+ CD4+ regulatory cells that control intestinal inflammation. J Exp Med 2000;192:295–302.

97. Griffin MD, Hong DK, Holman PO, Lee K-M, Whitters MJ, O'Herrin SM, Fallarino F, Collins M, Segal DM, Gajewski TF, Kranz DM, Bluestone JA. Blockage of T cell activation using a surface-linked single chain antibody to CTLA-4 (CD152). J Immunol 2000;164:4433–4442.

98. Hutloff A, Dittrich AM, Beier KC, Eljaschewitsch B, Kraft R, Anagnostopoulos I, Kroczek RA. ICOS is an inducible T-cell co-stimulator structurally and functionally related to CD28. Nature 1999;397:263–266.

99. Abbas AK, Sharpe AH. T-cell stimulation: an abundance of B7s. Nat Med 1999;5:1345–1346.

100. Dong H, Zhu G, Tamada K, Chen L. B7-H1, a third member of the B7 family, co-stimulates T-cell proliferation and interleukin-10 secretion. Nat Med 1999;5:1365–1369.

101. Hoyne G, Callow MG, Kup MC, Thomas WR. Inhibition of T-cell responses by feeding peptides containing major and cryptic epitopes: studies with the Der p1 allergen. Immunology 1994;83:190–195.

102. Hoyne GF, Jarnicki AG, Thomas WR, Lamb JR. Characterization of the specificity and duration of T cell tolerance to intranasally administered peptides in

mice: a role for intramolecular epitope suppression. Int Immunol 1997;9:1165–1173.

103. Hoyne GF, O'Hehir RE, Wraith DC, Thomas WR, Lamb JR. Inhibition of T cell and antibody responses to house dust mite allergen by inhalation of the dominant T cell epitope in naive and sensitised mice. J Exp Med 1993;178:1783–1788.

104. Hoyne GF, Askonas BA, Hetzel C, Thomas WR, Lamb, JR. Regulation of house dust mite responses by intranasally administered peptide: transient activation of CD4+ T cells precedes the development of tolerance in vivo. Int Immunol 1996;8:335–342.

105. Powrie F. T cells in inflammatory bowel disease: protective and pathogenic roles. Immunity 1995;3:171–174.

106. Powrie F, Carlino J, Leach MW, Mauze S, Coffman RL. A critical role for transforming growth factor β but not interleukin 4 in the suppression of T helper type 1–mediated colitis by CD45RB low CD4+ T cells. J Exp Med 1996;183:2669–2674.

107. Sakaguchi S. Regulatory T cells: key controllers of immunologic self-tolerance. Cell 2000;101:455–158.

108. Shevach EM. Regulatory T cells in autoimmunity. Annu Rev Immunol 2000;18:423–449.

109. Kitani A, Chua K, Nakamura K, Strober W. Activated self-MHC-reactive T cells have the cytokine phenotype of Th2/T regulatory cell 1 T cells. J Immunol 2000;165:691–702.

110. Thornton AM, Shevach EM. Suppressor effector function of CD4+ CD25+ immunoregulatory T cells is antigen nonspecific. J Immunol 2000;164:183–190.

111. Artavanis-Tsakonas S, Matsuno K, Fortini M. Notch signalling. Science 1995;268:225–232.

112. Simpson P. Notch signalling in development: on equivalence groups and asymmetric developmental potential. Curr Opin Genet Dev 1997;7:537–542.

113. Deftos ML, He YW, Ojala EW, Bevan MJ. Correlating notch signaling with thymocyte maturation. Immunity 1998;9:777–786.

114. Thornton AM, Shevach EM. CD4+ CD25+ immunoregulatory T cells suppress polyclonal T cell activation by inhibiting interleukin 2 production. J Exp Med 1998;188:287–296.

115. Lombardi G, Sidhus, Batchelor R, Lechler R. Anergic T cells suppress cells in vitro. Science 1994;264:1587–1589.

116. Hoyne GF, Le Roux I, Corsin-Jimenez M, Tan K, Dunne J, Forsyth LMG, Dallman MJ, Owen MJ, Ish-Horowicz D, Lamb JR. Serrate 1-induced notch signalling regulates the decision between immunity and tolerance made by peripheral CD4+ T cells. Int Immunol 2000;12:177–185.

9

Sensitization to Inhaled Allergen

SUSAN L. PRESCOTT

University of Western Australia
Perth, Western Australia, Australia

I. Introduction

As our understanding of asthma and allergic diseases evolves, so does the apparent complexity of these conditions and their pathogenesis. Allergic inflammation arises from inappropriate IgE-mediated immune responses to environmental allergens and typically develops in organs exposed to the environment (gut, respiratory tract, and skin). The resulting clinical manifestations probably represent heterogeneous conditions with varied genetic and environmental etiological influences. This has made the identification of causal factors more problematic.

The greatly increased rates of allergic diseases over the last 20–30 years in all racial groups highlights the urgent need to identify factors linked with progressive "westernization," which are unmasking an almost universal genetic predisposition. This chapter will explore the processes that lead to allergic sensitization (particularly to inhalants) and possible recent predisposing environmental changes.

II. Immune Responses to Inhaled Allergens and Atopic Inflammation

Extensive work in murine systems in the 1980s led to the recognition of different underlying cellular immune responses in atopic and non-atopic animals (1). Many of these differences have been also demonstrated in humans (2,3), mainly using in vitro culture systems. In both cases, production of excessive allergen-specific IgE is regulated by underlying T-helper (Th) cell responses. While

T-cell memory to inhalant allergens becomes almost universal in exposed individuals (4), most exposed non-atopic adult humans show interferon-γ (IFN-γ) dominated responses to allergens, similar to the murine Th type 1 (Th1) responses. Peripheral blood mononuclear cells from atopic adults instead produced a range of cytokines that inhibit IFN-γ responses, and favor IgE isotype switching [interleukin (IL)-4, IL-13] and allergic inflammation (IL-5, IL-9). This pattern of response closely resembles the murine type 2 (Th2) response, although the difference between atopic and non-atopic humans are less distinct (5).

For inhalant allergens the processes that lead to these mutually inhibitory cross-regulatory cytokine response patterns appear to be initiated in early life during first allergen encounter (6) and are consolidated with repeated exposure. Responses to food allergens show very different maturation patterns and are discussed elsewhere (7,8). There is considerable ongoing research to determine what factors favor Th2 differentiation and how these may be modified to prevent allergic sensitization.

III. Evolution of Allergen-Specific Immune Responses: Before Birth?

Exactly when T cells begin to respond to environmental allergens is unclear. Certainly, cells capable of responding to allergen are present in cord blood in sufficient numbers to produce positive lymphoproliferative responses and cytokine responses. Positive responses to allergens have been observed as early as 20–22 weeks (9,10). The magnitude of proliferation responses as well as T-cell expression of the activation marker CD25 and the memory marker CD45RO increase with gestational age (11). Allergen-specific proliferative responses were first demonstrated in term neonates by Kondo et al., who found that stimulation with ovalbumin or bovine serum albumin produced greater proliferative responses in newborns who went on to develop allergic disorders (12). Similar results have been obtained by other groups, not only with other food allergens (13) but also with inhaled allergens such as Der p1 and Lol p1 (14). More definitive evidence of allergen-specific fetal immune responses derives from microsatellite genotyping studies that demonstrate that responsive T cells are of fetal rather than maternal origin (15). In addition, neonatal (CBMC) responses to aeroallergens, such as home dust mite (HDM), show a typically Th2 skewed pattern cytokine response (15), indicating that the specific immune responses of the fetus are readily influenced by the pro-Th2 cytokine milieu of normal pregnancy (16). This is apparent in virtually all newborns, regardless of atopic risk (family history) and subsequent atopic history (6,15).

While neonatal responses to inhalant allergen have been seen in by many groups using varied culture systems, the significance, and the mechanisms of in utero priming are still not clear. The magnitude of CBMC responses is similar to the "memory" responses that characterize clonally expanded populations derived during repeated allergen exposure. These findings have led to speculation that the fetus may encounter allergens before birth. However, while the passage of allergen from the maternal to the fetal circulation is clearly established in animals (17), there is only indirect evidence in support of the operation of a comparable mechanism in humans (18). In a recent double-sided ex vivo perfusion model, both food proteins and inhaled allergens (Bet v1) crossed the human placenta (18). However, passage of aeroallergen was more selective and variable. One proposed mechanism for allergen transfer involves transplacental transport of allergen-specific IgG antibody and low levels of native or processed allergen from the maternal circulation (19).

Thus, while there is convincing evidence that the immune system is primed to respond to some environmental antigens before birth, including infectious (20,21) and possibly food allergens (12), inhalant-specific T-cell priming remains more controversial, as these allergens are likely to reach the fetus in extremely low levels. Some have suggested that CBMC responses may represent nonspecific reactivity (22) or cross-reactivity with other antigens.

Regardless of whether CBMC responses are the result of direct allergen stimulation or not, exactly how these antenatal responses affect evolving responses in the early postnatal period is still of great interest. It is certainly foreseeable that the characteristics of these expanding populations of seemingly "allergen-specific" T cells may affect responses during subsequent postnatal encounter with allergen. Differences in the neonatal responses of subsequently atopic infants compared with nonatopic infants further justify ongoing research in this area (discussed below).

IV. Implications of Exposure to Antigens/Allergens In Utero

Seen commonly, regardless of atopic risk, allergen-responsive cells in cord blood are not likely to be pathological. Rather than leading to inevitable allergic sensitization, these responses in utero may initiate normal tolerance mechanisms. While immature fetal T cells appear to be more readily activated, tolerized, or Th2 biased compared with adult cells, the processes that ultimately lead to tolerance or persistent T-cell reactivity are still not well understood.

Experimental animals show selective neonatal tolerance when their mothers are exposed to antigen (23) or allergens (24) during gestation. Offspring of women infected with filarial parasite during pregnancy have in vitro hyporesponsiveness to filarial but not other pathogens, compared with those born to uninfected mothers. This has been attributed to in utero tolerance mechanisms (25). In traditional models of tolerance, the fetus becomes tolerized to antigens encountered during this uniquely "immunoprivileged" environment, with "clonal deletion" of all self-reactive T cells (26). More recently, the "danger model" of tolerance (27) proposes that antigens do not evoke an immune responses without simultaneous activation of costimulatory (danger) signals. In this model, fetal self antigens do not elicit an immune response because they are not recognized as harmful, not because of "immune privilege." In each model, it is difficult to explain neonatal immune responsiveness to allergen (14,28,29) and other antigens (20) including autoantigens (30). It would be more logical to expect that presentation of allergen by immature fetal antigen-presenting cells (APC) in the absence of inflammatory signals may favor tolerance, as these cells are less capable of providing the costimulatory activation signals that prevent T-cell anergy.

It is now apparent that tolerance is an active process which is incomplete birth and ongoing in the postnatal period. These low-grade neonatal responses may be part of evolving tolerance mechanisms. Some responses will lead to sensitization, and others to tolerance. It takes normal infants a number of months or even years to develop food allergen (high-zone) tolerance. Aeroallergen tolerance (by low-zone tolerance) is further delayed. As these processes are driven by ongoing allergen exposure, early allergen avoidance strategies during this period (while practically impossible) may not be appropriate and have so far not been effective for allergy prevention (31).

V. Maturation of Inhalant Allergen Response in the Postnatal Period

In the early postnatal period, both humoral and cellular immune responses to inhaled allergens increase with age and correlate with exposure (6,23,33). Both atopic and non-atopic children show increasing lymphoproliferative responses to inhalant allergens with age (6) and declining responses to food allergens. Similarly, age-related increases in allergen-specific IgG levels occur in all exposed individuals and are not specific for atopy. In later childhood there are clear differences in allergen-specific antibody levels. IgG$_4$ subclass levels are higher in children with atopy (34), as observed in adults (35). This parallels the rise in aeroallergen-specific IgE after 2 years of age in atopic individuals (36) and reflects developing Th2 cytokine signaling. These differences in antibody responses are less evident in the early postnatal period before symptomatic allergy to inhalants; however, differences in the underlying cellular response to these allergens are already evident during this period.

Although normal in the neonatal period, Th2 responses to allergens are rapidly down-regulated in nonallergic infants over the first year of life (6,37), when there is progressive development of a reciprocal Th1-like pattern of immunity (38,39). This process is known as "low-zone tolerance" or "immune deviation" in murine systems, and involves cross-regulation between mutually antagonistic populations of Th1 and Th2 cells. In contrast, infants who subsequently develop atopy show consolidation of their neonatal patterns of Th2-polarized allergen-specific immunity to inhalant allergens (6,37,39).

These observations emphasize the importance of normal Th1 immune function in the early postnatal period (8). It appears that failure of this Th1-driven immune deviation leads to persistence and amplification of the neonatal allergen-specific Th2 response pattern, and subsequent Th2-mediated allergic disease. Clearly, immaturity of postnatal Th1 maturation may be implicated in allergic disease processes. Of note, although immaturities of Th1 function as measured by IFN-γ production capacity are universal in early life, IFN-γ defects are more marked in atopic individuals at birth (13,40–43). This has been proposed as a possible mechanism for impaired postnatal Th1 immune deviation. The preexistence of this Th1 "deficiency" at birth in atopic individuals suggests potential influences in the antenatal period. There is preliminary evidence that IFN-γ production capacity is also lower in infants of atopic mothers compared with those of atopic fathers (44), suggesting that mechanisms other than genetic factors could also play a role. However, this remains to be substantiated.

It has been suggested that factors that interfere with Th1 function in early life may be implicated in allergy pathogenesis (45). Immature Th1 (IFN-γ) responses in neonates appear largely due to immature signaling from (APCs) (46,47). The production of Th1-trophic IL-12 by mature APCs is a major factor determining Th1 differentiation in response to allergens (48,49). In the absence of mature IL-12 signaling the default response appears to be Th2 differentiation as seen in neonatal rodents (50). Although there are studies suggesting that children at high risk of atopy have less mature APC signaling (51), there is no direct evidence that delayed APC maturation underlies the perinatal Th1 immaturity associated with atopic disease.

VI. Environmental Influences on Immune Development

It is still not clear how events during gestation or the early postnatal period could favor subsequent Th2-polarized memory. It is possible that recent environmental changes may operate before birth to favor development of persistent Th2 immunity, particularly as the increased expression of clinical allergy is already apparent in infancy. The developing immune system is most susceptible to modulation during fetal life. Factors in the prenatal setting that could influence immune deviation include antigen exposure (dose, timing, and nature), maternal atopic status, the "bystander" effects of any ongoing maternal immune responses, the nature of antigen presentation, as well as numerous maternal exposures during gestation that could potentially affect immune responses. Early postnatal life also appears to be a "critical period" when numerous environmental and genetic factors interact to influence the pattern of postnatal immune development (52).

Pathological airway changes associated with asthma are seen in very early life and may predate the development of disease by years (53). There is preliminary evidence (54) that the altered airway remodeling seen in asthma may result from the inappropriate reactivation of embryological processes involved in airway morphogenesis. It is likely that antenatal factors also influence airway development, increase susceptibility to environmental damage, and predispose to altered patterns of subsequent airways response.

A. Influence of Timing, Route, and Dose of Allergen Exposure on Subsequent Inhalant Allergy

Although there are many reports suggesting that earlier exposure to allergens increases the risk of allergic sensitization (55), this area has been disappointing as a strategy for prevention (31). Many earlier studies suggested that pollen allergies are more common in individuals born during seasons (or years) when the pollen counts were highest (56–61). However, other groups have failed to show this association (62,63). For perennial inhalants a "threshold level" above which above which sensitization is more common has been documented (64). However, while higher levels of perennial allergens such as HDM (65) or cat (66) in early infancy have also been associated with early atopic sensitization, a number of recent reports suggest that this may protect from later atopy (67 and others).

The "dose" of antigen exposure may also influence the resulting *pattern* of T-helper cytokine responses. Smaller amounts of antigen promote increases in IL-4 secretion and inhibit proliferative responses in vitro (68), priming for Th2 differentiation. The role of this in the context of potential allergen exposure (in presumably small quantities) through breast milk (69) or during gestation is not clear.

Although exposure to an allergen in early life results in sensitization in a predisposed individual, this is not likely to be the result of the specific allergen encountered. Rather, sensitization appears to be due to an increased allergic propensity, dictated by multiple heterogeneous genetic and environmental interactions. Early exposure may affect this propensity, but atopy is not *caused* by allergens. Thus, in the absence of HDM exposure, at-risk children develop sensitivities to other prevalent allergens, such as *Alternaria* in the desert environment of Arizona (70). The pattern of allergen sensitivity is a reflection of patterns of environmental exposure (71), but it is likely that other factors (such as reduced pro-Th1 signals) may be important in the rising prevalence of allergy, by failing to counter the underlying Th2 immune default (45). Accordingly, current attempts to reduce levels of exposure to inhalant allergens in late pregnancy and early postnatal life have not significantly reduced subsequent risk of inhalant allergy.

Thus, it is now generally accepted that sensitization to allergens is the result of increased propensity for Th2 responses rather than primarily due to exposure to allergen.

B. Aeroallergen Characteristics That May Promote Allergic Sensitization

The immunogenicity of allergens may be largely the result of their capacity to initiate inflammatory "danger" signals, which up-regulate costimulatory molecules on APCs, and result in T-cell priming rather than anergy. It is now recognized that many allergens have "proinflammatory" biochemical activity (72,73). They may function as enzymes, enzyme inhibitors, transport proteins, or regulatory proteins (73). Many of the plant and mite allergens have hydrolytic enzyme activity (cysteine, serine, aspartate proteases, and metalloproteases) (74). Protease inhibitor (or amylase inhibitor) activity is seen in plant (wheat, barley) and pollen (ragweed, olive) allergens. Large amounts of enzyme activity can be detected in HDM samples (including trypsin, chymotrypsin, amylase, glucoamylase, elastase, cellulase, lipase, lysozyme, and alkaline phosphatase).

Through these biochemical activities it is conceivable that allergens may initiate local inflammation and epithelial disruption through non-IgE mechanisms. Mite allergens increase permeability of respiratory epithelium, induce cytokine release from epithelial cells, and increase their surface expression of intracellular adhesron molecule 1 (ICAM-1) and map-histocompatibility complex (MHC) class II. Some allergens enhance receptor mediated endocytosis by macrophages and other APCs, and those with intrinsic protease inhibitor activity bind directly to cell membrane proteases and signal cell proliferation (73). Allergens with carbohydrate moieties bind lectin receptors on macrophages releasing tumor necrosis factor-α (TNF-α) and other inflammatory mediators. Protease activity, which induces cytokine release, can direct the T-helper cell response to induce IgE production (75). These allergen properties add to immunogenicity (76) and perpetuate local immune responses (reviewed in 74). It is possible that atopic individuals lack the mechanisms to inactive these allergens and control the local inflammatory repair cycle (77).

It has been postulated that immunogenicity may not only reside in the allergen structure but in the MHC–antigen complex, and reactivity to some allergens is human leukocyte antigen (HLA) associated (78–82). It is also possible that allergens may dictate the way the T cell responds, possibly by affecting the way that the T-cell receptor (TCR) complex transduces signals for cell function. Evavold et al. (83) proposed mechanisms by which altered peptide ligands may function as either immunogenic peptides or antagonists when binding to TCRs. This area is still poorly understood.

C. Role of Microbial Products

The propensity of the immune system to mount Th2 responses to allergens may be potentially modified by strong Th1 stimulation. Microbial products produce strong activation signals that promote maturation of Th1 cell–mediated immunity (reviewed in 84). These effects are mediated through APC activation through many pathways including CD14 (receptor for bacterial lipopolysaccharide, LPS), which up-regulates the pro-Th-1 IL-12 pathway. It has been proposed that activation of these pathways offers some protection from Th2 differentiation (bystander effect) (84). Supporting this hypothesis, polymorphisms in the region of the CD14 gene have very recently been associated with total serum IgE levels (higher levels of soluble serum CD14 were associated with higher IFN-γ and lower IL-4 responses) (85).

While recurrent bacterial infections may enhance Th1 maturation, commensal organisms that colonize infants in the first days of life may play an equally (if not more) important role. Animals raised in a "germ-free" environment are predisposed to Th2 responses (86), and in humans there are differences in commensal microbial flora in atopic compared to non-atopic children (87), although this needs to be explored further.

It has been proposed that general improvements in public health and altered early childhood exposure to bacteria in Western cultures (loss of pro-Th-1 influences seen with recurrent bacterial infections) may have potentially unmasked Th2 propensity in predisposed individuals. While there is epidemiological evidence to support this association between reduced infection and higher rates of allergic disease in humans (88,89), there is little direct proof.

D. Other Environmental Influences

A number of other environmental exposures have the potential to modify developing immune responses to allergens.

Links between infant growth parameters and allergic sensitization suggest that nutritional factors may play a role (90–92). The anti-inflammatory benefits of specific dietary nutrients such as antioxidants and omega-3 polyunsaturated fatty acids (n-3 PUFAs) have also recently attracted interest. Both epidemiological and in vitro evidence suggests that these nutrients reduce allergic inflammation through a number of mechanisms (93–97). Declining n-3 PUFA and antioxidant intakes in Western diets may be associated with rising rates of allergic disease (98,99). A number of groups are investigating this association further, along with potential benefits of these nutrients in disease prevention.

Environmental pollutants have the capacity to promote allergic responses through direct immunological influence or by serving as adjuvants during allergen processing. Tobacco smoke and pollutants may modify epithelial integrity and mucosal permeability (100), facilitating the penetration and access of allergens to the immune system. Thus, exposure to these agents at critical stages in local tissue immune development may potentiate allergen sensitization.

While cigarette smoking is associated with increased serum IgE and a greater risk of atopy (101–103), including in children with passive smoke inhalation (104), the mechanisms are unclear. Children of non-atopic mothers who smoked in pregnancy also have higher cord blood IgE and greater atopic risk than those born to nonsmokers (105,106), indicating important antenatal effects. However, maternal smoking in pregnancy also affects fetal lung growth and development (107–111), increasing the risk of childhood wheezing due to smaller airway calibre (112).

Other environmental pollutants may also affect immune responses. There has been longstanding concern in the environmental sciences about the effect of persistent organic pollutants (POPs) derived from agricultural and industry. These highly lipid-soluble compounds such as the polychlorinated biphenyls (PCBs) persist in body tissues and are implicated in numerous disease processes (including immune dysfunction) in animals living in contaminated environments (113,114). These compounds are measurable in human tissue, cord blood, and breast milk, indicating exposure during early development. As well as altering T-helper cell function, some of these compounds have sex steroid properties (115) with the potential to alter Th1/Th2 differentiation. Of interest, one recent study has shown a significant correlation between PCB levels and IgE levels in cord blood (116). This area needs to be investigated further.

VII. Identifying Children Who Will Ultimately Develop Persistent Inhalant Allergy

Identifying children who will ultimately develop atopy also remains a problem for targeting future prevention. Decades of research failed to establish early markers that accurately predict atopy. Cord blood IgE was initially investigated for this purpose.

Although many studies have observed differences in cord blood IgE, Th1 (13,40–43) and Th2 (6,117) cytokine production, and cytokine receptors (118) at birth, none of these parameters has been of value in predicting atopic disease. An extensive search has also failed to identify genetic markers of disease, and it is likely that multiple varied genes will be implicated in the predisposition to allergic sensitization.

VIII. Interventions to Reduce Sensitization to Inhalants

There is a growing urgency to develop strategies that will help reverse that recent dramatic increase in the incidence of allergic sensitization. It is clear that a number of the early exposures previously discussed could influence sensitization to allergens and may therefore be candidate factors for disease prevention. To effectively prevent disease, intervention will be necessary before Th2 differentiation becomes established. To achieve this safely an improved understanding of the early life events and genetic factors that result in atopy is essential.

A. Allergen Avoidance Strategies

Despite numerous strategies to reduce allergen exposure in early life there has been no reduction in sensitization to inhaled allergens. A comprehensive review of allergen avoidance studies is now available from the Cochrane database (31). Although earlier studies of food allergen avoidance in pregnancy showed in a lower incidence of eczema in the first year of life (119–123), this benefit was only transient in longer term studies. Other studies failed to show a benefit of food allergen avoidance at any age (124,125) with no differences in the intervention versus control groups with respect to atopic dermatitis or asthma. Aeroallergen avoidance is more problematic and more difficult to achieve. There remain a number of ongoing studies examining the effects of avoiding inhalant allergens, including the Child Health Asthma Prevention Study (CHAPS) which focuses on intensive allergen avoidance during pregnancy and during the first year of life (11). The long-term effects of these interventions are awaited with great interest.

Thus, while studies of maternal dietary and inhalant allergen avoidance are inconclusive, it is difficult to recommend a specific approach to parents with a history of atopic disease.

B. "Vaccination" to Modify Immune Responses to Allergens

Two broad methods of "immunizing" infants to modify immune responses to allergens have been proposed. The first is not allergen specific, and involves administration of agents which provide a nonspecific Th-1 boost to the maturing immune system (as achieved normally by encounter with bacteria). Enhanced maturation of Th1 responses may thereby counter default Th2 responses to newly encountered allergens. The effect of the mycobacterial protein BCG as a source of strong Th1 activation in early infancy has been investigated by a number of groups. The results of two Swedish studies (126,127) failed to show any reduction of atopy in the vaccinated groups. However, a more recent study in Africa showed beneficial effects (128). It is likely that more appropriate agents will be identified with further research. Many remain concerned about the unpredictable long-term effects of immunmodulation in early life.

A proposed second allergen-specific method of "vaccination" involves controlled administration of inhalant allergens. In the murine models, administration of peptides through mucosal surfaces promotes tolerance (129). Holt (130) postulated that feeding or intranasal administration of allergenic peptides during childhood may be a way of controlling and accelerating immune maturation in a Th1 direction. Others have proposed coadministration with Th1 adjuvants, but these techniques are still in early development and the long-term effects unknown.

C. Other Interventions to Modify Immune Responses to Allergens

Other attempts to modify developing responses to allergens are ongoing. This includes modification of maternal diet in pregnancy (with antioxidants and n-3

PUFA supplementation) and modification of similar factors in the postnatal period.

At present, the most justified practical intervention is cessation of maternal smoking. There is ample evidence of the benefits of this intervention for lung development and function, and while the effects on immune development are less clear, many other benefits are evident.

IX. Conclusions

The focus of current research is toward the future possibility of preventative intervention for atopic diseases. While there are a number of proposed contrasting prevention strategies, too little is understood about normal immune development to predict the merits or longstanding implications of these strategies. Ideally, disease prevention will involve identification of infants at high risk of atopy, and introduction of safe, noninvasive strategies, which will effectively prevent the development of allergic immune responses while maintaining normal immunity. In order to achieve this there must be a more comprehensive understanding of how environmental and genetic factors influence normal immune development.

References

1. Mosmann TR, Coffman RL. Heterogeneity of cytokine secretion patterns and functions of helper T cells. Adv Immunol 1989; 46:111–147.
2. Corrigan CJ, Kay AB. T cells and eosinophils in the pathogenesis of asthma. Immunol Today 1992; 13(12):501.
3. Romagnani S. Human Th1 and Th2 subsets: doubt no more. Immunol Today 1991; 12:256–257.
4. Upham J, Holt B, Baron-Hay M et al. Inhalant allergen-specific T-cell reactivity is detectable in close to 100% of atopic and normal individuals: covert responses are unmasked by serum-free medium. Clin Exp Allergy 1995; 25:634.
5. Kapsenberg ML, Wierenga EA, Bos JD, Jansen HM. Functional subsets of allergen-reactive human CD4+ T cells. Immunol Today 1991; 12(11):392–395.
6. Prescott S, Macaubas C, Smallacombe T et al. Development of allergen-specific T-cell memory in atopic and normal children. Lancet 1999; 353(9148):196–200.
7. MacDonald TT. T cell immunity to oral allergens. Curr Opin Immunol 1998; 10:620–627.
8. Holt PG. Development of sensitization versus tolerance to inhalant allergens during early life. Pediatr Pulmonol Suppl 1997; 16:6–7.
9. Szepfalusi Z, Nentwich I, Gerstmayr M, Jost E, Toloran L. Prenatal allergen contact with milk proteins. Clin Exp Allergy 1997; 27:28–35.
10. Jones A, Miles E, Warner J, Colwell B, Bryant T, Warner J. Fetal peripheral blood mononuclear cell proliferative responses to mitogenic and allergenic stimuli during gestation. Pediatr Allergy Immunol 1996; 7:109–116.

11. Warner JA, Jones CA, Williams TJ, Warner JO. Maternal programming in asthma and allergy. Clin Exp Allergy 1998; 28:35–38.

12. Kondo N, Kobayashi Y, Shinoda S et al. Cord blood lymphocyte responses to food antigens for the prediction of allergic disorders. Arch Dis Child 1992; 67:1003–1007.

13. Warner JA, Miles EA, Jones AC, Quint DJ, Colwell BM, Warner JO. Is deficiency of interferon gamma production by allergen triggered cord blood cells a predictor of atopic eczema? Clin Exp Allergy 1994; 24:423–430.

14. Piccinni MP, Mecacci F, Sampognaro S et al. Aeroallergen sensitization can occur during fetal life. Int Arch Allergy Immunol 1993; 102:301–303.

15. Prescott S, Macaubas C, Holt B et al. Transplacental priming of the human immune system to environmental allergens: universal skewing of initial T-cell responses towards Th-2 cytokine profile. J Immunol 1998; 160:4730–4737.

16. Wegmann TG, Lin H, Guilbert L, Mosmann TR. Bidirectional cytokine interactions in the maternal-fetal relationship: is successful pregnancy a Th2 phenomenon? Immunol Today 1993; 14(7):353–356.

17. Dahl GM, Telemo E, Westrom BR, Jacobsson I, Karlson BW. The passage of orally fed proteins from mother to foetus in the rat. Comp Biochem Physiol 1984; 77A:199–201.

18. Szepfalusi Z, Loibichler C, Pichler J, Reisenberger K, Ebner C, Urbanek R. Direct evidence for transplacental allergen transfer. Pediatr Res 2000; 48:404–407.

19. Holt PG, O'Keeffe PO, Holt BJ et al. T-cell "priming" against environmental allergens in human neonates: sequential deletion of food antigen specificities during infancy with concomitant expansion of responses to ubiquitous inhalant allergens. Pediatr Allergy Immunol 1995; 6:85–90.

20. Dastur F, Shastry P, Iyer E et al. The fetal immune response to maternal tetanus toxoid immunization. JAPI 1993; 41:94–96.

21. Weil GJ, Hussain R, Kumaraswami V, Tripathy SP, Phillips KS, Ottesen EA. Prenatal allergic sensitization to helminth antigens in offspring of parasite-infected mothers. J Clin Invest 1983; 71:1124–1129.

22. Platts-Mills TA, Woodfolk JA. Cord blood proliferative responses to inhaled allergens: is there a phenomenon? J Allergy Clin Immunol 2000; 106:441–443.

23. Fazekas de St. Groth B, Basten A, Loblay R. Induction of memory and effector T suppressor cells by perinatal exposure to antigen. Eur J Immunol 1984; 14:228–235.

24. Nicklin S, MIller K. Naturally acquired tolerance to dietary antigen: effect of in utero and perinatal exposure on subsequent humoral immune competence in the rat. J Reprod Immunol 1987; 10:167–176.

25. Steel C, Guinea A, McCarthy J, Ottesen E. Long-term effect of prenatal exposure to maternal microfilaraemia on immune responsiveness to filarial parasite antigen. Lancet 1994; 343:890–893.

26. von-Boehmer H, Kisielow P. Self-nonself discrimination by T cells. Science 1990; 248(4961):1369–1373.

27. Matzinger P. Tolerance, danger and the extended family. Annu Rev Immunol 1994; 12:991.

28. Warner JA, Jones CA, Jones AC, Warner JO. Prenatal origins of allergic disease. J Allergy Clin Immunol 2000; 105(2 Pt 2):S493–498.

29. Warner J, Jones A, Miles E, Warner J. Prenatal sensitisation. Pediatr Allergy Immunol 1996; 7(Suppl 9):98–101.
30. Yu M, Fredrikson S, J JL, Link H. High numbers of autoantigen-reactive mononuclear cells expressing interferon-gamma (IFN-gamma), IL-4 and transforming growth factor-beta (TGF-beta) are present in cord blood. Clin Exp Immunol 1995; 101:190–196.
31. Kramer MS. Maternal antigen avoidance during pregnancy for preventing atopic disease in infants of women at high risk. Cochrane Database System Rev 2000; (2):CD000133.
32. Jenmalm M, Björksten B. Development of IgG subclass antibodies to ovalbumin, birch and cat during the first 8 years of life in atopic and nonatopic children. Submitted 1998.
33. Jenmalm M, Björksten B. Exposure to cow's milk during first three months of life is associated with high levels of IgG subclass antibodies to beta-lactoglobulin up to 8 years of age. Submitted 1998.
34. Jenmalm M, Holt P, Björkstén B. Maternal influence on IgG subclass antibodies to Bet vl during the first 18 months of life as detected with a sensitive ELISA. Int Arch Allergy Immunol 1997; 114:175–184.
35. Kemeny DM, Price JF, Richardson V, Richards D, Lessof MH. The IgE and IgG subclass antibody response to foods in babies during the first year of life and their relationship to feeding regimen and the development of food allergy. J Allergy Clin Immunol 1991; 87:920–929.
36. Van-Asperen PP, Kemp AS. The natural history of IgE sensitisation and atopic disease in early childhood. Acta Paediatr Scand 1989; 78:239–245.
37. Prescott SL, Macaubas C, Smallacombe T et al. Reciprocal age-related patterns of allergen-specific T-cell immunity in normal vs. atopic infants. Clin Exp Allergy 1998; 28 Suppl 5:39–44; discussion 50-1.
38. Yabuhara A, Macaubas C, Prescott SL et al. Th-2-polarised immunological memory to inhalant allergens in atopics is established during infancy and early childhood. Clin Exp Allergy 1997; 27(11):1261–1269.
39. Macaubas C, Sly PD, Burton P et al. Regulation of Th-cell responses to inhalant allergen during early childhood. Clin Exp Allergy 1999; 29:1223–1231.
40. Rinas U, Horneff G, Wahn V. Interferon-γ production by cord blood mononuclear cells is reduced in newborns with a family history of atopic disease and is independant from cord blood IgE levels. Pediatr Allergy Immunol 1993; 4:60–64.
41. Tang MLK, Kemp AS, Thorburn J, Hill D. Reduced interferon gamma secretion in neonates and subsequent atopy. Lancet 1994; 344:983–985.
42. Liao S, Liao T, Chiang B et al. Decreased production of IFNγ and decreased production of IL-6 by cord blood mononuclear cells of newborns with a high risk of allergy. Clin Exp Allergy 1996; 26:397–405.
43. Martinez F, Stern D, Wright A, Holberg C, Taussig L, Halonen M. Association of interleukin-2 and interferon-g production by blood mononuclear cells in infancy with parental allergy skin tests and with subsequent development of atopy. J Allergy Clin Immunol 1995; 96:652–660.
44. Prescott S, Jenmalm M, Bjorksten B, Holt P. Effects of maternal allergen-specific IgG in cordblood on early postnatal development of allergen-specific T-cell immunity. Allergy 2000; 55(5):470–475.

45. Holt P, Sly P, Bjorksten B. Atopic versus infectious diseases in childhood: a question of balance? Ped Allergy Immunol 1997; 8:56–58.
46. Wilson CB, Westall J, Johnston L, Lewis DB, Dower SK, Alpert AR. Decreased production of interferon gamma by human neonatal cells—intrinsic and regulatory deficiencies. J Clin Invest 1986; 77:860–867.
47. Lewis D, Yu C, Meyer J, English B, Kahn S, Wilson C. Cellular and molecular mechanisms for reduced interleukin 4 and interferon gamma production by neonatal T cells. J Clin Invest 1991; 87:194–202.
48. Romagnani S. Induction of Th1 and Th2 responses: a key role for the "natural" immune response? Immunol Today 1992; 13(10):379–381.
49. Manetti R, Gerosa F, Guidizi M et al. Interleukin-12 induces stable priming for interferon-g production during differentiation of human Th cells and transient interferon-g production in established Th2 cell clones. J Exp Med 1994; 179:1273–1283.
50. Ridge J, Fuchs E, Matzinger P. Neonatal tolerance revisited: turning on newborn T cells with dendritic cells. Science 1996; 271:1723–1726.
51. Pohl D, Bockelmann C, Forster K, Reiger C, Schauer U. Neonates at risk of atopy show impaired production of interferon-gamma after stimulation with bacterial products (LPS and SEE). Allergy 1997; 52:732–738.
52. Holt PG. Development of T-cell memory against inhalant allergens: risks for the future. Clin Exp Allergy 1999; 29:8–13.
53. Warner JO, Marguet C, Rao R, Roche WR, Pohunek P. Inflammatory mechanisms in childhood asthma. Clin Exp Allergy 1998; 28 Suppl 5:71–75; discussion 90-1.
54. Holgate S, Davies D, Lackie P, Howarth P, Roche W. Gene-Environment interactions at an epithelial interface in the pathogenesis of asthma. ACI Int 2000; Suppl 1:25–34.
55. Strachan D. Editorial: Is allergic disease programmed in early life? Clin Exp Allergy 1994; 24:603–605.
56. Björkstén F, Suoniemi I, Koski V. Neonatal birch pollen contact and subsequent allergy to birch pollen. Clin Allergy 1980; 10:585–591.
57. Björkstén F, Suoniemi I. Time and intensity of first pollen contacts and risk of subsequent pollen allergies. Acta Med Scand 1981; 209:299–303.
58. Pearson D, Freed D, Taylor G. Respiratory allergy and month of birth. Clin Allergy 1977; 7:29–33.
59. Rugtveit J. Environmental factors in the first months of life and the possible relationship to later development of hypersensitivity. Allergy 1990; 45:154–156.
60. Carosso A, Ruffino C, Bugiani M. The effect of birth season on pollenosis. Ann Allergy 1986; 56:301–303.
61. Businco L, Cantani A, Farinella F, Businco E. Month of birth and grass pollen or mite sensitisation in children with respiratory allergy: a significant relationship. Clin Allergy 1988; 18:269–274.
62. Morrison-Smith J, Springett V. Atopic disease and month of birth. Clin Allergy 1979; 9:153–157.
63. Kleiner H, Arkins JA, Lauwasser M. Correlation between date of birth and pollen sensitivity. Ann Allergy 1975; 34:310–314.

64. Lau S, Falkenhorst G, Weber A et al. High mite-allergen exposure increases the risk of sensitisation in atopic children and young adults. J Allergy Clin Immunol 1989; 84:718–725.

65. Sporik R, Holgate S, Platts-Mills T, Cogwell J. Exposure to house-dust mite allergen (Der p1) and development of asthma in childhood. N Engl J Med 1990; 323:502–507.

66. Suoniemi I, Bjorksten F, Haahtela T. Dependence on immediate hypersensitivity in the adolescent period on factors encountered in infancy. Allergy 1981; 36:263–268.

67. Hesselmar B, Aberg N, Aberg B, Eriksson B, Bjorksten B. Does early exposure to cat or dog protect against later allergy development? Clin Exp Allergy 1999; 29:611–617.

68. Secrist H, DeKruyff RH, Umetsu DT. Interleukin 4 production by CD4+ T cells from allergic individuals is modulated by antigen concentration and antigen presenting cell type. J Exp Med 1995; 181:1081–1089.

69. Kuroume T, Oguri M, Matsumura T et al. Milk sensitivity and soybean sensitivity in the production of eczematous manifestations in breast-fed infants with particular reference to intra-uterine sensitization. Ann Allergy 1976; 37:41–46.

70. Halonen M, Stern DA, Wright AL, Taussig LM, Martinez FD. Alternaria as a major allergen for asthma in children raised in a desert environment. Am J Respir Crit Care Med 1997; 155(4):1356–1361.

71. Martinez FD. Complexities of the genetics of asthma. Am J Respir Crit Care Med 1997; 156(4 pt 2):S117–122.

72. Stewart G, Thompson P. The biochemistry of common aeroallergens. Clin Exp Allergy 1996; 26:1020–1044.

73. Stewart G, McWilliam PT. Biochemical properties of aeroallergens: contributory factors in allergic sensitization? Pediatr Allergy Immunol 1993; 4:163–172.

74. Thompson P. Unique role of allergens and the epithelium in asthma. Eur Respir Rev 1998; in press..

75. Finkelman FD, Urban JF. Cytokines: making the right choice. Parasitol Today 1992; 8:311–314.

76. Lanzavecchia A. Receptor-mediated antigen uptake and its presentation to class II–restricted T lymphocytes. Annu Rev Immunol 1990; 8:773–793.

77. Mon L, Kleimberg I, Mancini C, Bellini A, Marini M, Mattoli S. Bronchial epithelial cells of atopic patients with asthma lack the ability to inactivate allergens. Biochem Biophys Res Commun 1995; 217:817–824.

78. Marsh D, Freidhoff L, Ehrlich-Kautzky E. Immune responsiveness to *Ambrosia artemisiifolia* (short ragweed) pollen allergen Amb a VI (Rae6) is associated with HLA-DR5 in allergic humans. Immunogenetics 1987; 26:230–236.

79. Marsh D, Hsu S, Roebber M et al. HLA-Dw2: a genetic marker for human immune response to short rag-weed pollen allergen Ra.5. I Response resulting primarily from natural antigenic exposure. J Exp Med 1982; 155:1439–1451.

80. Freidhoff LR, Ehrlich-Kautzky E, Meyers DA et al. Association of HLA-DR3 with human immune response to Lol p I and Lol p II allergens in allergic subjects. Tissue Antigens 1988; 31:211–219.

81. Ansari AA, Freidhoff LR, Meyers DA, Bias WB, Marsh DG. Human immune responsiveness to Lolium perenne grass pollen allergen Lol p III ia associated with HLA-DR3 and DR5. Hum Immunol 1989; 25:59–71.

82. Ansari AA, Shinomiya N, Zwollo P, Marsh DG. HLA-D gene studies in relation to immune responsiveness to a grass allergen, Lol p III. Immunogenetics 1991; 33:24–32.

83. Evavold BD, Sloan-Lancaster J, Allen PM. Tickling the TCR: selective T-cell functions stimulated by altered peptide ligands. Immunol Today 1993; 14 (12):602.

84. Holt P, Macaubas C, Prescott S, Sly P. Microbial stimulation as an aetiologic factor in atopic disease. Allergy 1999; 54 (Suppl 49):12–16.

85. Baldini M, Lohman IC, Halonen M, Erickson RP, Holt PG, Martinez FD. A Polymorphism in the 5′ flanking region of the CD14 gene is associated with circulating soluble CD14 levels and with total serum immunoglobulin E. Am J Respir Cell Mol Biol 1999; 20:976–983.

86. Sudo N, Sawamura S, Tananka K, Aiba Y, Kubo C, Koga Y. The requirement of intestinal bacterial flora for the development of an IgE production system fully susceptible to oral tolerance induction. J Immunol 1997; 159:1739–1745.

87. Bjorksten B, Naaber P, Sepp E, Mikelsaar M. The intestinal microflora in allergic Estonian and Swedish 2-year-old children. Clin Exp Allergy 1999; 29:342–346.

88. Strachan DP, Taylor EM, Carpenter RG. Family structure, neonatal infection, and hay fever in adolescence. Arch Dis Childh 1996; 74(5):422–426.

89. Shaheen S. Changing patterns of childhood infection and the rise in allergic disease. Lancet 1995; 25:1034–1037.

90. Oryszczyn MP, Annesi-Maesano I, Campagna D, Sahuquillo J, Huel G, Kauffmann F. Head circumference at birth and maternal factors related to cord blood total IgE. Clin Exp Allergy 1999; 29:334–341.

91. Fergusson DM, Crane J, Beasley R, Horwood LJ. Perinatal factors and atopic disease in childhood [see comments]. Clin Exp Allergy 1997; 27:1394–1401.

92. Godfrey KM, Barker DJP, Osmond C. Disproportionate fetal growth and raised IgE concentration in adult life. Clin Exp Allergy 1994; 24:641–648.

93. Grimble RF. Nutritional modulation of cytokine biology. Nutrition 1998; 14:634–640.

94. Soyland E, Nenseter MS, Braathen L, Drevon CA. Very long chain n-3 and n-6 polyunsaturated fatty acids inhibit proliferation of human T-lymphocytes in vitro [published erratum appears in Eur J Clin Invest 1993 Nov; 23(11):761]. Eur J Clin Invest 1993; 23:112–121.

95. Endres S, Meydani SN, Ghorbani R, Schindler R, Dinarello CA. Dietary supplementation with n-3 fatty acids suppresses interleukin-2 production and mononuclear cell proliferation. J Leukoc Biol 1993; 54:599–603.

96. Caughey GE, Mantzioris E, Gibson RA, Cleland LG, James MJ. The effect on human tumor necrosis factor alpha and interleukin 1 beta production of diets enriched in n-3 fatty acids from vegetable oil or fish oil. Am J Clin Nutr 1996; 63:116–122.

97. Khair-el-Din TA, Sicher SC, Vazquez MA, Wright WJ, Lu CY. Docosahexaenoic acid, a major constituent of fetal serum and fish oil diets, inhibits IFN gamma-induced Ia-expression by murine macrophages in vitro. J Immunol 1995; 154: 1296–1306.

98. Weiss S. Diet as a Risk Factor for Asthma, CIBA Foundation Symposium. New York: John Wiley and Sons, 1997.

99. Black P, Sharpe S. Dietary fat and asthma: Is there a connection? Eur Respir J 1997; 10:6–12.

100. Reidel F. Influence of adjuvant factors on development of allergy. Evidence from animal experiments. Pediatr Allergy Immunol 1991; 21:1–5.

101. Gerrard JW, Heiner DC, Ko CG, Mink J, Meyers A, Dosman J. Immunoglobulin levels in smokers and non-smokers. Ann Allergy 1980; 44:261–262.

102. Burrows S, Halonen M, Barbee RA, Lebowitz MD. The relationship of serum immunoglobulin E to cigarette smoking. Am Rev Respir Dis 1981; 124: 523–525.

103. Warren C, Holford-Stevens V, Wong C, Manfreda J. The relationship between smoking and total immunoglobulin E levels. J Allergy Clin Immunol 1982; 69:370–375.

104. Wjst M, Heinrich J, Liu P et al. Indoor factors and IgE levels in children. Allergy 1994; 49:766–771.

105. Ware J, Dockery D, Spiro F, Ferris B. Passive smoking, gas cooking and respiratory health of children living in six cities. Am Rev Respir Dis 1984; 129:366–374.

106. Magnusson C. Maternal smoking influences cord serum IgE and IgD levels and increases the risk for subsequent infant allergy. J Allergy Clin Immunol 1986; 78:898–904.

107. Hanrahan JP, Tager IB, Segal MR et al. The effect of maternal smoking during pregnancy on early infant lung function. Am Rev Respir Dis 1992; 145:1129–1135.

108. Brown RW, Hanrahan JP, Castille RG, Tager IB. Effect of maternal smoking during pregnancy on passive respiratory mechanics in early infancy. Pediatr Pulmonol 1995; 19:23–28.

109. Stick SM, Burton PR, Gurrin L, Sly PD, LeSouef PN. Effects of maternal smoking during pregnancy and a family history of asthma on respiratory function in newborn infants. Lancet 1996; 348:1060–1064.

110. Hoo A, Matthias H, Dezateux C, Costeloe K, Stocks J. Respiratory function among preterm infants whose mothers smoked during pregnancy. Am J Respir Crit Care Med 1998; 158:700–705.

111. Yuskel BA, Greenough F, Griffin F, Nocolaides KH. Tidal breathing parameters in the first week of life and subsequent cough and wheeze. Thorax 1996; 51:815–818.

112. Barker D, Godfrey K, Fall C, Osmond C, Winter P, Shaheen S. Relation of birthweight and childhood respiratory infection to adult lung function and death from chronic obstructive airways disease. Br Med J 1991; 303:671–675.

113. Ross PS, De Swart RL, Reijnders PJ, Van Loveren H, Vos JG, Osterhaus AD. Contaminant-related suppression of delayed-type hypersensitivity and antibody responses in harbor seals fed herring from the Baltic Sea. Environ Health Persp 1995; 103:162–167.

114. Ross PS, Vos JG, Birnbaum LS, Osterhaus AD. PCBs are a health risk for humans and wildlife [letter]. Science 2000; 289:1878–1879.

115. Battershill JM. Review of the safety assessment of polychlorinated biphenyls (PCBs) with particular reference to reproductive toxicity. Hum Exp Toxicol 1994; 13:581–597.

116. Reichrtova E, Ciznar P, Prachar V, Palkovicova L, Veningerova M. Cord serum immunoglobulin E related to the environmental contamination of human placentas with organochlorine compounds. Environ Health Persp 1999; 107:895–899.
117. Williams TJ, Jones CA, Miles EA, Warner JO, Warner JA. Fetal and neonatal IL-13 production during pregnancy and at birth and subsequent development of atopic symptoms. J Allergy Clin Immunol 2000; 105:951–959.
118. Upham JW, Hayes LM, Lundahl J, Sehmi R, Denburg JA. Reduced expression of hemopoietic cytokine receptors on cord blood progenitor cells in neonates at risk for atopy. J Allergy Clin Immunol 1999; 104:370–375.
119. Chandra RK, Puri S, Suraiya C, Cheema PS. Influence of maternal food antigen avoidance during pregnancy and lactation on incidence of atopic eczema in infants. Clin Allergy 1986; 16:563–569.
120. Hattevig G, Kjellman B, Sigurs N, Grodzinsky E, Hed J, Bjorksten B. The effect of maternal avoidance of eggs, cow's milk, and fish during lactation on the development of IgE, IgG, and IgA antibodies in infants. J Allergy Clin Immunol 1990; 85(1):108–115.
121. Sigurs N, Hattevig G, Kjellman B. Maternal avoidance of eggs, cow's milk, and fish during lactation: effect on allergic manifestations, skin-prick tests, and specific IgE antibodies in children at ag 4 years. Pediatrics 1992; 89(4):735–939.
122. Zeiger R, Heller S, Mellon M et al. Effect of combined maternal and infant food allergen avoidance on development of atopy in early infancy: a randomised study. J Allergy Clin Immunol 1989; 84:72–89.
123. Zeiger R, Heller S, Mellon M, Halsey J, Hamburger R, Sampson H. Genetic and environmental factors affecting the development of atopy through age 4 in children with atopic parents: a prospective radomised study of food allergen avoidance. Pediatr Allergy Immunol 1992; 3:110–127.
124. Falth-Magnusson K, Kjellman NIM. Development of atopic disease in babies whose mothers were receiving exclusion diet during pregnancy—a randomized study. J Allergy Clin Immunol 1987; 80:869–875.
125. Falth-Magnusson K, Kjellman N-I. Allergy prevention by maternal elimination diet during late pregnancy: a five year follow-up of a randomized trial. J Allergy Clin Immunol 1992; 89:709–713.
126. Strannegard IL, Larsson LO, Wennergren G, Strannegard O. Prevalence of allergy in children in relation to prior BCG vaccination and infection with atypical mycobacteria. Allergy 1998; 53:249–254.
127. Alm JS, Lilja G, Pershagen G, Scheynius A. Early BCG vaccination and development of atopy. Lancet 1997; 350(9075):400–403.
128. Aaby P, Shaheen SO, Heyes CB et al. Early BCG vaccination and reduction in atopy in Guinea-Bissau. Clin Exp Allergy 2000; 30:644–650.
129. O'Hehir RE, Hoyne GF, Thomas WR, Lamb JR. House dust mite allergy: from T cell epitopes to immune therapy. Eur J Clin Invest 1993; 23:763–772.
130. Holt PG. A potential vaccine strategy for asthma and allied atopic diseases during early childhood. Lancet 1994; 344:456–458.

10

Polarization of T-Helper Cells

**MARTIEN L. KAPSENBERG, EDDY A. WIERENGA,
PAWEL KALINSKI, and ESTHER C. De JONG**

Academic Medical Centre
University of Amsterdam
Amsterdam, The Netherlands

I. Introduction

As outlined in previous chapters, the development of allergic asthma is causally related to the activation of allergen-specific type 2 T-helper lymphocytes (Th2 cells). Here we review the recent progress in our understanding of the mechanisms that underlie the development of the various phenotypes of Th cells. We will also discuss some of the concepts explaining the predominant occurrence of allergen-specific Th2 cells in allergy.

Th1 and Th2 cells are essential for survival of infection with selective pathogens when natural immunity fails. They are effector T cells that develop from naive T cells upon activation by pathogen-derived antigens presented by antigen-presenting cells (APCs), in particular dendritic cells (DCs). The DCs reside as sentinel cells at the sites of pathogen entry. Upon activation by pathogens, DCs undergo a program of maturation into effector DCs that migrate to lymphoid organs and effectively activate naive T cells. Recent evidence indicates that pathogens evoke host protective responses by the commitment of maturing DCs to promote the development of either Th1 or Th2 cells, depending on the type of pathogen. The priming of sentinel DCs to become Th1- or Th2-promoting effector DCs probably follows from the different mechanisms by which bioactive molecules from pathogens activate DCs.

To date, the origin of the development of allergen-specific Th2 cells in allergic asthma is unclear. In most patients, allergic asthma is the consequence of the atopic state. A currently well-appreciated hypothesis is that development of atopy or atopic diseases early in life is related to a lower pressure of microbes or microbial compounds on specific immune cells, in particular DCs. This emerging knowledge may have important implications for designing strategies for preventing the development of asthma or for managing ongoing allergic asthma.

II. Polarized Effector T Cells

While most pathogens are efficiently cleared by innate phagocytes, survival from infection with certain pathogens eventually depends on the generation of specific immunity. Specific immunity is mediated by the activation of either type 1 or type 2 CD4$^+$ T-helper cells (Th1/Th2) specific for these pathogens (Fig. 1) (1,2). In fact, all pathogens evoke mixed Th1 and Th2 cell responses, but the balance varies with the type of pathogen.

Th1 cells develop predominantly in response to intracellular pathogens, such as microorganisms that hide in the endosomal compartment of host cells, e.g., mycobacteriae, salmonellae, and listeriae. While both Th1 and Th2 cells produce cytokines like granulocyte-macrophage colony-stimulating factor (GM-CSF), interleukin-3 (IL-3), and tumor necrosis factor-α (TNF-α), Th1 cells produce high levels of interferon-γ (IFN-γ) and no IL-4, IL-5, and IL-13. IFN-γ efficiently retards the intracellular proliferation and stimulates the killing of endosomal intracellular pathogens in phagocytic cells. In addition, protective Th1 cells develop in response to many virus types. These Th1 cells are protective as they support the development of cytotoxic CD8$^+$ T cells the are required for the killing of virus-infected host cells. During their development in the T-cell area of lymphoid organs, Th1 cells will express selected chemokine receptors (CCR1, CCR5, and CXCR3), which enable them to migrate to the inflamed tissues that are infected with intracellular pathogens. These tissues produce appropriate Th1 cell–attracting chemokines, such as IP-10 (3). Since this type of inflammatory response is mediated by Th1 cells, it may be referred to as a type 1 inflammatory response.

In contrast, Th2 cells, producing IL-4, IL-5, and IL-13, develop predominantly in response to extracellular microorganisms. Th2 cell cytokines support humoral immunity by promoting the production of opsonizing antibodies that bind to pathogens, which leads to their subsequent elimination by FcR-bearing phagocytosing cells (Fig. 1). The precise mechanisms of the Th cell–induced antibody isotype switches in B cells are not entirely clear, except that the IgE isotype switch is induced by IL-4 and/or IL-13 in the absence of certain other cytokines, a condition that is provided by highly polarized Th2 cells (see Chap. 4) (4). For instance, helminth infections are clearly associated with the development of helminth-specific Th-2 cells and high levels of IgE production (5).

Interestingly, helminth infections and helminth egg granuloma formation are also characterized by local infiltration of Th2 cells, indicating that Th2

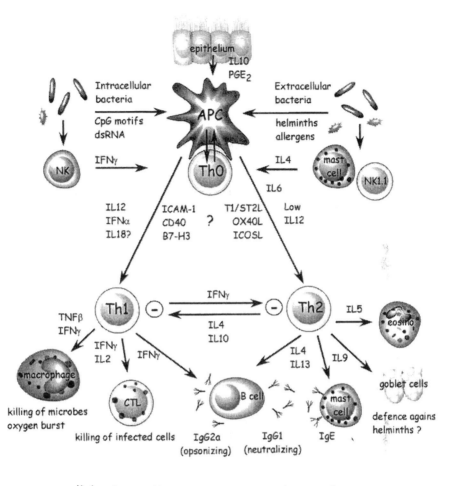

Figure 1 Polarization of Th0 cells. See text for explanation.

cells, like Th1 cells, can migrate to infected areas. To this aim, developing Th2 cells acquire a distinct set of chemokine receptors (CCR4 and CCR8), allowing them to migrate to helminth-infected tissues that produce the appropriate Th2 cell–attracting chemokines (3). Mouse studies showed that Th2 cells contribute to protection against the gut-dwelling helminths through IL-13-mediated activation of goblet and smooth muscle cells and fibroblasts in mucosal tissue and against tissue-dwelling helminths through IL-5-driven recruitment of eosinophils (5). In addition, Th2 cells against helminth egg antigens promote granuloma formation without the concomitant lethal pathology of Th1 cell–mediated inflammation. These findings in the mouse indicate that protection against different classes of pathogens require different inflammatory effector arms of the same type of Th2 cell–mediated (type 2) inflammation. Apparently, the superfluous effector arms of the inflammatory Th2 cells are well tolerated.

Clearly, the pathology of allergic asthma is based on this type of local activity of Th2 cells in the airways in response to airborne antigens (6). Studies in a mouse airway inflammation model (7) and clinical trials (8) suggested that IgE and eosinophils do not have a decisive role in the pathophysiology and symptoms of allergic asthma. More convincingly, the mouse models identified IL-13 as a cytokine crucial in allergen-induced airway hyperreactivity, mucus production, smooth muscle contraction, and connective tissue deposition (9). The cellular interplay between DCs, Th2 cells, and airway inflammation is discussed in more detail in Chapter 15.

Immunity by Th1 and Th2 cells can be counteracted by suppressor or "regulatory" $CD4^+$ T cells. At present two subsets have been identified, T_{reg} ($CD4^+$, $CD25^+$) and Tr1 cells. T_{reg} cells constitute about 10% of peripheral blood $CD4^+$ T cells and, even while they are quiescent, constitutively express CD25, the α chain of the IL-2 receptor. Mouse model studies have indicated that T_{reg} cells develop in the thymus (10) and are implicated in the prevention of organ-specific autoimmunity. To date it is unclear how T_{reg} are activated and whether they suppress antigen-specific immunity indirectly, by down-regulating the function of DC, or directly, by suppressing effector Th cells. Although T_{reg} cells produce IL-10, a cytokine implicated in down-regulation of the function of inflammatory immune cells, their suppressive effects seem to be exerted predominantly via a cognate interaction with APCs or Th cells, undefined thus far. Tr1 cells are cells that are generated in vitro form peripheral T cells in the presence of high levels of IL-10 (11) or a combination of immunosuppressive hormones (12). They produce high levels of IL-10 in combination of IFN-γ and IL-5, but no IL-4. In contrast to T_{reg} cells, Tr1 cells suppress the effector Th cells by virtue of their production of IL-10. Also Tr1 cells are implicated in the prevention of chronic inflammation, e.g., in Crohn's disease. Also, data are emerging that the condition of helminth egg granuloma formation is dominated, not only by Th2 cells but also by IL-10-producing suppressor T cells (12).

III. Th1/Th2-Cell-Polarizing Molecules

The chronicity of various infectious diseases, but also conditions such as autoimmunity, cancer, and allergy, have been linked to poor or aberrant Th cell polarization or, in some cases, to insufficient activity of suppressor cells. Therefore, it is important to study the mechanisms underlying the polarization of the T-cell response, i.e., how the response is optimally adapted to the type of invading microorganism as well as to the type of tissue (Fig. 1). For instance, the default response in airway-associated thoracic lymph nodes is Th2 biased and in the anterior chamber of the eye T suppressor cell biased. Th1 and Th2 cells are mature effector T cells that develop by functional polarization of naive Th cells after activation by APCs. In recent years, various molecules have been defined that polarize the cytokine profile of maturing T cells.

The best-studied identified Th1-driving factor is IL-12, which binds to the IL-12 receptor (13). Engagement of the IL-12 receptor costimulates Th cell proliferation and selectively up-regulates and primes for high IFN-γ production. Bioactive IL-12 p70 is almost exclusively produced by APC types, including DCs, upon activation by certain microbial products. IL-12 unresponsiveness in humans, due to mutations in the IL-12 receptor, is associated with chronic infections with various species of mycobacteriae, salmonellae, or toxoplasmae, but does not lead to increased susceptibility to virus infections (14). Also, IL-12-deficient mice, which have a strongly reduced frequency of Th1 cells in response to various endosomal pathogens, show normal Th1 cell development upon virus infection, indicating that IL-12 is indispensable for Th1 cell responses to endosomal pathogens, but redundant during Th1 responses against viruses (15). The Th1-polarizing activity of IL-12 is amplified by IL-18, of which the activity is strongly controlled by IL-18-binding protein. The full understanding of the importance of IL-18 as a skewer of Th1 responses is unclear as IL-18 may also amplify Th2 responses in the absence of IL-12 (16).

Another important set of Th1-driving factors are type I IFNs (17) produced by a variety of cell types, including APCs (18) and binding to type I IFN receptors. In this respect, murine cells are markedly different, as their IFN-mediated Th1 development mediated by IFN-γ, a type II IFN activating different signaling, and not by type I IFNs (19). This discrepancy strongly reduces the meaning of mouse model experiments on the role of IFNs in the development of specific immunity in the human. Both in mice and man, type I IFN production is strongly associated with viral infection and may be crucial in the development of protective Th1 immunity to viruses (20).

A variety of other Th1-polarizing molecules have been described of which the physiological role is not entirely clear. For instance, ICAM-1 is required in the interaction of naive T cells with APCs as an adhesion molecule, but also selectively primes for the production of type 1 cytokines (21). B7-H3 is a member of the B7 family of costimulatory molecules and drives Th1 cells, but the ligand molecule on the Th cells is unknown (22).

The most obvious Th2 cell–polarizing molecule is IL-4 (23). Although IL-4 can be produced in huge quantities by basophils, mast cells, and eosinophils, there is no evidence that these cells contribute to the polarization of specific immunity (24). Therefore, it is believed now that in the absence of initial Th1-driving signals IL-4 will drive the development of highly polarized Th2 cells via autocrine amplification. An impressive number of other Th2 cell–polarizing molecules have been described, predominantly in mouse models, including OX40L (25), ICOSL (26), T1/ST2 ligand (27), and MCP-1 (28).

Unfortunately, the various studies on OX40L (29) and ICOSL (30) are contradictory, suggesting that these are costimulatory molecules that favor the development of Th2 cells only under certain conditions, whereas the role for T1/ST2 and MCP-1 has not been confirmed in human cells. The physiological conditions required to obtain T_{reg} or Tr-1 cells are obscure.

IV. Intracellular Messengers of T-Cell Polarization

Cytokines act via specific membrane receptors expressed on selected sets of target cells, thereby inducing the cytoplasmic phosphorylation of so-called STAT (signal tranducer and activator of transcription) factors, which in turn migrate to the nucleus and mediate the cytokine-induced transcriptional control of sensitive genes (Fig. 2). The dominant Th cell–polarizing cytokines IL-12 and IL-4 lead to phosphorylation of the transcription factors STAT4 and STAT6, respectively, which are instrumental in the canonical Th cell polarization processes of which the underlying mechanisms are only gradually delineated. IL-12-induced phosphorylation of STAT4 in activated T cells increases the expression of the Th1-specific transcription factor T-bet (31). T-bet enhances IFN-γ production by remodeling the IFN-γ gene locus (32), making it accessible to the transcriptional machinery. As a positive-feedback effect, T-bet also increases expression of the signaling β_2 subunit of the IL-12 receptor (IL-12Rβ2) (32), perpetuating IL-12 responsiveness. In the human, but not in mice, IFN-α also increases IL-12Rβ2 expression through phosphorylation of STAT4 (33) and possibly through induction of T-bet. The importance of T-bet in Th1 development is underscored by the reversal of established Th2 cells by ectopically expressed T-bet, not only inducing the production of IFN-γ but also reducing the production of IL-4 (and IL-5) (31). Although STAT4 is essential for full-blown Th1 responses, disruption of the STAT4 gene does not totally block IFN-γ production nor does it prevent Th1 cell development (32).

IL-4 induces phosphorylation of STAT6, which in turn increases GATA-3 expression (34). GATA-3, like T-bet, is a chromatin remodeler and as such is responsible for opening the IL-4 locus (35). Upon activation of the DNA binding activity by CD28 costimulation, GATA-3 not only induces IL-4 production but also suppresses IL-12Rβ2 expression (34), thereby blocking IL-12-mediated Th1 development. Ectopic expression of STAT6 or GATA-3 conferred IL-4 production to non-IL-4-producing cells (36,37), indicating the powerful effects of these factors. However, in STAT6$^{-/-}$ mice, GATA-3 was still able to remodel chromatin at the IL-4 locus. In these mice, IL-4 could still be produced albeit at lower levels compared with wild-type mice (37).

In general, upon TCR/CD28 (co)stimulation, the IFN-γ and IL-4 loci are made accessible by T-bet and GATA-3. These processes are selectively accelerated by IL-12 (through STAT4) and IL-4 (through STAT6), respectively. Stabilizing feedback mechanisms are established by the autoinduction activities of GATA-3 (37) and T-bet (32), while the polarization processes are further

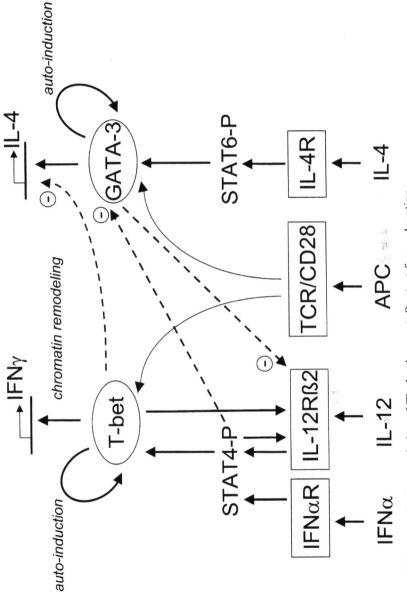

Figure 2 Molecular regulation of Th development. See text for explanation.

facilitated by suppression of the opposite phenotype, i.e., IL-12 inhibits GATA-3 expression (34), T-bet inhibits IL-4 (and IL-5) production (31), and IL-4 represses Th1 development by increasing GATA-3 expression, which inhibits IL-12Rβ2 expression and thus IL-12 responsiveness (34). Whether and how alternative polarizing factors interfere with these molecular mechanisms needs to be determined in most cases.

V. Dendritic Cells

Because APCs express many of the T-cell-polarizing molecules, discussed above, these cells play a pivotal role in the polarization of T-cell immunity. As reviewed in Chapter 2, the most important APCs are DCs that are present as immature sentinel antigen-trapping cells of myeloid origin at the potential sits of pathogen entry, in particular in the epithelia of the skin and mucosal tissues (38). DCs producing inflammatory mediators immediately upon tissue infection mediate early, innate immune responses. Furthermore, they initiate and regulate specific immunity by activating antigen-specific T-helper and cytotoxic cells. To this aim, sentinel DCs, like many other innate immune cells, express various receptors that enable them to recognize and endocytose microbes or their compounds, as discussed below, as well as stress factors released by surrounding infected cells. Remarkably, upon ligation of some of these receptors, sentinel DCs mature into effector cells that migrate to the draining lymphoid tissue and acquire the unique ability to stimulate native Th cells. The maturation process is required because at their sentinel stage resting DCs express little or no molecules required for antigen presentation to naive T cells, i.e., class I and II MHC molecules, the costimulatory molecules CD80 and CD86, chemokines that attract naive T cells, and chemokine receptors required to migrate to lymphoid organs (39).

Upon activation, sentinel DCs secrete inflammatory mediators like cytokines (TNF-α, IL-1β, IL-6, and IL-12), eicosanoids (PGE$_2$), and chemokines (IL-8, MDC, TARC), all of which contribute to local inflammation. At the same time, the DCs undergo the program of maturation including a transient up-regulation of their endocytic capacity and increased peptide loading of intracellular class I and II MHC molecules (40). Thereafter, DCs lose their endocytic capacity and redistribute their intracellular MHC molecules to the cell surface. They also change the expression of their chemokine receptors, which allows them to migrate to lymphoid organs. They also increase their expression of costimulatory molecules, adhesion molecules, and chemokines, all required to attract and facilitate the activation of naive T cells in the draining lymphoid organs (41).

Although DCs are all bone marrow derived, recent studies show a surprising heterogeneity. DCs not only show differential maturational stages, but can also belong to different lineages with different functions. Human myeloid

DCs are ontogenetically related to monocytes and express receptors for their growth factor GM-CSF. They represent the cells that populate the sites of potential pathogen entry. Immigration of these cells via peripheral blood and emigration via lymph in peripheral tissues is a continuous process that is strongly boosted by local inflammation. Plasmacytoid cells, on the other hand, are precursors of plasmacytoid dendritic cells (PDCs), which are considered to be lymphoid DCs because their development is related to the development of lymphocytes (41). These DCs grow in response to IL-3 instead of GM-CSF. PDCs are found at low numbers in peripheral lymphoid organs but are especially abundant in certain inflammatory conditions. For instance, they show up late after experimental out-of-season allergen challenge in patients with allergic rhinitis (42). The precise function of these PDCs as APCs is unknown to date, but they certainly are important as natural IFN-α-producing cells during viral infection (18).

The heterogeneity of DCs is more complex. Peripheral blood harbors at least five populations of precursor DCs, based not only on analysis of the expression of GM-CSF or IL-3 receptors, but also on the differential expression of CD11c, CD16, CD34, and DC-specific markers like MDC8 and BDCA-1 to 4 (43–45). In addition, DCs can be generated in vitro from peripheral blood monocytes in the presence of GM-CSF and IL-4 (40). Moreover, peripheral tissues harbor DCs with tissue-specific phenotypes, like Langerhans cells in epithelia of the skin, nose, and lung. Studies of the ontogenetic relationship between these tissue DCs and the peripheral blood precursors and their specific functions are emerging but are frustrated by the difficulties in isolating these cells, due to their low frequencies, lack of proliferation, and the inaccessibility of most tissues for functional analysis of the DCs.

Mouse model studies will be extremely helpful in this respect, albeit the heterogeneity of DCs in the mouse is slightly different from that in humans. Also in mice, myeloid and lymphoid DCs were found, and to some extent the expression of a CD8α homodimer is helpful in distinguishing between myeloid and lymphoid DCs (46). At present, also in the mouse IFN-α-producing plasmacytoid-like cells have been found, but as in humans their function as APCs has not been cleared (see Chap. 2).

VI. Polarized Effector Dendritic Cells

Mouse model experiments strongly suggest that DCs isolated from different tissues differentially polarize Th cells. DCs from spleen readily produce IL-12 and induce Th1 cells, in contrast to mucosal DCs freshly isolated from Peyer patches (47,48) or airway mucosa (49), that produce little or no of IL-12 but high levels of IL-10 and induce Th2, Th3, or Tr1 cell responses in vitro. However, upon culture thoracic DCs gain the ability to produce IL-12 and derive both Th1 and Th2 cell responses (48). Mouse skin DCs (Langerhans cells and dermal DCs) are able to produce IL-12 and are implicated in the differential development of Th1 cells in response to contact allergens as opposed to the lack of development of Th1 cells in UV-induced tolerance (50). Adding to the functional heterogeneity of the murine DCs, it was found that myeloid spleen DCs without CD8α expression show a poor ability for IL-12 production and readily induce Th2 cell responses, whereas CD8α$^+$ DCs produce IL-12 and bias for the development of Th1 cells (51).

All together the data discussed above suggest that DCs induce either Th1 or Th2 responses, depending on their lineage, their maturation stage, or the tissue in which they are dwelling. Only recently, it was realized that the potential of any DCs to induce Th1 or Th2 cell responses is flexible and strongly dependent on the condition of their maturation. When mature effector DCs engage T cells, they not only present pathogen-derived antigens (MHC-peptide complexes, signal 1) and costimulatory molecules (signal 2), but also express molecules that polarize the T cells (signal 3). The character of signal 3 strongly depends on the type of pathogen and the environmental conditions experienced by sentinel DCs during the onset of their final maturation (52). The character of signal 3 may be predetermined at their sentinel stage, but it will become fully available only upon engagement of T cells. The ligation of CD40 by CD40L expressed by activated T cells has an important role in this process. Naive T cells rapidly express CD40L upon their initial activation by the recognition of peptide-loaded MHC molecules and costimulation of CD28. Ligation of CD40, and perhaps a similar cross-talk between TRANCE-L on T cells and TRANCE on DCs, is the boost for DCs to fully express their profile of T-cell-polarizing molecules.

Thus, the type of T-cell response in lymphoid organs is adapted to the type of pathogen and the type of affected tissue through the priming of peripheral sentinel DC into functionally distinct effector cells that express their function upon the engagement of pathogen-specific naive T cells in the draining lymph nodes. Adaptation of DCs to pathogens is a consequence of both the direct impact of pathogen-derived compounds and the indirect effect of products from local tissue cells in reaction to these pathogens. This concept is supported by the finding that Th1 and Th2 cytokine profiles are found in draining lymph nodes of mice within 3 days, depending on the type of pathogen used during immunization in the hind footpads (53).

Support for this concept further follows from experiments with monocyte-derived sentinel-type DCs in vitro (52,54,55). Induction of maturation of these DCs, either by the combination of IL-1β and TNF-α ("maturation factors") or by LPS, induces highly immunogenic effector DCs that drive both Th1 and Th2 cells (DC0). By varying the condition of stimulation, effector DCs can be defined that selectively bias the development of either Th1 cells (DC1) or Th2 cells (DC2) (Fig. 3). For example, bacterial CpG-DNA motifs, pertussis toxin, and IFN-γ induce the development of type I DCs that promote the development of Th1 cells through elevated levels of IL-12. Interestingly, viral RNA (poly I:C) induces the development of another type 1 DC that preferentially polarizes Th1

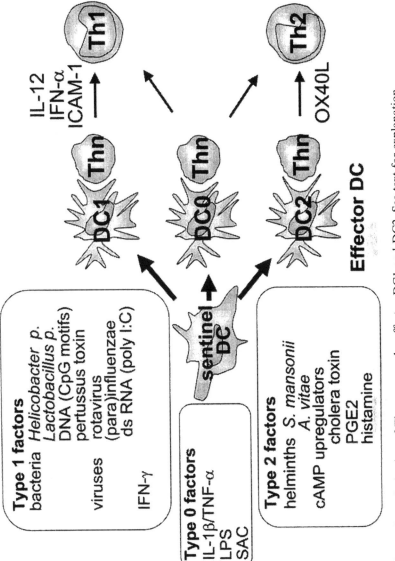

Figure 3 Polarization of Th responses by effector DC1 and DC2. See text for explanation.

cells, via unknown secreted molecules, not involving IL-12 nor IL-18 or type I IFN. These data are consistent with the data, discussed above, indicating that virus-induced Th1 cell development is independent of IL-12. On the other hand, secreted proteins from helminth eggs or worms (such as phosphorylcholine-containing glycoprotein ES-62) (55) induce type 2 DCs that promote the development of Th2 cells, mainly through the expression of OX40L. Compounds that up-regulate intracellular cAMP, such as cholera toxin, histamine, and PHE_2, also induce DC2 development but, although these DC2 also express OX40L required for costimulation, the Th2 cell polarization is dominated by an as-yet-unidentified soluble factor. All these DC subsets are genuine, stably committed effector cells because after final maturation their functional phenotype cannot be altered by the various modulators tested.

Similarly, activation of PDCs in vitro by CD40 ligation induces their maturation into effector DC2 cells, which promote the development of Th2 cells through an unknown mechanism, whereas viral activation of PDCs induces a DC1 effector phenotype with high levels of IFN-α (56,57). Thus, immature myeloid and lymphoid DCs both can become either Th1- or Th2-promoting immunogenic effector DCs, depending on the conditions triggering their maturation. The general rule is that pathogens evoke protective responses in the host by the conditional priming of immature DCs.

Mucosal DCs induce the generation of suppressor cells (47–49). Similarly, immature DCs lacking immunogenic costimulatory molecules are consequently tolerogenic by inducing the development of T_{reg}-like cells by activating naive Th cells in the absence of signals 2 and 3 (58). In addition, DCs arrested in an immature state by corticosteroids or IL-10 lack costimulatory molecules as well as cytokine production and, therefore, also induce the development of T_{reg} cells or, in certain conditions, anergic T cells (59). The conditions of induction of T-suppressor cells deserves much more attention and is actively explored by several research groups.

Therefore, in strict analogy to naive Th cells that adopt differentially polarized phenotype (Th1, Th3, Th3, Tr1), immature DCs react to their environment by adopting polarized DC1 or DC2 (and most likely additional) effector phenotypes.

VII. Pattern Recognition Molecules

The molecular basis of DC activation and polarization is gradually becoming clear. According to a concept originally coined by Janeway (60), DCs, like other innate immune cells, recognize pathogen-associated molecular patterns (PAMPs) through pattern recognition receptors (PRRs), including C-type lectins, selected scavenger receptors, and the newly defined family of Toll-like receptors (TLR1-10). Ligation of TLRs in DCs leads to production of inflammatory mediators and maturation. Ligands for some of the TLR have recently been identified (61): gram-negative bacteria express (LPSs) that signal via TLR4, whereas gram-positive bacteria express lipoteichoic acids (LTAs), which signal via TLR2. Bacteria also express and contain many other molecules that may activate innate immune cells, including flagellin signaling via TLR5, and CpG-DNA motifs, signaling via TLR9. Yeast and fungal cells express PAMPs in the form of mannans and β-glucans; retroviruses carry dsRNA; whereas protozoa express unique glycosylated proteins and lipids. All these molecules may trigger DCs in their own unique way.

To date, the data on how PRR signaling leads to the differential development of DC1 or DC2 is limited but interesting. Signaling via TLR9 leads to the development of DC1 with high IL-12 production (62). However, the expression of TLR9 is limited to endosomal membranes. This finding fits perfectly the knowledge that Th1-mediated protection to endosomal microorganisms is induced by IL-12. TLRs are not evenly distributed on myeloid and lymphoid DCs. TLR2 and TLR4 are mainly expressed in myeloid DCs and probably do not mediate DC polarization, whereas TLR9 is found predominantly in PDCs mediating INF-α production, which promotes the development of Th1 cells (62). Therefore, only myeloid DCs respond to LPS and LTA, whereas only PDCs react to CpG-DNA.

VIII. Alternative Pathways of T-Cell Polarization

Although no reliable studies using live pathogens are available, animal experiments with protein antigens indicate that the induction of Th1 versus Th2 profiles depends on the applies antigen dose. Although reliable data are lacking in the case of live pathogens, animal model experiments with protein antigen indicate that different isotype profiles of immunoglobulins versus delayed-type hypersensitivity profiles or Th1 versus Th2 profiles arise, depending on the applied antigen dose. Elegant experiments in vitro with peptide antigens suggest that at least one mechanism of this antigen dose-dependent Th1/Th2 polarization is related to the strength of the ligation of the TCR (63). At high peptide dose and with high-affinity peptides naive T cells preferentially develop into Th1 cells, whereas at low peptide dose or with low-affinity peptides the T cells develop into Th2 cells. Various explanatory mechanisms were proposed, including the level of the participation of CD4 in the MHC–TCR interaction (64) and the level of induction of CD40L (65). Another explanatory mechanism for the dose dependency of the Th1/Th2 balance is that at high antigen dose more lymphoid organs and more APC types are involved, including non-DC APC types, such as macrophages, that will have different expression profiles of Th cell–polarizing molecules.

The physiological meaning of differential Th1/Th2 responses to different numbers of live pathogens remains unclear. The optimal protection against pathogens will require either protective Th1 or Th2 responses depending on the type of pathogen, regardless of their numbers. For instance, if low-dose antigens induce Th2 responses and antibody production, it should be expected that each infection starts off with the antibody production, regardless of whether protection preferentially requires Th1 responses or not. This is unlikely, especially because Th2-driving antigen dose effects observed in vitro are easily overruled by the T-cell-polarizing effects of such pathogen-induced factors as IL-12 and IFN-α.

Th1/Th2 cell polarization can also occur in a DC-independent fashion. Although T cells probably do not express PPRs, they have receptors for hormones and are susceptible to pathogen-derived compounds utilizing alternative pathways of stimulation. A most convincing and important example is the bias for Th2 responses induced by progesterone that is produced by ovarian cells during pregnancy (66). This Th2 bias helps to prevent unnecessary elicitation of type 1 inflammatory responses detrimental to the fetus. This Th2 response is induced by the direct modulation of naive or memory T cells, whereas DCs are not susceptible. Certain toxins, like pertussis toxin and cholera toxin, can bias Th cells directly, although such biases may not necessarily be considered as protective responses. It is to be expected, however, that many other direct interactions of T cells and pathogens will prove to have a genuine role in the initiation of protective immunity.

IX. DC and Th2 Cells in Atopy

Th2 responses induce type 2 inflammation, which is protective against helminths but which is highly detrimental in allergic asthma and allergic rhinitis. To date, there is no clear explanation for the occurrence of atopy and atopic diseases. However, there is increasing appreciation for the concept that atopy and atopic diseases may be associated with a changed interaction with microorganisms. The prevalence of atopy and atopic diseases has steadily increased during the last decades in countries with a "Western" lifestyle. Intensive epidemiological studies made the improved diagnosis, enhanced industrial pollution or increased exposure to allergens, to be less likely causes. The relationships to maternal smoking, obesity, and, in particular, a hygienic lifestyle are still valid. The hygiene concept, originally formulated by David Strachan (67), puts forward that atopic disease is associated with a more hygienic lifestyle that reduces the number of cross-infections at an early age, as is evident in the conditions associated with higher social classes, smaller families, less day care, and less farming. The concept is supported by additional epidemiological studies indicating that atopics have undergone far fewer encounters with certain orofecal microorganisms (68), suggesting an important role for the microbial colonization of the gut.

The currently proposed mechanism underlying the hygiene hypothesis is that the default immune response at birth, as opposed to that in adulthood, is

Th2-cell biased and this bias disappears upon rapid contact with microbes or their compounds during the first months of life (69). Better hygiene has severely hampered the rate of gut colonization and in this way delayed the development of specific immunity. The restoration of the default Th1/Th2 response during the first months of life may be initiated by gut microbe–derived compounds, like toxins or lipoproteins, leaking into the body and driving the differentiation of DCs from the fetal phenotype into DCs with a phenotype associated with an enhanced ability to express Th1-driving molecules. A recently postulated alternative is that the colonization of the gut, especially with helminths, may eventually induce bystander suppressor cells that inhibit the development of any type of immunity against allergens (70). This hypothesis also explains why allergen-specific T-cell proliferation is low after successful immunotherapy.

The protective role of early encounters with pathogens or their compounds are substantiated in the mouse model of airway inflammation, indicating that *Mycobacterium* infection or its compound BCG prevent the development of inflammation upon allergen challenge in sensitized mice (71). It is tempting to speculate that DCs have a central role in the rebalancing or induction of bystander suppressor cells.

X. Concluding Remarks

Emerging data support a pivotal role of DCs in the initiation of protective immunity by polarizing Th cells in a pathogen- and tissue-matched fashion. In a strict analogy to naive Th cells, which develop into polarized Th cell subsets, immature DCs react to their environment, and to the different ways that pathogens induce their maturation, by adopting type 1- or type 2-polarized effector phenotypes, capable of inducing Th1 versus Th2 responses.

This knowledge generates a series of new, more detailed questions addressing which pathogen-associated molecules activate DC, as well as which receptors and signaling molecules, and which lineages of DC, are involved. These questions may often be difficult to answer. For instance, a single pathogen may require different types of protective immunity depending on the stage of its life cycle. In addition, within one species the required protective immune responses may vary (PK: unclear). Finally, many pathogens may evoke paradoxical responses, as each is equipped with an amazingly diverse array of tools to evade protective immunity.

An exciting perspective is that the development of atopy or atopic diseases might be treated by the prevention of the development of allergen-specific Th2 cells via modulation during the first weeks of life of the DC driving the fetal Th2 bias. Various current studies are focused on the possible beneficial effects of early vaccination or dietary supplementation. The additional effectiveness of common vaccination against childhood diseases in the prevention the development of allergy is still under debate. An initial study on probiotic supplementation showed that daily administration of *Lactobacillus* during the first half year of life reduced the development of atopic eczema with about 50%, a spectacular result (72). The effectiveness of immunotherapy of atopic disorders may also benefit from adjuvants such as bacterial DNA (CpG motifs), the efficacy of which approach is currently being tested (73).

References

1. Mosmann TR, Sad S. The expanding universe of T-cell subsets: Th1, Th2 and more. Immunol Today 1996; 17:138–146.
2. Romagnani S. The Th1/Th2 paradigm. Immunol Today 1997; 18:263–266.
3. D'Ambrosio D, Iellem A, Colantonio L, Clissi B, Pardi R, Sinigaglia F. Localization of Th-cell subsets in inflammation: differential thresholds for extravasation of Th1 and Th2 cells. Immunol Today 2000; 21:183–186.
4. Delprete G, Maggi E, Parronchi P, Chretien I, Tiri A, Macchia D, Ricci M, Banchereau J, De Vries J, Romagnani S. IL-4 is an essential factor for the IgE synthesis induce in vitro by human T cell clones and their supernatants. J Immunol 1988; 140:4193–4198.
5. Finkelman FDm Urban JF. The other side of the coin: the protective role of Th2 cytokines. J Allergy Clin Immunol 2001; 107:772–780.
6. Kay AB. T cells as orchestrators of the asthmatic response. CIBA Found Symp. 1997; 206:56–70.
7. Kips JC, Tournoy KG, Pauwels RA. Gene knockout models of asthma. Am J Respir Crit Care Med. 2000; 162:S66–S70.
8. Leckie MJ, ten Brinke A, Khan J, Diamant Z, O'Connor BJ, Walls CM, Mathur AK, Cowley HC, Chung KF, Djuganovic R, Hansel TT, Holgate T, Sterk PJ, Barnes PJ. Effects of an interleukin-5 blocking monoclonal antibody on eosinophils, airway hyper-responsiveness, and the late asthmatic response Lancet 2000; 356:2144–2148.
9. Wills-Karp M. IL-12/IL-13 axis in allergic asthma. J All Clin Immunol 2001; 107:9–18.
10. Shevach EM. Certified professionals: CD4(+)CD25(+) suppressor T cells. J Exp Med 2001; 193:F41–F45.
11. Roncarolo M-G, Levings MK. The role of different subsets of T regulatory cells in controlling autoimmunity. Curr Opin Immunol 2000; 12:676–683.
12. van den Biggelaar AHJ, van Ree R, Rodrigues LC, Lell B, Deelder AM, Kremsner PG, Yazdanbakhsh M. Decreased atopy in children infected with *Schistosoma haematobium*: a role for parasite-induced interleukin-10. Lancet 2000; 356:1723–1727.
13. Murphy KM, Ouyang W, Farrar JD, Yang JF, Ranganath S, Asnagli H, Afkarian M, Murphy TL. Signaling and transcription in T helper development. Annu Rev Immunol 2000; 18:451–494.
14. Jouanguy E, Doffinger R, Dupuis S, Pallier A, Altare F, Casanova JL. IL-12 and IFN-γ in host defence against mycobacteria and salmonella in mice and men. Curr Opin Immunol 1999; 11:346–351.

15. Schijns VECJ, Haagmans BL, Wierda CMH, Kruithof B, Heijnen IAFM, Alber G, Horzinek MC. Mice lacking IL-12 develop polarized Th1 cells during viral infection. J Immunol 1998; 160:3958–3964.

16. Nakanishi K, Yosimoto T, Tsutsui H, Okamura H. IL-18 regulates both Th1 and Th2 responses. Annu Rev Immunol 2001; 19:423–474.

17. Romagnani S. Biology of human Th1 and Th2 cells. J Clin Immunol 1995; 5:121–129.

18. Kadowaki N, Antonenko S, Lau JYN, Liu YJ. Natural interferon alpha/beta-producing cells link innate and adaptive immunity. J Exp Med 2000; 192:219–225.

19. Farrar JD, Murphy KM. Type I interferons and T helper development. Immunol Today 2000; 21:484–489.

20. Belardelli F, Gresser I. The neglected role of type I interferon in the T-cell response: implications for its clinical use. Immunol Today 1996; 17:369–372.

21. Salomon B, Bluestone JA. LFA-1 interaction with ICAM-1 and ICAM-2 regulates Th2 cytokine production. J Immunol 1998; 161:5138–5142.

22. Chapoval AI, Ni J, Lau JS, Wilcox RA, Files DB, Liu D, Dong HD, Sica GL, Zhu GF, Tamada K, Chen LP. B7-H3: a costimulatory molecule for T cell activation and IFN-γ production. Nat Immunol 2001; 2:269–274.

23. Paul WE, Melchers, Metcalf, Burgess, Strasser, Dexter, Nicola Interleukin 4: signal ling mechanisms and control of T cell differentiation. CIBA Found Symp 1997; 204:208–219.

24. Schmitz J, Thiel A, Kuhn R, Rajewski K, Muller W, Assenmacher M, Radbruch A. Induction of IL-4 expression in Th cells is not dependent on IL-4 form non-Th cells. J Exp Med 1994; 179:1349–1353.

25. Hutloff A, Dittrich AM, Beier KC, Eljaschewitsch B, Kraft R, Anagnostopoulos I, Kroczek RA. ICOS is an inducible T-cell co-stimulator structurally and functionally related to CD28. Nature 1999; 397:263–266.

26. Lane P. Role of OX40 signals in coordinating CD4 T cell selection, migration and cytokine differentiation in Th1 and Th2 cells. J Exp Med 2000; 191:201–205.

27. Lohning M, Stroehmann A, Coyle AJ, Grogan JL, Lin S, Gutiereres-Ramos JC, Levinson D, Radbruch A, Kamradt T. T1/ST2 is preferentially expressed on murine Th2 cells, independent of IL4, IL-5 and IL-10 and important for Th2 effector function. Prc Natl Acad Sci 1998; 95:6930–6935.

28. Gu L, Tseng S, Horner RM, Tam C, Loda M, Rollins BJ Control of T(H)2 polarization by the chemokine monocyte chemoattractant protein-1. Nature 2000; 404:407–411.

29. Chen AI, McAdam AJ, Buhlman JE, Scott S, Lupher ML, Brenfoeld EA, Baum PR, Fanslow WC, Calderhead DM, Freeman GL, Sharpe AH. OX40-ligand has a critical co-stimulatory role in dendritic cell: T cell interactions. Immunity 1999; 11:689–698.

30. Rottman JB, Smith T, Tonra JR, Ganley K, Bloom T, Silva R, Pierce B, Gutierrez-Ramos JC, Ozkaynak E, Coyle AJ. The costimulatory molecule ICOS plays an important role in immunopathogenesis of EAE. Nat Immunol 2001; 2:605–611.

31. Szabo SJ, Kim ST, Costa GL, Zhang X, Fathman CG, Glimcher LH. A novel transcription factor, T-bet, directs Th1 lineage commitment. Cell 2000; 100:655–669.

32. Mullen AC, High FA, Hutchins AS, Lee HW, Villarino AV, Livingston DM, Kung AL, Cereb N, Yao T-P, Yang SY, Reiner SL. Role of T-bet in commitment of TH1 cells before IL-12-dependent selection. Science 2001; 292:1907–1910.
33. Rogge L, Barberis-Maino L, Biffi M, Passini N, Presky DH, Gubler U, Sinigaglia F. Selective expression of an interleukin 12 receptor component by human T helper 1 cells. J Exp Med 1997; 185:825–831.
34. Ouyang W, Ranganath SH, Weindel K, Bhattacharya D, Murphy TL, Sha WC, Murphy KM. Inhibition of Th1 development mediated by GATA-3 through an IL-4-independent mechanism. Immunity 1998; 9:745–755.
35. Lee HJ, Takemoto N, Kurata H, Kamogawa Y, Miyatake S, O'Garra A, Arai N. GATA-3 induces T helper cell type 2 (Th2) cytokine expression and chromatin remodeling in committed Th1 cells. J Exp Med 2000; 192:105–116.
36. Kurata H, Lee HJ, O'Garra A, Arai N. Ectopic expression of activated STAT6 induces the expression of Th2-specific cytokines and transcription factors in developing Th1 cells. Immunity 1999; 11:677–688.
37. Ouyang W, Lohning M, Gao Z, Assenmacher M, Ranganath S, Radbruch A, Murphy KM. STAT6-independent GATA-3 autoactivation directs IL-4-independent Th2 development and commitment. Immunity 2000; 12:27–37.
38. Banchereau J, Steinman RM. Dendritic cells and the control of immunity. Nature 198; 392:245.
39. Sallusto F, Mackay CR, Lanzavecchia A. The role of chemokine receptors in primary, effector, and memory immune responses. Annu Rev Immunol 2000; 18:593–611.
40. Sallusto F, Lanzavecchia A. Efficient presentation of soluble antigen by cultured human dendritic cells is maintained by GM-CSF plus IL-4 and downregulated by TNF-alpha. J Exp Med 179:1109–1118.
41. Grouard G, Rissoan MC, Filgueira L, Durand I, Banchereau J, Liu YJ. The enigmatic plasmacytoid T cells develop into dendritic cells with interleukin (IL)-3 and CD40-ligand. J Exp Med 1997; 185:1101–1111.
42. Jahnsen FL, Lund-Johansen F, Dunne JF, Farkas L, Haye R, Brandtzaeg P. Experimentally induced recruitment of plasmacytoid (CD123(high)) dendritic cells in human nasal allergy. J Immunol 2000; 165:4062–4068.
43. Dzionek A, Fuchs A, Schmidt P, Cremer S, Zysk M, Miltenyi S, Buck DW, Schmitz J. BDCA-2, BDCA-3 and BDCA-4: three markers for distinct subsets of dendritic cells in human peripheral blood. J Immunol 2000; 165:6037–6046.
44. Schakel K, Poppe C, Mayer E, Federle C, Riethmuller G, Rieber EP. M-DC8+ leukocytes—novel human dendritic cell population. Pathobiology 1999; 67:287–290.
45. Summers KL, Hock BD, McKenzie JL, Hart DNJ. Phenotypic characterization of five dendritic cell subsets in human tonsils. Am J Pathol 2001; 159:285–295.
46. Shortman K. Dendritic cells: multiple subtypes, multiple origins, multiple functions. Immunol Cell Biol 2000; 78:161–165.
47. Iwasaki A, Kelsall BL. Freshly isolated Peyer's patch, but not spleen, dendritic cells produce interleukin 10 and induce the differentiation of helper type 2 cells. J Exp Med 1999; 190:229–239.
48. Weiner HL. The mucosal milieu creates tolerogenic dendritic cells and TRI and T(H)3 regulatory cells. Nat Immunol 2001; 2:671–672.

49. Stumbles PA. Regulation of T helper cell differentiation by respiratory tract dendritic cells. Immun Cell Biol 1999; 77:428–433.

50. Grabbe S, Schwarz T. Immunoregulatory mechanisms involved in elicitation of allergic contact hypersensitivity. Immunol Today 1998; 19:37–44.

51. Moser M, Murphy KM. Dendritic cell regulation of T(H)1-T(H)2 development. Nat Immunol 2000; 1:199–205.

52. Kalinski P, CMU Hilkens, EA Wierenga and ML Kapsenberg. T-cell priming by type-1 and type-2 polarized dendritic cells: the concept of a third signal. Immunol Today 1999; 20:561–569.

53. Toellner KM, Luther SA, Sze DMY, Choy RKW, Taylor DR, MacLennan ICM, Acha-Orbea H. T helper 1 (Th1) and Th2 characteristics start to develop during T cell priming and are associated with an immediate ability to induce immunoglobulin class switching. J Exp Med 1998; 187:1193–1204.

54. de Jong EC, Vieira P., Kalinski P, Schuitemaker JHN, Tanaka Y, Wierenga EA, Yazdanbakhsh M, Kapsenberg ML. Microbial compounds selectivity induce Th1-promoting or Th2-promoting dendritic cells with diverse Th-cell polarizing signals. J Immunol 2002; 168:1704.

55. Whelan M, Harnett MM, Houston KM, Patel V, Harnett W, Rigley KP. A filarial nematode–secreted product signals dendritic cells to acquire a phenotype that drives development of Th2 cells. J Immunol 2000; 164:6453–6460.

56. Cella M, Facchetti F, Lanzavecchia A, Colonna M. Plasmacytoid dendritic cells activated by influenza virus and CD40L drive a potent TH1 polarization. Nat Immunol 2000; 1:305–310.

57. Kadowaki N, Antonenko S, Lau JYN, Liu YJ. Natural interferon alpha/beta-producing cells link innate and adaptive immunity. J Exp Med 2000; 192:219–225.

58. Jonuleit H, Schmitt E, Steinbrink K, Enk AH. Dendritic cells as a tool to induce anergic and regulatory T cells. Trends Immunol 2001; 22:394–400.

59. Bellinghausen I, Brand U, Steinbrink K, Enk AH, Knopf J, Saloga J. Inhibition of human allergic T-cell responses by IL-10-treated dendritic cells: differences from hydrocortisone-treated dendritic cells. J All Clin Immunol 2001; 108:242–249.

60. Medzhitov R, Janeway C. Innate immune recognition: mechanisms and pathways. Immunol Rev 2000; 173:89–102.

61. Akira S, Takeda K, Kaisho T. Toll-like receptors: critical proteins linking innate and acquired immunity. Nat Immunol 2001; 2:675–680.

62. Wagner H. Toll meets bacterial CpG-DNA. Immunity 2001; 14:499–502.

63. O'Garra A, Arai N. The molecular basis of T helper 1 and T helper 2 cell differentiation. Trends Cell Biol 2000; 10:542–550.

64. Metz DP, Bottomly K. Low affinity TCR interactions of memory and naive CD4 T cells are differentially regulated by CD4-Associated p56lck. FASEB J 2000; 14:A991–A991.

65. Ruedl C, Bachmann MF, Kopf M. The antigen dose determines T helper subset development by regulation of CD40 ligand. Eur J Immunol 2000; 30:2056–2064.

66. Piccinni MP, Scaletti C, Maggi E, Romagnani S. Role of hormone-controlled Th1- and Th2-type cytokines in successful pregnancy. J Neuroimmunol 2000; 109:30–33.

67. Strachan DP. Hay-fever, hygiene, and household size. Br Med J 1989; 299:1259–1260.

68. Matricardi PM, Rosmini F, Riondino S, Fortini M, Ferrigno L, Rapicetta M, Bonini S. Exposure to foodborne and orofecal microbes versus airborne viruses in relation to atopy and allergic asthma: epidemiological study. Br Med J 2000; 320:412–417.
69. Martinez FD, Holt PG. Role of microbial burden in aetiology of allergy and asthma. Lancet 1999; 354:S12–S15.
70. Yazdanbakhsh M, van den Biggelaar A, Maizels RM. Th2 responses without atopy: immunoregulation in chronic helminth infections and reduced allergic disease. Trends Immunol 2001; 22:372–377.
71. Herz U, Lacy P, Renz H, Erb K. The influence of infections on the development and severity of allergic disorders. Curr Opin Immunol 2000; 12:632–640.
72. Kalliomaki M, Salminen S, Arvilommi H, Kero P, Koskinen P, Isolauri E. Probiotics in primary prevention of atopic disease: a randomised placebo-controlled trial. Lancet 2001; 357:1076–1079.
73. Krieg AM. From bugs to drugs: therapeutic immunomodulation with oligodeoxynucleotides containing CpG sequences from bacterial DNA. Antisense Nucl Acid Drug Dev 2001; 11:181–188.

11

CD28 and B7 Superfamily Members
Costimulation and Regulation of T-Cell Function

ANTHONY J. COYLE, STEPHEN MANNING, and JOSE-CARLOS GUTIERREZ-RAMOS

Millennium Pharmaceuticals
Cambridge, Massachusetts, U.S.A.

I. Contemporary Models of T-Cell Activation

In response to viral or bacterial infection, a series of highly regulated events are initiated to limit damage to the host and to provide long-term protection or immunity. However, this same protective response is also responsible for tissue destruction in response to self antigens resulting in autoimmunity or to innocuous soluble proteins that are recognized as harmful and induce allergic responses. Upon encountering foreign antigens, immature dendritic cells (DCs) migrate to colocalize with nonprimed antigen-specific T cells in the T-cell zone. At this site, T cells first become primed, in turn providing signals to mature and activate DCs. These primed T-helper precursor (THP) cells then migrate to the edge of the B-cell-rich follicle where they encounter antigen-bearing B cells that have also now accumulated in this area (1). These B cells then present peptide to primed T cells, which in turn secrete cytokines and deliver cognate signals to favor B-cell expansion and then either become immunoglobulin-expressing germinal center B cells or migrate to the red pulp and become antibody-producing plasma cells. Follicular dendritic cells (FDCs), also located in the germinal center, have the capacity to retain antigen for prolonged periods of time and are believed to have a role in selection of high-affinity clones and in the development of B-cell memory responses (2). A fraction of the activated T cells develop into memory cells, allowing for a fast and effective response once the specific antigen is reencountered. More than 30 years ago, Bretscher and Cohn proposed the two-signal hypothesis for T- and

B-lymphocyte activation (3). It has now become widely accepted that T cells require two distinct signals for optimal THP expansion. This model hypothesizes that peptides presented to antigen-specific T cells in the context of major histocompatability complex (MHC) class II molecules delivers signal 1, whereas a second or costimulatory signal through a distinct T-cell surface molecule triggers signal 2 (4). Signaling through signal 1 in the absence of costimulation leads to aborted activation and depletion of activated THP cells or a prolonged state of anergy or clonal unresponsiveness.

II. CD28/B7 Costimulatory Pathway

A. CD28 and CTLA-4 Regulate T-Cell Function

The molecular basis for the two-step costimulatory model was discovered almost 20 years after the original conceptual model was first proposed, by the cloning of an accessory costimulatory molecule, Tp44, subsequently referred to as CD28 (5). CD28 is a disulfide-linked homodimeric glycoprotein containing a single immunoglobulin variable-like domain. Signaling though CD28 with specific antibodies is required for optimal interleukin-2 (IL-2) production, IL-2 receptor expression, and cell cycle progression (6–8). T cells from mice deficient for CD28 also show strong impairment of proliferation in vitro after stimulation with antibodies to the T-cell receptor (TCR), allostimulation, and specific antigen (9–10). Similarly in vivo, CD28-deficient mice exhibit impaired T-helper B responses, although $CD8^+$ CTL induction appears to be normal (10). Recently, CD28 deficiency resulted in reduced severity in murine models of arthritis (11), experimental allergic encephalomyelitis (12), and mucosal lung inflammation (13).

In 1987, CTLA-4 was cloned from a subtracted cytolytic T-cell library as the second member of the CD28 family (14). In contrast to CD28, CTLA-4 is induced upon activation and delivers a negative signal to the activated T cell, opposing CD28-mediated costimulation (15). The importance of this pathway is further illustrated in mice deficient in CTLA-4, which exhibit profound lymphoproliferative defects characterized by polyclonal T-cell activation and a high frequency of cells expressing activation/memory T-cell antigens (16). More recently, CTLA-4 engagement was shown to augment antitumor immunity (17), to regulate autoimmune diabetes (18), and to provide an important signal leading to T-cell tolerance (19).

B. B7-1 and B7-2 Family

In 1982, a novel B-cell antigen was identified that was subsequently termed B7-1 and identified as the first ligand for CD28 (20,21). In 1993, a second CD28 ligand, B7-2, was identified (22). B7-1 (CD80) and B7-2 (CD86) belong to the Ig superfamily and exhibit 25% identity in the Ig-variable (v) and constant (c) extracellular domain, but exhibit pronounced differences in the amino acid sequence of their cytoplasmic domains. B7-1 binds CTLA-4 with the highest affinity whereas B7-2 binds to CD28 with the lowest affinity. The combination of B7-1-CD28 and B7-2-CTLA-4 binds with intermediate affinities. B7-2 is induced rapidly on B cells, DCs, and macrophages within hours, whereas B7-1 is up-regulated only at later times. These observations have led to the hypothesis that B7-2 interactions are required for the initial T-cell costimulation whereas B7-1-CD28 interactions are more involved in the sustained T-cell activation, but this remains to be substantiated. The interaction of B7-1 with CTLA-4 is one of the highest affinities described for cell surface molecules, and the more biologically relevant role of B7-1 may be to generate stable signaling complexes with CTLA-4 to terminate T-cell activation. This is supported by the observation that B7-1 transgenic mice exhibit markedly impaired immune responses (23), consistent with the ability of B7-1 to bind CTLA-4.

C. Differential Regulation of the Immune Response by B7-1 and B7-2

$CD4^+$ T cells have the capacity to differentiate to distinct effector populations characterized by their ability to produce different cytokines and surface receptors and, as a consequence, exhibit different functions. TH1 cells secrete interferon-γ (IFN-γ), IL-2, and tumor necrosis factor-α (TNF-α), and express the chemokine receptor CCR5 and the IL-18 receptor. Th2 cells produce IL-4, IL-5, and IL-10 and express the G-protein-coupled receptors CCR3, CCR4, and CRTH2, as well as the IL-1 receptor family member T1/ST2. Th1 cells influence the outcome following exposure to infectious agents and regulate autoimmune diseases, whereas Th2 cells are key effector cells in response to helminth infections and allergens.

One recent aspect of intense research in the area of costimulation was whether B7-1 and B7-2 have redundant roles in regulating the generation of effector cells or whether these molecules can deliver distinct signals required for THP function. Ligation of CD28 and CTLA-4 may directly regulate THP differentiation, as CD28 activation facilitates Th2 responses (24) whereas CTLA-4 inhibits Th2 responses (25). A large number of studies in vivo have attempted to address the importance of B7-1- and B7-2-mediated costimulation using a chimeric Fc protein consisting of the extracellular domain of CTLA-4 fused to human or mouse IgG Fc. This binds to B7-1 and B7-2 with high affinity and hence prevents both CD28 and CTLA-4 signaling. CTLA-4Ig inhibited IL-4 but not IFN-γ secretion during cutaneous leishmaniasis (26). Similar conclusions were drawn using NOD CTLA-4Ig transgenic mice, which developed enhanced autoimmune diabetes, associated with enhanced IFN-γ secretion, reduced IgG1 production, and diminished Th2 cytokine secretion (27). In contrast, B7 blockade suppresses Th1 cytokines, whereas IL-4 and IL-10 are increased after alloantigenic challenge (28). Similarly, studies using neutralizing antibodies to B7-1 or B7-2 in the induction of experimental autoimmune encephalomyelitis

(EAE) suggest that treatment with antibodies to B7-1 favors Th2 development and is associated with an amelioration of organ-specific disease, whereas antibodies to B7-2 augment Th1 responses and worsen disease (29). However, work in B7-1- and B7-2-deficient animals showed B7-2 to be the more critical molecule in EAE, whereas B7-1 does not have an important role (12).

D. Costimulation and T Regulatory Cell Function

Evidence is emerging that B7-1 and B7-2 provide an important signal to T regulatory cells that are present in the $CD25^+$ subset of $CD4^+$ T cells. Mice lacking B7-1 and B7-2 have a profound decrease in this population of T cells (as do CD28-deficient mice), which provides an explanation for the greatly increased severity and incidence of autoimmune diabetes in the NOD B7-deficient animals (30). Similarly, short-term inhibition of B7-1 and B7-2 using CTLA-4Ig also reduced the number of T regulatory cells. This suggests that homeostasis of this regulatory cell population is under the dynamic control of B7-1 and B7-2 and supports the concept that these cells are encountering an ongoing signal in the periphery to dampen down autoimmune responses. Recent in vitro experiments showed that the dependency on CD28-B7-mediated costimulation is greatly influenced by the antigenic experience of the T cell. Although antigen inexperienced $CD4^+$ T cells require B7-mediated signaling for IL-2 production, clonal expansion, and acquisition of effector function, optimal activation of recently activated T-helper subsets is B7 independent (31). While CTLA-4Ig is effective in inhibiting a number of immune responses in vivo when administered at the time of initial T-cell activation, delaying CTLA-4Ig treatment has sometimes been ineffective (32). Similarly, although CTLA-4Ig is effective in inhibiting a primary immune responses, some studies showed that secondary immune responses cannot be fully suppressed by administration of CTLA-4 Ig (33,34). Finally, recent data demonstrated that reactivation of memory cells is independent of both B7-1 and B7-2 (35).

III. The Expanding B7 Family

Largely as a consequence of the unraveling of the human genome, four new members of the B7 family have recently been identified, and their relationship by homology is shown in Fig. 1. Interestingly, these molecules are expressed on different cell types and are differentially regulated upon activation. While the function of these proteins remains to be fully understood, evidence is emerging that they exhibit distinct functions in regulating THP responses.

A. B7-Related Protein-1 (B7RP-1)

Swallow and colleagues using subtractive hybridization identified the third member of the B7 family, which they termed B7 homologue (B7h) (36). The

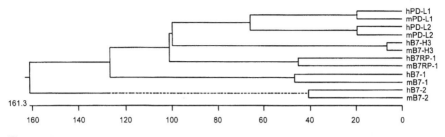

Figure 1 Phylogenetic tree of the B7 family members.

murine homologue of B7h was subsequently cloned from an intraepithelial lymphocyte library and termed B7-related protein-1 (B7RP-1) (37). B7RP-1 exhibits 20% homology to B7-1 and B7-2, and does not bind either CD28 or CTLA-4. B7RP-1 is expressed at low levels on monocytes and is up-regulated by IFN-γ, but not by TNF-α, lipopolysaccharide (LPS), or CD40 ligation (38). Resting B cells constitutively express B7RP-1, which is in contrast to the relatively low levels of B7-1 and 2. In situ analysis revealed that B7RP-1 is strongly expressed in the B-cell follicles of normal animals, in Peyer patches, and in thymus (39). Mice transgenic for B7RP-1Fc developed T-cell hyperplasia, plasmacytosis, and hypergammaglobulinemia (39).

B. ICOS, The Third Member of the CD28 Family

Recently, the T-cell counterpart of B7RP-1 has been identified as the third member of the CD28 family inducible costimulator (ICOS) (40,41). Unlike CD28, ICOS is induced with in 24–48 h of activation on all Th primed cells and is expressed on almost all CD45RO$^+$ cells in the tonsil (40,41). However, in vitro, in the presence of IL-12, ICOS is down-regulated resulting in the expression of a Th2-specific costimulatory molecule (41,42). In vitro, ICOS delivers a CD28-independent signal for IFN-γ and IL-4, but not for IL-2 production (39). Clearly, identification of ICOS has profound implications in the regulation of previously activated T cells and/or memory cells. Recent data suggest that B7RP-1–ICOS interactions play an essential role in T-cell-dependent B-cell activation, as IgG$_1$ and IgG$_{2a}$ titers are markedly diminished by disruption of B7RP-1-mediated signaling (41) and can provide a CD28-independent signal for viral immune responses (43). While the initial role of ICOS appeared to deliver a signal preferential to Th2 immune deviation, ICOS blockade also inhibits allograft rejection and the production of IFN-γ and IL-10 (44). Similarly, ICOS has an important role in the pathogenesis of EAE (45,46). Mice deficient in ICOS fail to generate germinal centers following immunization with soluble antigens, which is associated with a failure to up-regulate CD40L expression on T cells (47–49).

C. PD-1 Ligands—Negative Regulators of Immune Responses

The fourth member of the B7 family, termed B7 homologue 1 or B7-H, was identified among human cDNA expressed sequences in a search for B7-related proteins (50). B7-H1 shares 20% amino acid identity with the extracellular domains of B7-1 and only 15% with B7-2 (Fig. 1). Within the immune system, B7-H1 is constitutively expressed by DCs and is induced by IFN-γ and LPS on monocytes. B7-H1 was originally demonstrated to costimulate for IL-10 production by an IL-2 dependent mechanism and to facilitate T-cell proliferation (49). More recent observations have suggested that the principal function of B7-H1 is to inhibit T-cell proliferation and the production of IL-2, IFN-γ, and IL-10 (50). The ligand for B7-H1 is programmed death-1 (PD-1) (51). PD-1 is a 55-kD transmembrane protein that exhibits 24% amino acid homology in the extracellular domain to CTLA-4. Unlike the three other family members that possess a YxxM motif, PD-1 contains an inhibitory immunoreceptor (ITIM) motif in the cytoplasmic tail. PD-1, while being expressed on a minor population of thymocytes, is strongly induced on peripheral T cells upon activation (51). The fifth member of the B7 family was recently identified as a gene exhibiting 37% homology to B7-H1. This new member also binds PD-1 and has been termed PD-L2 (52). Both molecules have very similar functions in their ability to oppose T-cell activation and to attenuate cytokine production. Interestingly, PD-L2 is expressed constitutively on monocytes and is down-regulated upon activation, whereas PD-L1 is not present on resting cells and is inducible on activation (52). The relative importance of this differential expression remains to be determined, but suggest that PD-L1 and PD-L2 would play differing roles at various stages of the immune response. The importance of T-cell suppression mediated by PD-L1 and PD-L2 is supported by observations that mice deficient in PD-1 develop characteristic lupus-like disorders and glomerulonephritis (53). Thus, similar to CD28, PD-1 binds at least two ligands: PD-L1 and PD-L2. This raises the possibility that, in addition to CTLA-4:B7-1 or B7-2 interactions, PD-1:PD-L1 and PD-1:PD-L2 may be involved in the maintenance of peripheral self-tolerance by serving as a negative regulator of immune responses.

D. Identification of the Sixth Family Member: B7-Related Protein-2 (B7RP-2)/B7-H3

The sixth member of the family has recently been identified and cloned from a human DC library. The latest family member is most related to the ICOS ligand, and we have termed this gene B7RP-2. Unlike B7RP-1, which is expressed primarily on B cells, B7RP-2 mRNA is expressed at very high levels of immature DCs and upon stimulation with LPS is down-regulated on activation to a level comparable to B7-1. Despite its homology to other B7 family members this gene, also termed B7-H3, does not bind CD28, CTLA-4, ICOS, or PD-1, and the identity of its counterligand remains to be determined. B7-H3 costimulates both CD4$^+$ and CD8$^+$ T cells to proliferate and produce IFN-γ (54). Interestingly, B7-H3 also augments the generation of CTLs in vitro. However, whether this molecule has an important role in regulating cell mediated responses in vivo has not been determined.

IV. Regulation of T-Cell Function by the B7 Family

There is little doubt that CD28 ligation by B7-1 and B7-2 provides an important mechanism by which naive T cells produce IL-2 and undergo clonal expansion. Clearly in the absence of signal 2, the primary immune response, at least to soluble antigens, is severely impaired. So how does our recent awareness of multiple family members of the B7 family integrate in this two-step model? As shown in Fig. 2, for sustained T-cell proliferation it is likely that a continuous

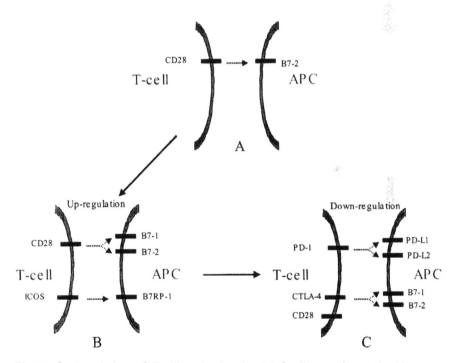

Figure 2 Regulation of T-cell activation by B7 family members. (A) Upon encountering an antigen-presenting cell (APC), the T-cell costimulatory molecule CD28 interacts with B7-2 causing the induction of B7-1, B7-2, and B7RP-1 on the APC, and the induction of ICOS on the T-cell. (B) The interactions of CD28 with B7-1 and B7-2 and ICOS with B7RP-1 lead to T-cell expansion and the induction of CTLA-4 and PD-1 on T cells, whereas PD-L1 and PD-L2 are induced on APCs. (C) The interactions of CTLA-4 with B7-1 and B7-2 and PD-1 with PD-L1 and PD-L2 lead to the downregulation of T-cell expansion.

supply of antigen-primed DCs are required to provide TCR ligation and B7 costimulation. B7RP-1 could provide this "step 2 of signal 2," and this would occur upon encounter with antigen-specific B cells that have endocytosed the same antigen for which the primed THP cells are antigen restricted, thus ensuring the specificity of the immune response (i.e., the cognate interaction). Shortly after antigen priming, DCs and macrophages expressing not only B7-1 and 2 would now inhibit T-cell activation via CTLA-4, but also PD-L1 and PD-L2. These ligands would be available to interact with PD-1 to suppress IFN-γ and IL-10 production and inhibit T-cell expansion.

V. Conclusions

Since the identification of the prototypic family member B7-1 about 20 years ago, our understanding of the mechanisms that govern the fate of THP cells has increased dramatically. However, with the identification of six members of the B7 family, the complexity of signals that regulate T-cell function has increased. These molecules appear to regulate the fate of previously primed THP cells rather than antigen-inexperienced cells (Fig. 2). An appreciation of the roles of these molecules will have important implications for understanding the pathogenesis of disorders characterized by inappropriate T-cell activation, including autoimmune and allergic diseases, transplant rejection, and regulation of tumor immunity.

References

1. Garside P, Ingulli E, Merica RR, Johnson JG, Noelle RJ, Jenkins MK. Visualization of specific B and T lymphocyte interactions in the lymph node. Science 1998; 281:96–99.
2. Klaus GGB, Humphret JH, Kunkl A, Dongworth DW. The follicular dendritic cell: its role in antigen presentation in the generation of immunological memory. Immunol Rev 1980; 53:3–28.
3. Bretscher PA, Cohn M. A theory of self and non self discrimination. Science 1970; 169:1042–1049.
4. Schwartz RH. A cell culture model for T lymphocyte clonal anergy. Science 1990; 4961: 1349–1356.
5. Aruffo A, Seed B. Molecular cloning of a CD28 cDNA by a high-efficiency COS cell expression system. Proc Natl Acad Sci USA 1987; 84:8573–8577.
6. June CH, Ledbetter JA, Gillespie MM, Lindsten T, Thompson CB. T-cell proliferation involving the CD28 pathway is associated with cyclosporine -resistant interleukin 2 gene expression. Mol Cell Biol 1987; 12:4472-81.
7. Harding FA, McArthur JG, Gross JA, Raulet DH, Allison JP. CD28-mediated signalling co-stimulates murine T cells and prevents induction of anergy in T-cell celones. Nature 1992; 6370:607–609.

8. Jenkins MK, Taylor PS, Norton SD, Urdahl KB. CD28 delivers a costimulatory signal involved in antigen-specific IL-2 production by human T cells. J Immunol 1991; 147:2461–2466.
9. Lucas PJ, Negishi I, Nakayama K, Fields LE, Loh DY. Naive CD28-deficient T cell can initiate but not sustain an in vitro antigen-specific immune response. J Immunol 1997; 154:5757–5768.
10. Shahinian A, Pfeffer K, Lee KP, Kundig TM, Kishihara A, Wakeham A, Kawai K, Ohashi PS, Thompson CB, Mak TW. Differential T cell costimulatory requirements in CD28-deficient mice. Science 1993; 261:609–612.
11. Tada Y, Nagasawa K, Ho A, Morito F, Ushiyama O, Suzuki N, Ohta H, Mak TW. CD28-deficient mice are highly resistant to collagen-induced arthritis. J Immunol 1999; 162:203-208.
12. Girvin AM, Dal Canto MC, Rhee L, Salomon B, Sharpe A, Bluestone JA, Miller SD. A critical role for B7/CD28 costimulation in experimental autoimmune encephalomyelitis: a comparative study using costimulatory molecule-deficient mice and monoclonal antibody blockade. J Immunol 2000; 164:136–143.
13. Mathur M, Hermann K, Qin Y, Gulmen F, Li X, Krimins R, Weinstock J, Elliott D, Bluestone JA, Padrid P. CD28 interactions with either CD80 or CD86 are sufficient to induce allergic airway inflammation in mice. Am J Respir Cell Mol Biol 1999; 21:498–509.
14. Brunet JF, Denizot F, Luciani MF, Roux-Dosseto M, Suzan M, Matei MG, Golstein P. A new member of the immunoglobulin superfamily—CTLA-4. Nature 1987; 328:267–270.
15. Walunas TL, Lenschow DJ, Bakker CY, Linsley PS, Freeman GJ, Geen JM, Thompson CB, Bluestone JA. CTLA-4 can function as a negative regulator of T cell activation. Immunity 1994; 1:405–413.
16. Tivol EA, Borriello F, Schweitzer AN, Lynch WP, Bluestone JA, Sharpe AH. Loss of CTLA-4 leads to massive lymphoproliferation and fatal multiorgan tissue destruction, revealing a critical negative regulatory role of CTLA-4. Immunity 1995; 3:541–547.
17. Leach DR, Krummel MF, Allison JP. Enhancement of antitumor immunity by CTLA-4 blockade. Science 1996; 271:1734–1736.
18. Luhder F, Hoglund P, Allison JP, Benoist C, Mathis D. Cytotoxic T lymphocyte-associated antigen 4 (CTLA-4) regulates the unfolding of autoimmune diabetes. J Exp Med 1998; 187:427–432.
19. Perez VL, Van Parijs L, Biuckians A, Zheng XX, Strom TB, Abbas AK. Induction of peripheral T cell tolerance in vivo requires CTLA-4 engagement. Immunity 1997; 4:411–417.
20. Yokochi T, Holly RD, Clark EA. B lymphoblast antigen (BB-1) expressed on Epstein Barr virus activated B cell blasts, b lymphoblastoid cell lines and Burkitts lymphomas. J Immunol 1982; 128:823–827.
21. Freedman AS, Freeman G, Horowitz JC, Daley J, Nadler. L. B7, a B-cell-restricted antigen that identifies preactivated B cells. J Immunol 1987; 139:3260–3267.
22. Freeman GJ, Borriello F, Hodes RJ, Reiser H, Hathcock KS, Laszlo G, McKnight AJ, Kim J, Du L, Lombard DB. Uncovering of functional alternative CTLA-4 counter-receptor in B7-deficient mice. Science 1993; 262: 907–909.

23. Sethna MP, van Parijs L, Sharpe AH, Abbas AK, Freeman GJ. A negative regulatory function of B7 revealed in B7-1 transgenic mice. Immunity 1994; 1: 415–421.

24. Khattri R, Auger JA, Griffin MD, Sharpe AH, Bluestone JA. Lymphoproliferative disorder in CTLA-4 knockout mice is characterized by CD28-regulated activation of Th2 responses. J Immunol 1999; 162:5784– 5791.

25. Oosterwegel MA, Mandelbrot DA, Boyd SD, Lorsbach RB, Jarrett DY, Abbas AK, Sharpe AH. The role of CTLA-4 in regulating Th2 differentiation. J Immunol 1999; 163:2634–2639.

26. Corry DB, Reiner SL, Linsley PS, Locksley RM. Differential effects of blockade of CD28-B7 on the development of Th1 or Th2 effector cells in experimental leishmaniasis. J Immunol 1994; 9:4142–4148.

27. Lenschow DJ, Herold KC, Rhee L, Patel B, Koons A, Qin HY, Fuchs E, Singh B, Thompson CB, Bluestone JA. CD28/B7 regulation of Th1 and Th2 subsets in the development of autoimmune diabetes. Immunity 1996; 3:285–293.

28. Sayegh MH, Akalin E, Hancock WW, Russell ME, Carpenter CB, Linsley PS, Turka LA. CD28-B7 blockade after alloantigenic challenge in vivo inhibits Th1 cytokines but spares Th2. J Exp Med 1995; 5:1869–1874.

29. Kuchroo VK, Das MP, Brown JA, Ranger AM, Zamvil SS, Sobel RA, Weiner HL, Nabavi N, Glimcher LH. B7-1 and B7-2 costimulatory molecules activate differentially the Th1/Th2 developmental pathways: application to autoimmune disease therapy. Cell 1995; 10:707–718.

30. Salomon B, Lenschow DJ, Rhee L, Ashourian N, Singh B, Sharpe A, Bluestone JA. B7/CD28 costimulation is essential for the homeostasis of the CD4+CD25+ immunoregulatory T cells that control autoimmune diabetes. Immunity 2000; 4:431–440.

31. Schweitzer AN, Sharpe AH. Studies using antigen-presenting cells lacking expression of both B7-1 (CD80) and B7-2 (CD86) show distinct requirements for B7 molecules during priming versus restimulation of Th2 but not Th1 cytokine production. J Immunol 1998; 6:2762–2771.

32. Corry DB, Reiner SL, Linsley PS, Locksley RM. Differential effects of blockade of CD28-B7 on the development of Th1 or Th2 effector cells in experimental leishmaniasis. J Immunol 1994; 9:4142–4148.

33. Tang A, Judge TA, Nickoloff BJ, Turka LA. Suppression of murine allergic contact dermatitis by CTLA4Ig. Tolerance induction of Th2 responses requires additional blockade of CD40-ligand. J Immunol 1996; 157:117–125.

34. Gause WC, Lu P, Zhou XD, Chen SJ, Madden KB, Morris SC, Linsley PS, Finkelman FD, Urban JF. Polygyrus: B7-independence of the secondary type 2 response. Exp Parasitol 1996; 84:264–273.

35. London CA, Lodge MP, Abbas AK. Functional responses and costimulator dependence of memory CD4+ T cells. J Immunol 2000; 164:265–272.

36. Swallow MM, Wallin JJ, Sha WC. B7h, a novel costimulatory homolog of B7.1 and B7.2, is induced by TNFalpha. Immunity 1999; 11:423–432.

37. Yoshinaga SK, Whoriskey JS, Khare SD, Sarmiento U, Guo J, Horan T, Shih G, Zhang M, Coccia MA, Kohno T, Tafuri-Bladt A, Brankow D, Campbell P, Chang D, Chiu L, Dai T, Duncan G, Elliott GS, Hui A, McCabe SM, Scully S, Shahinian A, Shaklee CL, Van G, Mak TW, Senaldi G. T-cell co-stimulation through B7RP-1 and ICOS. Nature 1999; 402:827–832.

38. Aicher A, Hayden-Ledbetter M, Brady WA, Pezzutto A, Richter G, Magaletti D, Buckwalter S, Ledbetter JA, Clark EA. Characterization of human inducible costimulator ligand expression and function. J Immunol 2000; 164:4689–4696.
39. Yoshinaga SK, Zhang M, Pistillo J, Horan T, Khare SD, Miner K, Sonnenberg M, Boone T, Brankow D, Dai T, Delaney J, Han H, Hui A, Kohno T, Manoukian R, Whoriskey JS, Coccia MA. Characterization of a new human B7-related protein: B7RP-1 is the ligand to the co-stimulatory protein ICOS. Int Immunol 2000; 10:1439–1447.
40. Hutloff A, Dittrich AM, Beier KC, Eljaschewitsch B, Kraft R, Anagnostopoulos I, Kroczek RA. ICOS is an inducible T-cell co-stimulator structurally and functionally related to CD28. Nature 1999; 6716:263–267.
41. Coyle AJ, Lehar S, Lloyd C, Tian J, Delaney T, Manning S, Nguyen T, Burwell T, Schneider H, Gonzalo JA, Gosselin M, Owen LR, Rudd CE, Gutierrez-Ramos JC. The CD28-related molecule ICOS is required for effective T cell–dependent immune responses. Immunity 2000; 95–105.
42. McAdam AJ, Chang TT, Lumelsky AE, Greenfield EA, Boussiotis Va, Duke-Cohan JS, Chernova T, Malenkovich N, Jabs C, Kuchroo VK, Ling V, Collins M, Sharpe AH, Freeman GJ. Mouse inducible costimulatory molecule (ICOS) expression is enhanced by CD28 costimulation and regulates differentiation of CD4(+) T cells. J Immunol 2000; 165:5035–5040.
43. Kopf M, Coyle AJ, Schmitz N, Barner M, Oxenius A, Gallimore A, Gutierrez-Ramos JC, Bachmann MF. Inducible costimulator protein (ICOS) controls T helper cell subset polarization after virus and parasite infection. J Exp Med 2000; 192:111–117.
44. Rottman JB, Smith T, Tonra JR, Ganley K, Bloom T, Silva R, Pierce B, Ozkaynak E, Coyle AJ. The costimulatory molecule ICOS plays an important role in the immunopathogenesis of EAE. Nature Immunol 2001; 2:605–611.
45. Dong C, Juedes AE, Temann U-A, Shresta S, Allison J, Ruddle NH, Flavell RA. ICOS costimulatory receptor is essential for T-cell activation and function. Nature 2001; 409:97–101.
46. Gonzalo JA, Tian J, Delaney T, Corcoran J, Rottman JB, Lora J, Al-Garawi A, Kroczek R, Gutierrez-Ramos JC, Coyle AJ. ICOS is critical for T helper cell–mediated lung mucosal inflammatory responses. Nat Immunol 2001: 2:597–604.
47. McAdam AJ, Greenwald RJ, Levin MA, Freeman GJ, Sharpe AH. ICOS is critical for CD40 mediated antibody class swithing. Nature 2001; 409:102–105.
48. Tafuri A, Shahinian A, Bladt F, Yoshinaga SK, Jordana M, Wakeham A, Boucher LM, Bouchard D, Chan VS, Duncan G, Odermatt B, Ho A, Itie A, Horan T, Whoriskey JS, Pawson T, Penninger JM, Ohashi PS, Mak TW. Essential role of ICOS in effective helper T cell responses. Nature 2001; 409:105–109.
49. Dong H, Zhu G, Tamada K, Chen L. B7-H1 a third member of the B7 family, costimulates T cell proliferation and interleukin 10 secretion. Nature Med 1999; 5:1365–1369.
50. Freeman GJ, Long AJ, Iwai Y, Bourque K, Chernova T, Nishimura H, Fitz LJ, Malenkovich N, Okazaki T, Byrne MC, Horton HF, Fouser L, Carter L, Ling V, Bowman MR, Carreno BM, Collins M, Wood CR, Honjo T. Engagement of the PD-1 immunoinhibitory receptor by a novel B7 family member leads to negative regulation of lymphocyte activation. J Exp Med 2000; 192:1027–1034.

51. Ishida Y, Agata Y, Shibahara K, Honjo T. Induced expression of PD-1, a novel member of the immunoglobulin gene superfamily, upon programmed cell death. EMBO J 1996; 11:3887–3895.
52. Latchman Y, Wood CR, Chernova T, Chaudhary D, Borde M, Chernova L, Iwai, Y, Long AJ, Brown JA, Nunes R, Greenfield, EA, Bourque K, Boussiotis VA, Carter LL, Carreno BM, Malenkovich N, Nishimura H, Honjo T, Sharpe AH, Freeman GJ. Nat Immunol (in press).
53. Nishimura H, Nose M, Hiai H, Minato N, Honjo T. Development of lupuslike autoimmune diseases by disruption of the PD-1 gene encoding an ITIM motif-carrying immunoreceptor. Immunity 1999; 11:141–151.
54. Chapoval AI, Ni JN, Lau JS, Wilcox RA, Flies DB, Liu D, Dong H, Sica GL, Tamada K, Chen L. B7-H3: A costimulatory molecule for T cell activation and IFN-γ production. Nature Immunol 2001; 2:1–6.

12

Control of Lymphocyte Trafficking Through the Lung

REINHARD PABST and THOMAS TSCHERNIG

Hannover Medical School
Hannover, Germany

I. Introduction

In general, lymphocytes are not sessile cells but travel throughout the body continuously using the blood and lymph as routes connecting lymphoid and nonlymphoid organs (1). At any given time point there are only about 2% of all lymphoid cells of the body in the blood (2) and the composition of lymphocytes in the organs differs greatly (3). Thus, a blood sample will only be representative of the situation in the lung, e.g., in asthma, if the alteration in numbers, subset composition, and activation in the bronchial wall is mirrored in qualitative and quantitative aspects in the blood (4). Minor changes in the rate of trafficking of lymphocytes to a specific area of the lung can eventually result in an impressive local accumulation without obvious effects on lymphocyte numbers in the blood. Before alterations of lymphocyte subsets in asthma can be interpreted meaningfully, the compartmentalization of lymphocyte subsets in the healthy lung has to be defined. In addition, not only the rate of entry into the lung but also the local proliferation, cell death, and, finally, the exit from the lung to the draining lymph nodes must be determined (5). In a recent review, immune dysregulation was suggested as a cause for allergic asthma, e.g., Th1 to Th2 reactions (6), but it remains to be shown whether specific subsets of lymphocytes are recruited or the cells enter at random but differentiate at a different tempo. The role of different regulatory factors, such as adhesion molecules, will be discussed using typical examples, and the major fields of future research in the dynamic situation and potential therapeutic implications will be outlined.

II. Heterogeneity of Lymphocyte Subsets

Lymphoid cells are characterized by their different origin and function (Fig. 1). Several subsets are found in the lung and it is necessary to know their origin, traffic, and life span. Very little is known about why certain cells are found at such a high frequency in the lung. For example, about 35% of all natural killer (NK) cells are localized in the lung at any given time (3). What is the reason for this preference? Neither the kinetics of the NK cells in the lung nor their compartmentalization has been studied in detail.

Another example of a subset neglected so far are the $\gamma\delta$ T cells (7). In a recent study it was documented that $\gamma\delta$ T cells can regulate airway function in a mouse asthma model in a manner independent of $\alpha\beta$ T cells, and this function has been proposed as a link with the innate immune system (8). For extrapolation to the situation in humans it is far too early because, in contrast to the mouse, there are very few $\gamma\delta$ T cells among the intraepithelial lymphocytes of the human bronchial wall (9). These examples are given to show the need for kinetic data of the different lymphocyte subsets, and after the rates of entry, transit, and exit have been studied the regulatory factors must be characterized.

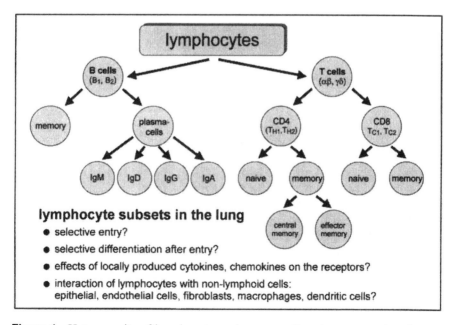

Figure 1   Heterogeneity of lymphocytes and open questions in respect to lymphocyte dynamics in the lung.

III. Techniques for Studying Lymphocyte Traffic to the Lung

Some technical aspects have to be considered when lymphocyte kinetics are studied (10). Experiments on lymphocyte traffic have been performed in vitro and also in vivo. The in vitro experiments can be of great help in defining the interactions of molecules on endothelial cells with those expressed on lymphocytes, e.g., adhesion of lymphocytes on monolayers of endothelial cells with or without flow conditions imitating the in vivo shear forces. However, the often used human umbilical vein endothelial cells (HUVECs) do not necessarily represent the different endothelial cells of the lung vascular bed. Lymphocytes have to be labeled so that they can be identified after injection in the lung. Different radioactive and fluorescent dyes have been used (see Ref. 11). These techniques include in vitro labeling procedures that might modify the migratory properties. Radioactive labels like ^{51}Cr have the advantage of affording a quick overview of radioactivity counting (12), but often only homogenized samples of the lung were measured; therefore, no localization in different compartments of the lung was possible. By using precursors of DNA synthesis, e.g., ^{3}H-TdR or the nonradioactive bromodesoxyuridine BrdU, the route of activated cells can be followed. Lymphocytes labeled with fluorescent dyes can be identified by fluorescence microscopy and in combination with surface markers the different subpopulations can also be identified.

In vitro labeling procedures with all their potentially harmful effects can be avoided when congenic animal strains are used, e.g., RT7a and RT7b rats (13). An even more laborious technique has been used by transplanting a single lung in congenic rats and identifying lymphocytes of the donor strain in the recipient, thus avoiding preparation of cell suspensions and in vitro labeling (14). Extremely critical aspects are that several time points have to be studied (11) to get meaningful data, and relative (e.g., percentage) and absolute data (e.g., lymphocytes/mg and per whole lung) must be given. For real comparison of lymphocyte migration data from different experiments many details have to be known, such as whether the animal was exsanguinated or the lung also perfused to wash out the blood including lymphocytes of the circulating and partially the marginal pool.

In conclusion, there is not one single technique that is most advantageous for all types of lymphocyte migration studies. In many cases a combination of several methods will be best. Conflicting data between different groups can often be resolved by taking into account the different techniques.

IV. Lymphocytes in the Lung Are Found in Different Compartments

Before the migratory routes of lymphocytes and the known and potential regulatory factors are discussed, the localization of lymphocytes in the lung will be described (Fig. 2). The different compartments and their subset compositions have been outlined in detail before, and the reader is referred to these reviews (5,15).

The mucosa-lined airways show three different lymphocyte compartments. First, there are lymphocytes in the epithelial layer, called intraepithelial lymphocytes (IELs). There are approximately 18 IELs per 100 epithelial cells in normal adults. They consist mainly of T cells but contain, in contrast to the gut, not almost exclusively CD8 T cells but also CD4 T cells. In contrast to the mouse, there are hardly any γδ cells among the IELs in humans. Second, in the lamina propria of the bronchi the CD4 T cells outnumber the CD8 T cells, and also B lymphocytes and plasma cells are found (for review, see Ref. 9). The third compartment is quite unique in containing the bronchus-associated lymphoid tissue (BALT), which has been discussed in detail recently (16). These aggregations of lymphocytes partly infiltrating the covering epithelium are not present at birth (in contrast to Peyer patches) and are found only in a certain proportion of children and adolescents but not in the lung of healthy adults (17,18). Lymphocytes can enter BALT via high endothelial venules (HEVs) in the T-cell area.

In the gas-exchange compartment of the lung there are three further lymphocyte compartments: the interstitial, intra-alveolar, and intravascular pool (Fig. 2). At first glance it might be surprising that the interstitial

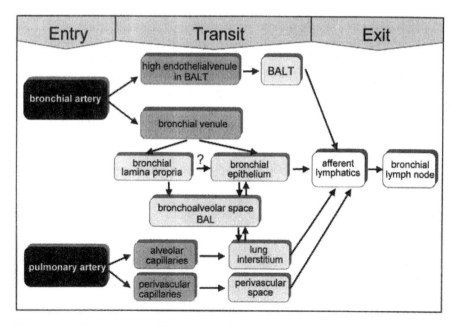

Figure 2 Different routes of lymphocytes into, through, and out of the compartments of the lung.

lymphocyte pool in humans is similar in size to the whole circulating blood pool (approximately 10×10^9) because the lung interstitium is very narrow (see Ref. 5). The lymphocytes in the branchoalveolar space are not impressive as a total pool in size, but this is the most easily accessible pool in humans by bronchoalveolar lavage (BAL), which is a routine clinical procedure. There are about 5–10% lymphocytes in the normal lavage fluid. The pool of lung lymphocytes often ignored are those found within the pulmonary vascular bed (see Ref. 5), the so-called marginated lymphocyte pool, which is of considerable size (19) and has a different migration pattern from that of lymphocytes from the blood (20) (Fig. 2).

Another unique aspect of lymphocyte kinetics in the lung is that lymphocytes transmigrate the covering epithelium into the airspace, return to the lung interstitium, and migrate via lymphatics to the draining bronchial lymph nodes. Thus, the lung is the only organ in which lymphocytes enter the lumen and are not destroyed as in the gut but return to the immune system in general via the bronchial lymph nodes (13,21). Little is known about the regulation of this route, e.g., where exactly these lymphocytes transmigrate the epithelium, which subsets use this route preferentially, and whether there are differences at different ages or in health and disease. Adhesion molecules such as ICAM-1, expressed on bronchial epithelium, and LFA-1 on the lymphocyte surface (22), might play a role. In each of these compartments of the lung the lymphocyte subset composition seems to be different as shown in the rat (23). Much less is known about the situation in humans. Such compartment-specific subset composition can be due to specific entry, local differentiation, and other reasons that could all be regulated differently. Even less is known about the compartmentalization of NK cells in the lung or the recruitment of these cells to the lung, although the lung contains a large proportion (approximately 35%) of all NK cells of the human body as mentioned above (3).

V. Lymphocyte Numbers in the Lung Depend Not Only on Entry from the Blood

When lymphocytes in a given compartment of the lung are counted, such as in a bronchial biopsy or BAL, this has to be taken as a snapshot of a very dynamic system. The number of lymphocytes always depends on the entry and exit, as well as local proliferation and local cell death, e.g., by apoptosis. In many experiments often only one of these parameters had been determined, leading to the erroneous conclusion that the lymphocyte traffic was altered. All of these different steps of lymphocyte kinetics in the different compartments might be regulated by heterogeneous factors, such as cytokines, chemokines, and adhesion molecules and their respective receptors and ligands. Therefore, several time points have to be studied to reach meaningful conclusions. For example, in recent experiments on the pulmonary clearance of *Haemophilus influenzae* after mucosal immunization, CD8 T-cell recruitment was evident at 30 min and increased over 24 h, whereas $\gamma\delta$ cells extravasated at 30 min and 1 h but were gone at 24 h (24).

VI. The Unique Double Blood Supply of the Lung Is of Great Relevance to Lymphocyte Traffic

The lung receives blood including lymphocytes via two routes: the function-associated pulmonary vessels and the bronchial vessels (vasa privata, nutritive vessels), as outlined in Fig. 2. The exit sites for lymphocytes are the pulmonary capillaries and in the bronchial system the postcapillary venules. An additional, neglected unique vascular bed of the lung seems to be the capillaries around larger pulmonary arteries and veins, which might play an important role as an entry site to the lung (25). Thus, these two different entrances for lymphocytes to the lung might be regulated separately.

VII. Lack of a Bronchial Blood Supply in the Mouse

The lung is unique in the two different routes by which lymphocytes can enter it. In the mouse, however, there is only a systemic blood supply to the trachea and mainstream bronchi but no bronchial arteries, capillaries, or veins within the bronchi in the lung parenchyma (26). The bronchial wall, consisting of the epithelium and the muscular layer but without cartilage and a real lamina propria, obviously depends on the oxygen from the air and on nutrients diffusing from alveolar capillaries. Therefore, the mouse cannot be used to study leukocyte traffic to the bronchial wall as an asthma model for species such as humans despite its great advantage due to transgenic and knockout technology.

VIII. Lessons Learned from Neutrophil Migration to the Lung

The transit of neutrophils through the pulmonary vascular bed has been studied in great detail (for review, see Refs. 27–29). Due to the diameter of lung capillaries and size of granulocytes the latter can only transit this capillary bed when they are able to deform. Consequently, young neutrophils only recently released from the bone marrow have a longer transit time because of their decreased deformability. Neutrophils, therefore, have a much slower transit time than the red blood cells, resulting in a 40–80 times higher concentration than in other blood vessels. This is called the pulmonary marginated neutrophil pool. It has been extrapolated that about one third of all granulocytes are contained in this pool and they can be mobilized by stress, resulting in stress leukocytosis. There is also a marginated pool for lymphocytes. The frequently described multistep cascade-type sequence of rolling, tethering, adhesion, and transmigration, all regulated by sequential interactions of different adhesion molecules on leukocytes and endothelial cells in postcapillary venules, does not happen in the pulmonary vascular system. A leukocyte cannot roll at this site because the diameter of the alveolar capillary is too small (30). These facts explain why adhesion molecules that are critical in leukocyte emigration in other organs, e.g., the pair ICAM-1 and LFA-1, play only a minor role in the lung vascular bed [as has been documented by Klemm et al. (22) using the isolated perfused rat lung]. It remains to be shown whether larger lymphoid cells such as lymphoid blasts or activated cells will transit even more slowly through the pulmonary bed, as these cells are much larger than a mature small lymphocyte (31). A further example of studies of neutrophil migration that could stimulate similar experiments on lymphocytes is the regulation of leukocyte transmigration of the epithelium in the basolateral to apical direction. This was dependent on Fc receptors and showed a mechanism for retention of neutrophils at the apical epithelial surface (32).

IX. Defensins as Chemoattractants for Lymphoid Cells in the Lung

As an example of the interaction between cells of the innate immune system and lymphoid cells in the lung (33,34) some recent data will be mentioned here. Defensins are low molecular weight antimicrobial peptides with a growing number produced by bronchial epithelial cells (35) and also by neutrophils. In a recent study, a human neutrophil defensin was documented to selectively attract naive T cells as well as immature dendritic cells in in vitro assays (36). An interesting aspect of these experiments was that $CD4^+$ and $CD8^+$ lymphocytes migrated similarly in the chemotaxis assay, but $CD4^+CD45 RO^+$ were attracted in a dose-dependent manner while naive Th lymphocytes ($CD4^+ CD45 RA^+$) were completely inactive. This is an interesting example of a defensin bridging innate and adaptive immunity.

X. Postnatal Increase of Lymphocytes in the BAL Fluid

In contrast to older children and adults, there are no leukocytes in the BAL fluid of healthy mature babies. Initially alveolar macrophages appear after birth, and from about 2 years of age "adult" numbers and ratios have been described (for review, see Ref. 37). There is some evidence that viral infections have a role in the age-related increase of lymphocytes in the bronchoalveolar space (38). Respiratory syncytial virus (RSV) infections in early childhood might be an important factor (39). Furthermore, the subset composition of lymphocytes in the BAL fluid differs with age: the CD4 to CD8 ratio was 0.6 in children (3 months to 10 years of age) in contrast to 2.7 in healthy young adults. The lower ratio in children seems to be due to a higher absolute number of CD8 T lymphocytes (40). It remains to be studied which factors regulate this postnatal increase of lymphocytes into the bronchoalveolar space and the accumulation of $CD4^+$ lymphocytes in older age (41). The exposure to inhaled dust or microbial antigen might result in the release of cytokines or chemokines from alveolar epithelial cells that work as chemoattractants for lymphocytes. The increase of lymphocytes with age in the BAL fluid can be influenced by a higher rate of local lymphocyte proliferation, less apoptosis, or reduced emigration. It remains to be studied whether an earlier postnatal "maturation" of the lymphocyte number and subset composition would be an advantage in fighting pulmonary infections in children. In a recently published study, very young mice were exposed to ambient particles and ovalbumin as an allergen. It was argued that the normal resistance to allergens was obviously disrupted by the airborne particles (42). In recent years it has often been stressed that early childhood seems to prime whether a child will become asthmatic a few years later (see, for example, Ref. 43). For ethical reasons such studies can hardly be done in young children, and therefore as a first step a relevant animal model has to be established.

Another area of research should be to find out why a certain percentage of children and adolescents have BALT, which is obviously included in the traffic routes of recirculating lymphocytes via HEVs (16). The following questions remain to be answered: could the development of BALT be induced, and would that have positive effects on the lung immune function in children and adults? Would the antigen uptake by the epithelium covering BALT result in protective immune reaction, or would tolerance develop? Will a Th1 or Th2 type of reaction be initiated? There are obviously more questions than answers so far, all depending on aspects of lymphocyte traffic to and through the lung. Constant et al. (44) recently stated that the lung per se favors Th differentiation toward the Th2 type.

XI. Adhesion Molecules in Lymphocyte Traffic

The different molecules involved in the interaction of leukocytes with endothelial cells have been characterized in great detail during the last few years. The cascade-type, sequential phenomena are normally described as tethering, rolling, activation, arrest, and transmigration (for review, see Refs. 45–47). The three great families of adhesion molecules—selectins, integrins, and the immunoglobulin superfamily—are all involved, and certain regional differences, such as the expression of MAdCAM-1 endothelial cells on the HEVs in the T-cell areas of Peyer patches and of PNAd on HEVs of peripheral lymph nodes, are often taken as examples for regional traffic differences. Using other techniques no difference between the entry of certain lymphocyte subsets into peripheral and mucosal lymphoid tissue could be found (summarized in Ref. 48). Bochner (49) recently compared the lymphocyte homing "to lymph nodes with that to the skin and lung" and stressed the many unsolved problems in the lung homing mechanisms. There is no doubt that adhesion molecules play an important role in directing lymphoid cells through the body. In vivo video microscopy experiments in the mouse are excellent techniques to study the steps of lymphocyte entry into the lymphoid organs (47). However, the transit through the organ will also be largely regulated by a sequence of adhesion and de-adhesion of lymphoid cells to the extracellular matrix and interstitial cells, and this phase can hardly be studied by video microscopy.

These basic mechanisms of a cascade-type interaction of lymphocytes with endothelial cells have often also been assumed for lymphocyte traffic through the lung (for review, see Refs. 50 and 51). One basic difference between lymph nodes and the lung has mostly been overlooked. In the lung interstitium there are no HEVs, and the leukocytes leave the vascular bed in the alveolar capillaries. Their diameter is smaller than that of a leukocyte. Therefore, there can be no rolling, but the leukocyte has to modify its shape and squeeze through this tight tube, as discussed for neutrophils above. In the vascular bed of the bronchial lamina propria venules with a normal venular endothelium are the site of lymphocyte emigration and also not HEVs. Therefore, it is not surprising that the role of adhesion molecules in the lung is not similar to that in lymph nodes. In reviews on lymphocyte traffic this unique situation of the lung often goes unmentioned, and too often phenomena studied on HEVs of lymph nodes are extrapolated to all other organs, including the lung.

The expression of adhesion molecules on the endothelial cells of pulmonary capillaries has been described in a few studies only. For example, ICAM-1 and ICAM-2 have been demonstrated on arteriolar, capillary, and venous endothelium in the human lung (52,53). In a mouse model of a T-cell-mediated immune reaction by the instillation of sheep red blood cells into the bronchoalveolar space, the expression of ICAM-1 on the luminal surface of lung endothelial cells and of the countermolecule LFA-1 on lymphocytes increased (54). The migration of lymphocytes to the lung incubated in vitro with anti-LFA-1 was reduced at 30 min and 2 h after intravenous injection (55). These data indicated a role of the interaction of LFA-1 with ICAM-1 in the lung. Using the isolated perfused rat lung and peripheral blood lymphocytes of congenic animals, preperfusion incubation of anti-LFA-1 led to an increase by 70% of lymphocytes recovered in the perfusate. Thus, this pair of adhesion molecules plays a role in lymphocyte migration to the lung (22). However, by video microscopy of the isolated perfused lung the blocking of ICAM-1 had no effect on lymphocyte trapping (56). In fibrotic lung disease induced by bleomycin a differential expression of ICAM-1 was shown on endothelial cells of arterioles, venules, and capillaries (57). The lung is interesting in another aspect because the bronchial epithelium also expresses ICAM-1, which is increased in rhinovirus infection and is not influenced by corticosteroid treatment (58). This might be relevant for lymphocytes returning from the airspace to the lung interstitium.

In allergic reactions of the lung the role of adhesion molecules might be different. Henderson et al. (59) blocked α_4-integrin by a local intranasal application of an antibody and this resulted in an inhibition of all signs of inflammation and IL-4 and IL-5 release. In contrast, α_4 blockage on circulating leukocytes only prevented eosinophilia. Lymphocyte migration had not been studied in that model. An example of interesting experiments that were done more often and for other questions are those of Hirata et al. (60). They incubated human bronchial biopsies in vitro with the appropriate antigen and demonstrated an up-regulation of the adhesion molecule VCAM-1 on the endothelial cells of lamina propria venules. These experiments show the up-regulation of an adhesion molecule induced by exposure to a specific antigen. In another interesting study bronchial biopsy specimens from asthmatics 6 h after segmental allergen challenge revealed increased ICAM-1 and E-selectin expression on the microvasculature correlating with the infiltration of eosinophils, mast cells, neutrophils, and T lymphocytes, whereas VCAM-1 was not detected on the endothelium at this time point (61). It is very likely that adhesion molecules regulate lymphocyte traffic to the lung, but the role of different adhesion molecules in the normal or allergic situation are only partly understood and therefore therapeutic intervention by antiadhesion molecules in asthma seems to be too early (Fig. 3). However, several studies have shown promising results on the role of adhesion molecules in the healthy and diseased lung in animal models (62–66). A future approach might be tissue engineering

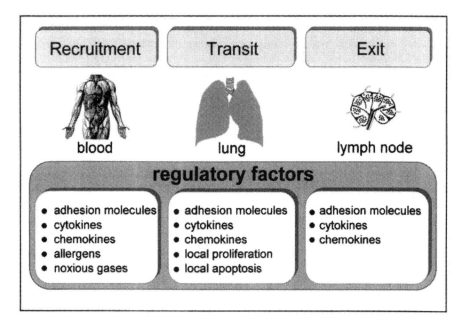

Figure 3 Regulatory factors and their potential therapeutic role in the recruitment, transit, and exit of lymphocytes in the lung.

of bronchial mucosa from controls and asthmatics to study cellular interactions in a standardized microenvironment (67).

XII. Chemokines in Lymphocyte Traffic to the Lung

Chemokines are a growing group of low molecular weight chemotactic cytokines (8–10 kD). Based on the position of one or two cysteine residues near the N terminus, four groups have been classified: CXC, CC, C, or CX3C. Many chemokines have several names, and it will take some time until the new nomenclature is generally accepted (68). For a general overview of the function of chemokines, the reader is referred to recent reviews (69–71). Several chemokines—in particular RANTES (CCL5)—have been shown to have a critical role in the recruitment of eosinophils in asthma (reviewed in Ref. 71). The study by Bless et al. (72) is a good example of different effects of the chemokines RANTES (CCL5), MCP-1 (CCL-2), and MIPIß (CCL-4) on neutrophil recruitment to the lung in an acute inflammatory reaction. Recently, a chemokine was described that was only expressed in bronchoepithelial cells and was therefore called "lungkine." This chemokine induced in vitro and in vivo migration of neutrophils, suggesting its role of lung-specific leukocyte migration (73). The role of chemokines in lymphocyte traffic, e.g., CCR7 in peripheral lymph node entry, CCR4 in inflamed skin, or CCR9 in lymphocyte migration to the lamina propria of the small intestine, has been summarized recently (74).

Much less is known about the relevance of chemokines and their receptors in lymphocyte migration to the lung. When in an allergic reaction the effect of RANTES was neutralized by the receptor agonist Met-RANTES not only the recruitment of eosinophils but also that of lymphocytes to the lung was suppressed (71). It is very likely that not only entry into the bronchial wall via bronchial venules but also into the lung parenchyma via alveolar capillaries is regulated by chemokines. In a recent study, an antibody against the secondary lymphoid tissue chemokine (SLC) was used in a lung inflammation model, and surprisingly the numbers of dendritic cells and neutrophils were increased but the numbers of CD4 T lymphocytes, including memory T cells, were decreased (75). These data document a potential therapeutic approach using antichemokine antibodies. The rapidly emerging knockout mice for the chemokines and their receptors will facilitate studies on this topic. As mentioned before, these mouse data should not be extrapolated without great caution to other species including humans when traffic to the bronchial wall is studied. In a recently published study, chemokine receptor expression was investigated on lymphocytes prepared by mincing human lung specimens and BAL samples. These lymphocytes expressed CCR5 and CXCR3 but not CCR9. There were no differences between lung T cells from normal versus asthmatic subjects (76). This single-sample study should not be overinterpreted as indicating specific lymphocyte traffic. Other pathways are cytokines released by macrophages or epithelial cells that also influence lymphoid cells in their direct neighborhood; that is, they regulate the microenvironment (77).

Thus, asthma models in animals (78) have to be carefully evaluated in terms of their relevance to the concept of airway inflammation (79), as well as asthma pathophysiology and future treatment concepts (80).

XIII. Conclusions

Lymphocytes consist of very heterogeneous subpopulations, and several compartments show a typical subset composition. These can be influenced (1) at the entry site, (i.e., the interaction between lymphoid and endothelial cell); (2) during transit through the lung interstitium; and (3) at the exit site into lymphatics draining to regional bronchial lymph nodes. Furthermore, lymphocytes can proliferate locally and/or undergo apoptosis. All the different phases of this dynamic traffic route can be regulated by cytokines, chemokines, adhesion molecules, and the respective receptors or ligands. A single biopsy or sample of one lung compartment can hardly be taken as representing the kinetics of lymphocyte traffic through the lung. Adequate animal models have to be used for many questions as serial samples from different lung compartments can hardly be taken from human volunteers or patients. In extrapolating from results in experimental animals to humans great caution must be taken and species differences considered.

The regulation of lymphocyte traffic through the lung is of utmost clinical relevance as it might provide different approaches for new therapeutic regimes (Fig. 3) in inflammatory and allergic diseases of the lung.

References

1. Pabst R, Miyasaka M. Lymphocyte migration: more than an interaction of lymphocytes with endothelial cells of the high endothelial venules via adhesion molecules. Immunologist 1999;7:29–32.
2. Westermann J, Pabst R. Lymphocytes in the blood. A diagnostic window on the lymphoid system? Immunol Today 1990;11:406–410.
3. Westermann J, Pabst R. Distribution of lymphocyte subsets and natural killer cells in the human body. Clin Invest 1992;70:539–544.
4. Lewis SA, Pavord ID, Stringer JR, Knox AJ, Weiss ST, Britton JR. The relation between peripheral blood leukocyte counts and respiratory symptoms, atopy, lung function, and airway responsiveness in adults. Chest 2001;119:105–114.
5. Pabst R. Mucosa-associated lymphoid tissue of the lung: localization, numbers and dynamics of lymphoid cells in the five different compartments. In: Busse WW, Holgate ST, eds. Asthma and Rhinitis. Oxford: Blackwell, 2000:543–556.
6. Lipscomb MF, Wilder JA. Immune dysregulation as a cause for allergic asthma. Curr Opin Pulmon Med 1999;5:10–20.

7. Hayday AC, Roberts S, Ramsburg E. Gamma delta cells and the regulation of mucosal immune responses. Am J Respir Crit Care Med 2000;162:S161–S163.
8. Lahn M, Kanehio A, Takeda K, Joetham A, Schwarze J, Köhler G, O'Brian R, Gelfand EW, Born W. Negative regulation of airway responsiveness that is dependent on gamma delta T cells and independent of alpha beta T cells. Nat Med 1999;5:1150–1156.
9. Erle DJ, Pabst R. Intraepithelial lymphocytes in the lung. A neglected lymphocyte population. Am J Respir Cell Mol Biol 2000;22:398–400.
10. Pabst R, Westermann J. Lymphocyte traffic to lymphoid and non-lymphoid organs in different species is regulated by several mechanisms. In: Hamann A, ed. Adhesion Molecules and Chemokines in Lymphocyte Trafficking. Amsterdam: Harwood Academic, 1997:21–37.
11. Pabst R, Binns RM, Rothkötter HJ, Westermann J. Quantitative analysis of lymphocyte fluxes in vivo. Curr Top Microbiol Immunol 1993;184:151–159.
12. Hamann A. Specific trafficking: which cells, which function. In: Hamann A, ed. Adhesion Molecules and Chemokines in Lymphocyte Trafficking. Amsterdam: Harwood Academic, 1997:1–19.
13. Lehmann C, Wilkening A, Leiber D, Markus A, Krug N, Pabst R, Tschernig T. Lymphocytes in the bronchoalveolar space reenter the lung tissue via the alveolar epithelium, migrate to regional lymph nodes, and subsequently rejoin the systemic immune system. Anat Rec 2001;264:229–236.
14. Tschernig T, Boeke K, Steinhoff G, Wonigeit K, Pabst R, Westermann J. The lung as a source and a target organ for T- and B-lymphocytes. Am J Respir Cell Mol Biol 1997;17:414–421.
15. Pabst R, Tschernig T. Lymphocytes in the lung: an often neglected cell. Numbers, characterization and compartmentalization. Anat Embryol 1995;192:293–299.
16. Tschernig T, Pabst R. Bronchus-associated lymphoid tissue (BALT) is not present in the normal adult lung but in different diseases. Pathobiology 2000;68:1–8.
17. Hiller AS, Kracke A, Tschernig T, Kasper M, Kleemann WJ, Tröger HD, Pabst R. Comparison of the immunohistology of mucosa-associated lymphoid tissue in the larynx and lungs in cases of sudden infant death and controls. Int J Legal Med 1997;110:316–322.
18. Hiller A, Tschernig T, Kleemann WJ, Pabst R. Bronchus-associated lymphoid tissue (BALT) and larynx-associated lymphoid tissue (LALT) are found at different frequencies in children, adolescents and adults. Scand J Immunol 1998;47:159–162.
19. Pabst R, Binns RM, Licence ST, Peter M. Evidence of a selective major vascular marginal pool of lymphocytes in the lung. Am Rev Respir Dis 1987;136:1213–1218.
20. Binns RM, Licence ST, Pabst R. Homing of blood, splenic and lung emigrant lymphoblasts: comparison with the behaviour of lymphocytes from these sources. Int Immunol 1992;4:1011–1019.
21. Pabst R, Binns RM. Lymphocytes migrate from the bronchoalveolar space to regional bronchial lymph nodes. Am J Respir Crit Care Med 1995;151:495–499.
22. Klemm A, Tschernig T, Ermert L, Althoff A, Merkle M, Gebert A, Ermert M, Seeger W, Pabst R. Blockade of leucocyte function-associated antigen-1 (LFA-1) decreases lymphocyte trapping in the normal pulmonary vasculature: studies in the isolated buffer-perfused rat lung. Clin Exp Immunol 2000;121:375–383.

23. Fliegert FG, Tschernig T, Pabst R. Comparison of lymphocyte subsets, monocytes and NK cells in three different lung compartments and peripheral blood in the rat. Exp Lung Res 1996;22:677–690.

24. Foxwell AR, Kyd JM, Karupiah G, Cripps AW. $CD8^+$ T cells have an essential role in pulmonary clearance of non-typeable *Haemophilus influenzae* following mucosal immunization. Infect Immun 2001;69:2636–2642.

25. Guntheroth WG, Luchtel DLKI. Pulmonary microcirculation: tubules rather than sheet and post. J Appl Physiol: Respir Environ Exerc Physiol 1982;53:510–515.

26. Mitzner W, Lee W, Georgakopoulos D, Wagner E. Angiogenesis in the mouse lung. Am J Pathol 2000;157:93–101.

27. Hogg JC, Doerschuk CM. Leukocyte traffic in the lung. Annu Rev Physiol 1995;57:97–114.

28. Doerschuk CM. Leukocyte trafficking in alveoli and airway passages. Respir Res 2000;1:136–140.

29. Wagner JG, Roth RA. Neutrophil migration mechanisms, with an emphasis on the pulmonary vasculature. Pharmacol Rev 2000;52:349–374.

30. Doerschuk CM. Neutrophil rheology and transit through capillaries and sinusoids. Am J Respir Crit Care Med 1999;159:1693–1695.

31. Luettig B, Kaiser M, Bode U, Bell EB, Sparshott SM, Bette M, Westermann J. Naive and memory T cells migrate in comparable numbers through the normal rat lung: only effector T cells accumulate and proliferate in the lamina propria of the bronchi. Am J Respir Cell Mol Biol 2001;25:69–77.

32. Reaves TA, Colgan SP, Selvaraj P, Pochet MM, Walsh S, Nusrat A, Liang TW, Madara JL, Parkos CA. Neutrophil transepithelial migration: regulation at the apical epithelial surface by Fc-mediated events. Am J Physiol Gastrointest Liver Physiol 2001;280:G746–G754.

33. Zhang P, Summer WR, Bagby GJ, Nelson S. Innate immunity and pulmonary host defense. Immunol Rev 2000;173:39–51.

34. Diamond G, Legarda D, Ryan LK. The innate immune response of the respiratory epithelium. Immunol Rev 2000;173:27–38.

35. Bals R, Wang X, Wu Z. Human beta-defensin 2 is a salt-sensitive peptide antibiotic expressed by human lung. J Clin Invest 1998;102:874–880.

36. Yang D, Chen Q, Chertov O, Oppenheim JJ. Human neutrophil defensins selectively chemoattract naive T and immature dendritic cells. J Leuk Biol 2000;68:9–14.

37. Grigg J, Riedler J. Developmental airway cell biology. The "normal" young child. Am J Respir Crit Care Med 2000;162:S52–S55.

38. Grigg J, Riedler J, Robertson CF. Bronchoalveolar lavage fluid cellularity and soluble intercellular adhesion molecule-1 in children with colds. Pediatr Pulmonol 1999;28:109–116.

39. Hussell T, Openshaw PJM. Intracellular IFN-gamma expression in natural killer cells precedes lung CD8+ T cell recruitment during respiratory syncytial virus infection. J Gen Virol 1998;79:2593–2601.

40. Ratjen F, Bredendiek M, Zheng L, Brendel M, Costabel U. Lymphocyte subsets in bronchoalveolar lavage fluid of children without bronchopulmonary disease. Am J Respir Crit Care Med 1995;152:174–178.

41. Meyer KC, Soergel P. Variation of bronchoalveolar lymphocyte phenotypes with age in the physiologically normal human lung. Thorax 1999;54:697–700.

42. Hamada K, Goldsmith CA, Goldman A, Kobzik L. Resistance of very young mice to inhaled allergen sensitization is overcome by coexposure to an air-pollutant aerosol. Am J Respir Crit Care Med 2000;161:1285–1293.

43. Holt PG, Sly PD. Prevention of adult asthma by early intervention during childhood: potential value of new generation immunomodulatory drugs. Thorax 2000;55:700–705.

44. Constant SL, Lee KS, Bottomly K. Site of antigen delivery can influence T cell priming: pulmonary environment promotes preferential Th2-type differentiation. Eur J Immunol 2000;30:840–847.

45. Springer TA. Traffic signals for lymphocyte recirculation and leukocyte emigration: the multistep paradigm. Cell 1994;76:301–314.

46. Butcher EC, Williams M, Youngman K, Rott L, Briskin M. Lymphocyte trafficking and regional immunity. Adv Immunol 1999;72:209–253.

47. Andrian von UH, Mackay CR. T-cell function and migration: two sides of the same coin. N Engl J Med 2000;343:1020–1034.

48. Westermann J, Bode U. Distribution of activated T cells migrating through the body: a matter of life and death. Immunol Today 1999;20:302–306.

49. Bochner BS. Road signs guiding leukocytes along the inflammation superhighway. J Allergy Clin Immunol 2000;106:817–828.

50. Delisser HM. The role and contribution of adhesion molecules to asthma and pulmonary disease. In: Busse WW, Holgate ST, eds. Asthma and Rhinitis. Oxford: Blackwell, 2000:691–701.

51. Stark JM. Leukocyte-endothelial adhesion. In: Busse WW, Holgate ST, eds. Asthma and Rhinitis. Oxford: Blackwell, 2000:702–720.

52. Steinhoff G, Behrend M, Richter N, Schlitt HJ, Cremer J, Haverich A. Distinct expression of cell–cell and cell–matrix adhesion molecules on endothelial cells in human heart and lung transplants. J Heart Lung Transplant 1995;14:1145–1155.

53. Southcott AM, Hemingway I, Lorimer S, Sugars K, Hellewell PG, Black CM, Jeffery PK, Gearing AJ, Haskard DO, du Bois RM. Adhesion molecule expression in the lung: a comparison between normal and diffuse interstitial lung disease. Eur Respir J 1998;11:91–98.

54. Ichikawa S, Goto Y, Uchino S, Kaltreider HB, Goetzl EJ, Sreedharan SP. Changes in adhesion molecule expression during patterns of immune cell migration in the inflamed lung. Arch Histol Cytol 1996;59:443–452.

55. Hamann A, Klugewitz K, Austrup F, Jablonski-Westrich D. Activation induces rapid and profound alterations in the trafficking of T cells. Eur J Immunol 2000;30:3207–3218.

56. Yamaguchi K, Nishio S, Sato N, Tsumura H, Ichihara A, Kudo H, Aoki T, Naoki K, Susuki K, Miyata A, Suzuki Y, Morooka S. Leukocyte kinetics in the pulmonary microcirculation: observations using real-time confocal luminescence microscopy coupled with high-speed video analysis. Lab Invest 1997;76:809–822.

57. Sato N, Suzuki Y, Nishio K, Suzuki K, Naoki K, Takeshita K, Kudo H, Miyao N, Tsumura H, Serizawa H, Suematsu M, Yamaguchi K. Roles of ICAM-1 for abnormal leukocyte recruitment in the microcirculation of bleomycin-induced fibrotic lung injury. Am J Respir Crit Care Med 2000;161:1681–1688.

58. Grünberg K, Sharon RF, Hiltermann TJN, Brahim JJ, Dick EC, Sterk PJ, van Krieken JHJM. Experimental rhinovirus 16 infection increases intercellular

adhesion molecule-1 expression in bronchial epithelium of asthmatics regardless of inhaled steroid treatment. Clin Exp Allergy 2000;30:1015–1023.

59. Henderson WR, Chi EY, Albert RK, Chu SJ, Lamm WJE, Rochon Y, Jonas M, Christie PE, Harlan JM. Blockade of CD49d (alpha4 integrin) on intrapulmonary but not circulating leukocytes inhibits airway inflammation and hyperresponsiveness in a mouse model. J Clin Invest 1997;100:3083–3092.

60. Hirata N, Kohrogi H, Iwagoe H, Goto E, Hamamoto J, Fujii K, Yamaguchi T, Kawano O, Ando M. Allergen exposure induces the expression of endothelial adhesion molecules in passively sensitized human bronchus. Time course and the role of cytokines. Am J Respir Cell Mol Biol 1998;18:12–20.

61. Montefort S, Gratziou C, Goulding D, Polosa R, Haskard DO, Howarth PH, Holgate ST, Caroll MP. Bronchial biopsy evidence for leukocyte infiltration and upregulation of leukocyte-endothelial cell adhesion molecules six hours after local allergen challenge of sensitized asthmatic airways. J Clin Invest 1994;93:1411–1421.

62. Toppila S, Paavonen T, Laitinen A, Laitinen LA, Renkonen R. Endothelial sulfated sialyl Lewis x glycans, putative L-selectin ligands, are preferentially expressed in bronchial asthma but not in other chronic inflammatory lung diseases. Am J Respir Cell Mol Biol 2000;23:492–498.

63. Ramos-Barbón D, Suzuki M, Taha R, Molet S, Issekutz TB, Hamid Q, Martin JG. Effect of alpha4-integrin blockade on CD4+ cell–driven late airway responses in the rat. Am J Respir Crit Care Med 2001;163:101–108.

64. Dixon AE, Mandac JB, Martin PJ, Hackman RC, Madtes DK, Clark JG. Adherence of adoptively transferred alloreactive Th1 cells in lung: partial dependence on LFA-1 and ICAM-1. Am J Physiol Lung Cell Mol Physiol 2000;279:L583–L591.

65. Kanehiro A, Takeda K, Joetham A, Tomkinson A, Ikemura T, Irvin CG, Gelfand EW. Timing of administration of anti-VLA-4 differentiates airway hyperresponsiveness in the central and peripheral airways in mice. Am J Respir Crit Care Med 2000;162:1132–1139.

66. Wolber FM, Curtis JL, Maly P, Kelly RJ, Smith P, Yednock TA, Lowe JB, Stoolman LM. Endothelial selectins and a4 integrins regulate independent pathways of T lymphocyte recruitment in the pulmonary immune response. J Immunol 1998;161:4396–4403.

67. Chakir J, Pagé N, Hamid Q, Laviolette M, Boulet LP, Rouabhia M. Bronchial mucosa produced by tissue engineering: a new tool to study cellular interactions in asthma. J Allergy Clin Immunol 2001;107:36–40.

68. Zlotnik A, Yoshie O. Chemokines: a new classification system and their role in immunity. Immunity 2000;12:121–127.

69. Moser B, Loetscher P. Lymphocyte traffic control by chemokines. Nat Immunol 2001;2:123–128.

70. Cyster JG. Chemokines and cell migration in secondary lymphoid organs. Science 1999;286:2098–2102.

71. Teran LM. CCL chemokines and asthma. Immunol Today 2000;21:235–241.

72. Bless NM, Huber-Lang M, Guo RF, Warner RL, Schmal H, Czermak BJ, Shanley TP, Crouch LD, Lentsch AB, Sarma V, Mulligan MS, Friedl HP, Ward PA. Role of CC chemokines (macrophage inflammatory protein-1ß, monocyte chemoattractant protein-1, RANTES) in acute lung injury in rats. J Immunol 2000;164:2650–2659.

73. Rossi DL, Hurst SD, Xu Y, Wang W, Menon S, Coffman RL, Zlotnik A. Lungkine, a novel CXC chemokine, specifically expressed by lung broncho-epithelial cells. J Immunol 1999;162:5490–5497.

74. Campbell JJ, Butcher EC. Chemokines in tissue-specific and microenvironment-specific lymphocyte homing. Curr Opin Immunol 2000;12:336–341.

75. Itakura M, Tokuda A, Kimura H, Nagai S, Yoneyama H, Onai N, Ishikawa S, Kuriyama T, Matsushima K. Blockade of secondary lymphoid tissue chemokine exacerbates *Propionibacterium acnes*-induced acute lung inflammation. J Immunol 2001;166:2071–2079.

76. Campbell JJ, Brightling CE, Symon FA, Qin S, Murphy KE, Hodge M, Andrew DP, Wu L, Butcher EC, Wardlaw AJ. Expression of chemokine receptors by lung T cells from normal and asthmatic subjects. J Immunol 2001;166:2842–2848.

77. Eghtesad M, Jackson HE, Cunningham AC. Primary human alveolar epithelial cells can elicit the transendothelial migration of CD14+ monocytes and CD3+ lymphocytes. Immunology 2001;102:157–164.

78. Vargaftig BB. What can we learn from murine models of asthma? Clin Exp Allergy 1999;29:9–13.

79. Larsen GL, Holt PG. The concept of airway inflammation. Am J Respir Crit Care Med 2000;162:S2–S6.

80. Bousquet J, Jeffery PK, Busse WW, Johnson M, Vignola AM. Asthma: from bronchoconstriction to airways inflammation and remodeling. Am J Respir Crit Care Med 2000;161:1720–1745.

13

Neuroimmune Interactions in the Pathogenesis of Allergic Asthma

ARMIN BRAUN

Fraunhofer Institute for Toxicology and
Aerosol Investigation
Hannover, Germany

**WOLFGANG A. NOCKHER
and HARALD RENZ**

University of Marburg
Marburg, Germany

I. Cellular Immunity and Airway Inflammation in Allergic Asthma

Allergic asthma is characterized by chronic airway inflammation that has been implied to have an important role in the development of airway hyperresponsiveness (AHR) and recurrent reversible airway obstruction. There is overwhelming evidence that T cells play a central role in allergic asthma (1). Strong evidence supports the notion that T-helper 2 (Th2) cells orchestrate allergic inflammation driven by effector functions of B cells, mast cells, and eosinophils. Differentiation of naive $CD4^+$ T cells (Th0) into Th1 or Th2 cells determines whether an antigen will raise a cellular or a humoral immune response. Delivery of foreign antigens to mucosal surfaces, such as the pulmonary airways, has been shown to preferentially induce a Th2-mediated response. Both the expansion of Th2 memory cells during the secondary exposure to allergen and the commitment of naive T cells to Th2 cells are required for the development of a Th2 immune response during allergic asthma. The availability of interleukin-12 (IL-12) and interferon-γ (IFN-γ) in contrast to IL-4 is decisive for the maturation of Th0 cells into Th1 or Th2 cells (2). Sources of IL-12 and IFN-γ are mainly macrophages and dendritic cells (DCs). Whereas cells responsible for the initial IL-4 production are less well defined and apparently include naive T cells themselves (3). In addition, the presentation of inhaled antigen to T cells by local antigen-presenting cells (APCs) is a critical step in triggering the local immune response toward a Th1 or Th2 type of immunity. Increasing evidence suggests that an already deviated Th1 or Th2 cell response can be reversed or further enhanced depending on the type of APCs responsible for restimulation and the subsequent secondary immune response (4). In early observations a regulation of Th1 and Th2 immune responses by dendritic cells has been found (5). However, recent data demonstrate that DCs in the respiratory tracts are specialized for initiating a Th2 immunity at the mucosal sites (6). By contrast, within the airways B cells do not appear to be essential as APCs, even though they support the induction and expansion of Th2 cells (7). Finally, the resident lung tissue macrophages play a pivotal role in initiating and development of a lung allergic immunity. They attenuate allergic inflammation and AHR by mounting Th1 responses in the bronchial mucosa that antagonizes Th2 responses to inhaled antigen (8). This Th1-promoting activity is an inherent property of lung macrophages and regulated by priming these cells with IFN-γ.

The importance of tissue macrophages during airway inflammation in allergic asthma has been further demonstrated by altered macrophage phenotype pattern. Alveolar macrophages from atopic asthmatics demonstrate changes in surface expression of coregulatory molecules and show CD83 expression, a marker of mature DCs (9,10). They also produce lower amounts of IL-12, which decreases Th2-type inflammation by stimulating Th1 cell differentiation and inhibition of IgE synthesis. Thus, suppressing coregulatory signals delivered by airway macrophages to Th2 cells are diminished, resulting in a profound shift to Th2 inflammation. In addition, an increased number of DCs further support the Th2 immune response in allergic asthma.

Th2 cells produce a cytokine profile that predominantly includes IL-4, IL-5, and IL-13. While IL-4 is involved in isotype switching in B cells toward IgE and propagation of Th2 cells, IL-5 has proinflammatory properties by its function on development, differentiation, recruitment, and survival of eosinophils. The importance of T cells or T-cell-driven processes is further underlined by the effectiveness of anti-inflammatory therapies, including glucocorticoids and several other mediators (11). This concept is currently leading to the development of novel drugs, including IL-5 or IgE inhibitors, which permits testing of this concept under in vivo conditions (12,13).

II. Airway Hyperresponsiveness

The success of anti-inflammatory therapy is not followed by a complete disappearance of symptoms (14), indicating long-lasting inflammation-induced effects. To date, no satisfying concept linking inflammation with persistent symptoms of asthma is available, but it is known that chronic inflammation is associated with clinical consequences, including nonspecific AHR. Nonspecific AHR may be defined as an increase in the ease in degree of airway narrowing in response to a wide range of bronchoconstrictor stimuli (15). The development of AHR in response to allergic inflammation is mediated by multiple independent and additive pathways working in concert (16–18). Several mechanisms have been identified to be involved in AHR. The airway changes leading to airway narrowing mainly include (1) altered neuronal regulation of airway tone, (2) increases in muscle content or function, and (3) increased epithelial mucus production and airway edema (15,18). Therefore, the mode of measuring AHR is critical for identifying the underlying mechanisms (Table 1). Depending on the method chosen for AHR measurement, different pathways can be distinguished. It has been previously shown that in vitro, electrical field stimulation of tracheal smooth muscle segments reflects specific neuronal airway dysfunction because the addition of both atropin (disruption of cholinergic pathways) and capsaicin (depletion of sensory neurons) completely blocks any reaction of the airway to electric field stimulation (19,20). By using specific stimuli, the measuring of lung function in animal models allows to distinguish between bronchoconstriction due to direct stimulation of airway smooth muscle and that due to alteration of sensory nerves (37,38). Capsaicin is a potent stimulant of sensory nerves and induces a characteristic modification of the normal breathing pattern. In contrast, methacholine acts via direct stimulation of airway smooth muscle cells. Other stimuli including histamine can affect both nerve and smooth muscle cells.

III. Innervation of the Lung

The human lung and airways are innervated via a complex system of autonomic nerve fibers with afferent and efferent effector functions. Neuronal control of airway function was originally thought to be solely dependent on a balance between cholinergic and adrenergic neurons. Results from experiments

Table 1 Assessment of Different Pathways of Airway Responsiveness in Allergic Bronchial Asthma

Stimulus	Effector cells	Acting through
Electrical field stimulation	Sensory neurons, motor neurons	Unspecific depolarization
Methacholine	Smooth muscle cells	M_3 receptors
Histamine	Smooth muscle cells, sensory neurons, motor neurons	H_1 receptors
Serotonin	Sensory neurons	$5\text{-}HT_1$ receptors
	Motor neurons	$5\text{-}HT_3$ receptors
Capsaicin	Sensory neurons	Vanilloid receptor
Hypotonic H_2O	Sensory neurons	Unspecific

Table 2 Innervation of the Lung

	Cholinergic system	Adrenergic system	Excitatory NANC system	Inhibitory NANC system
Major neurotransmitters	Acetylcholine	Noradrenaline (NA), adrenaline (A)	SP, NKA, NKB, CGRP	VIP, NO
Neuronal distribution	From upper tracheobronchial trees to small airways	Minor component of total nerve fibers in lung and airways	*SP fibers*: blood vessels, airway epithelium, (airway smooth muscle) *NKA fibers*: bronchial smooth muscle, blood vessels *CGRP fibers*: blood vessels, tracheobronchial smooth muscle, airway epithelium	Upper respiratory tract, vascular smooth muscle, bronchial glands
Receptors (R)	Muscarinic R M_1, M_2, M_3	α_1, α_2 (NA) β_1, β_2 (A)	NK-1 (SP) NK-2 (NKA) NK-3 (NKB)	VIP-R Guanylyl cyclase
R distribution	Parasympathetic ganglia (M_1), postganglionic cholinergic nerves (M_1, M_2), neg. autoreceptor (M_2), submucosal glands (M_1, M_3)	Cholinergic nerves (α_2, β_2), smooth muscle (β_2), blood vessel (α, β), mast cells (α_1), bronchial glands (α_1), epithelial and alveolar cells	Blood vessel (NK-1), smooth muscle (NK-2), cholinergic nerves (NK3)	Smooth muscle of small, but not large, airways; vascular smooth muscle submucosal glands
Key effects	Smooth muscle constriction, mucus secretion, bronchotransmission (autoreceptor) bronchodilatation (M_2)	Airway smooth muscle relaxation (β_2), suppression of cholinergic neurotransmission (α_2, β_2)	Neurogenic inflammation	Smooth muscle relaxation

performed about 100 years ago suggested the existence of a third innervation pathway. However, it was not until about 40 years ago that the existence of the nonadrenergic noncholinergic (NANC) system was established (21). The neurotransmitters involved in this system are of peptidergic nature and, therefore, this nervous system has been referred to as the peptidergic nervous system.

A. Parasympathetic Neurons

The parasympathetic nervous system plays an important role in maintaining bronchial smooth muscle tone by mediating bronchoconstrictory response. The key neurotransmitter in this system is acetylcholine, and the effects of the parasympathetic system can be blocked by atropine and augmented by acetylcholinesterase inhibitors (22,23). The parasympathetic neurons travel in the N. vagus. The afferent fibers originate from within and around the airway lumen and transmit the signals to the central nervous system. The efferent fibers innervate airway smooth muscle cells. The postganglionic fibers, carried in the N. vagus, extend from the upper tracheobronchial tree down to the small airways (24–26).

Acetylcholine exerts its functional activity via muscarinic receptors. Lung muscarinic receptors are present in high density, with distribution greatest in the large airways and least in the peripheral airways as revealed by radioligand binding and autoradiography studies (27–29). Five different muscarinic receptor subtypes have been sequenced and cloned (30,31). However, only three receptor subtypes have been identified based on pharmacological studies. They are termed M_1, M_2, and M_3, respectively (32–34). On human airway smooth muscle, the M_3 subtype is exclusively expressed. This receptor type is found in large and in some peripheral airways as well as in submucosal glands and is responsible for airway smooth muscle constriction and mucosecretion. The M_1 receptor is expressed in parasympathetic ganglia, facilitating vagal signal transmission, and on submucosal glands, where it is involved in the regulation of mucosecretion. Although both M_1 and M_3 receptors are expressed on submucosal glands, a much higher expression profile has been described for the M_3 subtype. The M_2 receptor is expressed on cholinergic nerves with negative regulatory effects and functions, and thus is an autoreceptor inhibiting acetylcholine (ACH) release. Although certainly the main effect of stimulating parasympathetic nerves is of excitatory nature and leads to bronchoconstriction, it must be emphasized that, in the case of M_2 receptor stimulation, the "paradox" effect of bronchoconstriction can be obtained (32–34).

B. Sympathetic Neurons

Compared with the parasympathetic neurons, the sympathetic nervous system is a minor component of the total nerve fibers in human airways and lung (25,26,35,36). There is only little evidence for direct sympathetic innervation of human airways. The efferent sympathetic neurons originate from the second to fourth toraxic preganglionic fibers, which end in the extrapulmonary stelate ganglia. Postganglionic fibers enter the lungs via the hili, accompanying the vagus nerves. It is important to note that there is considerable variation in sympathetic innervation among various species.

Based on the main effect of the sympathetic nervous system with regard to relaxation of bronchial smooth muscle, this system is termed the "inhibitory" system. Adrenaline and noradrenaline represent the major neurotransmitters. They act via stimulation of α and β receptors. In general, there is a much higher density of β than α receptors in the human lung (27,37). These receptors have been identified on a great variety of cell types, including airway smooth muscles, as well as alveolar and epithelial cells, with generally increasing numbers in the smaller airways of the peripheral lung (27,37–40).

The most important lung functions relevant to asthma are mediated via β_2 receptors. Although human lung contains both β_1 and β_2 receptors, a several-fold higher expression pattern of the β_2 receptors has been observed (38,39,41). Stimulation of the β_2 receptors results in airway smooth muscle relaxation (42), inhibition of antigen-induced mast cell mediator release (43–45), release of surfactant and others (46). In addition, stimulation of this receptor type inhibits cholinergic nerve activities, indirectly indicating expression of β_2 receptors on cholinergic neurons (47,48). The role of α receptors in this regard is not entirely clear. First, stimulation of α_1 receptors induces mucosecretion (49,50) and augments mast cell mediator release (51,52). Alternatively, stimulation of α_2 receptor has been demonstrated to inhibit both cholinergic and noncholinergic excitatory signaling (53–57). The former effects would result in a positive contribution of α_1 receptors to the pathogenesis of asthma, whereas the latter effects of α_2 receptors suggest a protective role.

C. NANC Neurons

The NANC system has been functionally subdivided into excitatory (e-NANC) and inhibitory (i-NANC) systems. Both systems exhibit their functional activity via a certain panel of neuropeptides. Stimulation of the e-NANC system results in marked bronchoconstriction. These effects are mediated by a group of neurotransmitters including substance P (SP), neurokinin A (NKA), neurokinin B (NKB), and calcitonin gene-related peptide (CGRP) (24–26,58–61). Afferent neurons of the NANC system are not strictly anatomically separated from vagus nerve. This group of mediators are referred to as the tachykinin family. Tachykinins bind to three distinct neurokinin receptors termed NK-1, NK-2 and NK-3, respectively. These three high-affinity tachykinin receptors bind a different kind of tachykinin with preference. NK-1 shows highest affinity for SP, NK-2 for NKA, and NK-3 for NKB, respectively.

Neurons of the e-NANC pathway have been identified in both human and animal lungs (62–66). They consist of nonmyelinated vagal afferent fibers.

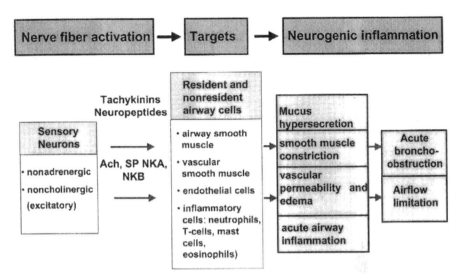

Figure 1 Interaction between neurons and immune cells in lung inflammation. (1). Lung and airways are innervated by adrenergic, cholinergic, and NANC (nonadrenergic noncholinergic) neurons. (2) Neurotrophins amplify the immunological response. (3) Neurons release tachykinins, neuropeptides, and neurotransmitters. (4) Resident and nonresident airway cells contribute to the inflammatory response. Altered neuronal function results in airway hyperresponsiveness.

Nerve endings of such nonmyelinated sensory C fibers have been identified in the airway epithelium. NK-2 receptor expression predominates on airway smooth muscle cells, whereas NK-1 receptors are mainly found on blood vessels. NK-3 receptors are expressed on particularly cholinergic nerves.

SP is synthesized in the vagal nodose ganglion and is retrogradually transported down the vagus, where it can be released from the afferent nerve fibers. SP immunoreactive nerve fibers are detected near blood vessels, airway epithelium, and, to a lesser extent, in airway smooth muscle (66,67). NKA is colocalized with SP in sensory airway nerves (68,69). NKA-immunoreactive nerves are predominantly found on airway smooth muscle cells around blood vessels. They are preferentially detected in the area of the larger airways and, to a lesser extent, in the trachea, bronchioles, and alveoli (69,70). In contrast, NKB has only little effect on human airways, at least in vitro (71,72).

CGRP is also colocalized with SP in airway nerves (73). In this regard, CGRP immunoreactivity coexists with that of other tachykinins in cell bodies of the nodose and jugular ganglia and in axons and nerve terminals within the airways. In the periphery, CGRP-positive nerves have been detected around blood vessels, within the tracheobronchial smooth muscle layers, and in the respiratory epithelium (73–75).

Inhibitory NANC neurons appear to be the predominant neural broncho-dilator system in humans since there is little evidence for sympathetic innervation of the human airways. Initial evidence for the existence of this system comes from experiments utilizing electrical field stimulation. When adrenergic and cholinergic receptors were blocked, field stimulation resulted in smooth muscle relaxation (25,26,35,36,76–78). Central neurotransmitters in this system are vasoactive intestinal peptide (VIP) and nitric oxide (NO) (79,80).

VIP-positive neurons often travel together with cholinergic nerves. Highest density of these nerves is greatest in the upper respiratory tract and least in bronchioli (81,82). Furthermore, they have been identified near airway smooth muscle, bronchial glands, and vascular smooth muscle. A variety of cell types express VIP receptors. They include pulmonary vascular smooth muscle, smooth muscle of larger but not small airways, airway epithelium, submucosal glands, and others.

D. The Axon Reflex

The axon reflex explains the possible role of the e-NANC in the pathophysiology of asthma. This concept has been originally proposed by Barnes (83). The axon reflex is initiated by direct stimulation of vagal afferent nerve endings in the airway epithelium. Any damage to airway epithelium causes such stimulation. A broad range of trigger factors have been identified, including infectious agents such as viral and bacterial infections, and inhaled environmental

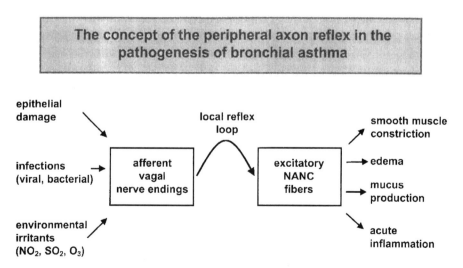

Figure 2 Peripheral axon reflex in the pathogenesis of asthma. Exitatory NANC fibers are activated in a local reflex loop by irritation of afferent neurons.

irritants such as NO_2, SO_2, ozone, and others. Futhermore, various inflammatory mediators released from airway inflammatory cells also stimulate vagal afferent nerve endings. Stimulation of such afferent nerve fibers results in a central reflex activity, leading to enhanced efferent cholinergic activities with the result of increased acetylcholine release. In parallel, there exists a "short-circuit" local reflex loop with the NANC efferent nerves. This peripheral reflex activity results in an increased release of neuropeptides and tachykinins, including SP, NKA, NKB, and CGRP. As a consequence, neuropeptide and tachykinin release causes airway smooth muscle restriction, mucus production, edema, and release of inflammatory mediators from various inflammatory cells (Figs. 1,2).

IV. Neuronal Changes in Allergic Asthma

In the last decade, growing evidence has indicated neuronal dysregulation on several levels in allergic asthma (84) (Table 3). Since cholinergic nerves represent the dominant bronchoconstrictory pathway and anticholinergic drugs are very effective bronchodilators in acute severe asthma, cholinergic mechanisms must be considered in the development of AHR. These possible mechanisms include enhanced cholinergic reflex activity, increased ACh release, enhanced sensitivity of smooth muscle to ACh, and increased density of muscarinic receptors on airway smooth muscle. In addition, sensory nerves are able to modulate cholinergic function. Cholinergic activity was shown to be increased

Table 3 Neuronal Alterations in Human Asthma and Animal Models of Asthma

Neuronal pathway	Mediators	Changes observed in BA	Species
Cholinergic innervation	Acetylcholine	• Increased acetylcholine release	Guinea pig, mouse
		• Loss of function of inhibitory M_2 muscarinic receptors	Guinea pig
NANC system	Tachykinins	• Increased levels in BAL fluid	Human, guinea pig
		• Up-regulation in cell bodies of ganglion nodosum	Guinea pig
		• Increased mechanosensitivity in sensory Aδ fibers	Guinea pig
		• Increased excitability of sensory neurons	Guinea pig
		• Increased response of sensory neurons to substance P	Guinea pig

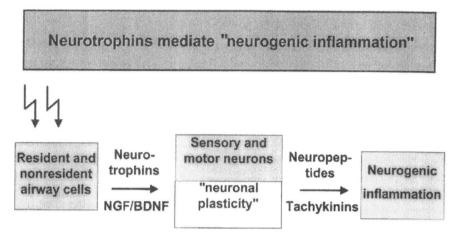

Figure 3 Neurotrophins control the "neurogenic inflammation". (1) Neurotrophins are produced by immune cells during allergic immune response. (2) Neurotrophins mediate "neuronal plasticity." (3) Direct immune modulatory effects of neurotransmitters (e.g., substance P and acetylcholine) on immune cells.

by tachykinins (85,86). Contraction of airway smooth muscle is mediated by M_3 muscarinic receptors on airway smooth muscle. There is no evidence, however, suggesting that AHR results from any alteration in the function of these M_3 muscarinic receptors. In contrast, there is clearly increased release of the neurotransmitter ACh in animal models of hyperresponsiveness and asthma (87). In addition, the loss of function of inhibitory M_2 muscarinic receptors on the airway parasympathetic nerves enhances vagally mediated bronchoconstriction and AHR following allergen challenges (88). The M_2 muscarinic receptors on the parasympathetic nerves in the lungs normally inhibit release of acetylcholine. When the receptors are blocked, the inhibitory effect is lost, leading to increases in ACh. Loss of M_2 receptor function has been shown as a result of eosinophilic mediators, resulting in AHR (89).

The sympathetic (adrenergic) nervous system is less prominent than the parasympathetic (cholinergic) nervous system in the human airways. It should be highlighted that there is a lack of sympathetic innervation of the human airway smooth muscle compared with other species (90–92). Its main neurotransmitters are noradrenaline (NA) and NPY. Guinea pig models indicate that antigen challenge induces a mast cell–mediated long-lasting increase in synaptic efficacy (93). In asthmatic airways, no difference in the number of NPY-immunoreactive nerves has been found as compared with healthy controls (94).

The e-NANC system exhibits a high degree of plasticity in inflammatory conditions. SP and NKA, preferentially released by sensory C fibers, are closely related members of the neuropeptide family termed *tachykinins*. These neuropeptides are synthesized preferentially in cell bodies of the sensory ganglia by a complex biosynthetic pathway. In addition, they are transferred via axonal transport not only to presynaptic axon endings in the spinal cord and the nucleus of the solitary tract, but also to peripheral sensory nerve endings (95). Upon exposure to mechanical, thermal, chemical (capsaicin, nicotine) or inflammatory stimuli (bradykinin, histamine, prostaglandins), tachykinins are released from nerve cells through a local (axon) reflex mechanism (83). Tachykinins act in a dual fashion, as afferent neurotransmitters to the central nervous system as well as efferent neurosecretory mediators diffusing into the peripheral tissue. Increased levels of the neuropeptide substance P (SP) have been detected in the high and low airways of asthmatic patients (94,96). Additionally, allergen challenge increased NKA levels in bronchoalveolar lavage (BAL) fluid of asthmatic patients (97). Nerve fibers containing SP have been described in and around bronchi, bronchioles, and the more distal airways, and occasionally extend to the alveolar wall. These fibers are located beneath and within the airway epithelium, around blood vessels and submucosal glands, within the bronchial smooth muscle layer, and around the local tracheobronchial ganglion cells (66). Although there is evidence for an increase in both the number and length of SP-immunoreactive nerve fibers in airways from subjects with bronchial asthma as compared with airways from healthy subjects (98), the study from Lilli et al. detected no difference in SP-like immunoreactivity (99). One reason for the latter finding may be that the nerves release SP due to continued stimulation. In a guinea pig model, it has been shown that sensory innervation of the airways is altered during allergic inflammation (100). The increase of SP and NKA in the lung in response to allergen challenges has been related to an increased production of these neuropeptides in neurons of the nodose ganglion (101). Impaired degradation of tachykinins could further enhance their local activity (102). Tachykinins are degraded and inactivated by neutral endopeptidase (NEP), a membrane-bound metallopeptidase located mainly on the surface of airway epithelial cells and also present in airway smooth muscle cells, submucosal glands, and fibroblasts. As a key role NEP limits the biological actions of mediators like tachykinins via enzymatic degradation. Allergen exposure, inhalation of cigarette smoke, and other respiratory irritants are associated with reduced NEP activity, thus enhancing the effects of tachykinins within the airways (103–105).

In addition, antigen-induced functional changes in sensory neurons, including depolarization of the resting membrane potential, changes in membrane resistance, increases in mechanosensitivity (of $A\delta$ vagal afferent airway nerves), and enhanced responses to SP, have been described (106,107). Since these neuronal alterations in asthma are associated with local inflammation, the concept that inflammatory mediators could be responsible for neuronal dysfunction was developed.

V. Effects of Inflammatory Mediators on Neurons

In addition to the neuroactive mediators that are released by lymphocytes, many mediators from effector cells, including mast cells, macrophages, and eosinophils, were shown to influence neuronal functions. Mast cells are localized at the interface of the internal and external environment and are often closely approximated to nerve endings within the lung where they respond to allergens and other exogenous stimuli. Upon stimulation, mast cells release neuroactive mediators, including histamine, arachidonic acid metabolites such as prostaglandin $D_2(PGD_2)$, and cysteinyl leukotrienes (LTC_4, LTD_4, and LTE_4), thromboxane A_2 (TxA_2) as well as an array of lipid mediators like platelet-activating factor (PAF) as well as growth factors, cytokines, and chemokines (108).

Inflammatory cells are also able to release certain proteinases (e.g., tryptase or trypsin), and apart from their role in protein degradation these enzymes are signaling molecules that regulate cells by cleaving proteinase-activated receptors (PARs), members of a family of G-protein-coupled receptors (109). Proteases cleave PARs within the extracellular domains to expose tethered ligands that bind and subsequently activate the cleaved receptor. PARs play an important role in response to inflammatory stimuli, and especially proteinase-activated receptor 2 (PAR2) mediates acute inflammation via a neurogenic mechanism (110). PAR2 has been shown to be expressed at peripheral and central terminals on a subset of afferent sensory neurons and PAR2 agonists to elicit neurogenic inflammation by release of SP and CGRP (110). Thus, neuropeptides and agonists of PAR2 have similar proinflammatory effects (111). Moreover, mast cells containing tryptase are located in close proximity to spinal afferent fibers containing SP and CGRP. Tryptase directly signals to neurons via PAR2 to stimulate release of these neuropeptides, which transmit the inflammatory signal of PAR2 through either the CGRP1 receptor or the NK-1 receptor on various target cells (e.g., endothelial cells, smooth muscle cells, or immune cells). Thus, activation of PARs contributes to a newly recognized pathway of neuroimmune interactions in peripheral tissues.

Cytokines produced by T cells or macrophages have a pivotal role in the pathogenesis of asthma, and up-regulation and/or increased expression has been shown in the airways of asthmatic patients (1,112,113). Many of these inflammatory mediators are implied to regulate and affect AHR in asthma. However, whether T-cell-derived cytokines (e.g., IL-4, IL-5, and IL-13) modulate neuronal smooth muscle innervation in a direct or indirect fashion, or whether they directly affect the smooth muscle cell itself, remains unclear. In contrast, cytokines, predominantly produced by macrophages, especially the neurotrophic cytokines including ciliary neurotrophic factor (CNTF), leukemia inhibitory factor (LIF), oncostatin M (OSM), IL-6, and cardiotrophin-1 (CT-1), were shown to influence sensory neurons (114,115).

Particularly IL-6 is known to affect peripheral sensory neurons and to support neuronal SP production and hypersensitivity (116,117). In addition, IL-1 and tumor necrosis factor-α (TNF-α) induce changes in sensory neurons and are involved in the inflammation-associated hyperalgesia (118,119).

VI. Putative Role of Neurotrophins in the Pathogenesis of Asthma

Some of the most effective mediators involved in inflammatory hyperalgesia are the neurotrophins nerve growth factor (NGF) and brain-derived neurotrophic factor (BDNF) (120–122). NGF is a mediator with functions on both immune and nerve cells (123). It is a well-studied example of a target-derived neurotrophic factor that is essential for development, differentiation, maintenance, and survival of peripheral sympathetic and neural crest–derived sensory nerve cells (124). NGF up-regulates expression of neuropeptides in sensory neurons (125) and contributes to inflammatory sensory hypersensitivity (120). In the central nervous system, NGF is a trophic factor for basal forebrain cholinergic neurons. The biological effects of neurotrophins are mediated by binding either to the specific high-affinity (kD-10^{-11}) glycoprotein receptors trkA (for NGF), trkB (for BDNF), and trkC (for NT-3) or the low-affinity (kD-10^{-9}) panneurotrophin receptor p75 (NTR). Neurotrophin receptors are widely expressed in the peripheral and central nervous systems as well as on cells of the immune system (126).

A. Sources of Neurotrophins in Allergic Disease

Based on their expression profile, neurotrophins are excellent candidates for mediating immune–nerve cell interactions. During the inflammatory processes, NGF is produced by a wide range of immune cells, including mast cells, macrophages, T cells, and B cells (for review, see 127). Analysis of a murine model of allergic airway inflammation revealed that T cells, B cells, and macrophages represent sources of enhanced NGF production (Table 4). In vitro, allergen stimulation of mononuclear cells from sensitized mice resulted in enhanced NGF synthesis (128). In addition, NGF production was enhanced by antigen stimulation in murine and human Th2 cell clones (129–131). BDNF synthesis has been detected in activated human T cells, B cells, macrophages, mast cells, and platelets (132–134). In addition to a constitutive production of BDNF by respiratory epithelial cells, we have demonstrated that activated murine macrophages and T cells, but not B cells, produce BDNF during allergic inflammation (133). Histological analysis of the inflamed lung revealed strong NGF and BDNF production by cells in the peribronchial inflammatory infiltrate (128,123). As of recently, there is also evidence for enhanced neurotrophin production in allergic patients.

Table 4 Neurotrophin Production by Inflammatory Cells in Lung and Airways

Cellular source	NGF	BDNF
Airway epithelium	Negative	Constitutively +, asthma ↑
Airway lumen		
Macrophages	Activated positive	Activated positive
T cells	Negative	Negative
Airway mucosa		
T cells	Activated positive	Activated positive
B cells	Activated positive	Negative

Patients with allergic asthma display increased levels of NGF in serum and BAL fluid (100,135,136). Increased neurotrophin production in response to allergen provocation was demonstrated in airways of subjects with allergic rhinitis and mild allergic asthma (137,138). After segmental allergen provocation in mildly asthmatic patients, the neurotrophin content in BAL fluid increased markedly in allergen-exposed lung segments, as opposed to saline-exposed control segments. Notably, this up-regulation was seen during the allergic late-phase response but not in the early phase (138).

B. Neuronal Plasticity and AHR in Response to Neurotrophins

Neuronal plasticity in the peripheral nervous system is not well characterized. For sensory neurons, the lowering of the activation threshold, changes in the processing of information, and altered neurotransmitter synthesis are possible mechanisms. To some extent inflammation-induced hyperalgesia shows remarkable similarities to AHR, particularly with respect to the effects of neurotrophins. Hyperalgesia can be defined by a decrease in the threshold for painful stimuli and heightened reflex pathways in sensory neurons (139). It is well established that neurotrophins play a central role in inflammation-induced hyperalgesia (140,141).

There is some evidence suggesting that sensory neurons innervating the lung are also responsive to neurotrophins because local increase of neurotrophins in the lung could mediate similar neuronal changes in animal models as seen during allergic inflammation (100,142). It has been well established that visceral sensory neurons localized in the nodose and dorsal root ganglia require neurotrophins for survival during development (143). In adults, functional properties of neurons are also affected by neurotrophins (144). NGF was shown to up-regulate neuropeptide production in sensory neurons and to contribute to inflammatory hypersensitivity (120). Though cultured nodose ganglion neurons do not require NGF for survival, their SP production is regulated by NGF (145). In transgenic mice overexpressing NGF in airway-restricted Clara cells, a marked sensory and sympathetic hyperinnervation and increased neuropeptide content was observed in projecting sensory neurons (146). In addition, these mice demonstrated AHR in response to capsaicin. In a guinea pig model, tracheal injection of NGF induced SP production in mechanically sensitive "Aδ" fibers that do not produce SP under physiological conditions (142). These NGF-mediated effects are comparable to neuronal changes observable during allergic inflammation (100). The induction of neuropeptides in mechanically sensitive neurons may lead to exaggerated reflex responses to innocuous stimuli (142). In a murine model of allergic airway inflammation, we were able to demonstrate that blocking of NGF by local treatment with anti-NGF antibodies prevented the development of AHR (128). Therefore, it is not surprising that NGF treatment induces AHR in the guinea pig. Along this line, de Vries and colleagues could block NGF-induced AHR to histamine with the NK-1-specific tachykinin antagonist SR140333, thus pointing again to the central role played by tachykinins in this condition (147). Taken together, these data provide further evidence that neurotrophins are central signaling molecules in immune–nerve cell communication as it occurs in pathophysiological conditions including asthma (148).

C. Immunological Plasticity in Response to Neurotrophins

In addition to the effects of neurotrophins on neuronal plasticity, there is growing evidence as well for a substained action of neurotrophins on immune cells involved in allergic inflammation, including mast cells, eosinophils, B cells, and T cells. One of the first reports demonstrating that neurotrophins can modulate immune cell activities came from Aloe et al. After injection of NGF into neonatal rats, they observed an increased number of mast cells in these animals (149). Further studies characterized NGF as an important growth and differentiation factor for mast cells and basophils (150–153). Since NGF is the best characterized neurotrophin, most of the available data pertain to it. NGF stimulates rapid degranulation of mast cells and basophils (154–156), promotes differentiation, activation, and cytokine production of mast cells, granulocytes, and macrophages (151,152,157,158), activates eosinophils (159), promotes proliferation of B- and T-cell subsets (160,161), enhances Th2 cytokine production and IgE synthesis in a murine asthma model (128), and induces differentiation of activated B cells in immunoglobulin-secreting plasma cells (162). It needs to be emphasized that the majority of NGF effects have been observed in preactivated cells. NGF by itself does not appear to activate the immune cells in physiologically relevant concentrations but rather modulates their threshold to other triggering stimuli (123). However, most of these investigations were performed in vitro. Therefore, the physiological function of NGF in vivo remains to be elucidated. Compared with NGF, there are few data available about possible functions of other neurotrophins in the immune system. The presence of a variety of neurotrophin receptors on developing and mature immune cells, however, suggests that the effects of other neurotrophins have to be considered as well (Table 5).

Recent studies demonstrated the expression of neurotrophins and their receptors in bone marrow and thymus cells. Since bone marrow and thymus are the preferential organs for immune cell maturation and differentiation, this suggests that neurotrophins have a role in immune cell differentiation as well (163, 164). Findings of higher neurotrophin transcript levels at fetal as compared with adult stages further support such a notion (164). Similar results were demonstrated in the thymus, where trkB on T cells inversely correlated with stages of maturation (165). Therefore, Maroder et al. hypothesized that stromal cell–derived neurotrophins have a direct influence on developing thymocytes (165).

Taken together these data provide evidence that NGF is involved in the development of "immunological plasticity." Immunological plasticity may be defined as a long-lasting change in immunological functions, including cell differentiation, mediator production and release, or sensitivity to activating stimuli. Since the immune and nervous system share many features, including recognition of and reaction to unknown stimuli, it is not surprising that both systems use similar mediators and mechanisms to perform their tasks.

VII. Effects of Neuropeptides on Immune Cells

A substantial number of studies provide evidence that neuropeptides and neuromediators released from nerve endings of the parasympathetic, sympathetic, and sensory systems directly influence immune cells and, thus, participate in immunomodulation (Table 6).

The major neurotransmitter of parasympathetic nerves is ACh, which exerts its biological activities via binding to the acetylcholine receptors. These receptors are classified as M_1 to M_3 on the basis of functional inhibition by

Table 5 NGF Receptor Expression and NGF Effects on Human Immune Cells

Cell type	trkA	p75NTR	Effects
T cells	+	−	c-fos transcription ↑, activation ↑, proliferation ↑, cytokine production ↑
B cells	+	+	Survival ↑, proliferation ↑, immunoglobulin production ↑
Monocytes/ macrophages	+	+/−	Respiratory burst ↑
Eosinophils	+	+	Viability ↑, chemotaxis ↑, cytotoxity ↑
Mast cells	+	−	Histamine release ↑, proliferation ↑, differentiation, cytokine production ↑
Basophils	+	−	Priming ↑

−, not detected; +, detected; +/−, conflicting data.

antagonists. The muscarinic receptors M_1 and M_2 are expressed on T cells, and their activation augments anti-CD3-induced mRNA expression of IL-2 and IL-2 receptors as well as T-cell proliferation (166). Macrophages express the M_3 receptor and subsequent stimulation with ACh triggers the release of chemotactic substances by alveolar macrophages (167).

Sympathetic nerves predominantly release NA and NPY. NA binds to α- and β-adrenergic receptor subtypes expressed on T cells, monocytes, and mast cells (168–170). In contrast to activation of muscarinic receptors, IL-2 production and thus T-cell proliferation are inhibited by β-adrenergic receptor activation (168). Catecholamine-induced release of IL-10 from unstimulated monocytes appears to be rapid and direct, without involvement

Table 6 Effect of Neuropeptides on Immune Cells

Neurotransmitter	Target	Effect
		Proinflammatory
ACh	T-cell	IL-2/IL-2R expression and IL-2 release, proliferation
	Macrophage	Mediator release
CGRP	Lymphocyte	Chemotaxis and adhesion
	Eosinophil	Chemotaxis and adhesion
NO	T cell	Stimulation of Th2 phenotype Inhibition of Th1 phenotype
SP	Lymphocyte	Stimulation
	T cell	Proliferation, chemotaxis, cytokine production, modulation of Th1/Th2 phenotype switching
	B cell	Differentiation, immunoglobulin switch
	Eosinophil	Migration, recruitment
	Neutrophil	Chemotaxis, superoxide production, adhesion
	Monocyte	TNF-α, IL-1, IL-6, and IL-10 release
		Anti-inflammatory
SOM	B cell	Inhibition of IgE production
	Basophil	Inhibition of mediator release
	T cell	Modulation of Th1/Th2 phenotype switching, adhesion
	Eosinophil	Increased adhesion and infiltration
NA	T cell	Inhibition of IL-2 release
	Monocyte	Stimulation IL-10 release
NPY	T cell	Th1/Th2 phenotype switching
VIP	T cell	Inhibition of IL-2, IL-4, and IL-10 production
	B cell	Inhibition of IgE secretion
	Mast cell	Inhibition of mediator release by mast cells
	Leukocyte	Chemotaxis

of immunological costimulation (170). Mast cells in the human lung bear the β_2-adrenergic receptor subtype (169). NPY serum levels have been demonstrated to be increased during acute exacerbation of asthma (171). NPY is capable of modulating immune cell functions such as T-cell adhesion to the extracellular fibronectin matrix which is mediated by integrin expression via NPY receptors (172). NPY was shown to induce Th2 cytokine release from a Th1 cell line and Th1 cytokines from a Th2 cell line, breaking the commitment of T-cell effector populations (173).

Immunoactive secretory products from the i-NANC system include mediators such as VIP and NO, which appear to be the major neurotransmitters in this system (174). Under normal conditions in mouse lungs, VIP receptors are localized on alveolar macrophages. Immunized and intratracheally challenged mice demonstrated elevated levels of VIP and its receptor expression on mononuclear cells and neutrophils in perivascular, peribronchiolar, and alveolar inflammatory infiltrates (175). Direct immunological effects of VIP include inhibition of T-cell proliferation; IL-2, IL-4, and IL-10 cytokine production; inhibition of IgE release by B cells; and inhibition of mediator release from mast cells (reviewed in 176). Once produced, NO passes membranes by simple diffusion and direct activation of soluble guanylate cyclase. A role of NO has been implied in skewing T lymphocytes toward a Th2 phenotype by inhibition of Th1 cells and their product IFN-γ (177).

e-NANC system–associated neuropeptides with immunomodulatory functions are somatostatin (SOM), CGRP, and the members of the tachykinin family, SP and NKA, which all act via G-protein-coupled receptors and thus share several effector functions. Specific receptors for CGRP and SOM have been demonstrated on monocytes, B cells, and T cells (178, 179). Similar to NPY, CGRP and SOM have the capacity to induce T-cell adhesion to fibronectin and to drive distinct Th1 and Th2 populations to an atypical expression pattern of Th2 or Th1 cytokines respectively and, therefore, break the commitment to a distinct T-helper phenotype (172,173).

SOM exerts various inhibitory functions on immune responses via specific receptor activation (reviewed in Ref. 179). SOM affects the suppression of Ig production in B cells, including IgE (180), modulation of lymphocyte proliferation (inhibitory effect at low concentrations or stimulatory effect at high concentrations), and reduction of (peritoneal) eosinophil infiltration in experimentally induced hypereosinophilia. Futhermore, SOM inhibits SP-induced mucus secretion in rats (181).

CGRP inhibits SP-induced superoxide production in neutrophils and the proliferation as well as the antigen presentation by peripheral mononuclear cells (182). It also stimulates chemotaxis and adhesion of lymphocytes (172) and causes eosinophilia in rat lung (183).

The tachykinin family includes neuropeptides such as SP, NKA, and NKB, and they exhibit their function via binding to the three neurokinin receptors NK-1 to NK-3. NK-1 receptor expression has been identified on immune cells such as B cells, T cells (184), monocytes, macrophages (185), eosinophils, and neutrophils (186). Like VIP receptor, NK-1 receptor expression by lung-infiltrating leukocytes in systemically and subsequently intratracheally allergen challenged mice is strongly elevated (175). Since SP binds to NK-1 with the highest affinity, it is the predominant mediator of immunomodulatory effects among tachykinins. The activities of SP on immune cells include a broad range of functional responses from neutrophils, eosinophils, mast cells, monocytes/macrophages, and lymphocytes (reviewed in Ref. 187). SP stimulates a number of neutrophil functions, including chemotaxis, superoxide production, and adherence to epithelium and endothelium. Most of these effects require high concentrations of SP, whereas at low doses SP primes the response to other stimuli that otherwise would be ineffective. SP has a degranulating effect on eosinophils and induces human eosinophil migration in vitro. In an in vivo study with allergic rhinitis patients, it was shown that SP administered after repeated allergen challenge enhanced the recruitment of eosinophils. It has been demonstrated that SP can cause histamine release from human lung mast cells (188). This is underlined by an in vitro model using trachea from the SP-hyperresponsive Fisher 344 rat, in which SP stimulation of mast cells represented a major factor leading to bronchoconstriction (189). Moreover, SP activates monocytes to release inflammatory cytokines, including TNF-α, IL-1, IL-6, and IL-10. In lymphocytes, SP inhibits glucocorticoid-induced thymocyte apoptosis (190); stimulates proliferation, cytokine production, chemotaxis (187), and a Th1/Th2 phenotype switch in T cells (172,173); and induces differentiation and Ig switching in B cells (184).

Taken together, the accumulated evidence now points to direct effects of neurotransmitters and neuropeptides on immune cells. A role of these neurogenic immunodulation in asthma is very likely, but since most of these data were obtained in vitro or in animal models, the clinical relevance of these observations requires further evaluation.

VIII. Conclusion

Lung and airways are predominantly innervated by a complex system of autonomic nerve fibers. There is emerging evidence that many cell types and mediators are involved in a bidirectional network between immune and nervous systems. It is well established that the cholinergic nervous system represents a major pathway responsible for acute and chronic airway obstruction due to smooth muscle constriction, edema, and inflammation. However, more recently it became evident that the NANC system also contributes to the pathogenesis of acute and chronic bronchial asthma to a significant extent. The NANC system activities are largely mediated via the release of neuropeptides and tachykinins. There is some evidence that in bronchial asthma enhanced production and/or release of such mediators occurs. On a functional level, this results in increased sensitivity of the NANC system in bronchial asthma. Production and/or release of tachykinins and neuropeptides is under close control of neurotrophins. The neurotrophins are produced in increased concentrations by both immune and nonimmune cells in the asthmatic patient. Neurotrophins are responsible for qualitative and/or quantitative changes in the functional activity and capacity of peripheral neurons, particularly of the NANC system. This effect is defined as *neuronal plasticity*. One important effect of neuronal plasticity is the enhanced production of neurotransmitters including neuropeptides following activation of the neurons.

One key result of these alterations is the development of AHR in bronchial asthma. In parallel, neurotrophins also exhibit profound effects on immune cells residing in airways and lung tissue. These effects are defined by the term *immunological plasticity*. In this regard, neurotrophins act as amplifiers of the locally occurring immune dysbalance. It is important to note that these effects of neurotrophins are not immediate but rather require some time to fully materialize. In this context, the proposed concept is to aggravate and amplify the pathology in bronchial asthma with all clinical consequences. Neurotrophins act as intermediate and long-term modulators of neuronal and immune functions. Amplification of the Th2-mediated inflammatory response occurs via direct action of neurotrophins on T cells, eosinophils, mast cells, and B cells. These effects are rather long lasting in comparison with the short-lasting effects of neuropeptides.

We are just beginning to unravel the complex interaction between the neural and immune systems. The above developed concepts await further exploration, particularly in suitable in vivo models. Ultimately, this concept must be proven using appropriate intervention strategies.

Acknowledgments

This work was supported by the Volkswagen Foundation and the Deutsche Forschungsgemeinschaft DFG.

References

1. Kay AB. Pathology of mild, severe, and fatal asthma. Am J Respir Crit Care Med 1996; 154(2 Pt 2):S66–69.
2. Constant SL, Bottomly K. Induction of Th1 and Th2 CD4+ T cell responses: the alternative approaches. Annu Rev Immunol 1997; 15:297–322.
3. Rincon M, Anguita J, Nakamura T, Fikrig E, Flavell RA. Interleukin (IL)-6 directs the differentiation of IL-4-producing CD4+ T cells. J Exp Med 1997; 185(3):461–469.

4. Desmedt M, Rottiers P, Dooms H, Fiers W, Grooten J. Macrophages induce cellular immunity by activating Th1 cell responses and suppressing Th2 cell responses. J Immunol 1998; 160(11):5300–5308.
5. Ronchese F, Hausmann B, Le Gros G. Interferon-gamma- and interleukin-4-producing T cells can be primed on dendritic cells in vivo and do not require the presence of B cells. Eur J Immunol 1994; 24(5):1148–1154.
6. Stumbles PA, Thomas JA, Pimm CL et al. Resting respiratory tract dendritic cells preferentially stimulate T helper cell type 2 (Th2) responses and require obligatory cytokine signals for induction of Th1 immunity. J Exp Med 1998; 188(11):2019–2031.
7. Korsgren M, Erjefalt JS, Korsgren O, Sundler F, Persson CG. Allergic eosinophil-rich inflammation develops in lungs and airways of B cell-deficient mice. J Exp Med 1997; 185(5):885–892.
8. Tang C, Inman MD, van Rooijen N, et al. Th type 1-stimulating activity of lung macrophages inhibits Th2-mediated allergic airway inflammation by an IFN-gamma-dependent mechanism. J Immunol 2001; 166(3):1471–1481.
9. Tang C, Ward C, Reid D, Bish R, O'Byrne PM, Walters EH. Normally suppressing CD40 coregulatory signals delivered by airway macrophages to TH2 lymphocytes are defective in patients with atopic asthma. J Allergy Clin Immunol 2001; 107(5):863–870.
10. Lensmar C, Prieto J, Dahlen B, Eklund A, Grunewald J, Roquet A. Airway inflammation and altered alveolar macrophage phenotype pattern after repeated low-dose allergen exposure of atopic asthmatic subjects. Clin Exp Allergy 1999; 29(12):1632–1640.
11. Wong WS, Koh DS. Advances in immunopharmacology of asthma. Biochem Pharmacol 2000; 59(11):1323–1335.
12. Kay AB. Allergy and allergic diseases. Second of two parts. N Engl J Med 2001; 344(2):109–113.
13. Kay AB. Allergy and allergic diseases. First of two parts. N Engl J Med 2001; 344(1):30–37.
14. Milgrom H, Fick RBJ, Su JQ, et al. Treatment of allergic asthma with monoclonal anti-IgE antibody. rhuMAb-E25 Study Group [see comments]. N Engl J Med 1999; 341(26):1966–1973.
15. Bousquet J, Jeffery PK, Busse WW, Johnson M, Vignola AM. Asthma. From bronchoconstriction to airways inflammation and remodeling. Am J Respir Crit Care Med 2000; 161(5):1720–1745.
16. Wilder JA, Collie DD, Wilson BS, Bice DE, Lyons CR, Lipscomb MF. Dissociation of airway hyperresponsiveness from immunoglobulin E and airway eosinophilia in a murine model of allergic asthma. Am J Respir Cell Mol Biol 1999; 20(6):1326–1334.
17. Herz U, Braun A, Ruckert R, Renz H. Various immunological phenotypes are associated with increased airway responsiveness. Clin Exp Allergy 1998; 28(5): 625–634.
18. Wills-Karp M. Immunologic basis of antigen-induced airway hyperresponsiveness. Annu Rev Immunol 1999; 17:255–281.
19. Andersson RG, Grundstrom N. The excitatory non-cholinergic, non-adrenergic nervous system of the guinea-pig airways. Eur J Respir Dis Suppl 1983; 131:141–157.

20. Ellis JL, Undem BJ. Antigen-induced enhancement of noncholinergic contractile responses to vagus nerve and electrical field stimulation in guinea pig isolated trachea. J Pharmacol Exp Ther 1992; 262(2):646–653.

21. Burnstock G, Cambell G, Bennett M. Inhibition of the smooth muscle of taenia coli. Nature 1963; 200:407.

22. Colebatch HJH, Halmagyui DFJ. Effect of vagotomy and vagal stimulation on lung mechanics and circulation. J Appl Physiol 1963; 18:881.

23. Olsen CR, Colebatch HJH, Mebel PE. Motor control of pulmonary airways studied by nerve stimulation. J Appl Physiol 1965; 20:202.

24. Casale TB. Neuromechanisms of asthma. Ann Allergy 1987; 59(6):391–398.

25. Richardson JB. Nerve supply to the lungs. Am Rev Respir Dis 1979; 119(5): 785–802.

26. Anderson HR. The epidemiological and allergic features of asthma in the New Guinea Highlands. Clin Allergy 1974; 4(2):171–183.

27. Barnes PJ, Basbaum CB, Nadel JA. Autoradiographic localization of autonomic receptors in airway smooth muscle. Marked differences between large and small airways. Am Rev Respir Dis 1983; 127(6):758–762.

28. Joad JP, Casale TB. [3H]quinuclidinyl benzilate binding to the human lung muscarinic receptor. Biochem Pharmacol 1988; 37(5):973–976.

29. Casale TB, Ecklund P. Characterization of muscarinic receptor subtypes on human peripheral lung. J Appl Physiol 1988; 65(2):594–600.

30. Bonner TI, Buckley NJ, Young AC, Brann MR. Identification of a family of muscarinic acetylcholine receptor genes. Science 1987; 237(4814):527–532.

31. Bonner TI, Young AC, Brann MR, Buckley NJ. Cloning and expression of the human and rat m5 muscarinic acetylcholine receptor genes. Neuron 1988; 1(5):403–410.

32. Barnes PJ. Muscarinic autoreceptors in airways. Their possible role in airway disease. Chest 1989; 96(6):1220–1221.

33. Barnes PJ. Muscarinic receptor subtypes: implications for lung disease. Thorax 1989; 44(3):161–167.

34. Mak JC, Barnes PJ. Autoradiographic visualization of muscarinic receptor subtypes in human and guinea pig lung. Am Rev Respir Dis 1990; 141(6):1559–1568.

35. Mann SP. The innervation of mammalian bronchial smooth muscle: the localization of catecholamines and cholinesterases. Histochem J 1971; 3(5):319–331.

36. Partanen M, Laitinen A, Hervonen A, Toivanen M, Laitinen LA. Catecholamine- and acetylcholinesterase-containing nerves in human lower respiratory tract. Histochemistry 1982; 76(2):175–188.

37. Spina D, Rigby PJ, Paterson JW, Goldie RG. Alpha 1-adrenoceptor function and autoradiographic distribution in human asthmatic lung. Br J Pharmacol 1989; 97(3):701–708.

38. Casale TB, Hart JE. (-)[125l]pindolol binding to human peripheral lung beta-receptors. Biochem Pharmacol 1987; 36(15):2557–2564.

39. Carstairs JR, Nimmo AJ, Barnes PJ. Autoradiographic visualization of beta-adrenoceptor subtypes in human lung. Am Rev Respir Dis 1985; 132(3):541–547.

40. Casale TB, Wood D, Wescott S, Kaliner M. Immunohistochemical identification of lung cells responsive to beta-stimulation with a rise in cAMP. J Appl Physiol 1987; 63(1):434–439.

41. Barnes PJ. Beta-adrenoceptors in lung tissue. In: Morley J, ed. Perspectives in Asthma, 1984.
42. Zaagsma J, van der Heijden PJ, van der Schaar MW, Bank CM. Comparison of functional beta-adrenoceptor heterogeneity in central and peripheral airway smooth muscle of guinea pig and man. J Recept Res 1983; 3(1–2):89–106.
43. Orange RP, Austen WG, Austen KF. Immunological release of histamine and slow-reacting substance of anaphylaxis from human lung. I. Modulation by agents influencing cellular levels of cyclic 3′,5′-adenosine monophosphate. J Exp Med 1971; 134(3):Suppl:136s+.
44. Orange RP, Kaliner MA, Laraia PJ, Austen KF. Immunological release of histamine and slow reacting substance of anaphylaxis from human lung. II. Influence of cellular levels of cyclic AMP. Fed Proc 1971; 30(6):1725–1729.
45. Butchers PR, Skidmore IF, Vardey CJ, Wheeldon A. Characterization of the receptor mediating the antianaphylactic effects of beta-adrenoceptor agonists in human lung tissue in vitro. Br J Pharmacol 1980; 71(2):663–667.
46. Brown LA, Longmore WJ. Adrenergic and cholinergic regulation of lung surfactant secretion in the isolated perfused rat lung and in the alveolar type II cell in culture. J Biol Chem 1981; 256(1):66–72.
47. Vermiere PA, Vanhoutte PM. Inhibitory effects of catecholamines in isolated canine bronchial smooth muscle. J Appl Physiol 1991; 46:787.
48. Rhoden KJ, Meldrum LA, Barnes PJ. Inhibition of cholinergic neurotransmission in human airways by beta 2-adrenoceptors. J Appl Physiol 1988; 65(2):700–705.
49. Culp DJ, McBride RK, Graham LA, Marin MG. Alpha-adrenergic regulation of secretion by tracheal glands. Am J Physiol 1990; 259(4 Pt 1):L198–205.
50. Lundgren JD, Shelhamer JH. Pathogenesis of airway mucus hypersecretion. J Allergy Clin Immunol 1990; 85(2):399–417.
51. Kaliner M, Orange RP, Austen KF. Immunological release of histamine and slow reacting substance of anaphylaxis from human lung. J Exp Med 1972; 136(3):556–567.
52. Moroni F, Fantozzi R, Masini E, Mannaioni PF. The modulation of histamine release by alpha-adrenoceptors: evidences in murine neoplastic mast cells. Agents Actions 1977; 7(1):57–61.
53. Starke K. Presynaptic receptors. Annu Rev Pharmacol Toxicol 1981; 21:7–30.
54. Grundstrom N, Andersson RG, Wikberg JE. Prejunctional alpha 2 adrenoceptors inhibit contraction of tracheal smooth muscle by inhibiting cholinergic neurotransmission. Life Sci 1981; 28(26):2981–2986.
55. Wikberg JE, Grundstrom N, Visnovsky P, Andersson RG. Pharmacology of B-HT 920 in some isolated smooth muscles of the guinea-pig. Acta Pharmacol Toxicol (Copenh) 1982; 50(4):266–271.
56. Grundstrom N, Andersson RG, Wikberg JE. Inhibition of the excitatory non-adrenergic, non-cholinergic neurotransmission in the guinea pig tracheobronchial tree mediated by alpha 2-adrenoceptors. Acta Pharmacol Toxicol (Copenh) 1984; 54(1):8–14.
57. Grundstrom N, Andersson RG. Inhibition of the cholinergic neurotransmission in human airways via prejunctional alpha-2-adrenoceptors. Acta Physiol Scand 1985; 125(3):513–517.

58. Casale TB, Little MM. Neuropeptides and allergic diseases. In: Middleton E Jr, et al., eds. Allergy: Principles and Practice, 3rd ed. St. Louis: Mosby-Year Book, 1989: 3.

59. Barnes PJ. Neural control of human airways in health and disease. Am Rev Respir Dis 1986; 134(6):1289–1314.

60. Barnes PJ. Neuropeptides in the lung: localization, function, and pathophysiologic implications. J Allergy Clin Immunol 1987; 79(2):285–295.

61. Casale TB. Airway neuropeptides. Am J Rhinol 1988; 2:121.

62. Lundberg JM, Saria A, Brodin E, Rosell S, Folkers K. A substance P antagonist inhibits vagally induced increase in vascular permeability and bronchial smooth muscle contraction in the guinea pig. Proc Natl Acad Sci USA 1983; 80(4):1120–1124.

63. Lundberg JM, Martling CR, Saria A. Substance P and capsaicin-induced contraction of human bronchi. Acta Physiol Scand 1983; 119(1):49–53.

64. Grundstrom N, Andersson RG, Wikberg JE. Pharmacological characterization of the autonomous innervation of the guinea pig tracheobronchial smooth muscle. Acta Pharmacol Toxicol (Copenh) 1981; 49(2):150–157.

65. Lundberg JM, Saria A. Bronchial smooth muscle contraction induced by stimulation of capsaicin-sensitive sensory neurons. Acta Physiol Scand 1983; 116(4):473–476.

66. Lundberg JM, Hokfelt T, Martling CR, Saria A, Cuello C. Substance P-immunoreactive sensory nerves in the lower respiratory tract of various mammals including man. Cell Tissue Res 1984; 235(2):251–261.

67. Wharton J, Polak JM, Bloom SR, Will JA, Brown MR, Pearse AG. Substance P-like immunoreactive nerves in mammalian lung. Invest Cell Pathol 1979; 2(1): 3–10.

68. Lundberg JM, Lundblad L, Martling CR, Saria A, Stjarne P, Anggard A. Coexistence of multiple peptides and classic transmitters in airway neurons: functional and pathophysiologic aspects. Am Rev Respir Dis 1987; 136(6 Pt 2): S16–22.

69. Lundberg JM, Saria A, Theodorsson-Norheim E. Multiple tachykinins in capsaicin-sensitive afferents: occurrence, release, and biological effects with special reference to irritation of the airways. In: Hakanson R, Sundler F, eds. Tachykinin Antagonists. Amsterdam: Elsevier Science, 1985.

70. Uchida Y, Nomura A, Ohtsuka M, et al. Neurokinin A as a potent bronchoconstrictor. Am Rev Respir Dis 1987; 136(3):718–721.

71. Barnes PJ. Neuropeptides in human airways: function and clinical implications. Am Rev Respir Dis 1987; 136(136):S77.

72. Naline E, Devillier P, Drapeau G, et al. Characterization of neurokinin effects and receptor selectivity in human isolated bronchi. Am Rev Respir Dis 1989; 140(3):679–686.

73. Martling CR, Saria A, Fischer JA, Hokfelt T, Lundberg JM. Calcitonin gene–related peptide and the lung: neuronal coexistence with substance P, release by capsaicin and vasodilatory effect. Regul Pept 1988; 20(2):125–139.

74. Palmer JB, Cuss FM, Mulderry PK, et al. Calcitonin gene-related peptide is localised to human airway nerves and potently constricts human airway smooth muscle. Br J Pharmacol 1987; 91(1):95–101.

75. Schimosegawa T, Said Sl. Pulmonary calcitonin gene-related peptide immunoreactivity: nerve-endocrine cell interrelationships. Am J Respir Cell Mol Biol 1991; 4(2):126–134.

76. Richardson J, Beland J. Nonadrenergic inhibitory nervous system in human airways. J Appl Physiol 1976; 41(5 Pt 1):764–771.

77. Ichinose M, Inoue H, Miura M, Takishima T. Nonadrenergic bronchodilation in normal subjects. Am Rev Respire Dis 1988; 138(1):31–34.

78. Coburn RF, Tomita T. Evidence for nonadrenergic inhibitory nerves in the guinea pig trachealis muscle. Am J Physiol 1973; 224(5):1072–1080.

79. Bult H, Boeckxstaens GE, pelckmans PA, Jordaens FH, Van Maercke YM, Herman AG. Nitric oxide as an inhibitory non-adrenergic non-cholinergic neurotransmitter. Nature 1990; 345(6273):346–347.

80. Boeckxstaens GE, Pelckmans PA, Bult H, De Man JG, Herman AG, Van Maercke YM. Non-adrenergic non-cholinergic relaxation mediated by nitric oxide in the canine ileocolonic junction. Eur J Pharmacol 1990; 190(1–2):239–246.

81. Dey RD, Shannon WA, Jr., Said SI. Localization of VIP-immunoreactive nerves in airways and pulmonary vessels of dogs, cat, and human subjects. Cell Tissue Res 1981; 220(2):231–238.

82. Laitinen A, Partanen M, Hervonen A, Pelto-Huikko M, Laitinen LA, VIP like immunoreactive nerves in human respiratory tract. Light and electron microscopic study. Histochemistry 1985; 82(4):313–319.

83. Barnes PJ. Asthma as an axon reflex. Lancet 1986; 1(8475):242–245.

84. Joos GF, Germonpre PR, Pauwels RA. Role of tachykinins in asthma. Allergy 2000; 55(4):321–337.

85. Mackay TW, Hulks G, Douglas NJ. Non-adrenergic, non-cholinergic function in the human airway. Respir Med 1988; 92(3):461–466.

86. Delaunois A, Gustin P, Segura P, Vargas M, Ansay M. Interactions between acetylcholine and substance P effects on lung mechanics in the rabbit. Fundam Clin Pharmacol 1996; 10(3):278–288.

87. Larsen GL, Fame TM, Renz H, et al. Increased acetylcholine release in tracheas from allergen-exposed IgE-immune mice. Am J Physiol 1994; 266:L263–L270.

88. Fryer AD, Adamko DJ, Yost BL, Jacoby DB. Effects of inflammatory cells on neuronal M2 muscarinic receptor function in the lung. Life Sci 1999; 64(6–7): 449–455.

89. Jacoby DB, Costello RM, Fryer AD. Eosinophil recruitment to the airway nerves. J Allergy Clin Immunol 2001; 107(2):211–218.

90. Barnes PJ. Overview of neural mechanisms in asthma. Pulm Pharmacol 1995; 8(4–5):151–159.

91. Casale TB. Neurogenic Control of Inflammation and Airway Function, Vol. 1. St. Louis:Mosby, 1996.

92. Joos GF, Germonpre PR, Pauwels RA. Neural mechanisms in asthma. Clin Exp Allergy 2000; 30 Suppl 1:60–65.

93. Weinreich D, Undem BJ, Taylor G, Barry MF. Antigen-induced long-term potentiation of nicotinic synaptic transmission in the superior cervical ganglion of the guinea pig. J Neurophysiol 1995; 73(5):2004–2016.

94. Howarth PH, Springall DR, Redington AE, Djukanovic R, Holgate ST, Polak JM. Neuropeptide-containing nerves in endobronchial biopsies from

asthmatic and nonasthmatic subjects. Am J Resp Cell Mol Biol 1995; 13(3): 288–296.

95. Brimijoin S, Lundberg JM, Brodin E, Hokfelt T, Nilsson G. Axonal transport of substance P in the vagus and sciatic nerves of the guinea pig. Brain Res 1980; 191(2):443–457.

96. Baumgarten CR, Witzel A, Kleine Tebbe J, Kunkel G. Substance P enhances antigen-evoked mediator release from human nasal mucosa. Peptides 1966; 17(1):25–30.

97. Heaney LG, Cross LJ, McGarvey LP, Buchanan KD, Ennis M, Shaw C. Neurokinin A is the predominant tachykinin in human bronchoalveolar lavage fluid in normal and asthmatic subjects. Thorax 1998; 53(5):357–362.

98. Ollerenshaw SL, Jarvis D, Sullivan CE, Woolcock AJ. Substance P immunoreactive nerves in airways from asthmatics and nonasthmatics. Eur Respir J 1991; 4(6):673–682.

99. Lilly CM, Bai TR, Shore SA, Hall AE, Drazen JM. Neuropeptide content of lungs from asthmatic and nonasthmatic patients. Am J Respir Crit Care Med 1995; 151(2 Pt 1):584–553.

100. Undem BJ, Hunter DD, Liu M, Haak-Frendscho M, Oakragly A, Fischer A. Allergen-induced sensory neuroplasticity in airways. Int Arch Allergy Immunol 1999; 118:150–153.

101. Fischer A, McGregor GP, Saria A, Philippin B. Kummer W. Induction of tachykinin gene and peptide expression in guinea pig nodose primary afferent neurons by allergic airway inflammation. J Clin Invest 1996; 98(10): 2284–2291.

102. van der Velden VHJ, Hulsmann AR. Peptidases: structure, function and modulation of peptide-mediated effects in the human lung. Clin Exp Allergy 1999; 29:445–456.

103. Tudoric N, Zhang M, Kljajic-Turkalj M, et al. Allergen inhalation challenge induces decrease of serum neutral endopeptidase (NEP) in asthmatics. Peptides 2000; 21(3):359–364.

104. Di Maria GU, Bellofiore S, Geppetti P. Regulation of airway neurogenic inflammation by neutral endopeptidase. Eur Respir J 1998; 12(6):1454–1462.

105. Sont JK, van Krieken JH, van Klink HC, et al. Enhanced expression of neutral endopeptidase (NEP) in airway epithelium in biopsies from steroid- versus nonsteroid-treated patients with atopic asthma. Am J Respir Cell Mol Biol 1997; 16(5):549–556.

106. Undem BJ, Hubbard W, Weinreich D. Immunologically induced neuromodulation of guinea pig nodose ganglion neurons. J Autonom Nerv Syst 1933; 44(1):35–44.

107. Weinreich D, Moore KA, Taylor GE. Allergic inflammation in isolated vagal sensory ganglia unmasks silent NK-2 tachykinin receptors. J Neurosci 1997; 17(20):7683–7693.

108. Holgate ST. The role of mast cells and basophils in inflammation. Clin Exp Allergy 2000; 30(Suppl 1):28–32.

109. Dery O, Corvera CU, Steinhoff M, Bunnett NW. Proteinase-activated receptors: novel mechanisms of signaling by serine proteases. Am J Physiol 1988; 274(6 Pt 1):C1429–1452.

110. Vergnolle N, Wallace JL, Bunnett NW, Hollenberg MD. Protease-activated receptors in inflammation, neuronal signaling and pain. Trends Pharmacol Sci 2001; 22(3):146–152.

111. Steinhoff M, Vergnolle N, Young SH, et al. Agonists of proteinase-activated receptor 2 induce inflammation by a neurogenic mechanism. Nat Med 2000; 6(2):151–158.

112. Virchow JC, Jr., Walker C, Hafner D, et al. T cells and cytokines in bronchoalveolar lavage fluid after segmental allergen provocation in atopic asthma. Am J Respir Crit Care Med 1995; 151(4):960–968.

113. Hamid QA, Minshall EM. Molecular pathology of allergic disease: I: Lower airway disease. J Allergy Clin Immunol 2000; 105(1 Pt 1):20–36.

114. Horton AR, Barlett PF, Pennica D, Davies AM. Cytokines promote the survival of mouse cranial sensory neurones at different developmental stages. Eur J Neurosci 1998; 10(2):673–679.

115. Horton AR, Bartlett PF, Pennica D, Davies AM. Cytokines promote the survival of mouse cranial sensory neurones at different developmental stages. Eur J Neurosci 1998; 10(2):673–679.

116. Murphy PG, Ramer MS, Borthwick L, Gauldie J, Richardson PM, Bisby MA. Endogenous interleukin-6 contributes to hypersensitivity to cutaneous stimuli and changes in neuropeptides associated with chronic nerve constriction in mice. Eur J Neurosci 1999; 11(7):2243–2253.

117. Thier M, Marz P, Otten U, Weis J, Rose-John S. Interleukin-6 (IL-6) and its soluble receptor support survival of sensory neurons. J Neurosci Res 1999; 55(4):411–422.

118. Ek M, Kurosawa M, Lundeberg T, Ericsson A. Activation of vagal afferents after intravenous injection of interleukin-1beta: role of endogenous prostaglandins. J Neurosci 1998; 18(22):9471–9479.

119. Woolf CJ, Allchorne A, Safieh-Garabedian B, Poole S. Cytokines, nerve growth factor and inflammatory hyperalgesia: the contribution of tumour necrosis factor alpha. Br J Pharmacol 1997; 121(3):417–424.

120. Donnerer J, Schuligoi R, Stein C. Increased content and transport of substance P and calcitonin gene-related peptide in sensory nerves innervating inflamed tissue: evidence for a regulatory function of nerve growth factor in vivo. Neuroscience 1992; 49(3):693–698.

121. Dmitrieva N, Shelton D, Rice AS, McMahon SB. The role of nerve growth factor in a model of visceral inflammation. Neuroscience 1977; 78(2):449–459.

122. Mannion RJ, Costigan M, Decosterd I, et al. Neurotrophins: peripherally and centrally acting modulators of tactile stimulus-induced inflammatory pain hypersensitivity. Proc Natl Acad Sci USA 1999; 96(16):9385–9390.

123. Levi Montalcini R, Skaper SD, Dal Toso R, Petrelli L, Leon A. Nerve growth factor: from neurotrophin to neurokine. Trends Neurosci 1996; 19(11):514–520.

124. Levi Montalcini R, Dal Toso R, della Valle F, Skaper SD, Leon A. Update of the NGF saga. J Neurol Sci 1995; 130(2):119–127.

125. Lindsay RM, Harmar AJ. Nerve growth factor regulates expression of neuropeptide genes in adult sensory neurons. Nature 1989; 337(6205):362–364.

126. Lewin GR, Barde YA. Physiology of the neurotrophins. Annu Rev Neurosci 1996; 19:289–317.

127. Braun A. Neurotrophins a new family of cytokines. Mod Asp Immunobiol 2001; 1(1):8–9.

128. Braun A, Appel E, Baruch R et al. Role of nerve growth factor in a mouse model of allergic airway inflammation and asthma. Eur J Immunol 1998; 28(10): 3240–3251.

129. Lambiase A, Bracci Laudiero L, Bonini S et al. Human CD4+ T cell clones produce and release nerve growth factor and express high-affinity nerve growth factor receptors. J Allergy Clin Immunol 1997; 100(3):408–414.

130. Otten U, Scully JL, Ehrhard PB, Gadient RA. Neurotrophins: signals between the nervous and immune systems. Prog Brain Res 1994; 103:293–305.

131. Otten U, Gadient RA. Neurotrophins and cytokines—intermediaries between the immune and nervous systems. Int J Dev Neurosci 1995; 13(3–4):147–151.

132. Kerschensteiner M, Gallmeier E, Behrens L et al. Activated human T cells, B cells, and monocytes produce brain-derived neurotrophic factor in vitro and in inflammatory brain lesions: a neuroprotective role of inflammation? J Exp Med 1999; 189(5):865–870.

133. Braun A, Lommatzsch M, Mannsfeldt A et al. Cellular sources of enhanced brain-derived neurotrophic factor (BDNF) production in a mouse model of allergic inflammation. Am J Respir Cell Mol Biol 1999; 21:537–546.

134. Radka SF, Holst PA, Fritsche M, Altar CA. Presence of brain-derived neurotrophic factor in brain and human and rat but not mouse serum detected by a sensitive and specific immunoassay. Brain Res 1996; 709(1):122–301.

135. Bonini S, Lambiase A, Bonini S et al. Circulating nerve growth factor levels are increased in humans with alergic diseases and asthma. Proc Natl Acad Sci USA 1996; 93(20):10955–10960.

136. Bonini S, Lambiase A, Bonini S, Levi-Schaffer F, Aloe L. Nerve growth factor: an important molecule in allergic inflammation and tissue remodelling. Int Arch Allergy Immunol 1999; 118(2–4):159–162.

137. Sanico AM, Stanisz AM, Gleeson TD et al. Nerve growth factor expression and release in allergic inflammatory disease of the upper airways. Am J Respir Crit Care Med 2000; 161(5):1631–1635.

138. Virchow JC, Julius P, Lommatzsch M, Luttmann W, Renz H, Braun A. Neurotrophins are increased in bronchoalveolar lavage fluid after segmental allergen provocation. Am J Respir Crit Care Med 1998; 158(6):2002–2005.

139. Carr MJ, Hunter DD, Undem BJ. Neurotrophins and asthma. Curr Opin Pulmon Med 2001; 7(1):1–7.

140. Safieh-Garabedian B, Poole S, Allchorne A, Winter J, Woolf CJ. Contribution of interleukin-1 beta to the inflammation-induced increase in nerve growth factor levels and inflammatory hyperalgesia. Brit J Pharmacol 1995; 115(7):1265–1275.

141. Woolf CJ, allchorne A, Safieh-Garabedian B, Poole S. Cytokines, nerve growth factor and inflammatory hyperalgesia: the contribution of tumour necrosis factor alpha. B J Pharmacol 1997; 121(3):417–424.

142. Hunter DD, Myers AC, Undem BJ. Nerve growth factor–induced phenotypic switch in guinea pig airway sensory neurons. Am J Respir Crit Care Med 2000; 161:1985–1990.

143. Snider WD. Functions of the neurotrophins during nervous system development: what the knockouts are teaching us. Cell 1994; 77(5):627–638.

144. Chalazonitis A, Peterson ER, Crain SM. Nerve growth factor regulates the action potential duration of mature sensory neurons. Proc Natl Acad Sci USA 1987; 84(1):289–293.

145. MacLean DB, Lewis SF, Wheeler FB. Substance P content in cultured neonatal rat vagal sensory neurons: the effect of nerve growth factor. Brain Res 1988; 457(1):53–62.

146. Hoyle GW, Graham RM, Finkelstein JB, Nguyen KP, Gozal D, Friedman M. Hyperinnervation of the airways in transgenic mice overexpressing nerve growth factor. Am J Respir Cell Mol Biol 1998; 18(2):149–157.

147. de Vries A, Dessing MC, Engels F, Henricks PA, Nijkamp FP, Nerve growth factor induces a neurokinin-1 receptor- mediated airway hyperresponsiveness in guinea pigs. Am J Respir Crit Care Med 1999; 159(5 Pt 1):1541–1544.

148. Braun A, Lommatzsch M, Renz H. The role of neurotrophins in allergic bronchial asthma. Clin Exp Allergy 2000; 30(2):178–186.

149. Aloe L, Levi Montalcini R. Mast cells increase in tissues of neonatal rats injected with the nerve growth factor. Brain Res 1977; 133(2):358–366.

150. Bürgi B, Otten UH, Ochensberger B et al. Basophil priming by neurotrophic factors. Activation through the trk receptor. J Immunol 1996; 157(12): 5582–5588.

151. Kannan Y, Matsuda H, Ushio H, Kawamoto K, Shimada Y. Murine granulocyte-macrophage and mast cell colony formation promoted by nerve growth factor. Int Arch Allergy Immunol 1993; 102(4):362–367.

152. Matsuda H, Kannan Y, Ushio H et al. Nerve growth factor induces development of connective tissue-type mast cells in vitro from murine bone marrow cells. J Exp Med 1991; 174(1):7–14.

153. Tam SY, Tsai M, Yamaguchi M, Yano K, Butterfield JH, Galli SJ. Expression of functional TrkA receptor tyrosine kinase in the HMC-1 human mast cell line and in human mast cells. Blood 1997; 90(5):1807–1820.

154. Horigome K, Pryor JC, Bullock ED, Johnson EM, Jr. Mediator release from mast cells by nerve growth factor. Neurotrophin specificity and receptor mediation. J Biol Chem 1993; 268(20):14881–14887.

155. Horigome K, Bullock ED, Johnson EM, Jr. Effects of nerve growth factor on rat peritoneal mast cells. Survival promotion and immediate-early gene induction. J Biol Chem 1994; 269(4):2695–2702.

156. Bischoff SC, Dahinden CA. Effect of nerve growth factor on the release of inflammatory mediators by mature human basophils. Blood 1992; 79(10):2662–2669.

157. Susaki Y, Shimizu S, Katakura K et al. Functional properties of murine macrophages promoted by nerve growth factor. Blood 1996; 88(12):4630–4637.

158. Welker P, Grabbe J, Grutzkau A, Henz BM. Effects of nerve growth factor (NGF) and other fibroblast-derived growth factors on immature human mast cells (HMC-1). Immunology 1998; 94(3):310–317.

159. Hamada A, Watanabe N, Ohtomo H, Matsuda H. Nerve growth factor enhances survival and cytotoxic activity of human eosinophils. Br J Hematol 1996; 93(2): 299–302.

160. Otten U, Ehrhard P, Peck R. Nerve growth factor induces growth and differentiation of human B lymphocytes. Proc Natl Acad Sci USA 1989; 86(24): 10059–10063.

161. Thrope LW, Perez Polo JR. The influence of nerve growth factor on the in vitro proliferative response of rat spleen lymphocytes. J Neurosci Res 1987; 18(1): 134–139.

162. Brodie C, Gelfand EW. Regulation of immunoglobulin productioin by nerve growth factor: comparison with anti-CD40. J Neuroimmunol 1994; 52(1):87–96.

163. Laurenzi MA, Beccari T, Stenke L, Sjolinder M, Stinchi S, Lindgren JA. Expression of mRNA encoding neurotrophins and neurotrophin receptors in human granulocytes and bone marrow cells–enhanced neurotrophin-4 expression induced by LTB4. J Leukocyte Biol 1998; 64(2):228–234.

164. Labouyrie E, Dubus P, Groppi A et al. Expression of neurotrophins and their receptors in human bone marrow. Am J Pathol 1999; 154(2):405-15.

165. Maroder M, Bellavia D, Meco D et al. Expression of trKB neurotrophin receptor during T cell development. Role of brain derived neurotrophic factor in immature thymocyte survival. J Immunol 1996; 157(7):2864–2872.

166. Fujino H, Kitamura Y, Yada T, Uehara T, Nomura Y. Stimulatory roles of muscarinic acetylcholine receptors on T cell antigen receptor/CD3 complex-mediated interleukin-2 production in human peripheral blood lymphocytes. Mol Pharmacol 1997; 51(6):1007–1014.

167. Sato E, Koyama S, Okubo Y, Kubo K, Sekiguchi M. Acetylcholine stimulates alveolar macrophages to release inflammatory cell chemotactic activity. Am J Physiol 1998; 274(6 pt 1):L970–L979.

168. Kammer GM. The adenylate cyclase-cAMP-protein kinase A pathway and regulation of the immune response. Immunol Today 1988; 9(7–8):222–229.

169. Carstairs JR, Nimmo AJ, Barnes PJ. Autoradiographic visualization of beta-adrenoceptor subtypes in human lung. Am Rev Respir Dis 1985; 132(3):541–547.

170. Woiciechowsky C, Asadullah K, Nestler D, et al. Sympathetic activation triggers systemic interleukin-10 release in immunodepression induced by brain injury [see comments]. Nat Med 1998; 4(7):808–813.

171. Cardell LO, Uddman R, Edvinsson L. Low plasma concentrations of VIP and elevated levels of other neuropeptides during exacerbations of asthma. Eur Respir J 1994; 7(12):2169–2173.

172. Levite M, Cahalon L, Hershkoviz R, Steinman L, Lider O. Neuropeptides, via specific receptors, regulate T cell adhesion to fibronectin. J Immunol 1998; 160(2):993–1000.

173. Levite M. Neuropeptides, by direct interaction with T cells, induce cytokine secretion and break the commitment to a distinct T helper phenotype. Proc Natl Acad Sci USA 1998; 95(21):12544–12549.

174. Belvisi MG, Stretton CD, Yacoub M, Barnes PJ. Nitric oxide is the endogenous neurotransmitter of bronchodilator nerves in humans. Eur J Pharmacol 1992; 210(2):221–222.

175. Kaltreider HB, Ichikawa S, Byrd PK et al. Upregulation of neuropeptides and neuropeptide receptors in a murine model of immune inflammation in lung parenchyma. Am J Respir Cell Mol Biol 1997; 16(2):133–144.

176. Bellinger DL, Lorton D, Brouxhon S, Felten S, Felten DL. The significance of vasoactive intestinal polypeptide (VIP) in immunomodulation. Adv Neuroimmunol 1996; 6(1):5–27.

177. Taylor-Robinson AW, Liew FY, Severn A et al. Regulation of the immune response by nitric oxide differentially produced by T helper type 1 and T helper type 2 cells. Eur J Immunol 1994; 24(4):980–984.

178. McGillis JP, Humphreys S, Reid S. Characterization of functional calcitonin gene-related peptide receptors on rat lymphocytes. J Immunol 1991; 147(10):3482–3489.

179. van Hagen PM, Krenning EP, Kwekkeboom DJ et al. Somatostatin and the immune and haematopoetic system; a review. Eur J Clin Invest 1994; 24(2):91–99.

180. Kimata H, Yoshida A, Ishioka C, Mikawa H. Differential effect of vasoactive intestinal peptide, somatostatin, and substance P on human IgE and IgG subclass production [published erratum appears in Cell Immunol 1993 Jul;149(2):450]. Cell Immunol 1992; 144(2):429–442.

181. Wagner U, Fehmann HC, Bredenbroker D, Yu F, Barth PJ, von Wichert P. Galanin and somatostatin inhibition of substance P–induced airway mucus secretion in the rat. Neuropeptides 1995; 28(1):59–64.

182. Tanabe T, Otani H, Zeng XT, Mishima K, Ogawa R, Inagaki C. Inhibitory effects of calcitonin gene-related peptide on substance-P-induced superoxide production in human neutrophils [published erratum appears in Eur J Pharmacol 1997 Feb 19;321(1):137-41]. Eur J Pharmacol 1996; 314(1–2):175–183.

183. Bellibas SE. The effect of human calcitonin gene-related peptide on eosinophil chemotaxis in the rat airway. Peptides 1996; 17(3):563–564.

184. Braun A, Wiebe P, Pfeufer A, Gessner R, Renz H. Differential modulation of human immunoglobulin isotype production by the neuropeptides substance P, NKA and NKB. J Neuroimmunol 1999; 97(1–2):43–50.

185. Ho WZ, Lai JP, Zhu XH, Uvaydova M, Douglas SD. Human monocytes and macrophages express substance P and neurokinin-1 receptor. J Immunol 1997; 159(11):5654–5660.

186. Iwamoto I, Nakagawa N, Yamazaki H, Kimura A, Tomioka H, Yashida S. Mechanism for substance P-induced activation of human neutrophils and eosinophils. Regul Peptides 1993; 46(1–2):228–230.

187. van der Velden VH, Hulsmann AR. Autonomic innervation of human airways: structure, function, and pathophysiology in asthma. Neuroimmunomodulation 1999; 6(3):145–159.

188. Heaney LG, Cross LJ, Stanford CF, Ennis M. Substance P induces histamine release from human pulmonary mast cells. Clinical and experimental allergy 1995; 25(2):179–186.

189. Joose GF, Lefebvre RA, Bullock GR, Pauwels RA. Role of 5-hydroxytryptamine and mast cells in the tachykinin-induced contraction of rat trachea in vitro. Eur J Pharmacol 1997; 338(3):259–268.

190. Dimri R, Sharabi Y, Shoham J. Specific inhibition of glucocorticoid-induced thymocyte apoptosis by substance P. J Immunol 2000; 164(5):2479–2468.

14

Immunopathology of Atopic and Nonatopic Asthma

MARC HUMBERT

Hôpital Antoine Béclère
Assistance Publique— Hôpitaux de Paris
Clamart, France

**SUN YING and
DOUGLAS S. ROBINSON**

National Heart and Lung Institute
Imperial College School of Medicine
London, England

I. Introduction

Atopy is a disorder characterized by sustained, inappropriate IgE responses to common environmental antigens ("allergens") encountered at mucosal surfaces (1). Atopy is a very common feature in asthmatics: atopic asthma is characterized by infiltration of the bronchial mucosa with eosinophils and Th2-type cells, circulating specific IgE antibodies and positive skin tests to common aeroallergens, and airway hyperresponsiveness (2). Stimulation of IgE synthesis by B cells and mobilization of eosinophils is believed to be driven by a complex network of cytokines and chemokines, including interleukin-4 (IL-4) and IL-5 (3). Since Rackeman's clinical classification of asthma, it has been widely accepted that a subgroup of asthmatic patients are not demonstrably atopic—the "intrinsic" variant of the disease (4). Intrinsic asthmatics show negative skin tests and there is no history of allergy (4,5). Furthermore, serum total IgE concentrations are within the normal range and there is no evidence of specific IgE antibodies directed against common allergens (5). These patients are usually older than their allergic counterparts and have onset of symptoms in later life, often with a more severe clinical course (4,5). There is a preponderance of females, and the association of nasal polyps and aspirin sensitivity occurs more frequently in the nonatopic form of the disease (4,5). Whereas some authors suggest that around 10% of asthmatics have the intrinsic form of the disease, the Swiss SAPALDIA survey (8357 adults, 18–60 years old) found that one-third of total asthmatics were nonallergic (intrinsic) (6).

Ever since the first description of intrinsic asthma there has been debate about the relationship of this variant of the disease to atopy (7). Our recent studies support the concept that although intrinsic asthma has a different clinical profile from extrinsic asthma, it does not appear to be a distinct immunopathological entity (5). In this chapter we will review the current literature on the immunopathology of atopic and nonatopic asthmatics.

II. Eosinophilic Airways Inflammation

Eosinophils are potent inflammatory cells that secrete a number of lipid mediators and proteins relevant to the pathophysiology of asthma, including leucotrienes (LT) C_4, D_4, and E_4, platelet-activating factor (PAF), and basic proteins [major basic protein (MBP), eosinophil-derived neurotoxin (EDN), eosinophil cationic protein (ECP), and eosinophil peroxidase (EPO)] (8). Basic proteins induce a direct damage to the airway epithelium and promote bronchial hyperresponsiveness (9,10). Eosinophils are also able to produce pro-inflammatory cytokines and thereby amplify the inflammatory reaction [transforming growth factor-β (TGF-β), tumor necrosis factor-α (TNF-α), interleukin-4 (IL-4), IL-5, IL-6, IL-8, granulocyte-macrophage colony-stimulating factor (GM-CSF), RANTES, eotaxin, etc.] (8,11).

Derived from myeloid progenitors in the bone marrow, mature eosinophils circulate briefly in the peripheral blood and home to the site of inflammation under the action of several factors, including cytokines and chemokines (8). Eosinophil production and maturation are regulated by the eosinophil-active cytokines IL-5, IL-3, and GM-CSF (8,12).

Eosinophils, although classically associated with "allergic" inflammation, are also abundant in the bronchial submucosa of intrinsic asthmatics, perhaps in even greater numbers than in atopic asthmatics for a given degree of disease severity (5,13,14) (Fig. 1). This is explicable in both groups of patients, at least in part, by local expression of the pro-eosinophilic cytokines IL-3, IL-5 and GM-CSF, and chemokines interacting with the eotaxin receptor CCR3 which recruit, activate and prolong the survival of circulating eosinophils (see below). Irrespective of atopy, blood and sputum eosinophilia are commonly associated with asthma: the numbers of eosinophils in peripheral blood, bronchoalveolar lavage (BAL) fluid, and bronchial biopsies are elevated in asthma, as compared with normal controls, and it is possible to demonstrate an increasing degree of eosinophilia with clinical severity (13). Furthermore, immunostaining of the bronchial mucosa of patients who had died from severe asthma revealed the presence of large numbers of activated eosinophils (15). Correlations were found between the concentrations of MBP and the numbers of denuded epithelial cells in BAL fluid (16). In atopic asthmatics, late-phase bronchoconstriction is accompanied by an influx of eosinophils in BAL fluid (17). This is not observed in individuals developing an isolated early-phase

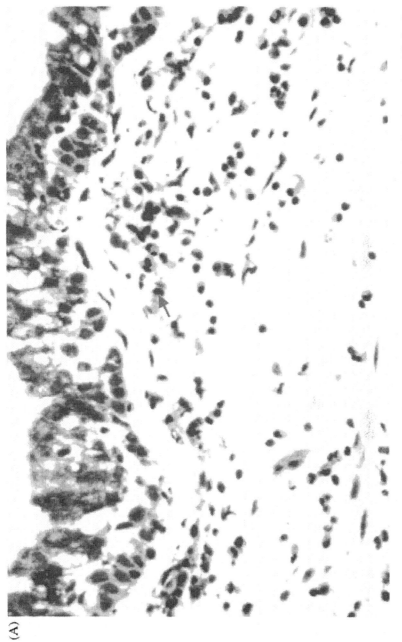

Figure 1 Eosinophilic inflammation in atopic and nonatopic asthma. (A) Congo red staining showing eosinophils in the bronchial mucosa from a nonatopic asthmatic subject (arrows). (B) Counts of cells stained by immunohistochemistry using the monoclonal antibody EG-2, which recognizes the eosinophil cationic protein (ECP), in bronchial biopsies from atopic and nonatopic asthmatics and control subjects. Immunohistochemistry was developed with fast red counterstain and cells enumerated per millimeter of basement membrane.

(B)

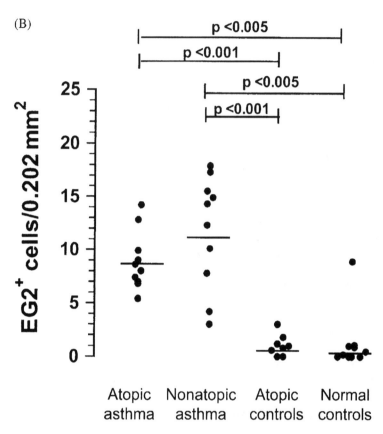

Figure 1 Continued.

response. Last, airway eosinophils are very sensitive to corticosteroid therapy, and their disappearance is associated with an improvement of bronchial hyperresponsiveness (18).

III. T Lymphocytes

T cells have a central role to play in an antigen-driven inflammatory process because they are the only cells capable of recognizing antigenic material after processing by antigen-presenting cells (APCs) (19). $CD4^+$ and $CD8^+$ T lymphocytes activated in this manner elaborate a wide variety of protein mediators including cytokines, which have the capacity to orchestrate the differentiation, recruitment, accumulation, and activation of specific granulocytes at mucosal surfaces. T-cell-derived products can also influence immunoglobulin production by plasma cells. There now exists considerable support for the hypothesis that atopic and non-atopic asthma represent specialized forms of cell-mediated immunity in which cytokines secreted predominantly by activated T-cells (but also by other leukocytes, such as mast cells and eosinophils) bring about the specific accumulation and activation of eosinophils (14). T-cells producing IL-4, IL-5, and IL-10 but not interferon-γ (IFN-γ) are referred to as T-helper 2 (Th2) cells (20,21). These cells provide B-cell help for isotype switching to IgE, and eosinophil maturation, survival, and activation. T-lymphocyte activation and expression of Th2-type cytokines is believed to contribute to tissue eosinophilia and local IgE-dependent events in allergic diseases and asthma (14).

The demonstration of primed circulating blood T lymphocytes in acute severe asthma is interesting as it presumably reflects the presence of activated cells in the bronchial mucosa, the major site of the asthmatic inflammatory process (22). In allergic individuals, circulating blood $CD4^+$ T lymphocytes produce high level of Th2-type cytokines including IL-5, GM-CSF, and IL-3 and may therefore promote eosinophilic inflammation (23). In the airways, the numbers of activated $CD25^+$ lymphocytes are equally elevated in atopic and non-atopic asthma compared with controls (24). Moreover, elevated numbers of $CD4^+$ T lymphocytes expressing IL-5 mRNA have been demonstrated in the airways from asthmatics compared to nonasthmatic controls (25,26). More precisely, a Th2-like cytokine profile has been identified in bronchial samples from atopic and nonatopic asthma (26,27) (Fig. 2). This is in agreement with the demonstration that $CD4^+$ and, to a lesser extent, $CD8^+$ T-cell lines grown from BAL cells from atopic asthmatics produce more IL-5 protein than in control subjects (28).

IV. B Lymphocytes

In contrast with the general agreement that eosinophils and activated T lymphocytes may play a role in asthma in both clinical settings, the possible role of IgE and IgE-mediated mechanisms, especially (but not exclusively) in intrinsic asthma, is less clear (5). Based on the relationship, at the population level, between total serum IgE concentrations and the incidence of asthma/AHR, some authors have questioned the existence of intrinsic asthma, suggesting that all asthmatics have an IgE-dependent component to their disease (7). However, this relationship need not be causal and could equally well reflect the possibility that individuals who have a propensity to develop asthma also have a predisposition to produce IgE inappropriately. We and others have confirmed that nonatopic asthmatics have mildly elevated total serum IgE concentrations as compared with nonatopic controls, despite the fact that, as a group, nonatopic asthmatics tend to be older than their allergic counterparts and that IgE serum concentrations tend to decline with age (5,25).

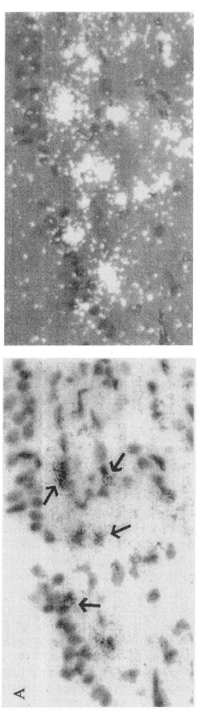

Figure 2 In situ hybridization for interleukin-4 (IL-4) and IL-5 messenger ribonucleic acid (mRNA) in bronchial biopsies from atopic and nonatopic asthmatics. (A) Photomicrographs of in situ hybridization localizing IL-4 mRNA containing cells in bronchial biopsies from patients with nonatopic asthma. Hybridization signals from radiolabeled probes were developed to show dark silver grains, or white dots (darkfield illumination, right-hand panel). (B) Cell counts for IL-4 and IL-5 mRNA- and protein-positive cells in bronchial biopsies from atopic and nonatopic asthmatic and control subjects (25,26).

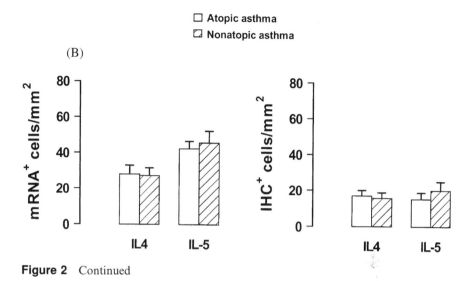

(B)

Figure 2 Continued

Th2-type cytokine-induced B-cell activation and subsequent IgE production is believed to be a critical characteristic of patients with atopy. Interaction of environmental allergens with cells sensitized by binding of surface Fc receptors to allergen-specific IgE is assumed to play a role in the pathogenesis of atopic asthma. IL-4 or IL-13 is absolutely required for IgE switching in B cells, a prerequisite for elevated IgE synthesis, and thus atopy (see Chap. 4) (29,30). Evidence for local IgE synthesis has been demonstrated in CD20$^+$ B cells in the nasal mucosa of patients with hayfever (31). In patients with bronchial asthma, as compared with normal controls, despite comparable numbers of CD20$^+$ B lymphocytes within the bronchial mucosa, we detected elevated numbers of cells expressing the ε germline gene transcript (Iε) and cells expressing Cε, which detects either the sterile transcript or mature ε heavy-chain messenger RNA (Fig. 3). These elevations were detected in biopsies from both atopic and non-atopic asthmatics but not in biopsies from atopic nonasthmatics compared with those from nonatopic normal healthy control subjects (32). Furthermore, there was an association between the number of Cε$^+$ and Iε$^+$ cells and the number of cells expressing IL-4 mRNA, indicating that these changes may be at least in part under the regulation of IL-4 (32). This suggests that local bronchial mucosal IgE production may indeed occur in so-called intrinsic asthma. This, along with the elevated numbers of cells expressing FcεRI in these patients (33), suggests the possibility of local IgE-mediated processes in the absence of detectable systemic IgE production. Thus, nonatopic as well as atopic asthma may be associated with production of IgE directed against as-yet-unidentified allergens or antigens. These results are also compatible with a possible role for virus-specific IgE (34) or IgG autoantibodies of FcεRI in non-atopic asthma, as

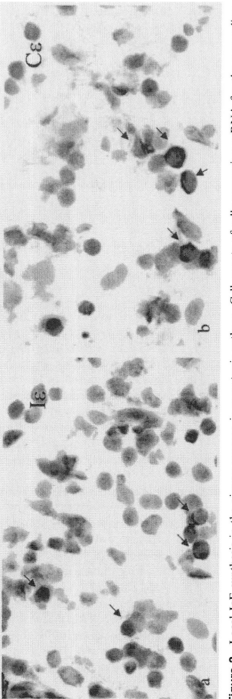

Figure 3 Local IgE synthesis in the airway mucosa in nonatopic asthma. Cell counts of cells expressing mRNA for the ε germline transcripts (Iε) and mature IgE heavy chain (Cε) in bronchial biopsies from atopic and nonatopic asthmatics. (From Ref. 32.).

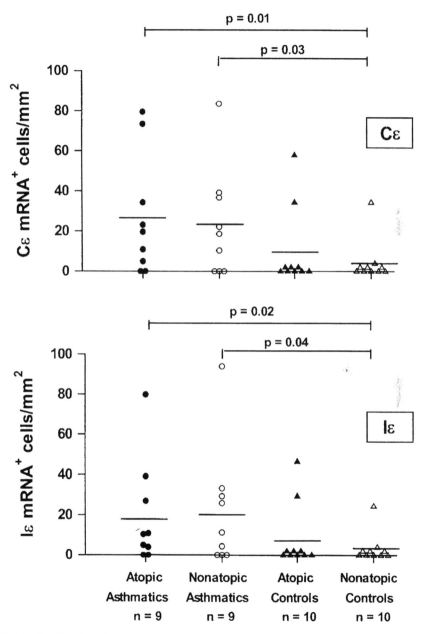

Figure 3 Continued.

previously suggested in chronic idiopathic urticaria, a disease characterized by basophil and mast cell release of histamine and other vasoactive mediators in the absence of any clear allergic, infectious, drug-induced, or physical cause (35). Other autoantibodies have been detected in intrinsic asthmatics, including a circulating IgG autoantibody directed against a common 55-kD antigen shared by platelets and cultured endothelial cells (36). Its role in pathophysiology of asthma has not been elucidated.

V. Mast Cells and Basophils

Mast cells and basophils have long been recognized as major effector cells of allergic reactions by virtue of their high-affinity surface receptors for IgE (FcεRI). The early-phase bronchoconstrictor response to allergen challenge of sensitized atopic asthmatics can probably be accounted for by mast cell and basophil products, mostly histamine. Mast cells can produce and store several cytokines that may play a role in the chronic asthmatic process, including TNF-α, IL-4, IL-5, and IL-6 (37). Mast cells are also believed to be responsible, at least in part, for airway remodeling through fibroblast activation. Mast cells have been observed in the airways of asthmatics and, although not necessarily increased in numbers, are in activated state (degranulated) (38). BBl$^+$ basophils were identified in baseline bronchial biopsies of atopic as well as nonatopic asthmatics, although eosinophils and mast cells were 10-fold higher (39,40). Similarly, basophils increased after allergen inhalation in atopic asthma, but again basophils were less than 10% of eosinophils (39).

VI. Macrophages

Macrophages are phagocytic cells derived from bone marrow precursors. They have a fundamental role as accessory cells and also produce several mediators and cytokines promoting chronic inflammation. Macrophages infiltrate the asthmatic airways, especially in nonatopic patients, but also in atopics where allergen challenge activates macrophages (24,41). This cell type may also play a role in airway remodeling through the production of growth factors such as PDGF, bone fibroblast growth factor (bFGF), and TGF-β (2).

In contrast to the many similarities between atopic and nonatopic asthma, particularly in regard to the expression of Th2-type cytokines, CC chemokines, and IgE, there is a potentially important difference, i.e., the markedly elevated numbers of CD68$^+$ cells expressing the GM-CSF receptor α subunit in non-atopic asthma (42). Do these findings support some form of abnormal macrophage activation in this variant of asthma? Many of these cells were FcεRI$^+$ (33), suggesting that there may be enhanced IgE-dependent antigen presentation in the bronchial mucosa of patients with so-called intrinsic asthma. Macrophage activation may also reflect the existence of an ongoing infectious (viral?)

or autoimmune process in these nonatopic individuals. On the other hand, the nonatopic asthmatics were older than their atopic counterparts, and so the increase in macrophage activity could simply have been a reflection of a longer duration of disease. Further studies are needed to analyze the role and function of macrophages in the nonatopic variant of the disease (43).

VII. Cytokines and Chemokines

A. Proeosinophilic Cytokines

Accumulating evidence tends to show that the combined effects of a wide array of cytokines produced by different cell types, including activated T lymphocytes, could play a major part in regulating the successive steps leading to a characteristic eosinophil-rich airways inflammation (2,5,14). It is well established that tissue recruitment of eosinophils from the bloodstream requires rolling and firm adhesion of circulating cells under the control of cytokine-induced adhesion molecules (mostly of selection and integrin families), and migration following a gradient of chemotactic substances in which the newly described family of chemokines are of utmost importance (44,45). In addition, eosinophils can be activated by several environmental factors, including eosinophil-active cytokines (IL-5, GM-CSF, and IL-3) (46–48). As a result, tissue damage is due at least in part to the release of toxic granule proteins from activated infiltrating eosinophils (8–10).

Eosinophil-Active Cytokines (IL-5, GM-CSF, IL-3)

T lymphocytes are though to orchestrate eosinophilic inflammation in asthma through the release of cytokines, including "eosinophil-active" cytokines (IL-5, GM-CSF, and IL-3) which promote eosinophil maturation, activation, hyperadhesion, and survival (3,14,26). The relevance of IL-5 to asthma has been highlighted by the demonstration of elevated numbers of bronchial mucosal activated (EG2$^+$) eosinophils expressing the IL-5 receptor α-chain mRNA in asthmatics and by positive correlations between the numbers of cells expressing IL-5 mRNA and markers of asthma severity, such as bronchial hyperresponsiveness and asthma symptom (Aas) score (49,50). In both variants of asthma, using double immunohistochemistry and in situ hybridization, 71% of IL-5 mRNA$^+$ signals colocalized to CD3$^+$ T cells, the majority of which (>70%) were CD4$^+$, although CD8$^+$ cells also expressed IL-5 (26). The remaining signals colocalized to mast cells and eosinophils (26). In contrast, double immunohistochemistry showed that IL-5 immunoreactivity was predominantly associated with eosinophils and mast cells (26). However, numbers of IL-5$^+$ cells detected by immunohistochemistry were relatively low, raising the possibility that insufficient protein accumulated within T cells to enable detection by immunohistochemistry (26).

GM-CSF and IL-3 are also thought to participate to the bronchial pro-eosinophilic cytokine network in asthma (51). T-cell lines grown from BAL cells in patients with atopic asthma have the capacity of producing elevated quantities of GM-CSF (28). Bronchial mucosal inflammatory cells expressing GM-CSF and IL-3 have been demonstrated in atopic and non-atopic asthma, with a trend for a more pronounced production of these cytokines in non-atopic asthma (51). Interestingly, this paralleled the marked bronchial mucosal eosinophilic inflammation observed in intrinsic asthma (51). Others have shown that bronchial epithelial cells are also capable of participating in production of GM-CSF in asthma, emphasising that noninflammatory cells can participate actively in the local inflammatory process (52–54). Interestingly, inhaled corticosteriod attenuates both epithelial cell GM-CSF expression and the numbers of epithelial activated eosinophils, suggesting that inhaled corticosteroids could attenuate airway inflammation partly by down-regulating epithelial cell cytokine expression (53,54). Last, GM-CSF could also act on macrophages, as suggested by elevated α-GM-CSF receptor expression on CD68$^+$ macrophages in nonatopic asthmatics (5,42).

Eosinophil Chemokines

The past few years have seen the discovery of a group of chemoattractive cytokines (termed chemokines) with similarities in structure whose principal activities appear to include chemoattraction and activation of leukocytes, including granulocytes, monocytes, and T lymphocytes (see Chap. 16) (45). Chemokines are polypeptides of relatively small molecular weight (8–14 kD) that have been assigned to different subgroups by structural criteria. The α and β chemokines, which contain four cysteines, are the largest families. The α chemokines have their first two cysteines separated by one additional amino acid ("CXC chemokines": IL-8, etc.), whereas these cysteines are adjacent to each other in the β-chemokine subgroup ("CC chemokines": eotaxins, MCPs, RANTES, etc.). Interestingly, chemokines are distinguished from classical chemoattracants by a certain cell–target specificity: the CXC chemokines tend to act more on neutrophils, whereas the CC chemokines tend to act more on monocytes and, in some cases, basophils, lymphocytes, and eosinophils (55). Owing to the effects of some CC chemokines on basophils and eosinophils, their ability to attract and activate monocytes, and their potential role in lymphocyte recruitment, these molecules have emerged as the most potent stimulators of effector cell accumulation and activation in allergic inflammation (45). The CC chemokines interacting with the "eotaxin receptor" CCR3 (eotaxin-1, eotaxin-2, RANTES, MCP-3, MCP-4, etc.) are potent pro-eosinophilic cytokines that are believed to play an important role in asthma (55). Since eosinophil chemokines all stimulate eosinophils via CCR3, this receptor is potentially a prime therapeutic target in asthma and other diseases involving eosinophil-mediated tissue damage. Antagonizing CCR3 may be particularly relevant to asthma, as this receptor is also expressed by several cell types playing a pivotal role in this condition, including Th2-type cells, basophils, and mast cells (56).

Eotaxin mediates eosinophil (but not neutrophil) accumulation in vivo. Recently, eotaxin and CCR3 mRNA and protein product have been identified in the bronchial submucosa of atopic and non-atopic asthmatics (40,57). Moreover, eotaxin and CCR3 expression correlate with airway responsiveness (40,57). Cytokeratin-positive epithelial cells and CD31$^+$ endothelial cells were the major source of eotaxin mRNA, whereas CCR3 colocalized predominantly to eosinophils (40). These data are consistent with the hypothesis that damage to the bronchial mucosa in asthma involves secretion of eotaxin by epithelial and endothelial cells, resulting in eosinophil infiltration mediated via CCR3.

RANTES, MCP-3, and MCP-4 have all the properties that are needed to mobilize and activate basophils and eosinophils, and currently available evidence suggests their primary role in allergic inflammation (45). A combined expression of eosinophil chemokines (eotaxins, MCPs, and RANTES) together with eosinophil-active cytokines (IL-5, GM-CSF, and IL-3) has been demonstrated in both variants of asthma, indicating that these cytokines could act in synergy to promote the elaboration of an eosinophil-rich bronchial mucosal infiltrate (40) (Fig. 4). Indeed, priming eosinophils with IL-5 increases the chemotactic properties of RANTES on eosinophils (51,58). The cell sources of RANTES and MCPs in asthma also include primarily epithelial and endothelial cells, as well as macrophages, T lymphocytes, and eosinophils (40).

B. Proatopic Cytokines

Ever since the first description of intrinsic asthma, there has been debate about the relationship of this variant of the disease to atopy (4–7). One suggestion is that intrinsic asthma represents a form of autoimmunity, or autoallergy, triggered by infection as a respiratory influenza–like illness often precedes onset. Other authors have suggested that intrinsic asthmatics are allergic to an as-yet undetected allergen. Our viewpoint is that although intrinsic asthma has a different clinical profile from extrinsic asthma, it does not appear to be a distinct immunopathological entity (5). This concept is supported by the demonstration of elevated numbers of activated eosinophils, Th2-type lymphocytes, and cells expressing FcεRI in bronchial biopsies from atopic and nonatopic asthmatics, together with epidemiological evidence indicating that serum IgE concentrations relate closely to asthma prevalence regardless of atopic status (5).

In addition to promoting IgE synthesis IL-4 is the major factor orienting T-helper cells towards a Th2 phenotype (59). Moreover, vascular cell adhesion molecule-1 (VCAM-1) expression is up-regulated by several cytokines, including IL-4 and IL-13, highlighting a possible role for IL-4 and IL-13 (60,61). IL-4 expression is a feature of asthma, irrespective of its atopic status, providing further evidence for similarities in the immunopathogenesis of

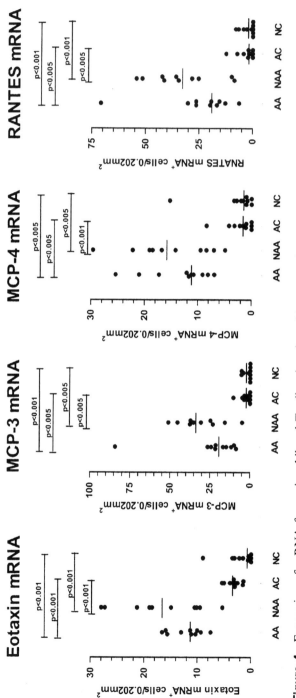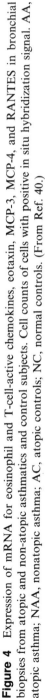

Figure 4 Expression of mRNA for eosinophil and T-cell-active chemokines, eotaxin, MCP-3, MCP-4, and RANTES in bronchial biopsies from atopic and non-atopic asthmatics and control subjects. Cell counts of cells with positive in situ hybridization signal. AA, atopic asthma; NAA, nonatopic asthma; AC, atopic controls; NC, normal controls. (From Ref. 40.)

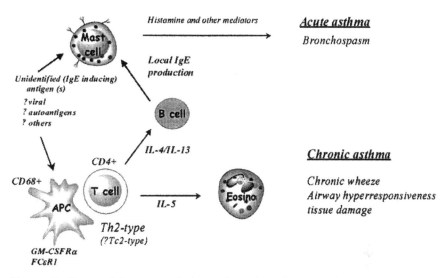

Figure 5 Proposed immunopathology of atopic and nonatopic asthma. Unknown antigens and inflammation induce CD68$^+$ macrophages to express GM-CSF receptor and high-affinity IgE receptor (FcεRI), and these cells activate a Th2-type (or Tc-2 type) T-cell response leading to synthesis of IL-4, IL-5, and IL-13. These cytokines switch local mucosal B cells to IgE synthesis (some that recognize the unknown inciting antigen), which then associates with FcεRI on both mast cells and additional antigen-presenting cells, thus leading to acute asthma symptoms and amplifying local T-cell-driven inflammation via eosinophils and other effector cells.

atopic and nonatopic asthma (5,25,26) (Fig. 2). As previously indicated for IL-5, IL-4 mRNA bronchial mucosal expression in asthma is mainly CD4$^+$ T-cell derived (26). These data are at variance with those of Walker et al. who found that IL-4 protein concentrations were elevated in concentrated BAL fluid from atopic, but not nonatopic, asthmatics in comparison with controls (62). The reasons for this apparent discrepancy are unclear but may reflect methodological problems (variable protein recovery following concentration of BAL fluid or the possible presence of inhibitors that interfere with the protein assay). In addition, we have reported elevated expression of IL-13 mRNA in the bronchial mucosa of so-called atopic and nonatopic asthma (63). Therefore, although intrinsic asthmatics have no demonstrable atopy, they have a biological pattern of airway inflammation strongly suggesting a possible "atopic-like" status that may be restricted to the bronchial submucosa (5).

Expression of IL-4 receptor α chain mRNA and protein is also significantly elevated in the epithelium and subepithelium of biopsies from atopic and nonatopic asthmatics compared with atopic controls (64). However, compared with their allergic counterparts, these patients have fewer cells

Table 1 Summary of Immunopathological Similarities and Differences Between Atopic and Nonatopic Asthma

Factor	Atopic asthma	Nonatopic asthma
Phenotypic cell surface markers		
CD45$^+$	→	→ or ↑
CD3	→	→ or ↑
CD4	→	→ or ↑
CD8	→	→
CD25	↑	↑
EG2$^+$ eosinophils	↑	↑
BBl$^+$ basophils	↑	↑
CD68$^+$ macrophages	→	↑
Th2 and eosinophil-associated cytokines		
IL-3	↑	↑
IL-4	↑[a]	↑
IL-5	↑	↑
IL-13	↑	↑
GM-CSF	↑	↑
CC chemokines		
Eotaxin	↑	↑
Eotaxin-2	↑	↑
RANTES	↑	↑
MCP-3	↑	↑
MCP-4	↑	↑
Cytokine receptors		
IL-4Rα	↑	↑
IL-5Rα	↑	↑
GM-CSFRα	→	↑
CCR3	↑	↑
IgE/FcεRI		
FcεRI$^+$ cells	↑	↑
I$_\varepsilon$/C$_\varepsilon$	↑	↑

[a]Elevated in AC compared with NC by RT-PCR, not in situ hybridization (8).
BBl, a basophil granule–specific marker monoclonal antibody; EG2, cleaved form of eosinophil cationic protein; GM-CSF, granulocyte-macrophage colony-stimulating factor; IL, interleukin; MCP, monocyte chemotactic protein; RANTES, regulated on activation normal T cell expressed and secreted; →, no difference compared with atopic controls (AC) and nonatopic controls (NC); ↑, elevated when compared with AC and NC.

expressing the IL-4 receptor α chain (64). Therefore, Christodoupoulos and colleagues suggested that a deficiency in the IL-4 signaling pathway could be implicated in nonatopic asthma (65). The transcription factors GATA-3 and cMAF mediate IL-4 and IL-5 synthesis, whereas STAT6 is critical for IL-4 receptor signaling (65). These authors showed an up-regulation of GATA-3 and cMAF in both variants of asthma and suggested that reduced IL-4R signaling, because of lower STAT6 expression, might be a feature of nonatopic asthma (65). Despite this possible decrease in IL-4R signaling, we showed that local IgE synthesis in CD20$^+$ B cells could be demonstrated in the bronchial submucosa of patients with atopic and nonatopic asthma (32).

VIII. Conclusion

In conclusion, recent findings suggest that atopic and nonatopic (intrinsic) asthmatics are characterized by a broadly conserved bronchial mucosal pro-eosinophilic cytokine network in which IL-5 appears to play a key role (Fig. 5). Moreover inappropriate IgE-mediated mechanisms might occur in asthma, irrespective of its atopic status, as suggested by elevated serum IgE concentrations and bronchial mucosal expression of cells positive for FcεRI, IL-4, IL-13, I$_ε$, and C$_ε$. In general, these findings support the concept that these subtypes of asthma, despite showing distinct clinical features, share many common immunopathological mechanisms. Promising future directions of research regarding intrinsic asthma include the possible identification of novel allergens or antigens, the detailed description of local bronchial mucosal IgE production, and the understanding of a possible macrophage dysfunction. In addition, a role for infectious (viral?) or autoimmune processes has yet to be firmly identified.

References

1. Pepys J. Atopy. In: Gill PGH, Coombs RRA, Cochmann PJ, eds. Clinical Aspects of Immunology, 3rd ed. Oxford: Blackwell Scientific, 1975:877–902.
2. Bousquet J, Jeffery PK, Busse WW, Johnson M, Vignola AM. Asthma: from bronchoconstriction to airways inflammation and remodeling. Am J Respir Crit Care Med 2000; 161:1720–1745.
3. Robinson DS, Hamid Q, Ying S, Tsicopoulos A, Barkans J, Bentley AM, Corrigan CJ, Durham SR, Kay AB. Predominant T$_{H2}$-like bronchoalveolar T-lymphocyte population in atopic asthma. N Engl J Med 1992; 326:298–304.
4. Rackeman FM. A working classification of asthma. Am J Med 1947; 3:601–606.
5. Humbert M, Menz G, Ying S, Corrigan CJ, Robinson DS, Durham SR, Kay AB. Extrinsic (atopic) and intrinsic (non-atopic) asthma: more similarities than differences. Immunol Today 1999; 20:528–533.
6. Würthrich B, Schindler C, Leuenberger P, Ackermann-Liebrich U. Prevalence of atopy and pollinosis in the adult population of Switzerland (SAPALDIA study). Int Arch Allergy Immunol 1995; 106:149–156.
7. Burrows B, Martinez FD, Halonen M, Barbee RA, Cline MG. Association of asthma with serum IgE levels and skin-test reactivity to allergens. N Engl J Med 1989; 320:271–277.

8. Wardlaw AJ, Moqbel R, Kay AB. Eosinophils: biology and role in disease. Adv Immunol 1995; 60:151–266.

9. Motojima S, Frigas E, Loegering DA, Gleich GJ. Toxicity of eosinophil cationic protein for guinea pig tracheal epithelium. Am Rev Respir Dis 1989; 139:801–805.

10. Gundel RH, Letts LG, Gleich GJ. Human eosinophil major basic protein induces airway constriction and airway responsiveness in primates. J Clin Invest 1991; 87:1470–1473.

11. Broide DH, Paine MM, Firestein GS. Eosinophils express interleukin-5 and granuloctye macrophage colony-stimulating factor mRNA at sites of allergic inflammation in asthmatics. J Clin Invest 1992; 90:1414–1424.

12. Lopez AF, Sanderson CJ, Gamble JR, Campbell HD, Young IG, Vadas MA. Recombinant interleukin 5 is selective activator of human eosinophil function. J Exp Med 1988; 167:219–224.

13. Bousquet J, Chanez P, Lacoste J-Y, Barnèon G, Ghanavian N, Enander I, Venge P, Ahlstedt S, Simony-Lafontaine J, Godard P, Michel F-B. Eosinophilic inflammation in asthma. N Engl J Med 1990; 323:1033–1039.

14. Corrigan CJ, Kay AB. T cells and eosinophils in the pathogenesis of asthma. Immunol Today 1992; 13:501–507.

15. Azzawi M, Johnston PW, Majumbar S, Kay AB, Jeffery PK. T lymphocytes and activated eosinophils in airway mucosa in fatal asthma and cystic fibrosis. Am Rev Respir Dis 1992; 145:1477–1482.

16. Wardlaw AJ, Dunnette S, Gleich GJ, Collins JV, Kay AB. Eosinophils and mast cells in bronchoalveolar lavage in mild asthma: relationship to bronchial hyperreactivity. Am Rev Respir Dis 1988; 137:62–69.

17. Till S, Durham SR, Rajakulasingam K, Humbert M, Huston D, Dickason R, Kay AB, Corrigan CJ. Allegen-induced proliferation and interleukin-5 production by bronchoalveolar lavage and blood T cells after segmental allergen challenge. Am J Respir Crit Care Med 1998; 158:404–411.

18. Robinson D, Hamid Q, Ying S, Bentley A, Assoufi B, Durham S, Kay AB. Prednisolone treatment in asthma is associated with modulation of bronchoalveolar lavage cell interleukin-4, interleukin-5, and interferon-cytokine gene expression. Am Rev Respir Dis 1993; 148:401–406.

19. Germain RN. Antigen processing and presentation. In: Paul WE, ed. Fundamental Immunology, 3rd ed. New York: Raven Press, 1993:629–676.

20. Mossmann TR, Coffman RL. Two types of mouse helper T cell clone: implication for immune regulation. Immunol Today 1987; 8:223–227.

21. Mossmann TR, Sad S. The expanding universe of T-cell subjects: Th1, Th2 and more. Immunol Today 1996; 17:138–146.

22. Corrigan CJ, Kay AB. CD4 T-lymphocyte activation in acute severe asthma: relationship to disease activity and atopic status. Am Rev Respir Dis 1990; 141:970–977.

23. Romagnani S. Lymphokine production by human T cells in disease states. Annu Rev Immunol 1994; 12:227–257.

24. Bentley AM, Menz G, Storz C, Robinson DS, Bradley B, Jeffery PK, Durham SR, Kay AB. Identification of T lymphocytes, macrophages, and activated eosinophils in the bronchial mucosa of intrinsic asthma: relationship to symptoms and bronchial responsiveness. Am Rev Respir Dis 1992; 146:500–506.

25. Humbert M, Durham SR, Ying S, Kimmitt P, Barkans J, Assoufi B, Pfister R, Menz G, Robinson DS, Kay AB, Corrigan CJ. IL-4 and IL-5 mRNA and protein in bronchial biopsies from atopic and non-atopic asthmatics: evidence "intrinsic" asthma being a distinct immunopathological entity. Am J Respir Crit Care Med 1996; 154:1497–1504.

26. Ying S, Humbert M, Barkans J, Corrigan CJ, Pfister R, Menz G, Larche M, Robinson DS, Durham SR, Kay AB. Expression of IL-4 and IL-5 mRNA and protein product by CD4$^+$ and CD8$^+$ T cells, eosinophils, and mast cells in bronchial biopsies obtained from atopic and nonatopic (intrinsic) asthmatics. J Immunol 1997; 158:3539–3544.

27. Ying S, Durham SR, Corrigan C, Hamid Q, Kay AB. Phenotype of cells expressing mRNA for TH2 type (IL-4 and IL-5) and TH1 type (IL-2 and IFN-gamma) cytokines in bronchoalveolar lavage and bronchial biopsies from atopic asthmatics. Am J Respir Cell Mol Biol 1944.

28. Till S, Li B, Durham S, Humbert M, Assoufi B, Huston D, Dickason R, Jeannin P, Kay AB, Corrigan C. Secretion of the eosinophil-active cytokines (IL-5, GM-CSF and IL-3) by bronchoalveolar lavage CD4$^+$ and CD8$^+$ T cell lines in atopic asthmatics and atopic and non-atopic controls. Eur J Immunol 1995; 25:2727–2231.

29. Del Prete G, Maggi E, Parronchi P, Chretien I, Tiri A, Macchia D, Ricci M, Banchereau J, De Vries J, Romagnani S. IL-4 is an essential co-factor for the IgE synthesis induced in vitro by human T cell clones and their supernatants. J Immunol 1988; 140:4193–4198.

30. Minty A, Chalon P, Derocq JM, Dumont X, Guillemot JC, Kaghad M, Labit C, Leplatois P, Liauzun P, Miloux B. Interleukin-13 is a new human lymphokine regulating inflammatory and immune responses. Nature 1993; 362:248–250.

31. Durham SR, Gould HJ, Thienes CP, Jacobson MR, Masuyama K, Rak S, Lowhagen O, Schotman E, Cameron L, Hamid QA. Expression of epsilon germ-line gene transcripts and mRNA for the epsilon heavy chain of IgE in nasal B cells and the effects of topical corticosteriod. Eur J Immunol 1997; 27:2899–2906.

32. Ying S, Humbert M, Meng Q, Pfister R, Menz G, Gould HJ, Kay AB, Durham SR. Local expression of epsilon germline gene transcripts and RNA for the epsilon heavy chain of IgE in the bronchial mucosa in atopic and nonatopic asthma. J Allergy Clin Immunol 2001; 107:686–692.

33. Humbert M, Grant JA, Taborda-Barata L, Durham SR, Pfister R, Menz G, Barkans J, Ying S, Kay AB. High affinity IgE receptor (FcεRI)-bearing cells in bronchial biopsies from atopic and non-atopic asthma. Am J Respir Crit Care Med 1996; 153:1931–1937.

34. Welliver RC, Wong DT, Sun M, Middleton Jr E, Vaughan RS, Ogra PL. The development of respiratory syncytial virus–specific IgE and the release of histamine in nasopharyngeal secretions after infection. N Engl J Med 1981; 305:841–846.

35. Hide M, Francis DM, Grattan CEH, Hakimi J, Kochan JP, Greaves MW. Autoantibodies against the high-affinity IgE receptor as a cause of histamine release in chronic urticaria. N Engl J Med 1993; 328:1599–1604.

36. Lassalle P, Delneste Y, Gosset P, Gras-Masse H, Wallaert B, Tonnel A-B. T and B cell immune response to a 55-kDa endothelial cell-derived antigen in severe asthma. Eur J Immunol 1993; 23:796–803.

37. Bradding P, Roberts JA, Britten KM, Montefort S, Djukanovic R, Mueller R, Heusser CH, Howarth PH, Holgate ST. Interleukin-4, -5, and -6 and tumor necrosis factor-α in normal and asthmatic airways: evidence for the human mast cell as a source of these cytokines. Am J Respir Cell Mol Biol 1995; 10:471–480.

38. Djukanovic R, Wilson JW, Britten KM. Mucosal inflammation in asthma. Am Rev Respir Dis 1990; 142:434–457.

39. Macfarlane AJ, Kon OM, Smith SJ, Zeibecoglou K, Khan LN, Barata LT, McEuen AR, Buckley MG, Walls AF, Meng Q, Humbert M, Barnes NC, Robinson DS, Ying S, Kay AB. Basophils in atopic and non-atopic asthma and late allergic reactions. J Allergy Clin Immunol 2000; 105:99–107.

40. Ying S, Meng Q, Zeibecoglou K, Robinson DS, Macfarlane A, Humbert M, Kay AB. Eosinophil chemotactic chemokines (eotaxin, eotaxin-2, RANTES, monocyte chemotactic protein-3 (MCP-3), and MCP-4), and C-C chemokine receptor 3 expression in bronchial biopsies from atopic and nonatopic (intrinsic) asthmatics. J Immunol 1999; 163:6321–6329.

41. Gosset P, Tsicopoulos A, Wallaert B, Vannimenus C, Joseph M, Tonnel AB, Capron A. Increased secretion of tumor necrosis factor-alpha and interleukin-6 by alveolar macrophages consecutive to the development of the late asthmatic reaction. J Allergy Clin Immunol 1991; 88:561–571.

42. Kotsimbos TC, Ghaffar O, Minshall EM, Humbert M, Durham SR, Pfister R, Menz G, Kay AB, Hamid QA. Upregulation of αGM-CSF-receptor in non-atopic but not in atopic asthma. J Allergy Clin Immunol 1997; 99:666–672.

43. Poulter LW, Janossy G, Power C, Sreenan S, Burke C. Immunological/Physio-Physiological relationships in asthma: potential regulation by lung macrophages. Immunol Today 1994; 15:258–261.

44. Springer TA. Traffic signals for lymphocyte recirculation and leukocyte emigration: the multistep paradigm. Cell 1994; 76:301–314.

45. Baggiolini M, Dahinden CA. CC chemokines in allergic inflammation. Immunol Today 1994; 15:127–133.

46. Walsh GM, Hartnell A, Wardlaw AJ, Kurihara K, Sanderson CJ, Kay AB. IL-5 enhances the in vitro adhesion of human eosinophils, but not neutrophils, in a leucocyte integrin (CD11/18)-dependent manner. Immunology 1990; 71:258–265.

47. Warringa RAJ, Koenderman L, Kok PTM, Krehnict J, Bruijneel PLB. Modulation and induction of eosinophil chemotaxis by granulocyte-monocyte colony stimulating factor and interleukin 3. Blood 1991; 77:2694–2700.

48. Rothenberg ME, Owen Jr WF, Silberstein DS, Woods J, Soberman RJ, Austen KF, Stevens RL. Human eosinophils have prolonged survival, enhanced functional properties and become hypodense when exposed to human interleukin 3. J Clin Invest 1988; 81:1986–1692.

49. Yasruel Z, Humbert M, Kotsimbos TC, Ploysongsang Y, Minshall E, Durham SR, Pfister R, Menz G, Tavernier J, Kay AB, Hamid Q. Expression of membrane-bound and soluble interleukin-5 alpha receptor mRNA in the bronchial mucosa of atopic and non-atopic asthmatics. Am J Respir Crit Care Med 1997; 155:1413–1418.

50. Humbert M, Corrigan CJ, Durham SR, Kimmitt P, Till SJ, Kay AB. Relationship between bronchial mucosal interleukin-4 and interleukin-5 mRNA expression and disease severity in atopic asthma. Am J Respir Crit Care Med 1997; 156:704–708.

51. Humbert M, Ying S, Corrigan C, Menz G, Barkans J, Pfister R, Meng Q, Van Damme J, Opdenakker G, Durham SR, Kay AB. Bronchial mucosal gene expression of the CC chemokines RANTES and MCP-3 in symptomatic atopic and non-atopic asthmatics: relationship to the eosinophil-active cytokines IL-5, GM-CSF and IL-3. Am J Respir Cell Mol Biol 1997; 16:1–8.
52. Hoshi H, Ohno I, Honma M, Tanno Y, Yamauchi K, Tamura G, Shirato K. IL-5, IL-8 and GM-CSF immunostaining of sputum cells in bronchial asthma and chronic bronchitis. Clin Exp Allergy 1995; 25:720–728.
53. Sousa AR, Poston RN, Lane SJ, Nakhosteen JA, Lee TH. Detection of GM-CSF in asthmatic bronchial epithelium and decrease by inhaled corticosteroids. Am Rev Respir Dis 1993; 147:1557–1561.
54. Davies RJ, Wang JH, Trigg CJ, Devalia JL. Expression of granulocyte/macrophage-colony-stimulating factor, interleukin-8 and RANTES in the bronchial epithelium of mild asthmatics is down-regulated by inhaled beclomethasone dipropionate. Int Arch Allergy Immunol 1995; 107:428–429.
55. Schall TJ, Bacon KB. Chemokines, leukocyte trafficking, and inflammation. Curr Opin Immunol 1994; 6:865–873.
56. Menzies-Gow A, Robinson DS. Eosinophil chemokines and their receptors: an attractive target in asthma. Lancet 2000; 355:1741–1743.
57. Ying S, Robinson DS, Meng Q, Rottman J, Kennedy R, Ringler DJ, Mackay CR, Daugherty BL, Springer MS, Durham SR, Williams TJ, Kay AB. Enhanced expression of eotaxin and CCR3 mRNA and protein in atopic asthma. Association with airway hyperresponsiveness and predominant co-localization of eotaxin mRNA to bronchial epithelial and endothelial cells. Eur J Immunol 1997; 27:3507–3516.
58. Collins PD, Marleau S, Griffiths-Johnson DA, Jose PJ, Williams TJ. cooperation between interleukin-5 and the chemokine eotaxin to induce eosinophil accumulation in vivo. J Exp Med 1995; 182:1169–1174.
59. Chomarat P, Banchereau J. Interleukin-4 and interleukin-13: their similarities and discrepancies. Int Rev Immunol 1998; 17:1–52.
60. Schleimer RP, Sterbinsky SA, Kaiser J, Bickel CA, Klunk DA, Tomioka K, Newman W, Luscinskas FW, Gimbrone MA Jr, McIntyre BW. IL-4 induces adherence of human eosinophils and basophils but not neutrophils to endothelium: association with expression of VCAM-1. J Immunol 1992; 148:1086–1092.
61. Bochner BS, Klunk DA, Sterbinsky SA, Coffman RL, Schleimer RP. IL-13 selectively induces vascular cell adhesion molecule-1 expression in human endothelial cells. J Immunol 1995; 154:799–803.
62. Walker C, Bode E, Boer L, Hansel TT, Blaser K, Virchow Jr J-C. Allergic and non-allergic asthmatics have distinct patterns of T-cell activation and cytokine production in peripheral blood and bronchoalveolar lavage. Am Rev Respir Dis 1992; 146:109–115.
63. Humbert M, Durham SR, Kimmitt P, Powell N, Assoufi B, Pfister R, Menz G, Kay AB, Corrigan CJ. Elevated expression of mRNA encoding interleukin-13 in the bronchial mucosa of atopic and non-atopic asthmatics. J Allergy Clin Immunol 1997; 99:657–665.
64. Kotsimbos TC, Ghaffar O, Minshall EM, Humbert M, Durham SR, Pfister R, Menz G, Kay AB, Hamid Q. Expression of interleukin-4 receptor-subunit is

increased in bronchial biopsies from atopic and non-atopic asthmatics. J Allergy Clin Immunol 1998; 102:859–866.

65. Christodoupoulos P, Cameron L, Nakamura Y, Lemière C, Muro S, Dugas M, Boulet L-P, Laviolette M, Olivenstein R, Hamid Q. Th2 cytokine-associated transcription factors in atopica and nonatopic asthma: evidence for differential signal transducer and activator of transcription 6 expression. J Allergy Clin Immunol 2001; 107:586–591.

15

Immunology of Eosinophilic Airway Inflammation
What the Animal Models Teach Us

BART N. LAMBRECHT, LEONIE S. VAN RIJT,
and HARMJAN KUIPERS

Erasmus University Medical Centre
Rotterdam, The Netherlands

I. Human Asthma as a Th2-Driven Disorder?

Asthma is a chronic disorder of the airways in which symptoms such as short-ness of breath, cough, and dyspnea are primarily related to airway obstruction. Increased airway responsiveness to provocative stimuli, termed airway hyper-responsiveness (AHR), and mucus hypersecretion by goblet cells are two of the principal causes of airway obstruction observed in asthma patients. Although asthma is a very complex disorder, our understanding of the pathogenesis of this disease has evolved substantially over the past decade. Following bronchial allergen exposure in atopic individuals, cross-linking of IgE on mast cells leads to immediate degranulation of mast cells and to synthesis of prostaglandins, leukotrienes, and cytokines (Fig. 1). Mast cells release a variety of preformed mediators known to directly constrict bronchial smooth muscle, irritate local nerve endings, dilate blood vessels, and increase leakage of plasma into the air-ways, leading to the occurrence of airway narrowing within 15 min after chal-lenge. This form of IgE-mediated allergy is classically called type I immediate hypersensitivity according to the classification of Gell and Coombs. In about 50% of challenged individuals, this early response is followed by a second, late bronchoconstrictive response that occurs 4–8 h after challenge and is char-acterized by tissue infiltration with mononuclear cells, T cells, and eosinophils (Fig. 2). It is now believed that this late-phase response (LPR) of cellular inflammation is mediated by T lymphocytes. Cytokines produced by T-helper (Th) cells promote the activation of inflammatory cells and their recruitment to

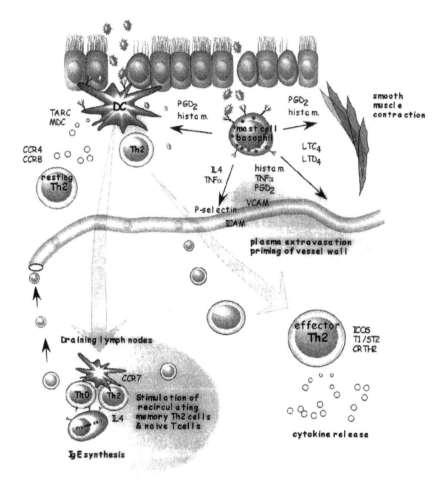

Figure 1 Events during the early-phase response to allergen. Allergens cross-link IgE receptors on mast cells, leading to degranulation of these cells and release of preformed mediators, and synthesis of new mediators and cytokines. The result is bronchial smooth muscle contraction, plasma extravasation, and mucosal edema. Some mast cell mediators also up-regulate the expression of cell adhesion molecules on the vessel wall so that it becomes primed to allow leukocyte rolling and extravasation. During this early-phase response, allergen is also recognized by IgE on airway DCs. These cells can attract tissue dwelling Th2 cells by expression of MDC and TARC, and can locally activate these cells to become full effector cells regulating airway eosinophilia. As this process involves the novel synthesis of cytokines, it occurs later in time and is therefore called the late-phase response. At the same time, DCs also carry the allergen to the draining lymph nodes where they present it to recirculating nonpolarized central memory T cells as well as to naive T cells that can then proliferate and differentiate into Th2 effector cells. These effector cells are now fully armed to extravasate at the primed vessel wall and can contribute to the late-phase response.

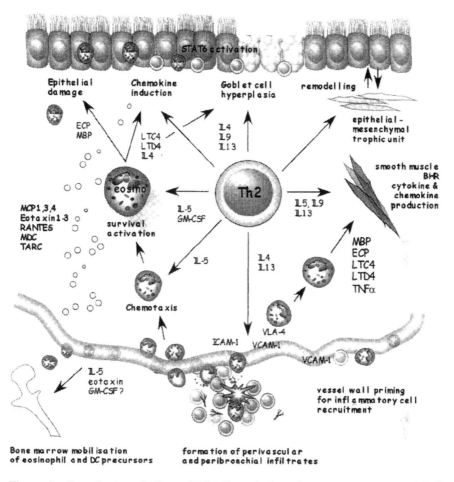

Figure 2 Contribution of effector Th2 cells to the late-phase response, as a model of chronic asthma. See text for explanation.

late-phase reaction inflammatory sites. In contrast to delayed-type hypersensitivity (DTH, type IV hypersensitivity), in which Th1 cytokines are clearly involved, the LPR is controlled by Th2 cells. The Th lymphocyte responses can indeed be operationally divided on the basis of the cytokines produced after encounter of antigen-specific T cells with antigen. Th1 lymphocytes predominantly secrete interleukin-2 (IL-2), interferon-γ (IFN-γ), and tumor necrosis factor-β (TNF-β) to activate macrophages and to induce a strong cellular immune response typical of the DTH reaction. Conversely, Th2 lymphocytes secrete IL-4, IL-5, IL-6, IL-9, IL-10, and granulocyte-macrophage colony-stimulating factor (GM-CSF) to induce a humoral immune response and possibly to induce antiparasitic defense mechanisms (1). Th2 cytokines have also been implicated in the pathophysiology of the LPR; IL-4 leads to up-regulation of cell adhesion molecules on inflammatory endothelium, leading to the recruitment of inflammatory cells, and stimulates the production of IgE by B cells (2); IL-5 is important for the growth, differentiation, and activation of tissue eosinophils and can directly activate airway smooth muscle (3,4); IL-9 is important for mast cell growth and activation, bronchial hyperreactivity, and goblet cell hyperplasia (5); IL-13 is important for bronchial hyperreactivity, goblet cell hyperplasia, and IgE synthesis (6,7); GM-CSF stimulates the growth and survival of eosinophils and the activation of antigen-presenting cells (APCs). Moreover, cytokines produced by Th2 cells and inflammatory cells can affect the (myo)fibroblast, epithelia, and smooth muscle cells in the lungs directly or indirectly stimulating other inflammatory cells to secrete mediators and chemokines.

It is currently held that the changes observed during the LPR after allergen challenge are closely related to the pathophysiology of chronic asthma. Endobronchial biopsy and bronchoalveolar lavage (BAL) studies in patients with chronic and intermittent asthma have indeed revealed eosinophilic mucosal inflammation and have also identified activated CD4$^+$ Th lymphocytes producing a defined set of Th2 cytokines. As revealed in Chapter 14 biopsy studies have demonstrated that the mRNA and/or the protein for IL-3, IL-4, IL-5, IL-9, IL-11, IL-13, IL-16, and GM-CSF are found in increased amounts in the airways of both atopic and nonatopic asthmatics, the signals colocalizing mainly with T-cell markers and/or mast cells, basophils, and eosinophils (8–11). Moreover, recent studies also found increased presence of Th2-associated T-cell transcription factors c-maf, GATA-3, and STAT6 in patients with both forms of asthma, as well as a reduced level of the Th1-associated transcription factor T-bet in patients with atopic asthma (12,13). However, there has probably been too much emphasis on asthma being an exclusively Th2-driven disorder. Indeed, closer analysis reveals that the prototypical cytokine IFN-γ is also increased in the serum of patients with severe acute asthma attacks and in the BAL fluid and cytoplasm of CD4$^+$ T cells following allergen exposure in stable atopic asthmatics (14,15).

II. Use of Murine Models of Eosinophilic Airway Inflammation

Whereas studies in humans have shown only an association between the asthma phenotype and increased numbers of CD4+ T cells secreting Th2 cytokines, animal models of the disease offer the possibility of showing cause and effect. Experimental models to study the development and function of the immune and inflammatory response have focused mainly on the mouse and have generated a large amount of reagents such as monoclonal antibodies directed against immune cells, cytokines, chemokines, and (anti-)inflammatory mediators.

This, together with the availability of inbred wild-type (WT), mutant, gene knockout ($-/-$), as well as transgenic (Tg) strains in which the expression of these molecules is genetically altered, has made mouse the most widely used animal species to study the pathogenesis of asthma (16). Murine models of allergen-induced pulmonary inflammation share many features with human asthma, including the development of antigen-induced pulmonary eosinophilia, AHR, antigen-specific cellular and antibody response, elaboration of Th2 cytokines (IL-4 and IL-5), and expression of chemokines with activity for eosinophils. Of the various antigens, ovalbumin (OVA) is the most widely used antigen to induce eosinophilic airway inflammation, although some investigators have used the more relevant house dust mite (HDM) or cockroach allergens. The different models reported in the literature vary widely in the strain of mice used, in the method in which sensitization to and challenge with OVA is performed, and, finally, in the time point after exposure when mice are sacrificed for analysis (for review, see Refs. 16–18). However minor at first sight, differences in the genetic strain of mice used, in the route of sensitization and challenge, and in the time point of observation can have a dramatic influence on the outcome of a manipulation (Table 1). This partly explains much of the discrepancy between the results of identical manipulations by different investigators in a seemingly identical mouse model. In its simplest form, OVA is injected intraperitoneally with or without a Th2 skewing adjuvant, such as alum. This period of "sensitization" to inhaled antigen is followed 10–14 days later by a period of OVA "challenge" to the airways, either in the form of single or repeated inhalation of OVA aerosol or intranasal application of soluble OVA (Fig. 3). Before final analysis of airway inflammation by either immunohistology or cellular analysis of BAL fluid, some investigators have been able to demonstrate bronchial hyperreactivity to inhaled or intravenous bronchoconstrictive agents such as metacholine, serotonin, or carbachol, using either invasive or noninvasive (plethysmographic) measurements.

There is ongoing debate as to whether murine models are relevant to the study of mechanisms of human asthma. A major drawback of the murine model is the observation that plasma extravasation and mucosal edema are not a prominent feature of challenged airways, in contrast to human asthma (19). Moreover, murine eosinophils fail to localize in the airway epithelium and do not seem to degranulate upon encounter with allergen, questioning their role in the induction of bronchial hyperreactivity and induction of tissue damage to the airway mucosa (20). Strikingly, mice with genetic disruption of major basic protein (MBP) or eosinophil peroxidase (EPO), the toxic granule proteins of esoinophils, develop AHR and airway inflammation, as do their wild-type littermates (21,22). Moreover, most models use fairly acute exposure to inhaled OVA, leading to a form of acute inflammation that may not be relevant to chronic asthma of which airway remodeling is a prominent feature (23). The measurement of AHR in mice is at best suboptimal and is largely influenced by the genetic strain of mice used (24). Various measurements of respiratory

Table 1

Variable	Most common variations	Remarks
Mouse strain		
	Balb/c	Genetic influence can be marked,
	C57BL/6	especially when related to degree
	A/J	of Th2 cytokine production,
	C3H	cellular inflammation, and AHR.
Sensitization		
Antigen	Ovalbumin	Most naturally occurring allergens
	Sheep red blood cells	have enzymatic activity. OVA and
	Dermatophagoides pteronyssinus	sheep red blood cells are inert.
	Nippostrongyloides	
Route	Intraperitoneal	Depending on the route, different
	Inhalational	APCs present the Ag to naive
	Epicutaneous	T cells. Cytokine milieu differs
	Subcutaneous	depending on route.
Adjuvant	Alum	Adjuvants stimulate the maturation
	Ricin	and migration of DCs. Most
	None	adjuvants used skew the response to Th2.
Schedule	Single injection	Booster usually 1 week after first
	Booster injection	injection.
Challenge		
Exposure	15, 30, 60 min	Models on chronic exposure to
	Single	allergen are lacking.
	Repeated (3–7 days)	
Route	Aerosol	Aerosol particle size can vary.
	Nasal aspiration	Low volumes required.
Endpoint analysis		
Time point	3, 6, 24, 48 h after last exp.	Marked effect on cell recovery by BAL.
Eosinophilia	BAL fluid cell count	DiffQuick stain, May-Grunwald-Giemsa.
	EPO levels BAL	Can be measured by ELISA.
	Flow cytometry	Also allows detection of T, B, DC, macrophages.
	Histology	H&E stain, cyanide-resistant peroxidase, MBP moAb.
AHR	Invasive measurement	R_L or APTI index.
	Body plethysmograph	P_{enh} value or forced oscillation
	In vitro tracheal rings	technique.
Cytokine levels	BAL fluid	Levels in BAL fluid can be low.
	Mediastinal lymph nodes	Three day culture w/o or w OVA.
	Intracellular	Intracellular staining allows single cell analysis.

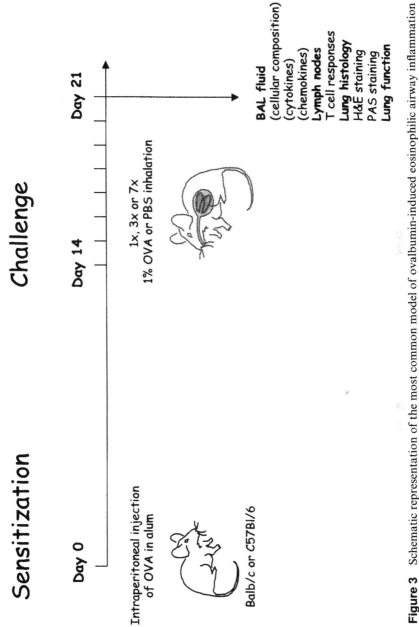

Figure 3 Schematic representation of the most common model of ovalbumin-induced eosinophilic airway inflammation in the mouse. See Table 1 for variations in the various parameters used to induce and measure the airway response.

function, such as lung resistance (R_L), dynamic compliance (C_{dyn}), and enhanced pause (P_{enh}), reflect different aspects of central versus peripheral airway inflammation and are used in various models by various authors to compare identical manipulations, adding a lot of confusion to the field (25,26).

Despite these drawbacks, murine models of eosinophilic airway inflammation have in a reductionist manner elucidated parts of the complex inflammatory processes of asthmatic airways and have provided us with an important tool to help identify the potential contribution of individual inflammatory molecules and cells to specific pathophysiological processes. In the remainder of this chapter, special attention will be given to the interaction between antigen-presenting dendritic cells (DCs) and Th2 cells that ultimately leads to infiltration of the airways with eosinophils.

III. Role of Antigen-Presenting Cells in the Induction of Airway Eosinophilia in the Mouse

A. Antigen Presentation by DCs Is Essential to T-Cell Activation in the Lung

The recognition of allergen by (APCs) is the first step of immune recognition that eventually leads to the formation of Th2 immunity to inhaled allergen and development of asthma (see Chap. 2). A number of professional APCs, such as DCs, B cells, and macrophages, are present in the airways, but it is increasingly clear that the network of DCs is particularly important for inducing sensitization (27). DCs are bone marrow–derived cells that continuously patrol the mucosae, skin, and internal organs of our body in search of foreign antigens. These cells are specialized to induce primary immune responses (28). Studies in rodents have demonstrated that the majority of cells expressing major histocompatibility complex (MHC) class II in the lungs are airway and interstitial DCs that capture inhaled soluble OVA (29). Upon recognition of foreign antigens in the airway mucosa they migrate to the T-cell area of draining lymph nodes and report their antigenic cargo to naive T cells, at the same time providing essential costimulatory molecules (CD80, CD86, intercellular adhesion molecule-1) for inducing the primary immune response (30,31).

Most investigators have used the intraperitoneal route of injection of OVA with alum adjuvant to sensitize mice systemically to OVA, leading to accumulation of OVA antigen in the spleen and mediastinal lymph nodes, draining the peritoneal cavity as well as the lungs (Fig. 3). The rationale for using adjuvant is that it leads to activation and maturation of local DCs and their migration into lymph nodes draining the site of injection (32). Realizing that this may not be the relevant route for naturally occurring sensitization, others have tried to induce sensitization by inhalation of antigen, with variable success (33). Primary aerosolization with the protein antigen OVA is, however, a tolerogenic event that leads to down-regulation of the IgE response and eosinophilic airway inflammation. Although suppressor cells that express the γδ T-cell receptor and/or regulatory Th cells have been implicated in this antigen-specific down-regulation of the immune response, the precise mechanisms are unknown (34,35). One explanation could be that under baseline conditions, airway DCs are in a quiescent state and fail to be properly activated by OVA in the absence of adjuvant, leading to the induction of tolerance to inhaled OVA (36). The group of Jordana et al. have very elegantly shown that adenoviral-mediated expression of the DC maturation cytokine GM-CSF into the airway mucosa increases the numbers and activation status of airway DCs, rendering mice sensitive to primary OVA aerosol and leading to the abolition of inhalational tolerance and to development of Th2-dependent airway eosinophilia (37,38). Similarly, up-regulation of airway DC function was clearly associated with the augmentation of OVA sensitization by influenza A virus infection in adult mice and by exposure to the particulate air pollutant residual oil fly ash in neonatal mice (39–41). Together these findings suggest that local activation of DCs seems to be a requisite for induction of sensitization.

To directly prove that airway DCs can induce sensitization to inhaled antigen, we have injected OVA-pulsed myeloid DCs into the airways of naive animals and have observed the occurrence of a naive immune response in the draining lymph nodes (31,42,43). As soon as 12 h after intratracheal injection, DCs migrated into the draining mediastinal lymph nodes (MLNs) inducing division only in those T cells specific for antigen (Fig. 4). There was no migration beyond this first draining lymph node station, illustrating the compartmentalization of the primary immune response induced by DCs in the lung. It was only between 72 and 92 h after injection that divided Ag-specific effector T cells emigrated from the draining MLN into the bloodstream and the peripheral tissues and spleen (31). When OVA-DC–immunized animals were challenged with an aerosol of OVA 14 days after primary immunization, they developed peribronchial and perivascular infiltrates of eosinophils, T cells, and mono-nuclear cells as well as goblet cell hyperplasia (Fig. 5) (42). Intracellular cytokine staining of individual $CD4^+$ and $CD8^+$ T cells within the BAL fluid compartment revealed that $CD4^+$ cells produced IL-4 and IL-5 but also IFN-γ, whereas $CD8^+$ T cells exclusively produced IFN-γ, reflecting the mixed Th1/Th2 balance also observed in human asthma (Fig. 6). In an identical model, others have since demonstrated that OVA-pulsed DCs also induce bronchial hyperreactivity (44).

B. Cytokines Involved in the Induction of Sensitization by DCs

Interleukin-12

Dendritic cells have been shown to induce both Th1 and Th2 types of responses upon transfer in vivo, depending on a variety of factors, of which the level of IL-12 production seems to be the most important (Fig. 1) (see Chap. 10). IL-12 is essential for stimulating the innate immune system, e.g., natural killer (NK)

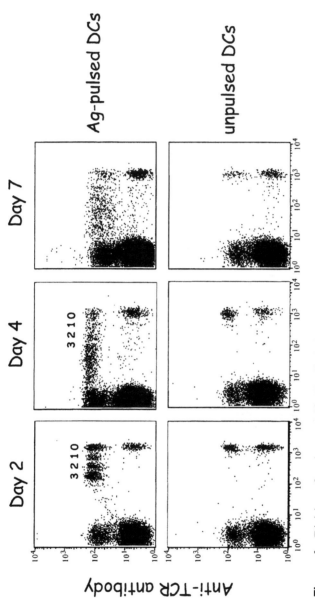

Figure 4 Division of antigen-specific T cells following intratracheal injection of DCs. On day -2, mice received TCR transgenic T cells labeled with the division-sensitive dye CFSE. On day 0 they received either 1×10^6 antigen pulsed DCs (top panels) or 1×10^6 unpulsed DCs (lower panels) via the trachea. On day 2, 4, and 7 draining mediastinal lymph nodes were collected, stained with anti-CD4 and anti-TCR Tg antibody. Division can be seen in Tg^+ T cells as sequential halving of the CFSE signal. In the unpulsed group, there is no T-cell division.

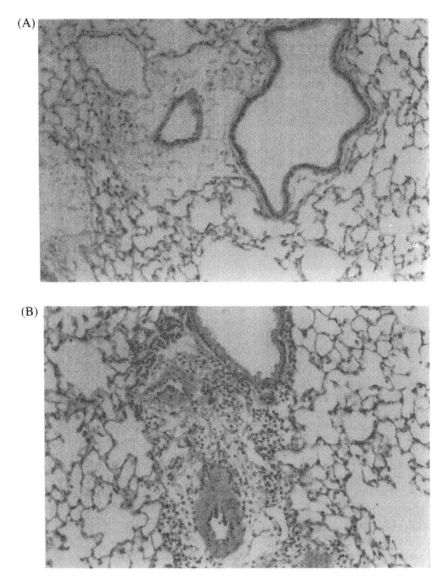

Figure 5 Airway histology of mice immunized with PBS-pulsed DCs (A) or OVA-pulsed DCs (B and C) and subsequently exposed to OVA aerosol. (A) There are no peribronchial or perivascular changes in animals exposed to OVA when animals were immunized with control PBS-DC (400 ×). (B) Actively immunized mice demonstrate peribronchial and perivascular infiltrates that contain mononuclear cells, eosinophils, and T cells. Some inflammatory cells adhere to the vessel wall (400 ×). (C) On higher magnification, there is a marked increase in the number of goblet cells and the height of the airway epithelial cells in actively immunized mice (1000 ×).

(C)

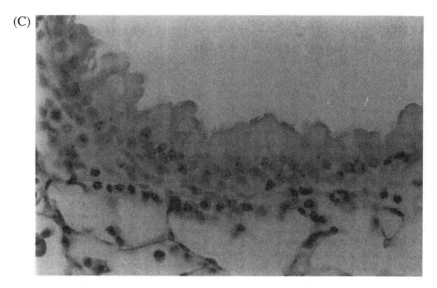

Figure 5 Continued.

cells, for IFN-γ production and for the development of a Th1 response, as evidenced by the lack of DTH responses in IL-12-deficient mice (45). Numerous studies have demonstrated the importance of IL-12 in preventing Th2 immune responses (46). Keane-Myers et al. demonstrated that endogenous blockade of IL-12 in a normally nonresponsive murine strain resulted in development of Th2 immune responses to allergen exposure, accompanied by a shift of Th1 cytokines toward Th2 cytokines (47). Also, IL-12-deficient mice show enhanced Th2 responses to inhaled OVA. Therefore, lack of IL-12 production in airway DCs could be the reason behind the development of default Th2 responses to inhaled antigen. It was shown that resting respiratory tract DCs in rodents produce little if any IL-12 (48). It has been suggested that the level of IL-12 production in DCs could be genetically determined and may vary between atopics and non-atopics (46). One striking observation in murine asthma models was the identification of a gene locus that determines IL-12 production in susceptible and resistant mouse strains, by determining levels of the complement factor C5, a known stimulus for IL-12 production by APCs (49). Another possibility is that the environment of the lung favors the development of Th2 responses by down-regulating the production of IL-12 in DCs (50). Of the possible candidate factors involved in this process, IL-10 and prostaglandin E_2 (PGE_2) are produced by airway epithelial cells and known to down-regulate IL-12 production. In the presence of these factors, DCs induce Th2 responses (51,52). Models of intraperitoneal OVA and airway immunization have also demonstrated that exogenous administration of recombinant IL-12 can markedly suppress Th2 sensitization and subsequent airway eosinophilia in an

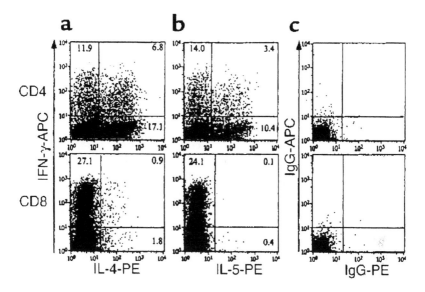

Figure 6 Intracellular staining for Th2 and Th1 cytokines in CD4 and CD8 T cells in the BAL fluid of mice with eosinophilic airway inflammation. Cells were obtained from BAL, stained with anti CD4 and anti CD8 antibodies, followed by fixing and permeabilization to allow staining with IL-4/IFH-γ (left panel), IL-5/IFN-γ (middle), or isotype controls (right panel). Percentages indicate percentage of cells expressing a particular cytokine.

IFN-γ-dependent manner (53,54). Moreover, factors known to increase the levels of IL-12 within APCs, such as unmethylated CpG motifs within bacterial DNA, heat-killed *Listeria monocytogenes* microorganisms, and *Mycobacterium bovis*–bacillus Calmette-Guérin, are capable of inhibiting sensitization to inhaled OVA (55–57). Thus, it seems that the level of IL-12 during the interaction of DCs and naive T cells is critical for determining Th polarization.

Interleukin-4 and Interleukin-13

Despite the fact that absence of IL-12 might predispose to Th2 development, the prototypical Th2 cytokine IL-4 is essential for Th2 development, as evidenced by strongly reduced Th2 responses and airway eosinophilia in anti-IL4 antibody treated mice, IL-4 deficient mice, IL-4 receptor α chain (IL-4Rα) deficient mice or mice deficient in the critical downstream signal transducer and activator of transcription 6 (STAT6) (2,7,58–60). Closer analysis of these various knock-out mouse strains has, however, suggested that there may be IL-4R and STAT6 dependent, but IL-4-independent mechanisms to generate IL-5 producing CD4$^+$ T cells, IL-13 being a likely candidate for Th2 development in the absence of IL-4 (6,7,61–64). One important caveat is the fact that IL-13 receptors have not been directly detected on murine T cells. It is interesting to observe that the importance of IL-13 in inducing Th2 development might be related to the route of immunization and the genetic background of the mouse strain. In this regard, sensitization of C57Bl/6 mice to OVA via the skin, where the network of Langerhans cells is operative, seems to depend exclusively on IL-13, whereas sensitization via the airways or the peritoneum depends on IL-4 (65).

Elegant mouse experiments by DeKruyff's group have used a congenic mouse strain approach to localize the genetic trait responsible for AHR in the Balb/c strain and resistance in the DBA/2 strain. These BALB/c congenic mice contained a part of chromosome 11 from the AHR-resistance DBA/2 mouse strain. The part of chromosome 11 was synthenic to the known human asthma susceptibility locus 5q23-35. By careful genetic analysis, a single locus called *Tapr* (T-cell and airway phenotype regulator) was identified and found to be associated with protection against AHR and associated with low levels of IL-4 production being carried into the Balb/c genome. Subsequently, they identified the *Tim1* and *Tim3* gene (T-cell immunoglobulin and mucin domain) products. Among various mouse strains, significant polymorphisms in the *Tim1* gene, correlate with high levels of IL-4 production by primary-activated T cells, but also with AHR. Therefore, signaling through T-cell-expressed TIM-1 and subsequent IL-4 production is closely linked to development of allergy and AHR (66). The human homologue of TIM-1 is the hepatitis A virus cellular receptor-1, which is located in the asthma susceptibility locus 5q23-35 and demonstrates wide polymorphisms in the general population.

The important role of IL-4 and/or IL-13 in the development of Th2 sensitization immediately raises the question of what cell type initially produces these cytokines. Although DCs do not produce IL-4, some recent reports have demonstrated that human immature DCs can produce IL-13 (67). However our recent studies demonstrated that murine DCs fail to induce Th2-dependent airway eosinophilia when transferred into IL-4 deficient C57Bl/6 mice (42). Alternatively, the source of initial IL-4 production could be found in cells of the innate immune system. A population of NK1.1$^+$ cells (NK cells, or NK T cells), is known to produce large amounts of this cytokine in vivo (68). However, sensitized β_2-microglobulin-deficient or CD1d-deficient mice, which lack functional NK1.1 T cells, have normal Th2-dependent eosinophilic responses to inhaled OVA (68–70). Despite this, depleting NK1.1 antibodies given before sensitization abolish the Th2 response to OVA, suggesting that NK cells may be important (68). It has been shown that DCs can directly interact with NK cells, but the relevance of this interaction for initial IL-4 production and allergic sensitization remains to be determined (71). Alternatively, T cells expressing the $\gamma\delta$ T-cell receptor (TCR) could be an early source of initial IL-4, as mice lacking these cells have deficient Th2 responses to OVA (72,73). Mast cells can also be an early source of IL-4 and/or IL-13, but are rarely detected in mouse T-cell area, the site of initial priming of T cells by DCs. Also, the release of cytokines by these cells is grately facilitated by cross-linking of the FcεRI receptor by IgE bound to antigen. Thus, Th2 sensitization (i.e., IgE production) would already have occured before mast cells can contribute to Th2 polarization.

The most likely source of initial IL-4 is the naive T cell itself. Under conditions where IL-12 production is low, naive T cells polarize toward IL-4 production in the absence of exogenous IL-4 (74,75). Exposure to inhaled allergens occurs at low concentrations, generating a low MHC-peptide density on the DC. A number of experimental systems suggest that low Ag doses and low avidity interactions between T cells and DCs favor the development of a Th2 response (76). Also, chronic exposure to low levels of allergen might lead to low numbers of DCs continuously reaching the draining lymph nodes. Sustained TCR activation at low stimulator DC/responder T cell ratios independently favors the development of a Th2 response (77,78).

C. Costimulatory Molecules Involved in the Induction of Sensitization by DCs

It has been suggested that the particular expression of costimulatory molecules on APCs is critical for Th2 differentiation from naive T cells (79). DCs in the lung express high levels of CD80 and CD86, compared with B cells and macrophages (80). Airway DC-induced Th2 responses in the lung fail to develop in the absence of CD28, the receptor for CD80 and CD86 expressed on T cells (42). Models of intraperitoneal sensitization to OVA have highlighted that administration of CTLA4-Ig or blocking antibodies to either CD80 and/or CD86 can inhibit airway eosinophilia when given during primary immunization (81–83). Although CD86 preferentially stimulates Th2 and CD80 stimulates Th1 formation in some disease models, the situation is far from clear in the murine asthma model, CD80 and CD86 having redundant roles (84,85). Hammad recently proposed that the particular expression of CD80 or CD86 on DCs in response to Der p1 HDM allergen is determined by the atopic state of the donor. DCs from non-atopic donors express predominantly CD80, which leads to Th1 cytokine induction in syngeneic T cells, whereas DCs from HDM-allergic donors express CD86 and induce Th2 responses in syngeneic T cells (86). We have recently found that a ligand for the newly described Th2-associated type I IL-1 receptor family member T1/ST2 is expressed on DCs and critically contributes to Th2 induction in the lung (42,87). It will also be interesting to learn whether the newly described CD28-related molecule *inducible costimulator* (ICOS) ligands B7-related protein B7rp-1 and the Th2-associated TNF receptor family member OX40L have direct effects on Th polarization induced by DCs in the lung (88,89). Interestingly, OX40 and ICOS-deficient mice do not develop OVA-induced airway eosinophilia, goblet cell hyperplasia, and AHR (90).

IV. Role of Antigen-Presenting Cells in the Maintenance of Airway Eosinophilia in Sensitized Animals

A. Role of Antigen-Presenting Cells During the Effector Response to Inhaled Antigen

In addition to their contribution to the primary immune response leading to sensitization, DCs are likely to contribute to the chronic secondary Th2 immune response that occurs in the airways of asthmatics. Bronchial biopsies have revealed increased numbers of CD1a$^+$ MHC class II$^+$ DCs in the epithelium and in the subepithelial lamina propria of nonsmoking atopic asthmatics compared with nonatopic controls (91,92). Similarly, Hammad et al. demonstrated that human PBMCs of HDM-allergic donors that were injected into severe combined immunodeficiency mice (humanized SCID model) developed into DCs after inhalation exposure to allergen and were present within inflammatory airway lesions (93). We observed a 60-fold increase in the number of airway and BAL fluid DCs in OVA-sensitized and -exposed rats with eosinophilic airway inflammation (94). This massive increase is accompanied by an increased output of CD31$^+$ Ly6C$^-$ DCs from the bone marrow, Indeed, allergen challenge in sensitized animals induces an increase in the earliest GM-CSF-responsive precursor for DCs in the bone marrow and an increase in circulating DCs (van Rijt et al., unpublished, and Ref. 94). This increase in DC cell number strongly suggested that DCs are functionally important for generating airway eosinophilia. In support of this, it was recently shown that CD11b$^+$ CD11c$^+$ airway DCs retain antigen for several weeks after exposure and have the potential to present this antigen for several weeks to T-cell lines ex vivo (95). To address the functional contribution of DCs to eosinophilic airway inflammation in sensitized animals in vivo, we have used transgenic mice in which the suicide gene thymidine kinase is preferentially expressed in cells of the DC lineage (96). Using this transgenic strain, treatment with the antiviral drug ganciclovir selectively depleted DCs, but not macrophages, B cells, or T cells, from the airways of OVA-sensitized mice (Fig. 7A and B). In sensitized animals treated with ganciclovir, there was a complete disappearance of eosinophilic airway inflammation and goblet cell hyperplasia induced by OVA (Fig. 7C and D). These findings strongly suggest that memory/effector CD4$^+$ Th2 cells were not properly activated in the absence of DCs. Indeed, the levels of the Th2 cytokines IL-4 and IL-5 in the airways were suppressed in animals lacking DCs. Moreover, there was no allergen-induced boosting of OVA-specific IgE levels in the absence of DCs. These findings suggest that DCs are essential not only for generating Th2 cells during the primary sensitization phase but also for the generation of effector function during the secondary challenge phase.

The reasons behind this could be that memory T cells in vivo need much more costimulation than has been appreciated from in vitro data and therefore rely on professional APCs that can provide these stimuli. Indeed, allergen-induced IL-4 and IL-13 production in bronchial explants and in peripheral

Figure 7 Role of dendritic cells in the effector response to inhaled antigen in sensitized mice. (A) Thymidine kinase transgenic mice given PBS have normal numbers of airway DCs, as revealed by MHC class II staining on tracheal whole mounts. (B) Thymidine kinase transgenic mice treated with ganciclovir for 6 days have a dramatic reduction in airway DCs. (C) Sensitized transgenic mice treated with PBS and subsequently challenged with OVA aerosol develop peribronchial and perivascular eosinophilic inflammation. (D) Sensitized transgenic mice treated with ganciclovir to deplete DCs and subsequently challenged with OVA aerosol have a complete absence of peribronchial and perivascular eosinophilic inflammation. These data imply that DCs are necessary to generate effector cells controlling eosinophilic airway inflammation.

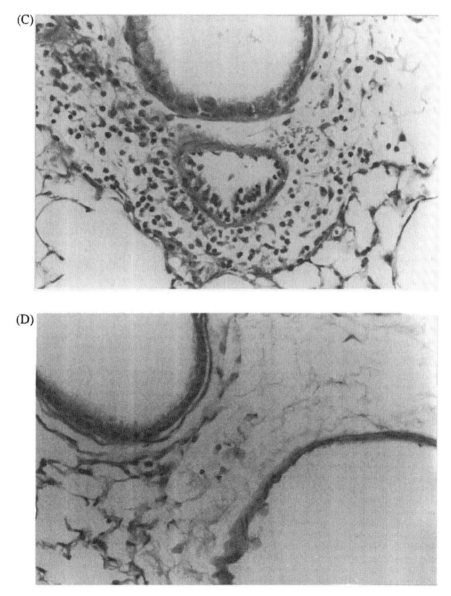

Figure 7 Continued.

blood cells from asthmatics is dependent on delivery of costimulation via the CD80/CD86 pathway (97). Similarly, animal models have shown that eosinophilic airway inflammation in sensitized mice can be suppressed by blocking the CD80/CD86-CD28 pathway during challenge (42,81–83,85). It could be that CD80 and/or CD86 signals are specifically required to induce cytokine production from effector Th2 cells, while homing of Th2 cells in the lung or even proliferation of memory effector Th2 cells is independent of these molecules (42,98,99). By analogy, it was recently shown that the stimulation of ICOS by its ligand B7-rp1 is critical for the generation of effector function in Th2 lymphocytes in several models of airway eosinophilia and AHR (89,100–102). Similarly blocking the Th2-restricted T1/ST2 molecule suppresses Th2 effector function and airway eosinophilia in the lung (42,87). The latter finding is of particular therapeutic interest as it was recently found that increased levels of soluble T1/ST2 are detected during asthma exacerbations, the levels correlating with the severity of the disease (103). Alternatively, migratory DCs might be essential to stimulate recirculating resting memory unpolarized Th cells in the draining lymph nodes to divide and become Th2 effectors (99). These central memory T cells have recently been shown to recirculate exclusively via the lymph nodes, not via peripheral tissues. Therefore, activation of these cells requires a migratory APC such as a DC. In this scenario, during the early-phase response, DCs might recognize allergen and carry it to the draining node to stimulate these resting cells to become memory effector Th2 cells that can subsequently orchestrate the LPR (Fig. 1) (99,104).

B. Other Antigen-Presenting Cell Types Are of Less Importance in the Murine Model

Studies in B-cell-deficient mice have revealed that B cells do not play an important role in the sensitization process to inhaled antigen, nor do they seem to contribute significantly to the secondary immune response and the development of airway eosinophilia, although they might contribute to plasma extravasation during the early-phase response to OVA aerosol and to bronchial hyperreactivity (see below). Similarly, macrophages were unable to induce sensitization to inhaled OVA when adoptively transferred into naive animals (43). Both alveolar and interstitial macrophages actively suppress the activation and proliferation of naive and memory T cells in the lung by their direct inhibitory effects via nitric oxide and transforming growth factor-1 (TGF-β) on T-cell proliferation and DC activation (99,105,106). As a consequence, alveolar macrophage elimination in vivo using clodronate-filled liposomes is associated with an increase in the primary and secondary pulmonary immune response to inhaled antigen in mice, associated with an enhancement of Th2 responses and airway inflammation (107,108). Recently, it was also shown that airway eosinophils express MHC class II and the costimulatory molecules CD80 and CD86, effectively contributing to the stimulation of effector Th2 cells in the lungs and

lymph nodes of sensitized mice (85,109,110). However, sensitized IL-5-defi-
cient and anti-IL-5-treated mice that lack eosinophils in the airways demonstrate normal Th2 responses in the draining lymph nodes (111). Therefore,
eosinophils might have an enhancing role in antigen presentation but do not
seem to be essential for mounting the Th2 effector response.

V. Role of CD4 Cells and Their Cytokine Products in Inducing Eosinophilic Airway Inflammation and Airway Hyperreactivity

A. Role of CD4⁺ Th2 Cells in Mouse Models of Asthma

The essential role of $CD4^+$ Th2 cells in regulating airway eosinophilia is suggested by the finding that eosinophilic airway inflammation and its accompanying bronchial hyperreactivity(BHR) is associated with increased amounts
of CD4 T cells producing IL-4, IL-5, and/or IL-13 being recovered from the
airways of asthmatics and challenged mice (8,42,59,112,113). Recent studies
using antigen-MHC-dimer molecules to detect antigen-specific T cells suggest
that Th2 cells remain present in the BAL fluid compartment for prolonged
periods following antigen challenge in sensitized mice (95). Moreover, administration of OVA-specific $CD4^+$ Th2 cells from OVA TCR Tg mice or from OVA-
sensitized mice to naive mice was able to transfer the development of airway
eosinophilia, BHR, and goblet cell hyperplasia upon exposure to OVA aerosol
(114–117). Finally, and most importantly, elimination of $CD4^+$ T cells by injecting depleting anti-CD4 monoclonal antibodies or absence of $CD4^+$ T cells in
MHC class II $^{-/-}$ mice abolishes eosinophilic airway inflammation, AHR, and
goblet cell hyperplasia induced by OVA aerosol (118–121).

B. Role of Individual Th2 Cytokines

Although it is clear that $CD4^+$ T cells mediate many of the asthmatic features,
the individual roles of Th2 cytokines IL-4, IL-5, IL-6, IL-9, and IL-13 are less
clearly defined and vary depending on the type of experimental protocol, mouse
strain, as well as the parameter (eosinophilia or AHR or goblet cell hyperplasia)
that is being studied (for an overview, see Fig. 2).

Interleukin-4

The prototypical Th2 cytokine IL-4 induces polarization of Th0 cells into Th2
cells, enhances mast cell activation, induces IgE class switching in B cells,
enhances the expression of vascular cell adhesion molecule-1 (VCAM-1) on
endothelial cells and induces expression of the mucin 5AC and eotaxin genes in
epithelial cells. In agreement, all of the typical features of asthma, such as
eosinophilia, AHR, and goblet cell hyperplasia, are absent in IL-4$^{-/-}$,
IL4R$\alpha^{-/-}$, and STAT6$^{-/-}$ mice (see above). It is difficult to study whether the

changed phenotype of these mice is due to defective Th2 development (i.e., with defective IL-5 and IL-13 production) or to direct deficiency of IL-4 as an effector molecule. In most, but not all, animal models of asthma it seems that IL-4 is most important for inducing the Th2 response, having a more redundant function during the challenge period of the airways. Indeed, it was shown that AHR and airway eosinophilia were not abolished when antibodies to IL-4 were given during challenge of the airways (58,59,63,121). The transcription factor GATA-3 is a molecular master switch that determines Th2 polarization and cytokine secretion. Interestingly, mice treated with local intranasal administration of GATA-3 antisense oligonucleotides during challenge to OVA had strongly diminished asthma features, suggesting that IL-4 has effector functions (122). Conversely, overexpression of GATA-3 in CD4 T cells does not enhance airway inflammation (123). One of the major effector functions of IL-4 during allergic inflammation might be enhanced up-regulation of VCAM-1, the counterreceptor on endothelial cells for recruiting *very late antigen-4* (VLA-4)-4–positive eosinophils (124). Alternatively, studies of adoptive transfer of in vitro differentiated IL-4$^{-/-}$ Th2 cells into IFN-γ R$^{-/-}$ mice have shown that the major effector role of IL-4 during the challenge phase of eosinophilia is suppression of IFN-γ, known to down-regulate airway—but not tissue—eosinophilia (125). Transgenic expression of IL-4 in the airways induces some mild degree of peribronchial eosinophilic inflammation, up-regulates expression of the mucin 5AC gene, but does not induce AHR, illustrating that IL-4 is not sufficient to cause all aspects of the asthmatic phenotype (126,127).

Interleukin-13

IL-13 is secreted by T cells, NK cells, mast cells, and eosinophils and has a critical role in IgE responses and Th2 development and function in mice, by signaling through the IL4Rα and STAT6, a mechanism shared with IL-4 (64,128). Indeed, studies using the antagonist sIL-13Rα2-IgFc have shown that IL-13 is a major cytokine regulating AHR and mucus cell hypersecretion, independently of tissue eosinophilia or IL-4 (6,7,46). Transgenic expression and administration of IL-13 in the lung of naive mice leads to tissue infiltration with eosinophils and mononuclear cells, goblet cell hyperplasia, subepithelial fibrosis, and importantly AHR to metacholine (6,129,130). Adoptive transfer experiments have shown that IL-13 could be the factor responsible for mucus hypersecretion, goblet cell hyperplasia, and AHR induced by adoptive transfer of IL-4$^{-/-}$ CD4^{+} T cells and seems to be the most essential Th2-derived cytokine for inducing eotaxin expression in the lung (130–132). Most of the cellular effects of IL-13 are mediated trough the downstream signaling molecule STAT6 in epithelial cells, leading to the secretion of chemokines, attraction of inflammatory cell types, and, finally, to development of AHR. However, adoptive transfer of IL-13-producing Th cells into IL-4R$\alpha^{-/-}$ mice still induces eosinophilia and AHR, suggesting that phosphorylation of STAT6 occurs independently of the

IL-4Rα chain, and identifying a new signaling pathway by which IL-13 exerts its effects in the lung (130).

Interleukin-5

The importance of IL-5 in regulating lung eosinophilia is underscored in IL-5$^{-/-}$ and in mice treated with blocking anti-IL-5 antibodies that show strongly reduced blood and tissue eosinophilia (3,133). When IL-5$^{-/-}$ CD4$^+$ Th2 cells were transferred into naive mice, they failed to induce airway eosinophilia yet induced normal mucus hypersecretion (131). Studies in IL-5$^{-/-}$ mice have shown that IL-5 is required for growth and differentiation of eosinophils in the bone marrow and that it cooperates with eotaxin to generate a chemotactic signal that attracts eosinophils into the lung (133–135). Consistent with this, administration of IL-5 to the lung and transgenic expression of IL-5 in the lung leads to profound airway eosinophilia (136–138). Despite the fact that IL-5 is critical for eosinophilia, it has been a very complex issue to study whether IL-5 and its ensuing eosinophilic response is critical for the establishment of AHR in mice. Models of administration or transgenic expression of IL-5 to the lung have shown either no effect or an increase in AHR (136–138). Depending on the mouse strain, antigen, and protocol used to study the involvement of IL-5, AHR has been shown to be dependent or independent of IL-5 and eosinophils. Studies in the OVA model in C57BL/6 mice have highlighted that IL-5$^{-/-}$ mice and mice treated with anti-IL-5 moAbs have reduced eosinophilia and abolished AHR, whereas those using certain parasite antigens or HDMs have shown an independence (3,61,117,139,140). Studies in the OVA model using Balb/c mice have suggested two pathways to generate AHR. One is dependent on IL-5 and eosinophils (111,141,142); the other is independent of IL-4, IL-5, and eosinophils, but clearly dependent on CD4$^+$ T cells and IL-13 (59,63,121,130,143). Treatment of IL-4$^{-/-}$ mice with blocking anti-IL-5 completely reduced airway eosinophilia but did not abolish AHR (121). In contrast, treatment of IL-13$^{-/-}$ mice with blocking anti-IL-5 abolished eosinophilia and AHR, suggesting that airway eosinophilia is linked to the mechanism underlying AHR only in the absence of IL-13 (63). The fact that eosinophils seem to be of minor importance for AHR could be related to the fact that in some mouse models eosinophils do not degranulate upon recognition of allergen (20–22). In this scenario, the airways and smooth muscle are not exposed to MBP and eosinophil peroxidase. However, eosinophils are an important source of cysteinyl leukotrienes, known to contribute to AHR, airway leakiness, and mucus cell hyperplasia (144).

Interleukin-6

The Th2 cytokine IL-6 has effects on B-cell IgE production and enhances Th2 formation in the presence of IL-4, but also has some anti-inflammatory actions (145). This cytokine is increased in the draining lymph nodes and BAL fluid of

OVA-exposed mice and transgenic overexpression in the lung leads to impressive subepithelial fibrosis and lymphocytic infiltration, without inducing tissue eosinophilia. When these mice were challenged to OVA aerosol, the eosinophilic response and AHR were diminished. Moreover, sensitized IL-$6^{-/-}$ have increased eosinophilic responses, increased chemokine production, and enhanced AHR in response to OVA compared with their WT littermates (146). Therefore, the role of IL-6 in the murine asthma model is mainly anti-inflammatory.

Interleukin-9

Interleukin-9 is another Th2-associated cytokine that stimulates mast cell growth and differentiation, eosinophil survival and differentiation, goblet cell hyperplasia, and IgE production by B cells (5,147). IL-9 induces the expression of eosinophil-selective chemokines and directly stimulates MUC5AC gene expression leading to mucus hypersecretion, probably due to induction of IL-13 production (148–151). A genetic trait that determines baseline AHR in mice maps to the IL-9 locus on chromosome 13, suggesting that IL-9 might affect bronchial smooth muscle directly. Atopic asthmatics and nasal polyposis patients with BHR, but not those without BHR, have greatly increased expression IL-9 within airway T cells and eosinophils, and the degree of expression correlates well with the degree of BHR (5). This has led to the proposition that IL-9 might be an asthma susceptibility gene. In support of this, transgenic mice systemically overexpressing IL-9 had exaggerated tissue eosinophilia, IgE responses, and AHR in response to *Aspergillus fumigatus* challenge (152). Selective and doxycycline regulated overexpression of the IL-9 gene within the lungs of transgenic mice resulted in massive eosinophilic airway inflammation, mast cell hyperplasia, mucus cell hypersecretion, and marked AHR in response to metacholine (151,153). Airway eosinophilia, goblet cell hyperplasia, AHR, and IgE levels were suppressed by daily injections of antimurine IL-9 during the challenge phase with OVA in OVA-sensitized mice (154). Recently, however, it was shown that OVA-sensitized IL-$9^{-/-}$ develop a robust Th2 response to inhaled OVA and display similar airway eosinophilia, goblet cell hyperplasia, AHR, and IgE synthesis, compared with their WT littermates (155). Conversely, IL-$9^{-/-}$ mice have reduced mastocytosis and goblet cell hyperplasia in a Th2 pulmonary granuloma model (149). This again illustrates that the type of antigen and the use of blocking antibodies versus knockout mice is important in determining the role of a particular cytokine in a particular mouse model.

Interleukin-11

IL-11 is closely related to IL-6 and its expression is increased in the airways of asthmatics, correlating with asthma severity (10,156). Transgenic overexpression of IL-11 induced subepithelial fibrosis, lymphocytic infiltration, and AHR in the absence of airways eosinophilia, or goblet cell hyperplasia (157).

However, transgenic overexpression of IL-11 in mice was shown to inhibit OVA-induced tissue eosinophilia, Th2-cytokine expression, and VCAM-1 expression, suggesting that the observed increase in asthmatics may serve to dampen ongoing severe inflammation (158).

C. Is There a Role for Th1 Cytokines in the Effector Response to Inhaled Allergen?

Interferon-γ

Studies in humans have suggested that $CD4^+$ T cells producing IFN-γ are also found in increased amounts in the airways of asthmatics and that increased levels are found during acute asthma attacks (15). Similarly, when studied at the single-cell level using intracellular staining, it is clear from a number of murine asthma models that $CD4^+$ T cells producing either IFN-γ exclusively or in combination with IL-4 and/or IL-5 can be recovered from the BAL fluid and lungs of OVA-challenged mice (42,153). In addition, CD8 cells producing INF-γ exclusively are attracted to the airways of challenged mice. This raises the important question of whether IFN-γ derived from $CD4^+$ and/or $CD8^+$ cells contributes to the asthmatic phenotype. Administration of IFN-γ or Th1 cells during allergen challenge has been shown to reduce airway eosinophilia and AHR by reducing the recruitment of eosinophils, by down-regulating eotaxin, or by direct engagement of the IFN-γ receptor on eosinophils (116,125,159,160). Moreover, IFN-γ receptor–deficient mice have a reduced clearance of airway eosinophilia following discontinuation of OVA challenge (161). However, in some models, IFN-γ does not seem to suppress tissue eosinophilia whereas airway eosinophilia assessed by BAL is markedly suppressed (125). T-Bet, a Th1-specific T-box transcription factor, transactivates the IFN-γ gene in Th1 cells and has the unique capacity to redirect fully polarized Th2 cells into Th1 cells. Mice with a targeted deletion of the T-bet gene and SCID mice receiving $CD4^+$ cells from $T\text{-bet}^{-/-}$ mice spontaneously demonstrated AHR and eosinophilic airway inflammation characteristic of asthma, in the absence of allergen exposure. In this regard it is intriguing that the mouse T-bet gene is located on chromosome 11 in a region that has been linked to AHR in mice and humans. These findings were supported by the finding of reduced expression of T-bet in airway biopsies from asthmatic subjects (13).

Despite this evidence for a protective role of Th1 cytokines in asthma, some investigators have suggested that endogenous IFN-γ is essential for the establishment of AHR following OVA challenge in OVA-sensitized mice, independent of eosinophilia (162). One recent report has shown that IFN-γ synergizes with IL-13 to induce AHR and goblet cell hyperplasia when administered together by increasing the numbers of NK cells and DCs in the airways (163). Moreover, adoptive transfer of OVA-specific Th1 cells together with Th2 cells enhances damage to the airways in some models (114,164,165).

Interleukin-12

Other Th1-promoting cytokines such as IL-12 also influence eosinophilia. When IL-12 was given during challenge of the airways, there was a reduction in IL-4 and IL-5, airway eosinophilia, and AHR that was independent of IFN-γ or IL-10 (53,54,166). By analogy, neutralization of IL-12 during challenge in sensitized mice led to enhanced Th2 cytokine production and AHR, and IL-12 knockout mice had increased airway eosinophilia in one model of asthma (47,167). In the absence of IL-12 and/or IFN-γ, unmethylated CpG oligonucleotides are less effective in down-regulating airway responses to OVA (168). However, studies in IL-12 knockout mice suggest that under certain circumstances endogenous IL-12 might also have some proinflammatory effects by increasing the expression of VCAM-1 on airway vascular endothelium (169).

Interleukin-18

The precise contribution of the Th1-enhancing cytokine IL-18 remains elusive. It was shown that exogenous IL-18 cooperates with IL-12 to reduce tissue eosinophilia, IgE, and AHR in one model of asthma, whereas IL-18 enhanced these parameters in other models (170–172). It was shown that IL-18$^{-/-}$ mice had enhanced airway responses to OVA (173). The most likely explanation for these discrepancies is that IL-18 is less of a Th1-skewing factor than initially thought and that effects of this cytokine might depend on the timing of administration (174). In this regard it was interesting to note that IL-18 administration to the lung led to primary sensitization to OVA via the airways (172). Also, IL-18 directly stimulates IgE synthesis by B cells (175). Although unproven, one likely explanation could be that locally administered IL-18 enhances the function of airway DCs.

From these data it appears that CD4^{+} Th1 cells might contribute to asthma depending on the model studied, and one should be very cautious on the use of a Th1-inducing vaccine to treat patients with asthma.

D. Is There a Role for CD4^{+} Regulatory Th3 Cells in Asthma?

Inhalational Tolerance

One explanation that has been put forward to explain the pathophysiology of asthma is that the aberrant Th2 immune response to inhaled allergen is a failure of the normal tolerance mechanism to inhaled antigen (176). Inhalational tolerance has been extensively studied in the mouse and is transferable by T lymphocytes derived from the spleen or draining lymph nodes into naive animals. Th3 cells are regulatory cells producing high amounts of IL-10 and/or TGF-β and have been implicated in regulation of both oral and inhalational tolerance. Regulatory T cells are induced by immature DCs and modulate both Th1 and Th2 effector responses (177). It was recently shown that IL-10-producing airway DCs induce inhalation tolerance to OVA (36).

Interleukin-10

Although IL-10 is a prototypical Th2 cytokine in the mouse and enhances the formation of Th2 cells by down-regulating IL-12 in DCs and other APCs, its effects during challenge of the airways are mainly anti-inflammatory. Consistent with this, administration of IL-10 during challenge was shown to reduce airway eosinophilia, infiltration with DCs, and Th1 and Th2 cytokine production (178–180). However, studies using IL-10$^{-/-}$ mice are somewhat inconsistent, reflecting the dual role of IL-10 in allergy, enhancing Th2 responses when given during priming while suppressing them when given during challenge. Indeed, it was shown that allergen challenge of IL-10$^{-/-}$ mice results in either enhanced, unaffected, or decreased airway eosinophilia compared with IL-10$^{+/+}$ controls, with varying effects on AHR (181–183).

Transforming Growth Factor-β

TGF-β is also produced by Th3 cells and could be very important in down-regulating mucosal immune responses. It was shown that adoptive transfer of OVA-specific T cells producing TGF-β could diminish eosinophilic airway inflammation and AHR (184). By analogy, overexpression in T cells of the transcription factor Smad7, an intracellular antagonist of TGF-β signaling, enhanced eosinophilic airway inflammation and AHR (185). Others have shown that oral tolerance to OVA could suppress airway eosinophilia in a TGF-β-independent fashion (186).

VI. Role of CD8 Cells and Their Cytokine Products in Regulating Eosinophilic Airway Inflammation and Airway Hyperreactivity

The discussion so far has mainly focused on CD4$^+$ Th cells. Increased amounts of CD8$^+$ lymphocytes producing IFN-γ are recovered from the airways of challenged mice in the OVA model (42,113). Although it was shown that (virus-specific) CD8$^+$ cells can be induced to produce IL-4 and IL-5 within an IL-4-rich environment (therefore called Tc2 cells), the production of these cytokines in the OVA model is absent (Fig. 6) (187,188). It was shown that CD8-deficient and β$_2$-microglobulin-deficient mice that lack CD8$^+$ T cells and NK1.1 T cells develop normal eosinophilic responses to inhaled OVA in some models, whereas others have shown that depletion of CD8$^+$ cells using moAbs led to the disappearance of IL-5 production, eosinophilia, and AHR (69,189–191). Part of the explanation might be that CD8 depletion also depletes other CD8$^+$ cells such as γδ T cells or CD8$^+$ DCs.

The role of CD8$^+$ αβ TCR T cells in the regulation of IgE responses in the mouse and rat is fairly established (see Chap. 4).

VII. Do Mast Cells and IgE Have an Extended Role Beyond the Early Asthmatic Response by Orchestrating Airway Eosinophilia?

A. Mast Cells

Mast cells participate in the initial early phase response after exposure to allergen (see Fig. 1), but their importance in orchestrating eosinophilia during the LPR is uncertain. After IgE-triggered activation, mast cells may promote the LPR and inflammation of the airways with eosinophils by producing inflammatory mediators (e.g., IL-1, IFN-α, and leukotrienes) and eosinophil-directed cytokines (IL-4, IL-5, and IL-13) (144). Mast cell mediators, in turn, induce chemokines that attract eosinophils. One very important mediator of mast cells is the major cyclooxygenase metabolite of arachidonic acid prostaglandin D2 (PGD_2), which signals through the prostaglandin D and the Th2-selective CRTH2 receptors. PGD_2 is a bronchoconstrictor and vasodilator that serves as a marker for mast cell degranulation in the acute-phase response. The CRTH2 receptor is expressed on murine and human Th2 cells and eosinophils (192). The expression of prostaglandin D, but not CRTH2, is increased in the airways of mice with OVA-induced airway eosinophilia. Mice lacking the prostaglandin D receptor have severely diminished AHR, eosinophilia, and goblet cell hyperplasia, but intact IgE responses (193). Supporting these data, mice overexpressing the human lipocalin-type PGD synthase have increased airway levels of PGD_2, concomitant with increased levels of Th2 cytokines, eotaxin, and airway eosinophils (194). Despite these findings that PGD_2 is also critical for the LPR to allergen, studies in mast cell–deficient W/W^v mice suggested that mast cells do not appear to be required for eosinophilia and/or AHR in some animal models of allergic disease in which adjuvant is used to prime Th2 responses (120,195,196). In protocols in which weaker Th2 responses are induced by injection of OVA in the absence of adjuvant, mast cells are clearly necessary for chronic eosinophilia and AHR in response to inhaled OVA (197,198).

B. Immunoglobulin E

Although IgE has an established role in mediating mast cell degranulation and the early-phase response after allergen challenge, it is questionable whether IgE is needed to mediate the enhancing effects of mast cells on airway eosinophilia and AHR, and again depends on the model studied. In allergen-sensitized mice with a targeted deletion for the gene for IgE or treated with anti-IgE antibodies, the recruitment of eosinophils into the lungs and AHR was not impaired after allergen challenge (111,199). If IgE has a function in chronic eosinophilic inflammation, it is most likely via formation of IgE immune complexes and its enhancing effects of allergen recognition and presentation by DCs and B cells, either via an FcϵRI or CD23 mechanism (see Chap. 4) (200–202).

VIII. Downstream Events That Contribute to the Asthmatic Phenotype in Mice

In the above paragraphs, we have described the various immune cells and their mediators that are involved in the regulation of airway eosinophilia and AHR. It is increasingly clear that an extremely complex inflammatory cascade is induced by the various actions of DCs, Th2 cells, and mast cells that leads to airway eosinophilia, AHR, and mucus hypersecretion.

A. Extravasation of Leukocytes Is Controlled by Cell Adhesion Molecules

Extravasation of eosinophils into inflammatory sites is a multistep process characterized by initial intravascular rolling and firm adhesion to endothelium, followed by sequential eosinophil diapedesis between endothelial cells and chemotaxis into tissues. Rolling of eosinophils on endothelium is mediated via endothelial-expressed P-selectin and, accordingly, P-selectin deficient mice have reduced numbers of eosinophils in challenged airways (203). Lymphocyte *f*unction *a*ntigen-1 (LFA-1) interacting with endothelial ICAM-1, or, more importantly VLA-4 interacting with VCAM-1 mediates firm adhesion of eosinophils. Accordingly, ICAM-1$^{-/-}$ mice, but not ICAM-2$^{-/-}$ mice, have reduced tissue eosinophilia and AHR upon allergen challenge (203–205). T lymphocytes and IL-4/IL-13 are important for regulating the expression of VCAM-1 on endothelial cells, in conjunction with TNF-α. The expression of VCAM-1 is highly increased on endothelial cells of challenged mice (206). Mice deficient in VCAM-1 or treated with anti-VCAM-1, anti-VLA-4, or anti-α_4 integrin (CD49d) antibodies had strongly reduced tissue eosinophilia and AHR (189,206,207). It appears that VLA-4 and LFA-1 are also highly expressed on a population of CD11c$^+$ putative DCs, explaining part of the effectiveness of these antibodies in inhibiting the response to OVA (207).

B. Extravasation of Leukocytes Is Regulated by Chemokines and Their Receptors

It cannot be overemphasized that the regulated production of chemokines has an important role in this downstream chain of events (see Chap. 16). Although many immune cells produce chemokines that contribute to the asthmatic phenotype, a dominant source of these molecules are the epithelial cells, endothelial cells, and fibroblasts of the lung (132,189). Of the various CC chemokines, eotaxin-1 and -2, *m*onocyte *c*hemotactic *p*roteins (MCPs) 1 and 5, *m*onocyte-*d*erived *c*hemokine (MDC), and *r*egulated upon *a*ctivation *n*ormal *T* cell *e*xpressed and *s*ecreted (RANTES) seem to be most important for regulating tissue eosinophilia and AHR, sometimes in conjunction with IL-5 (Fig. 2) (134,189,208,209). Lloyd et al. have convincingly demonstrated that signaling through CCR3 via eotaxin is important for recruiting Th2 cells and eosinophils early in the response, whereas signaling through CCR4 via the MDC or *thymus activated and regulated chemokine* (TARC) ligand is more important for recruiting Th2 cells and eosinophils during repeated challenge (210). It is also increasingly clear that chemokines are involved not only in regulating the trafficking of inflammatory cells, but also in regulating their development in the bone marrow, and that they regulate such fundamental parameters as Th1/Th2 differentiation. It will be important to study the asthmatic phenotype of the various chemokine (receptor) knockout mice.

IX. Concluding Remarks

Over the years there has been an explosion of research on the use of murine models of eosinophilic airway inflammation to study the role of a particular cell or mediator in the pathogenesis of asthma. When Koch's postulates are applied, a model emerges in which DCs are crucial cells in the induction and maintenance of T-cell reactivity to inhaled allergen (Fig. 5). Effector $CD4^+$ T cells and mast cells elaborate cytokines that induce the Th2 phenotype (IL-4), tissue eosinophilia (IL-5), mucus hypersecretion (IL-4, IL-13, IL-9), and AHR (IL-5 and IL-13). These studies have identified these cells and mediators as crucial targets for the therapy of asthma.

Acknowledgments

This work was supported by grants 3.2.99.37 and 32.00.45 of the Dutch Asthma Foundation.

References

1. Abbas AK, Murphy KM, Sher A. Functional diversity of helper T lymphocytes. Nature 1996; 383:787–793.
2. Brusselle GG, Kips JC, Joos GF, Bluethmann H, Pauwels RA. Allergen-induced airway inflammation and bronchial responsiveness in wild-type and interleukin-4-deficient mice. Am J Respir Cell Mol Biol 1995; 12:254–259.
3. Foster PS, Hogan SP, Ramsay AJ, Matthaei KI, Young KI. Interleukin 5 deficiency abolishes eosinophilia, airways hyperreactivity and lung damage in a mouse asthma model. J Exp Med 1996; 183:195–201.
4. Hakonarson H, Maskeri N, Carter C, Chuang S, Grunstein MM. Autocrine interaction between IL-5 and IL-1beta mediates altered responsiveness of atopic asthmatic sensitized airway smooth muscle. J Clin Invest 1999; 104:657–667.
5. Soussi-Gounni A, Kontolemos M, Hamid Q. Role of IL-9 in the pathophysiology of allergic diseases. J Allergy Clin Immunol 2001; 107:575–582.
6. Wills-Karp M, Luyimbazi J, Xu X, Schofield B, Neben TY, Karp CL, Donaldson DD. Interleukin-13: central mediator of allergic asthma. Science 1998; 282: 2258–2261.

                                                                  Lambrecht et al.

7. Grunig G, Warnock M, Wakil AE, Venkayya R, Brombacher F, Rennick DM, Sheppard D, Mohrs M, Donaldson DD, Locksley RM, Corry DB. Requirement for IL-13 independently of IL-4 in experimental asthma [see comments]. Science 1998; 282:2261–2263.
8. Humbert M, Menz G, Ying S, Corrigan CJ, Robinson DS, Durham SR, Kay AB. The immunopathology of extrinsic (atopic) and intrinsic (nonatopic) asthma: more similarities than differences. Immunol Today 1999; 20:528–533.
9. Shimbara A, Christodoulopoulos P, Soussi-Gounni A, Olivenstein R, Nakamura Y, Levitt RC, Nicolaides NC, Holroyd KJ, Tsicopoulos A, Lafitte JJ, Wallaert B, Hamid QA. IL-9 and its receptor in allergic and nonallergic lung disease: increased expression in asthma. J Allergy Clin Immunol 2000; 105:108–115.
10. Minshall E, Chakir J, Laviolette M, Molet S, Zhu Z, Olivenstein R, Elias JA, Hamid Q. IL-11 expression is increased in severe asthma: association with epithelial cells and eosinophils. J Allergy Clin Immunol 2000; 105:232–238.
11. Laberge S, Pinsonneault S, Varga EM, Till SJ, Nouri-Aria K, Jacobson M, Cruikshank WW, Center DM, Hamid Q, Durham SR. Increased expression of IL-16 immunoreactivity in bronchial mucosa after segmental allergen challenge in patients with asthma. J Allergy Clin Immunol 2000; 106:293–301.
12. Christodoulopoulos P, Cameron L, Nakamura Y, Lemiere C, Muro S, Dugas M, Boulet LP, Laviolette M, Olivenstein R, Hamid Q. TH2 cytokine-associated transcription factors in atopic and nonatopic asthma: evidence for differential signal transducer and activator of transcription 6 expression. J Allergy Clin Immunol 2001; 107:586–591.
13. Finotto S, Neurath MF, Glickman JN, Qin S, Lehr HA, Green FH, Ackerman K, Haley K, Galle PR, Szabo SJ, Drazen JM, De Sanctis GT, Glimcher LH. Development of spontaneous airway changes consistent with human asthma in mice lacking T-bet. Science 2002; 295:336–338.
14. Busse WW, Lemanske RF. Advances in Immunology. Asthma. N Engl J Med 2001; 344:350–362.
15. Krug N, Madden AE, Redington AE, Lackie P, Djukanovic R, Schauer U, Holgate ST, Frew AJ, Howarth PH. T-cell cytokine profile evaluated at the single cell level in BAL and blood in allergic asthma. Am J Respir Cell Mol Biol 1996; 14:319–326.
16. Lloyd CM, Gonzalo JA, Coyle AJ, Gutierrez-Ramos JC. Mouse models of allergic airway disease. Adv Immunol 2001; 77:263–295.
17. van Rijt LS, Lambrecht BN. Role of dendritic cells and Th2 lymphocytes in asthma:lessons from eosinophilic airway inflammation in the mouse. Microsc Res Tech 2001; 53:256–272.
18. Lee NA, Gelfand EW, Lee JJ. Pulmonary T cells and eosinophils: coconspirators or independent triggers of allergic respiratory pathology? J Allergy Clin Immunol 2001; 107:945–957.
19. Erjefalt JS, Andersson P, Gustafsson B, Korsgren M, Sonmark B, Persson CG. Allergen challenge-induced extravasation of plasma in mouse airways. Clin Exp Allergy 1998; 28:1013–1020.
20. Stelts D, Egan RW, Falcone A, Garlisi CG, Gleich GJ, Kreutner W, Kung TT, Nahrebne DK, Chapman RW, Minnicozzi M. Eosinophils retain their granule

major basic protein in a murine model of allergic pulmonary inflammation. Am J Respir Cell Mol Biol 1998; 18:463–470.

21. Denzler KL, Farmer SC, Crosby JR, Borchers M, Cieslewicz G, Larson KA, Cormier-Regard S, Lee NA, Lee JJ. Eosinophil major basic protein-1 does not contribute to allergen-induced airway pathologies in mouse models of asthma. J Immunol 2000; 165:5509–5517.

22. Denzler KL, Borchers MT, Crosby JR, Cieslewicz G, Hines EM, Justice JP, Cormier SA, Lindenberger KA, Song W, Wu W, Hazen SL, Gleich GJ, Lee JJ, Lee NA. Extensive eosinophil degranulation and peroxidase-mediated oxidation of airway proteins do not occur in a mouse ovalbumin-challenge model of pulmonary inflammation. J Immunol 2001; 167:1672–1682.

23. Temelkovski J, Hogan SP, Shepherd DP, Foster PS, Kumar RK. An improved murine model of asthma: selective airway inflammation, epithelial lesions and increased methacholine responsiveness following chronic exposure to aerosolised allergen. Thorax 1998; 53:849–856.

24. De Sanctis GT, Daheshia M, Daser A. Genetics of airway hyperresponsiveness. J Allergy Clin Immunol 2001; 108:11–20.

25. Takeda K, Haczku A, Lee JJ, Irvin CG, Gelfand EW. Strain dependence of airway hyperresponsiveness reflects differences in eosinophil localization in the lung. Am J Physiol Lung Cell Mol Physiol 2001; 281:L394–402.

26. Kanehiro A, Takeda K, Joetham A, Tomkinson A, Ikemura T, Irvin CG, Gelfand EW. Timing of administration of anti-VLA-4 differentiates airway hyperresponsiveness in the central and peripheral airways in mice. Am J Respir Crit Care Med 2000; 162:1132–1139.

27. Lambrecht BN. The dendritic cell in allergic airway diseases: a new player to the game. Clin Exp Allergy 2001; 31:206–218.

28. Banchereau J, Steinman RM. Dendritic cells and the control of immunity. Nature 1998; 392:245–252.

29. Holt PG. Regulation of immune responses at mucosal surfaces: allergic respiratory disease as a paradigm. Immun Cell Biol 1998; 76:119–124.

30. Vermaelen KY, Carro-Muino I, Lambrecht BN, Pauwels RA. Specific migratory dendritic cells rapidly transport antigen from the airways to the thoracic lymph nodes. J Exp Med 2001; 193:51–60.

31. Lambrecht BN, Pauwels RA, Fazekas De St Groth B. Induction of rapid T cell activation, division, and recirculation by intratracheal injection of dendritic cells in a TCR transgenic model. J Immunol 2000; 164:2937–2946.

32. Guery JC, Ria F, Adorini L. Dendritic cells but not B cells present antigenic complexes to class II-restricted T cells after administration of protein in adjuvant. J Exp Med 1996; 183:751–757.

33. Renz H, Smith HR, Henson JE, Ray BS, Irvin CG, Gelfand EW. Aerosolized antigen exposure without adjuvant causes increased IgE production and increased airway responsiveness in the mouse. J Allergy Clin Immunol 1992; 89:1127–1138.

34. McMenamin C, Pimm C, McKersey M, Holt PG. Regulation of IgE responses to inhaled antigen in mice by antigen-specific gamma delta T cells. Science 1994; 265:1869–1871.

35. Seymour BWP, Gershwin LJ, Coffman RL. Aerosol-induced immunoglobulin (Ig)-E unresponsiveness to ovalbumin does not require CD8(+) or T cell receptor (TCR)-gamma/delta(+) T cells or interferon (IFN)-gamma in a murine model of allergen sensitization. J Exp Med 1998; 187:721–731.

36. Akbari O, DeKruyff RH, Umetsu DT. Pulmonary dendritic cells producing IL-10 mediate tolerance induced by respiratory exposure to antigen. Nat Immunol 2001; 2:725–731.

37. Stampfli MR, Wiley RE, Scott Neigh G, Gajewska BU, Lei XF, Snider DP, Xing Z, Jordana M. GM-CSF transgene expression in the airway allows aerosolized ovalbumin to induce allergic sensitization in mice. J Clin Invest 1998; 102: 1704–1714.

38. Wang J, Snider DP, Hewlett BR, Lukacs NW, Gauldie J, Liang H, Xing Z. Transgenic expression of granulocyte-macrophage colony-stimulating factor induces the differentiation and activation of a novel dendritic cell population in the lung. Blood 2000; 95:2337–2345.

39. Yamamoto N, Suzuki S, Shirai A, Suzuki M, Nakazawa M, Nagashima Y, Okubo T. Dendritic cells are associated with augmentation of antigen sensitization by influenza A virus infection in mice. Eur J Immunol 2000; 30:316–326.

40. Yamamoto N, Suzuki S, Suzuki Y, Shirai A, Nakazawa M, Suzuki M, Takamasu T, Nagashima Y, Minami M, Ishigatsubo Y. Immune response induced by airway sensitization after influenza A virus infection depends on timing of antigen exposure in mice. J Virol 2001; 75:499–505.

41. Hamada K, Goldsmith CA, Goldman A, Kobzik L. Resistance of very young mice to inhaled allergen sensitization is overcome by coexposure to an air-pollutant aerosol. Am J Respir Crit Care Med 2000; 161:1285–1293.

42. Lambrecht BN, De Veerman M, Coyle AJ, Gutierrez-Ramos JC, Thielemans K, Pauwels RA. Myeloid dendritic cells induce Th2 responses to inhaled antigen, leading to eosinophilic airway inflammation. J Clin Invest 2000; 106:551–559.

43. Lambrecht BN, Peleman RA, Bullock GR, Pauwels RA. Sensitization to inhaled antigen by intratracheal instillation of dendritic cells. Clin Exp Allergy 2000; 30:214–224.

44. Sung S, Rose CE, Jr., Fu SM. Intratracheal priming with ovalbumin- and ovalbumin 323–339 peptide-pulsed dendritic cells induces airway hyperresponsiveness, lung eosinophilia, goblet cell hyperplasia, and inflammation. J Immunol 2001; 166:1261–1271.

45. Magram J, Connaughton SE, Warrier RR, Carvajal DM, Wu C, Ferrante J, Stewart C, Sarmiento U, Faherty DA, Gately M. IL-12-deficient mice are defective in IFN-γ production and type 1 cytokine responses. Immunity 1996; 4:471–481.

46. Wills-Karp M. IL-12/IL-13 axis in allergic asthma. J Allergy Clin Immunol 2001; 107:9–18.

47. Keane-Myers A, Wysocka M, Trinchieri G, Wills-Karp M. Resistance to antigen-induced airway hyperresponsiveness requires endogenous production of IL-12. J Immunol 1998; 161:919–926.

48. Stumbles PA, Thomas JA, Pimm CL, Lee PT, Venaille TJ, Proksch S, Holt PG. Resting respiratory tract dendritic cells preferentially stimulate T helper cell type 2 (Th2) responses and require obligatory cytokine signals for induction of Th1 immunity. J Exp Med 1998; 188:2019–2031.

49. Karp CL, Grupe A, Schadt, Ewart SL, Keane-Moore M, Cuomo PJ, Kohl J, Wahl L, Kuperman D, Germer S, Aud D, Peltz G, Wills-Karp M. Identification of complement factor 5 as a susceptibility locus for experimental allergic asthma. Nat Immunol 2000; 1:221–226.

50. Constant S, Lee KS, Bottomly K. Site of antigen delivery can influence T cell priming: pulmonary environment promotes preferential Th2-type differentiation. Eur J Immunol 2000; 30:840–847.

51. DeSmedt T, Vanmechelen M, DeBecker G, Urbain J, Leo O, Moser M. Effect of interleukin-10 on dendritic cell maturation and function. Eur J Immunol 1997; 27:1229–1235.

52. Kalinski P, Schuitemaker JHN, Hilkens CMU, Kapsenberg ML. Prostaglandin E2 induces the final maturation of IL-12-deficient CD1a$^+$ CD83$^+$ dendritic cells: the levels of IL-12 are determined during the final DC maturation and are resistant to further modulation. J Immunol 1998; 161:2804–2809.

53. Kips JC, Brusselle GG, Joos GF, Peleman RA, Tavernier J, Devos R, Pauwels RA. Interleukin-12 inhibits antigen-induced airway hyperresponsiveness in mice. Am J Respir Crit Care Med 1996; 153:535–539.

54. Stampfli MR, Scott Neigh G, Wiley RE, Cwiartka M, Ritz SA, Hitt MM, Xing Z, Jordana M. Regulation of allergic mucosal sensitization by interleukin-12 gene transfer to the airway. Am J Respir Cell Mol Biol 1999; 21:317–326.

55. Kline JN, Waldschmidt TJ, Businga TR, Lemish JE, Weinstock JV, Thorne PS, Krieg AM. Modulation of airway inflammation by CpG oligodesoxynucleotides in a murine model of asthma. J Immunol 1998; 160:2555–2559.

56. Hansen G, Yeung VP, Berry G, Umetsu DT, Dekruyff RH. Vaccination with heat-killed listeria as adjuvant reverses established allergen-induced airway hyperreactivity and inflammation: role of CD8+ T cells and IL-18. J Immunol 2000; 164:223–230.

57. Erb KJ, Holloway JW, Sobeck A, Moll H, Le Gros G. Infection of mice with Mycobacterium bovis-bacillus Calmette-Guerin (BCG) suppresses allergen-induced airway eosinophilia. J Exp Med 1998; 187:561–569.

58. Coyle AJ, Le Gros G, Bertrand C, Tsuyuki S, Heusser CH, Kopf M, Anderson GP. Interleukin-4 is required for the induction of lung Th2 mucosal immunity. Am J Respir Cell Mol Biol 1995; 13:54–59.

59. Corry DB, Folkesson HG, Warnock ML, Erle DJ, Matthay MA, Wiener-Kronish JP, Locksley RM. Interleukin 4, but not interleukin 5 or eosinophils, is required in a murine model of acute airway hyperreactivity [see comments] [published erratum appears in J Exp Med 1997 May 5; 185(9):1715]. J Exp Med 1996; 183:109–117.

60. Kuperman D, Schofield B, Wills-Karp M, Grusby MJ. Signal transducer and activator of transcription factor 6 (Stat6)-deficient mice are protected from antigen-induced airway hyperresponsiveness and mucus production. J Exp Med 1998; 187:939–948.

61. Hogan SP, Mould A, Kikutani H, Ramsay AJ, Foster PS. Aeroallergen-induced eosinophilic inflammation, lung damage, and airways hyperreactivity in mice can occur independently of IL-4 and allergen-specific immunoglobulins. J Clin Invest 1997; 99:1329–1339.

62. Tomkinson A, Kanehiro A, Rabinovitch N, Joetham A, Cieslewicz G, Gelfand EW. The failure of STAT6-deficient mice to develop airway eosinophilia and airway hyperresponsiveness is overcome by interleukin-5. Am J Respir Crit Care Med 1999; 160:1283–1291.

63. Webb DC, McKenzie AN, Koskinen AM, Yang M, Mattes J, Foster PS. Integrated signals between IL-13, IL-4, and IL-5 regulate airways hyperreactivity. J Immunol 2000; 165:108–113.

64. McKenzie GJ, Emson CL, Bell SE, Andeson S, Fallon P, Zurawski G, Murray R, Grencis R, McKenzie ANJ. Impaired development of Th2 cells in IL-13-deficient mice. Immunity 1998; 9:423–432.

65. Herrick Ca, MacLeod H, Glusac E, Tigelaar RE, Bottomly K. The responses induced by epicutaneous or inhalational protein exposure are differentially dependent on IL-4. J Clin Invest 2000; 105:765–775.

66. McIntire JJ, Umetsu SE, Akbari O, Potter M, Kuchroo VK, Barsh GS, Freeman GJ, Umetsu DT, Dekruyff RH. Identification of Tapr (an airway hyperreactivity regulatory locus) and the linked Tim gene family. Nat Immunol 2001; 2:1109–1116.

67. Johansson B, Ingvarsson S, Bjorck P, Borrebaeck CA. Human interdigitating dendritic cells induce isotype switching and IL-13-depending IgM production in CD40-activated naive B cells. J Immunol 2000; 164:1847–1854.

68. Korsgren M, Persson CGA, Sundler F, Bjerke T, Hansson T, Chambers BJ, Hong S, Van Kaer L, Ljunggren HG, Korsgren O. Natural killer cells determine development of allergen-induced eosinophilic airway inflammation in mice. J Exp Med 1999; 189:553–562.

69. Zhang Y, Rogers KH, Lewis DB. β2-microglobulin-dependent T cells are dispensable for allergen-induced T helper 2 responses. J Exp Med 1996; 184: 1507–1512.

70. Daser A, Gerstner B, Hansen R, Bulfone-Paus S, Renz H. Impaired NK1.1+ T cells do not prevent the development of an IgE-dependent allergic phenotype [see comments]. Clin Exp Allergy 1998; 28:950–955.

71. Kadowaki N, Antonenko S, Ho S, Rissoan MC, Soumelis V, Porcelli S, Lanier LL, Liu YJ. Distinct cytokine profiles of neonatal natural killer T cells after expansion with subsets of dendritic cells. J. Exp Med 2001; 193:1221–1226.

72. Zuany-Amorim C, Ruffie C, Haile S, Vargaftig BB, Pereira P, Pretolani M. Requirement for gammadelta T cells in allergic airway inflammation. Science 1998; 280:1265–1267.

73. Schramm CM, Puddington L, Yiamouyiannis CA, Lingenheld EG, Whiteley HE, Wolyniec WW, Noonan TC, Thrall RS. Proinflammatory roles of T-cell receptor (TCR)gammadelta and TCRalphabeta lymphocytes in a murine model of asthma. Am J Respir Cell Mol Biol 2000; 22:218–215.

74. Ohshima Y, Delespesse G. T cell-derived IL-4 and dendritic cell-derived IL-12 regulate the lymphokine-producing phenotype of alloantigen-primed naive human CD4 T cells. J Immunol 1997; 158:629–636.

75. Croft M, Swain SL. Recently activated naive CD4 T cells can help resting B cells, and can produce sufficient autocrine IL-4 to drive differentiation to secretion of Th-2 type cytokines. J Immunol 1995; 154:4269–4282.

76. Constant SL, Bottomly K. Induction of Th1 and Th2 CD4+ T cell responses: the alternative approaches. Annu Rev Immunol 1997; 15:297–322.
77. Tanaka H, Demeure C, Rubio M, Delespesse G, Sarfati M. Human monocyte-derived dendritic cells induce naive T cell differentiation into T helper cell type 2 (Th2) or Th1/Th2 effectors: role of stimulator/responder ratio. J Exp Med 2000; 192:405–411.
78. Lanzavecchia A, Sallusto F. From synapses to immunological memory: the role of sustained T cell stimulation. Curr Opin Immunol 2000; 12:92–98.
79. Schweitzer N, Borriello F, Wong RCK, Abbas AK, Sharpe AH. Role of costi-mulators in T cell differentiation. Studies using antigen-presenting cells lacking expression of CD80 or CD86. J Immunol 1997; 158:2713–2722.
80. Masten BJ, Lipscomb MF. Comparison of lung dendritic cells and B cells in stimulating naive antigen-specific T cells. J Immunol 1999; 162:1310–1317.
81. Tsuyuki S, Tsuyuki J, Einsle K, Kopf M, Coyle AJ. Costimulation through B7-2 (CD86) is required for the induction of a lung mucosal T helper cell 2 (TH2) immune response and altered airway responsiveness. J Exp Med 1997; 185: 1671–1679.
82. Harris N, Peach R, Naemura J, Linsley PS, Le Gros G, Ronchese F. CD80 costimulation is essential for the induction of airway eosinophilia. J Exp Med 1997; 185:177–182.
83. Haczku A, Takeda K, Redai I, Hamelmann E, Cieslewicz G, Joetham A, Loader J, Lee JJ, Irvin C, Gelfand EW. Anti-CD86 (B7.2) treatment abolishes allergic airway hyperresponsiveness in mice. Am J Respir Crit Care Med 1999; 159: 1638–1643.
84. Mark DA, Donovan CE, De Sanctis GT, Krinzman SJ, Kobzik L, Linsley PS, Sayegh MH, Lederer J, Perkins DL, Finn PW. Both CD80 and CD86 co-stimulatory molecules regulate allergic pulmonary inflammation. Int Immunol 1998; 10:1647–1655.
85. Mathur M, Herrmann K, Qin Y, Gulmen F, Li X, Krimins R, Weinstock J, Elliott D, Bluestone JA, Padrid P. CD28 interactions with either CD80 or CD86 are sufficient to induce allergic airway inflammation in mice. Am J Respir Cell Mol Biol 1999; 21:498–509.
86. Hammad H, Charbonnier AS, Duez C, Jacquet A, Stewart GA, Tonnel AB, Pestel J. Th2 polarization by Der p 1–pulsed monocyte-derived dendritic cells is due to the allergic status of the donors. Blood 2001; 98:1135–1141.
87. Coyle AJ, Lloyd C, Tian J, Nguyen T, Erikkson C, Wang L, Ottoson P, Persson P, Delaney T, Lehar S, Lin S, Poisson L, Meisel C, Kamradt T, Bjerke T, Levinson D, Gutierrez-Ramos JC. Crucial role of the interleukin 1 receptor family member T1/ST2 in T helper cell type 2-mediated lung mucosal immune responses. J Exp Med 1999; 190:895–902.
88. Yoshinaga SK, Whorisky JS, Khare SD, Sarmiento U, Guo J, Horan T, Shih G, Zhang M, Coccia MA, Kohno T, Tafuri-Bladt A, Brankow D, Campbell P, Chang D, Chiu L, Dai T, Duncan G, Elliot GS, Hui A, McCabe SM, Scully S, Shahinian A, Shaklee CL, Van G, Mak TW, Senaldi G. T-cell co-stimulation through B7RP-1 and ICOS. Nature 1999; 402:827–832.

89. Gonzalo JA, Tian J, Delaney T, Corcoran J, Rottman JB, Lora J, A1-Garawi A, Kroczek R, Gutierrez-Ramos JC, Coyle AJ. ICOS is critical for T helper cell-mediated lung mucosal inflammatory responses. Nat Immunol 2001; 2:597–604.

90. Hiwot-Jember AG, Zuberi RI, Liu F-T, Croft M. Development of allergic inflammation in a murine model of asthma is dependent on the costimulatory receptor OX40. J Exp Med 2001; 193:387–392.

91. Moller GM, Overbeek SE, VanHeldenMeeuwsen CG, VanHaarst JMW, Prens EP, Mulder PG, Postma DS, Hoogsteden HC. Increased numbers of dendritic cells in the bronchial mucosa of atopic asthmatic patients: downregulation by inhaled corticosteroids. Clin Exp Allergy 1996; 26:517–524.

92. Tunon de Lara JM, Redington AE, Bradding P, Church MK, Hartley JA, Semper AE, Holgate ST. Dendritic cells in normal and asthmatic airways: expression of the alfa subunit of the high affinity immunoglobulin E receptor. Clin Exp Allergy 1996; 26:648–655.

93. Hammad H, Duez C, Fahy O, Tsicopoulos A, Andre C, Wallaert B, Lebecque S, Tonnel AB, Pestel J. Human dendritic cells in the severe combined immunodeficiency mouse model: their potentiating role in the allergic reaction. Lab Invest 2000; 80:605–614.

94. Lambrecht BN, Carro-Muino I, Vermaelen K, Pauwels RA. Allergen-induced changes in bone-marrow progenitor and airway dendritic cells in sensitized rats. Am J Respir Cell Mol Biol 1999; 20:1165–1174.

95. Julia V, Hessel EM, Malherbe L, Glaichenhaus N, O'Garra A, Coffman R. A restricted subset of dendritic cells captures airborne antigen and remains able to activate specific T cells long after antigen exposure. Immunity 2002; 16:271–283.

96. Lambrecht BN, Salomon B, Klatzmann D, Pauwels RA. Dendritic cells are required for the development of chronic eosinophilic airway inflammation in response to inhaled antigen in sensitized mice. J. Immunol 1998; 160:4090–4097.

97. Djukanovic R. The role of co-stimulation in airway inflammation. Clin Exp Allergy 2000; 30:S46–S50.

98. Harris N, Prout M, Peach R, Fazekas De St Groth B, Ronchese F. CD80 costimulation is required for Th2 cell cytokine production but not for antigen-specific accumulation and migration into the lung. J Immunol 2001; 166:4908–4914.

99. Harris NL, Watt V, Ronchese F, Le Gros G. Differential T cell function and fate in lymph node and nonlymphoid tissues. J Exp Med 2002; 195:317–326.

100. Coyle AJ, Lehar S, Lloyd C, Tian J, Delaney T, Manning S, Nguyen T, Burwell T, Shchreider H, Gonzalo JA, Gosselin M, Owen LR, Rudd Ce, Gutierrez-Ramos J. The CD28-related molecule ICOS is required for effective T-cell dependent immune responses. Immunity 2000; 13:95–105.

101. Guo J, Stolina M, Bready JV, Yin S, Horan T, Yoshinaga SK, Senaldi G. Stimulatory effects of B7-related protein-1 on cellular and humoral immune responses in mice. J Immunol 2001; 166:5578–5584.

102. Tesciuba AG, Subudhi S, Rother RP, Faas SJ, Frants AM, Elliot D, Weinstock J, Matis LA, Bluestone JA, Sperling AI. Inducible costimulator regulates Th2-mediated inflammation, but not Th2 differentiation, in a model of allergic airway disease. J Immunol 2001; 167:1996–2003.

103. Oshikawa K, Kuroiwa K, Tago K, Iwahana H, Yanagiswawa K, Ohno S, Tominaga S, Sugiyama Y. Elevated soluble ST2 protein levels in sera of patients with asthma with an acute exacerbation. Am J Respir Crit Care Med 2000; 164:277–281.

104. Sallusto F, Langenkamp A, Geginat J, Lanzavecchia A. Functional subsets of memory T cells identified by CCR7 expression. Curr Top Microbiol Immunol 2000; 251:167–171.

105. Holt PG, Schon-Hegrad MA, Oliver J. MHC class II antigen-bearing dendritic cells in pulmonary tissues of the rat (regulation of antigen presentation activity by endogenous macrophage populations). J Exp Med 1988; 167:262–274.

106. Lee SC, Jaffar ZH, Wan KS, Holgate ST, Roberts K. Regulation of pulmonary T cell responses to inhaled antigen: role in Th1- and Th2-mediated inflammation. J Immunol 1999; 162:6867–6879.

107. Thepen T, McMenamin C, Girn B, Kraal G, Holt PG. Regulation of IgE production in pre-sensitized animals: in vivo elimination of alveolar macrophages preferentially increases IgE responses to inhaled allergen. Clin Exp Allergy 1992; 22:1107–1114.

108. Thepen T, Van Rooijen N, Kraal G. Alveolar macrophage elimination in vivo is associated in vivo with an increase in pulmonary immune responses in mice. J Exp Med 1989; 170:494–509.

109. Korsgren M, Erjefält JS, Korsgren O, Sundler F, Persson CGA. Allergic eosinophil-rich inflammation develops in lungs and airways of B cell-deficient mice. J Exp Med1997; 185:885–892.

110. Shi HZ, Humbles A, Gerard C, Jin Z, Weller PF. Lymph node trafficking and antigen presentation by endobronchial eosinophils. J Clin Invest 2000; 105: 945–953.

111. Hamelmann E, Cieslewicz G, Schwarze J, Ishizuka T, Joetham A, Heusser C, Gelfand EW. Anti-interleukin 5 but not anti-IgE prevents airway inflammation and airway hyperresponsiveness. Am J Respir Crit Care Med 1999; 160: 934–941.

112. Garlisi CG, Falcone A, Billah MM, Egan RW, Umland SP. T cells are the predominant source of interleukin-5 but not interleukin-4 mRNA expression in the lungs of antigen-challenged allergic mice. Am J Respir Cell Mol Biol 1996; 15:420–428.

113. Winterrowd GE, Chin JE. Flow cytometric detection of antigen-specific cytokine responses in lung T cells in a murine model of pulmonary inflammation. J Immunol Meth 1999; 226:105–118.

114. Hansen G, Berry G, Dekruyff RH, Umetsu DT. Allergen-specific Th1 cells fail to counterbalance Th2 cell–induced airway hyperreactivity but cause severe airway inflammation. J Clin Invest 1999; 175–183.

115. Cohn L, Tepper JS, Bottomly K. IL-4-independent induction of airway hyperresponsiveness by Th2, but not Th1, cells. J Immunol 1998; 161:3813–3816.

116. Cohn L, Homer RJ, Niu N, Bottomly K. T helper 1 cells and interferon gamma regulate allergic airway inflammation and mucus production. J Exp Med 1999; 190:1309–1318.

117. Hogan SP, Koskinen A, Matthaei KI, Young IG, Foster PS. Interleukin-5-producing CD4 T cells play a pivotal role in aeroallergen-induced eosinophilia,

bronchial hyperreactivity, and lung damage in mice. Am J Respir Crit Care Med 1998; 157:210–218.

118. Nakajima H, Iwamoto I, Tomoe S, Matsumura R, Tomioka H, Takatsu K, Yoshida S. CD4+ T-lymphocytes and interleukin-5 mediate antigen-induced eosinophil infiltration into the mouse trachea. Am Rev Respir Dis 1992; 146: 374–377.

119. Gavett SH, Chen X, Finkelman F, Wills-Karp M. Depletion of murine CD4+ T lymphocytes prevents antigen-induced airway hyperreactivity and pulmonary eosinophilia. Am J Respir Cell Mol Biol 1994; 10:587–593.

120. Brusselle GG, Kips JC, Tavernier J, Van Der Heyden JG, Cuvelier CA, Pauwels RA, Bluethmann H. Attenuation of allergic airway inflammation in IL-4 deficient mice. Clin Exp Allergy 1994; 24:73–80.

121. Hogan SP, Matthaei KI, Young JM, Koskinen A, Young IG, Foster PS. A novel T cell-regulated mechanism modulating allergen-induced airways hyperreactivity in BALB/c mice independently of IL-4 and IL-5. J Immunol 1998; 161:1501–1509.

122. Finotto S, De Sanctis GT, Lehr HA, Herz U, Buerke M, Schipp, Bartsch B, Atreya R, Schmitt E, Galle PR, Renz H, Neurath MF. Treatment of allergic airway inflammation and hyperresponsiveness by antisense-induced local block-ade of GATA-3 expression. J Exp Med 2001; 193:1247–1260.

123. Nawijn MC, Dingjan GM, Ferreira R, Lambrecht BN, Karis A, Grosveld F, Savelkoul H, Hendricks RL. Enforced expression of GATA-3 in transgenic mice inhibits Th1 differentiation and induces the formation of a T_1/ST_2 expressing Th2-committed T cell compartment in vivo. J Immunol 2001; 167:724–732.

124. Cohn L, Homer RJ, Marinov A, Rankin J, Bottomly K. Induction of airway mucus production By T helper 2 (Th2) cells: a critical role for interleukin 4 in cell recruitment but not mucus production. J Exp Med 1997; 186:1737–1747.

125. Cohn L, Herrick C, Niu N, Homer RJ, Bottomly K. IL-4 promotes airway eosinophilia by suppressing IFNγ production: defining a novel role for IFNγ in the regulation of allergic inflammation. J Immunol 2001; 166:2760–2767.

126. Temann UA, Prasad B, Gallup MW, Basbaum C, Ho SB, Flavell RA, Rankin JA. A novel role for murine IL-4 in vivo: induction of MUC5AC gene expression and mucin hypersecretion. Am J Respir Cell Mol Biol 1997; 16:471–478.

127. Rankin JA, Picarella DE, Geba GP, Temann UA, Prasad B, DiCosmo B, Tarallo A, Stripp B, Whitsett J, Flavell RA. Phenotypic and physiologic characterization of transgenic mice expressing interleukin 4 in the lung: lymphocytic and eosi-nophilic inflammation without airway hyperreactivity. Proc Natl Acad Sci USA 1996; 93:7821–7825.

128. Corry DB. IL-13 in allergy: home at last. Curr Opin Immunol 1999; 11:610–614.

129. Zhu Z, Homer RJ, Wang Z, Chen Q, Geba GP, Wang J, Zhang Y, Elias JA. Pulmonary expression of interleukin-13 causes inflammation, mucus hyperse-cretion, subepithelial fibrosis, physiologic abnormalities, and eotaxin production. J Clin Invest 1999; 103:779–788.

130. Mattes J, Yang M, Siqueira A, Clark K, MacKenzie J, McKenzie AN, Webb DC, Matthaei KI, Foster PS. IL-13 induces airways hyperreactivity inde-pendently of the IL-4Rα chain in the allergic lung. J Immunol 2001; 167:1683–1692.

131. Cohn L, Homer RJ, MacLeod H, Mohrs M, Brombacher F, Bottomly K. Th2-induced airway mucus production is dependent on IL-4Ralpha, but not on eosinophils. J Immunol 1999; 162:6178–6183.

132. Li L, Xia Y, Nguyen A, Lai YH, Feng L, Mosmann TR, Lo D. Effects of Th2 cytokines on chemokine expression in the lung: IL-13 potently induces eotaxin expression by airway epithelial cells. J Immunol 1999; 162:2477–2487.

133. Kung TT, Stelts DM, Zurcher JA, Adams GK, Egan RW, Kreutner W, Watnick AS, Jones H, Chapman RW. Involvement of IL-5 in a murine model of allergic pulmonary inflammation: Prophylactic and therapeutic effect of an anti-IL-5 antibody.Am J Respir Cell Mol Biol 1995; 13:360–365.

134. Mould AW, Ramsay AJ, Matthaei KI, Young IG, Rothenberg ME, Foster PS. The effect of IL-5 and eotaxin expression in the lung on eosinophil trafficking and degranulation and the induction of bronchial hyperreactivity. J Immunol 2000; 164:2142–2150.

135. Wang J, Palmer K, Lotvall J, Milan S, Lei XF, Matthaei KI, Gauldie J, Inman MD, Jordana M, Xing Z. Circulating, but not local lung, IL-5 is required for the development of antigen-induced airways eosinophilia. J Clin Invest 1998; 102:1132–1141.

136. Van Oosterhout AJ, Fattah D, Van Ark I, Hofman G, Buckley TL, Nijkamp FP. Eosinophil infiltration precedes development of airway hyperreactivity and mucosal exudation after intranasal administration of interleukin-5 to mice. J Allergy Clin Immunol 1995; 96:104–112.

137. Lee JJ, McGarry MP, Farmer SC, Denzler KL, Larson KA, Carrigan PE, Brenneise IE, Horton MA, Haczku A, Gelfand EW, Leikauf GD, Lee NA. Interleukin-5 expression in the lung epithelium of transgenic mice leads to pulmonary changes pathognomonic of asthma. J Exp Med 1997; 185:2143–2156.

138. Lefort J, Bachelet CM, Leduc D, Vargaftig BB. Effect of antigen provocation of IL-5 transgenic mice on eosinophil mobilization and bronchial hyperresponsiveness. J Allergy Clin Immunol 1996; 97:788–799.

139. Coyle AJ, Kohler G, Tsuyuki S, Brombacher F, Kopf M. Eosinophils are not required to induce airway hyperresponsiveness after nematode infection. Eur J Immunol 1998; 28:2640–2647.

140. Tournoy KG, Kips JC, Schou C, Pauwels RA. Airway eosinophilia is not a requirement for allergen-induced airway hyperresponsiveness. Clin Exp Allergy 2000; 30:79–85.

141. Cieslewicz G, Tomkinson A, Adler A, Duez C, Schwarze J, Takeda K, Larson KA, Lee JJ, Irvin CG, Gelfand EW. The late, but not early, asthmatic response is dependent on IL-5 and correlates with eosinophil infiltration. J Clin Invest 1999; 104:301–308.

142. Karras JG, McGraw K, McKay RA, Cooper SR, Lerner D, Lu T, Walker C, Dean NM, Monia BP. Inhibition of antigen-induced eosinophilia and late phase airway hyperresponsiveness by an IL-5 antisense oligonucleotide in mouse models of asthma. J Immunol 2000; 164:5409–5415.

143. Wilder JA, Collie DD, Wilson BS, Bice DE, Lyons CR, Lipscomb MF. Dissociation of airway hyperresponsiveness from immunoglobulin E and airway eosinophilia in a murine model of allergic asthma. Am J Respir Cell Mol Biol 1999; 20:1326–1334.

144. Henderson WR, Jr., Lewis DB, Albert RK, Zhang Y, Lamm WJ, Chiang GK, Jones F, Eriksen P, Tien YT, Jonas M, Chi EY. The importance of leukotrienes in airway inflammation in a mouse model of asthma. J Exp Med 1996; 184:1483–1494.

145. Rincon M, Anguita J, Nakamura T, Fikrig E,Flavell RA, Interleukin-6 directs the differentiation of IL-4-producing CD4$^+$ T cells. J Exp Med 1997; 185:461–469.

146. Wang J, Homer RJ, Chen Q, Elias JA. Endogenous and exogenous IL-6 inhibit aeroallergen-induced Th2 inflammation. J Immunol 2000; 165:4051–4061.

147. Louahead J, Zhou Y, Maloy WL, Rani PU, Weiss C, Tomer Y, Vink A, Renauld J, Van Snick J, Nicolaides NC, Levitt RC, Haczku A. Interleukin 9 promotes influx and local maturation of eosinophils. Blood 2001; 97:1035–1042.

148. Louahed J, Toda M, Jen J, Hamid Q, Renauld JC, Levitt RC, Nicolaides NC. Interleukin-9 upregulates mucus expression in the airways [see comments]. Am J Respir Cell Mol Biol 2000; 22:649–656.

149. Townsend JM, Fallon GP, Matthews JD, Smith P, Jolin EH, McKenzie NA. IL-9-deficient mice establish fundamental roles for IL-9 in pulmonary mastocytosis and goblet cell hyperplasia but not T cell development. Immunity 2000; 13:573–583.

150. Dong Q, Louahed J, Vink A, Sullivan CD, Messler CJ, Zhou Y, Haczku A, Huaux F, Arras M, Holroyd KJ, Renauld JC, Levitt RC, Nicolaides NC. IL-9 induces chemokine expression in lung epithelial cells and baseline airway eosinophilia in transgenic mice. Eur J Immunol 1999; 29:2130–2139.

151. Temann UA, Ray P, Flavell RA. Pulmonary overexpression of IL-9 induces Th2 cytokine expression, leading to immune pathology. J Clin Invest 2002; 109:29–39.

152. McLane MP, Haczku A, van de Rijn M, Weiss C, Ferrante V, MacDonald D, Renauld JC, Nicolaides NC, Holroyd KJ, Levitt RC. Interleukin-9 promotes allergen-induced eosinophilic inflammation and airway hyperresponsiveness in transgenic mice. Am J Respir Cell Mol Biol 1998; 19:713–720.

153. Temann UA, Geba GP, Rankin JA, Flavell RA. Expression of interleukin 9 in the lungs of transgenic mice causes airway inflammation, mast cell hyperplasia, and bronchial hyperresponsiveness. J Exp Med 1998; 188:1307–1320.

154. Kung TT, Luo B, Crawley Y, Garlisi CG, Devito K, Minnicozzi M, Egan RW, Kreutner W, Chapman RW. Effect of anti-mIL-9 antibody on the development of pulmonary inflammation and airway hyperresponsiveness in allergic mice. Am J Respir Cell Mol Biol 2001; 25:600–605.

155. McMillan SJ, Bishop B, Townsend MJ, McKenzie AN, Lloyd CM. The absence of interleukin 9 does not affect the development of allergen-induced pulmonary inflammation nor airway hyperreactivity. J Exp Med 2002; 195:51–57.

156. Zheng T, Zhu Z, Wang J, Homer RJ, Elias JA. IL-11: insights in asthma from overexpression transgenic modeling. J Allergy Clin Immunol 2001; 108:489–496.

157. Kuhn C, 3rd, Homer RJ, Zhu Z, Ward N, Flavell RA, Geba GP, Elias JA. Airway hyperresponsiveness and airway obstruction in transgenic mice. Morphologic correlates in mice overexpressing interleukin (IL)-11 and IL-6 in the lung. Am J Respir Cell Mol Biol 2000; 22:289–295.

158. Wang J, Homer RJ, Hong L, Cohn L, Lee CG, Jung S, Elias JA. IL-11 selectively inhibits aeroallergen-induced pulmonary eosinophilia and Th2 cytokine production. J Immunol 2000; 165:2222–2231.

159. Iwamoto I, Nakajima H, Endo H, Yoshida S. Interferon gamma regulates antigen-induced eosinophil recruitment into the mouse airways by inhibiting the infiltration of CD4+ T cells. J Exp Med 1993; 177:573–576.

160. Li XM, Chopra RK, Chou TY, Schofield, Wills-Karp M, Huang SK. Mucosal IFN-gamma gene transfer inhibits pulmonary allergic responses in mice. J Immunol 1996; 157:3216–3219.

161. Coyle AJ, Tsuyuki S, Bertrand C, Huang S, Aguet M, Alkan SS, Anderson GP. Mice lacking the IFN-gamma receptor have impaired ability to resolve a lung eosinophilic inflammatory response associated with a prolonged capacity of T cells to exhibit a Th2 cytokine profile. J Immunol 1996; 156:2680–2685.

162. Hessel EM, Van Oosterhout AJ, Van Ark I, Van Esch B, Hofman G, Van Loveren H, Savelkoul HF, Nijkamp FP. Development of airway hyperresponsiveness is dependent on interferon-gamma and independent of eosinophil infiltration. Am J Respir Cell Mol Biol 1997; 16:325–334.

163. Ford JG, Rennick D, Donaldson DD, Venkayya R, McArthur C, Hansell E, Kurup VP, Warnock M, Grunig G. IL-13 and IFN-gamma: interactions in lung inflammation. J Immunol 2001; 167:1769–1777.

164. Randolph DA, Stephens R, Carruthers CJ, Chaplin DD. Cooperation between Th1 and Th2 cells in a murine model of eosinophilic airway inflammation. J Clin Invest 1999; 104:1021–1029.

165. Randolph DA, Carruthers CJ, Szabo SJ, Murphy KM, Chaplin DD. Modulation of airway inflammation by passive transfer of allergen-specific Th1 and Th2 cells in a mouse model of asthma. J Immunol 1999; 162:2375–2383.

166. Gavett SH, O'Hearn DJ, Li X, Huang SK, Finkelman FD, Wills-Karp M. Interleukin 12 inhibits antigen-induced airway hyperresponsiveness, inflammation, and Th2 cytokine expression in mice. J Exp Med 1995; 182:1527–1536.

167. Zhao LL, Linden A, Sjostrand M, Cui ZH, Lotvall J, Jordana M. IL-12 regulates bone marrow eosinophilia and airway eotaxin levels induced by airway allergen exposure. Allergy 2000; 55:749–756.

168. Kline JN, Krieg AM, Waldschmidt TJ, Ballas ZK, Jain V,Businga TR. CpG oligodeoxynucleotides do not require TH1 cytokines to prevent eosinophilic airway inflammation in a murine model of asthma. J Allergy Clin Immunol 1999; 104:1258–1264.

169. Wang S, Fan Y, Han X, Yang J, Bilenki L, Yang X. IL-12-dependent vascular cell adhesion molecule-1 expression contributes to airway eosinophilic inflammation in a mouse model of asthma-like reaction. J Immunol 2001; 166:2741–2749.

170. Hofstra CL, Van Ark I, Hofman G, Kool M, Nijkamp FP, Van Oosterhout AJ. Prevention of Th2-like cell responses by coadministration of IL-12 and IL-18 is associated with inhibition of antigen-induced airway hyperresponsiveness, eosinophilia, and serum IgE levels. J Immunol 1998; 161:5054–5060.

171. Kumano K, Nakao A, Nakajima H, Hayashi F, Kurimoto M, Okamura H, Saito Y, Iwamoto I. Interleukin-18 enhances antigen-induced eosinophil recruitment into the mouse airways. Am J Respir Crit Care Med 1999; 160:873–878.

172. Wild JS, Sigounas A, Sur N, Siddiqui MS, Alam R, Kurimoto M, Sur S. IFN-gamma-inducing factor (IL-18) increases allergic sensitization, serum IgE, Th2

cytokines, and airway eosinophilia in a mouse model of allergic asthma. J Immunol 2000; 164:2701–2710.

173. Kodama T, Matsuyama T, Kuribayashi K, Nishioka Y, Sugita M, Akira S, Nakanishi K, Okamura H. IL-18 deficiency selectively enhances allergen-induced eosinophilia in mice. J Allergy Clin Immunol 2000; 105:45–53.

174. Nakanishi K, Yoshimoto T, Tsutsui H, Okamura H. Interleukin-18 is a unique cytokine that stimulates both Th1 and Th2 responses depending on its cytokine milieu. Cytokine Growth Factor Rev 2001; 12:53–72.

175. Yoshimoto T, Mizutani H, Tsutsui H, Noben-Trauth N, Yamanaka K, Tanaka M, Izumi S, Okamura H, Paul WE, Nakanishi K. IL-18 induction of IgE: dependence on CD4+ T cells, IL-4 and STAT6. Nat Immunol 2000; 1:132–137.

176. Tsitoura DC, Blumenthal RL, Berry G, DeKruyff RH, Umetsu DT. Mechanisms preventing allergen-induced airway hyperreactivity: role of tolerance and immune deviation. J Allergy Clin Immunol 2000; 106:239–246.

177. Roncarolo MG, Levings MK, Traversari C. Differentiation of T regulatory cells by immature dendritic cells. J Exp Med 2001; 193:F5–F10.

178. Zuany-Amorim C, Haïlé S, Leduc D, Dumarey C, Huerre M, Vargaftig BB, Pretolani M. Interleukin 10 inhibits antigen-induced cellular recruitment into the airways of sensitized mice. J Clin Invest 1995; 95:2644–2651.

179. van Scott MR, Justice JP, Bradfield JF, Enright E, Sigounas A, Sur S. IL-10 reduces Th2 cytokine production and eosinophilia but augments airway reactivity in allergic mice. Am J Physiol Lung Cell Mol Physiol 2000; 278:L667–674.

180. Stampfli MR, Cwiartka M, Gajewska BU, Alvarez D, Ritz SA, Inman MD, Xing Z, Jordana M. Interleukin-10 gene transfer to the airway regulates allergic mucosal sensitization in mice. Am J Respir Cell Mol Biol 1999; 21:586–596.

181. Tournoy KG, Kips JC, Pauwels RA. Endogenous interleukin-10 suppresses allergen-induced airway inflammation and nonspecific airway responsiveness. Clin Exp Allergy 2000; 30:775–783.

182. Makela MJ, Kanehiro A, Borish L, Dakhama A, Loader J, Joetham A, Xing Z, Jordana M, Larsen GL, Gelfand EW. IL-10 is necessary for the expression of airway hyperresponsiveness but not pulmonary inflammation after allergic sensitization. Proc Natl Acad Sci USA 2000; 97:6007–6012.

183. Yang X, Wang S, Fan Y, Han X. IL-10 deficiency prevents IL-5 overproduction and eosinophilic inflammation in a murine model of asthma-like reaction. Eur J Immunol 2000; 30:382–391.

184. Hansen G, McIntire JJ, Yeung VP, Berry G, Thorbecke GJ, Chen L, Dekruyff RH, Umetsu DT. CD4(+) T helper cells engineered to produce latent TGF-beta1 reverse allergen-induced airway hyperreactivity and inflammation. J. Clin Invest 2000; 105:61–70.

185. Nakao A, Miike S, Hatano M, Okumura K, Tokuhisa T, Ra C, Iwamoto I. Blockade of transforming growth factor beta/Smad signaling in T cells by overexpression of Smad7 enhances antigen-induced airway inflammation and airway reactivity. J Exp Med 2000; 192:151–158.

186. Russo M, Nahori MA, Lefort J, Gomes E, de Castro Keller A, Rodriguez D, Ribeiro OG, Adriouch S, Gallois V, de Faria AM, Vargaftig BB. Suppression of asthma-like responses in different mouse strains by oral tolerance. Am J Respir Cell Mol Biol 2001; 24:518–526.

187. Coyle AJ, Erard F, Bertrand C, Walti S, Pircher H, Le Gros G. Virus-specific CD8+ cells can switch to interleukin 5 production and induce airway eosinophilia. J Exp Med 1995; 181:1229–1233.

188. Erard F, Wild MT, Garcia-Sanz JA, Le Gros G. Switch of CD8 T cells to noncytolytic CD8-CD4- cells that make TH2 cytokines and help B cells. Science 1993; 260:1802–1805.

189. Gonzalo JA, Lloyd CM, Kremer L, Finger E, Martinez-A C, Siegelman MH, Cybulsky M, Gutierrez-Ramos JC. Eosinophil recruitment to the lung in a murine model of allergic inflammation. The role of T cells, chemokines, and adhesion receptors. J Clin Invest 1996; 98:2332–2345.

190. Hamelmann E, Oshiba A, Paluh J, Bradley K, Loader J, Potter TA, Larsen GL, Gelfand EW. Requirement for CD8+ T cells in the development of airway hyperresponsiveness in a murine model of airway sensitization. J Exp Med 1996; 183:1719–1729.

191. Schwarze J, Makela M, Cieslewicz G, Dakhama A, Lahn M, Ikemura T, Joetham A, Gelfand EW. Transfer of the enhancing effect of respiratory syncytial virus infection on subsequent allergic airway sensitization by T lymphocytes. J Immunol 1999; 163:5729–5734.

192. Hirai H, Tanaka K, Yoshie O, Ogawa K, Kenmotsu K, Takamori Y, Ichimasa M, Sugamura K, Nakamura M, Takano S, Nagata K. Prostaglandin D2 selectively induces chemotaxis in T helper type 2 cells, eosinophils, and basophils via seven-transmembrane receptor CRTH2. J Exp Med 2001; 193:255–261.

193. Matsuoka T, Hirata M, Tanaka H, Takahashi Y, Murata T, Kabashima K, Sugimoto Y, Kobayashi T, Ushikubi F, Aze Y, Eguchi N, Urade Y, Yoshida N, Kimura K, Mizoguchi A, Honda Y, Nagai H, Narumiya S. Prostaglandin D2 as a mediator of allergic asthma. Science 2000; 287:2013–2017.

194. Fujitani Y, Kanaoka Y, Aritake K, Uodome N, Okazaki-Hatake K, Urade Y. Pronounced eosinophilic lung inflammation and Th2 cytokine release in human lipocalin-type prostaglandin D synthase transgenic mice. J Immunol 2002; 168:443–449.

195. Takeda K, Hamelmann E, Joetham A, Shultz LD, Larsen GL, Irvin CG, Gelfand EW. Development of eosinophilic airway inflammation and airway hyperresponsiveness in mast cell-deficient mice J Exp Med 1997; 186:449–454.

196. Kobayashi T, Miura T, Haba T, Sato M, Serizawa I, Nagai H, Ishizaka K. An essential role of mast cells in the development of airway hyperresponsiveness in a murine asthma model. J Immunol 2000; 164:3855–3861.

197. Kung TT, Stelts D, Zurcher JA, Jones H, Umland SP, Kreutner W, Egan RW, Chapman RW. Mast cells modulate allergic pulmonary eosinophilia in mice. Am J Respir Cell Mol Biol 1995; 12:404–409.

198. Williams CM, Galli SJ. Mast cells can amplify airway reactivity and features of chronic inflammation in an asthma model in mice. J Exp Med 2000; 192:455–462.

199. Mehlhop PD, van de Rijn M, Goldberg AB, Brewer JP, Kurup VP, Martin TR, Oettgen HC. Allergen-induced bronchial hyperreactivity and eosinophilic inflammation occur in the absence of IgE in a mouse model of asthma. Proc Natl Acad Sci USA 1997; 94:1344–1349.

200. Coyle AJ, Wagner K, Bertrand C, Tsuyuki S, Bews J, Heusser C. Central role of immunoglobulin E in the induction of lung eosinophil infiltration and T helper 2

cell cytokine production: inhibition by a non-anaphylactogenic anti-IgE antibody. J Exp Med 1996; 183:1303–1310.

201. Zuberi RI, Apgar JR, Chen SS, Liu FT. Role for IgE in airway secretions: IgE immune complexes are more potent inducers than antigen alone of airway inflammation in a murine model. J Immunol 2000; 164:2667–2673.

202. Tumas DB, Chan B, Werther W, Wrin T, Vennari J, Desjardin N, Shields RL, Jardieu P. Anti-IgE efficacy in murine asthma models is dependent on the method of allergen sensitization. J Allergy Clin Immunol 2001; 107:1025–1033.

203. Broide DH, Sullivan S, Gifford T, Sriramarao P. Inhibition of pulmonary eosinophilia in P-selectin- and ICAM-1-deficient mice. Am J Respir Cell Mol Biol 1998; 18:218–225.

204. Wolyniec WW, De Sanctis GT, Nabozny G, Torcellini C, Haynes N, Joetham A, Gelfand EW, Drazen JM, Noonan TC. Reduction of antigen-induced airway hyperreactivity and eosinophilia in ICAM-1-deficient mice. Am J Respir Cell Mol Biol 1998; 18:777–785.

205. Gerwin N, Gonzalo JA, Lloyd C, Coyle AJ, Reiss Y, Banu N, Wang B, Xu H, Avraham H, Engelhardt B, Springer TA, Gutierrez-Ramos JC. Prolonged eosinophil accumulation in allergic lung interstitium of ICAM-2 deficient mice results in extended hyperresponsiveness. Immunity 1999; 10:9–19.

206. Nakajima H, Sano H, Nishimura T, Yoshida S, Iwamoto I. Role of vascular cell adhesion molecule 1/very late activation antigen 4 and intercellular adhesion molecule 1/lymphocyte function-associated antigen 1 interactions in antigen-induced eosinophil and T cell recruitment into the tissue. J Exp Med 1994; 179:1145–1154.

207. Henderson WR, Chi EY, Albert RK, Chu S, Lamm WJ, Rochon Y, Jonas M, Christie PE, Harlan JM. Blockade of CD49d on intrapulmonary but not circulating leukocytes inhibits airway inflammation and hyperresponsiveness in a mouse model of asthma. J Clin Invest 1998; 100:3083–3092.

208. Gonzalo JA, Llyod CM, Wen D, Albar JP, Wells TN, Proudfoot A, Martinez-A C, Dorf M, Bjerke T, Coyle AJ, Gutierrez-Ramos JC. The coordinated action of CC chemokines in the lung orchestrates allergic inflammation and airway hyperresponsiveness. J Exp Med 1998; 188:157–167.

209. Gonzalo JA, Pan Y, Lloyd CM, Jia GQ, Yu G, Dussault B, Powers CA, Proudfoot AE, Coyle AJ, Gearing D, Gutierrez-Ramos JC. Mouse monocyte-derived chemokine is involved in airway hyperreactivity and lung inflammation. J Immunol 1999; 163:403–411.

210. Llyod CM, Delaney T, Nguyen T, Tian J, Martinez-A C, Coyle AJ, Gutierrez-Ramos JC. CC chemokine receptor (CCR)3/Eotaxin is followed by CCR4/Monocyte- derived chemokine in mediating pulmonary T helper lymphocyte type 2 recruitment after serial antigen challenge In vivo. J Exp Med 2000; 191:265–274.

16

Regulation of Cellular Traffic in the Asthmatic Lung

CLARE M. LLOYD

Imperial College
London, England

**JOSE-CARLOS
GUTIERREZ-RAMOS**

Millennium Pharmaceuticals
Cambridge, Massachusetts, U.S.A.

I. Introduction

As outlined in previous chapters, one of the characteristic features of the asthmatic reaction is the accumulation of leukocytes in the lung. These leukocytic infiltrates are composed of a variety of different cells of the immune system. Their accumulation in the lung necessitates their travel from the peripheral circulation, through the vascular endothelium, through the lung parenchymal areas and, ultimately, via the bronchial epithelium to the bronchiolar spaces. This journey involves the complex interplay of a series of molecules that mediate migration to the sites of inflammation. This chapter will discuss the processes by which leukocytes are recruited to the various areas of the lung and the families of molecules that coordinate these processes.

II. Inflammatory Infiltrates

One of the most prominent cells observed within bronchiolar lavage (BAL) and biopsies from patients following allergen challenge is the eosinophil. Eosinophils are thought to be responsible for the tissue damage that leads to the disruption of the bronchial epithelium, enhanced bronchial responsiveness, and bronchial obstruction. Endobronchial allergen challenge studies in mild atopics have shown that eosinophils appear in the submucosa as early as 6 h following allergen challenge. By 24 h the majority of these eosinophils have migrated through the bronchial epithelium into the airways where they sit in the bronchiolar epithelial lining fluid, and can be collected during BAL. Although eosinophils are the predominant leukocytes to appear in the lavage, it is recognized that mast cells and basophils are also present during the early phases following allergen challenge, playing an important role in the acute phase. Increasingly the importance of T cells in controlling the allergic reaction is also being recognized. Pulmonary infiltrates during asthma are composed of eosinophils in conjunction with lymphocytes, macrophages, and, to a lesser extent, neutrophils. The time course for recruitment of each of these different cell types is different and is dependent on a series of molecules that control and coordinate this complex series of events.

III. Leukocyte Recruitment

In order to reach sites of inflammation circulating leukocytes must exit the bloodstream by crossing the vascular endothelium (Fig. 1). Leukocytes attach to the apical surface of the endothelium in the postcapillary venules where the shear stress tends to be at its lowest. The first step in the process of leukocyte transmigration is the generation of transient selectin-mediated interactions that cause tethering and then rolling of the leukocyte along the endothelial surface (1). The relatively slow velocity of the rolling leukocyte on the selectins ensures interaction with chemokines that are presented on the apical surface of the endothelium by glycosaminoglycans (2). Chemokines bind their respective receptor expressed on the leukocyte surface leading to alteration of β_2-integrin avidity, particularly CD11b/CD18, on the leukocyte cell membrane (3). The β_2-integrins bind to their Ig counterligands such as intercellular adhesion molecule-1 (ICAM-1), ICAM-2, or ICAM-3, which have been up-regulated on the endothelial surface by proinflammatory cytokines. These interactions provide firm attachment for the leukocytes to the endothelium and facilitate transendothelial migration of the leukocytes.

IV. The Chemokine Family

Chemokines are small, secreted, heparin-binding proteins that mediated leukocyte recruitment. This family of molecules can be distinguished from classical chemoattractant molecules such as bacterial derived N-formyl peptides, complement fragment peptides C3a and C5a, and lipid molecules such as leukotriene B_4 and platelet-activating factor on the basis of shared structural similarities. Members of the chemokine family have four conserved cysteine residues that form disulfide bonds critical to the tertiary structures of the proteins. Chemokines are classified into four subclasses according to the position of the first two cysteines, which are either adjacent (CC), or separated by one amino acid (CXC). Two other subclasses have been identified with, as yet, one

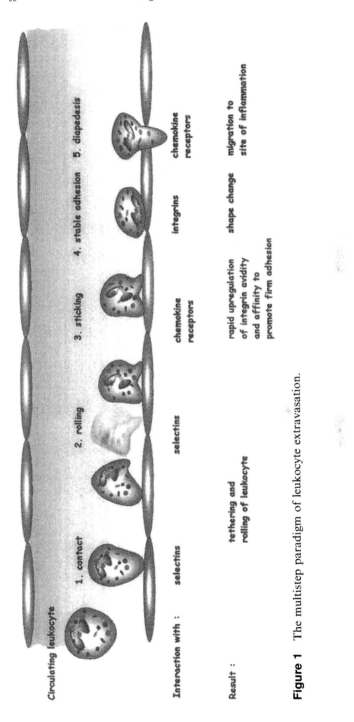

Figure 1 The multistep paradigm of leukocyte extravasation.

member in each. The C class has only two cysteines instead of four and has lymphotactin as its member, whereas the CX3C subclass has three amino acids between the first two cysteines and a mucin stalk at the N-terminal end, and incorporates fractalkine/neurotactin (4,5). Chemokines have a short amino-terminal domain preceding the first cysteine, a backbone made of β strands and the connecting loops found between the second and fourth cysteines, and a carboxy-terminal α helix of 20–30 amino acids. To date there are 23 human CC chemokines, 14 human CXC chemokines, and one member of both the CX3C and C subclasses—making a total of 39 known human chemokines. The major chemokines thought to be involved in the inflammatory response during allergic asthma are shown in Table 1. To counteract the confusion arising from many chemokines having more than one name, a new nomenclature has been established (6) whereby L (ligand) is added with a corresponding number for each group (CXCL, CCL, CL, and CXXXCL).

V. The Chemokine Receptor Family

The specific biological effects of the chemokines are mediated via interactions with heterotrimeric, seven-transmembrane, G-protein-coupled receptors (GPCRs). These chemokine receptors are part of a much bigger superfamily of GPCRs that include receptors for hormones, neurotransmitters, paracrine substances, inflammatory mediators, certain proteinases, taste and deodorant molecules, and even photons and calcium ions (7). Chemokine receptors

Table 1 Chemokines and Receptors Involved in Asthma

Chemokine	Cognate receptor	Target cell in asthma
Eotaxin (CCL11)	CCR3	Eosinophils, basophils, mast cells
Eotaxin-2 (CCL24)	CCR3	Eosinophils, basophils, mast cells
RANTES (CCL5)	CCR1, CCR3, CCR5	Eosinophils, monocytes, activated T cells
MCP-1 (CCL2)	CCR2	Monocytes, basophils, activated T cells
MCP-3 (CCL7)	CCR1, CCR2, CCR3	Eosinophils, basophils, monocytes, activated T cells
MCP-4 (CCL13)	CCR2, CCR3	Eosinophils, basophils, monocytes, activated T cells
MDC (CCL22)	CCR4	Monocytes, Th2 cells
MIP-la (CCL3)	CCR1, CCR5	Eosinophils, monocytes, activated T cells
IL-8 (CXCL8)	CXCR1, CXCR2	Neutrophils

measure approximately 350 amino acids in length and require the introduction of few gaps in the primary sequence to ensure alignment to other chemokine receptors. Each has a short extracellular N terminus that is acid overall and may be sulfated on tyrosine residues and contain N-glycosylation sites, an intracellular C terminus containing serine and threonine residues that act as phosphorylation sites for receptor regulation. Receptors have seven α-helical transmembrane domains, with three intracellular and three extracellular connecting loops composed of hydrophilic amino acids that are oriented perpendicularly to the plasma membrane; a disulfide bond links highly conserved cysteines in extracellular loops 1 and 2. G proteins are coupled through the C-terminal segment and possibly through the third intracellular loop.

To date 18 human chemokine receptors have been identified (6,8). Chemokine receptors CXCR1–CXCR5 bind the CXC family of chemokines, whereas the CC family consists of 10 receptors CCR1–CCR10. Receptors for lymphotactin (XCR1) and fractalkine/neurotactin (CX3CR1) have been identified and cloned. Another receptor, known as the Duffy antigen receptor for chemokines (DARC), has been shown to bind promiscuously to both CXC and CC chemokines. Interestingly, there is a certain amount of promiscuity in the chemokine superfamily, with many ligands binding different receptors and vice versa.

Interaction of chemokines with their counterreceptors mediates a series of effects, which ultimately result in the directional movement of the leukocyte. Perhaps the most impressive effect is the change in shape that occurs within seconds of addition of chemokine to a leukocyte suspension. Polymerization and breakdown of actin leads to formation and retraction of lamellipodia that function as the limbs of the migrating cells. Stimulation also induces up-regulation and activation of integrins, which then enable the leukocyte to adhere more firmly to the vascular endothelial cell wall before migrating through to other tissues. Several other rapid and transient responses are characteristic of the activation of leukocytes by chemokines, such as the rise in intracellular free calcium concentration; the production of microbicidal oxygen radicals and bioactive lipids; and the release of the contents of the cytoplasmic storage granules, such as proteases from neutrophils and monocytes, histamine from basophils, and cytotoxic proteins from eosinophils.

VI. Chemokines in Allergy

Since one of the hallmarks of the asthmatic reaction is a prominent mixed leukocytic infiltrate, it is perhaps unsurprising that a multitude of chemokines and receptors are expressed in lavage samples and biopsies from patients, as well as in animal models. A summary of the predominant cellular sources for chemokines during allergic responses is shown in Table 2.

Table 2 Cellular Source of Chemokines in the Allergic Lung

Chemokine	Cellular source in the lung
Eotaxin (CCL11)	Epithelial cell, alveolar macrophage, endothelial cell, smooth muscle cell, fibroblast, eosinophil, lymphocyte
Eotaxin-2 (CCL24)	Unknown
RANTES (CCL5)	Epithelial cell, smooth muscle, eosinophil
MCP-1 (CCL2)	Epithelial cell, fibroblast, alveolar macrophage
MCP-3 (CCL7)	Epithelial cell
MCP-4 (CCL13)	Epithelial cell
MDC (CCL22)[a]	Smooth muscle cell, alveolar macrophage
TARC (CCL17)	Epithelial cell
MIP-1α (CCL3)	Alveolar macrophage
IL-8 (CXCL8)	Alveolar macrophage

[a]In a mouse model.

A. Eotaxins

There are three chemokines with eosinophilic chemotactic activity, including eotaxin (CCL11), eotaxin-2 (CCL24), and eotaxin-3 (CCL26). Although these peptides are structurally distinct, they share the ability to specifically chemoattract eosinophils.

Eotaxin was originally identified in the BAL fluid of allergen-sensitized guinea pigs (9). Thereafter, the mouse and human genes were cloned, with the human gene exhibiting 58% identity with the guinea pig and mouse genes (10–12). All of these chemokines exert their effects via interactions with CCR3. Eotaxin mRNA expression is increased in bronchial biopsies of mild asthmatics and in BAL cells obtained 6 h after segmental allergen challenge (13–15). Eotaxin protein has also been demonstrated in biopsies from atopic and non-atopic asthmatics using immunohistochemistry (16). Moreover, soluble eotaxin has been measured in serum of asthmatics, and eotaxin levels correlated with disease severity—especially during acute asthma (17). Studies of the kinetics of eotaxin production have found that the release of this chemokine in BAL fluid of asthmatics is similar to that of other key, proasthmatic chemokines such as RANTES, macrophage inflammatory protein-1α (MIP-1α), and monocyte chemotactic protein-1 (MCP-1). Eotaxin levels peaked at 4 h following allergen challenge and decreased by 24 h. Interestingly, IL-5 has been found to have a different pattern of release. Levels of IL-5 increase gradually in BAL fluid after allergen challenge, peaking at 24 h after challenge, suggesting that while eotaxin initiates eosinophil recruitment, IL-5 maintains lung eosinophilia (18). The main cell types found to express eotaxin are epithelial cells (19,20), but macrophages, T cells, and mast cells have also shown positive expression.

Eotaxin-2 was originally termed CKβ6 and was identified by random sequencing of expressed sequence tags (EST) in an activated monocyte cDNA library (21). After an early categorization as an inhibitory factor for myeloid proliferation, its potent chemoattractant activity for eosinophils was demonstrated (22,23). Although eotaxin and eotaxin-2 are functionally similar, they share only 39% identity at the amino acid level and differ almost completely at the N-terminal region. Eotaxin-2 is also chemotactic for basophils and induces release of both histamine and leukotriene C_4 (LTC_4) from IL-3-primed basophils. Intradermal injection of eotaxin-2 into rhesus monkeys elicits eosinophil recruitment at the injection site (23). Increased mRNA for eotaxin has been exhibited in skin biopsies isolated during the allergen-induced late-phase cutaneous response (24), and in bronchial biopsies derived from non-atopic and atopic asthmatics (25). Eotaxin-2 protein has not yet been demonstrated in asthmatic airways. However, a functional role for eotaxin-2 in allergic inflammation has been postulated in studies showing that glucocorticoids downregulate eotaxin-2 mRNA expression in nasal polyps (24).

Eotaxin-3 has only 36% and 32% identity with eotaxin and eotaxin-2, respectively, yet has considerable functional identity (25,26). Eotaxin-3 is chemotactic for eosinophils and basophils, but is 10-fold less potent than the other two eotaxins. Eotaxin-3 is constitutively expressed in the heart and ovary, and mRNA expression is induced in endothelial cells by IL-4 and IL-3. Injection of eotaxin-3 into cynomolgus monkeys induces eosinophils recruitment at the injection site (26), but the role of this chemokine in asthma remains unproven.

B. Rantes (CCL5)

RANTES (regulated on activation, normal T cell expressed, and secreted) was originally described as a lymphocyte and monocyte chemoattractant, and was later identified as the first potent eosinophilic chemokine. While looking at the production of eosinophil activity by lymphocytes RANTES was identified as the major eosinophil chemoattractant produced by contaminating platelets (27). Direct evidence for a role in eosinophil recruitment came from in vivo studies where intradermal injection of RANTES in both atopic and nonatopic volunteers induces recruitment of both eosinophils and lymphocytes to the injection site. RANTES has also been identified as a prominent eosinophil attractant in BAL fluid of asthmatics exposed to allergen challenge (28). In this study, concentrations of BAL RANTES as low as 0.5 ng/mL induced eosinophil chemotaxis and levels of RANTES correlated with eosinophil numbers in BAL fluid, suggesting a direct role for RANTES in the recruitment of eosinophils during the late-phase reaction. Consistent with this observation, increased RANTES mRNA expression has been demonstrated in bronchial biopsies isolated from patients with atopic and nonatopic asthma (16). Levels of RANTES, together with MIP-1α and MCP-1, appears in BAL fluid at 4 h, slightly earlier than eotaxin, but levels return to baseline by 24 h (29). RANTES immunoreactivity has also been found in nasal biopsies taken from atopic and nonatopic patients suffering from nasal polyposis (30).

C. Monocyte Chemotactic Proteins (MCPs)

A number of MCPs have been described, including MCP-1 (CCL2), MCP-2 (CCL8), MCP-3 (CCL7), MCP-4 (CCL13), and MCP-5 (CCL12). The MCPs share relatively high homology at the amino acid level and have varied functional characteristics. All of the MCPs are chemotactic for monocytes, but MCP-3 and MCP-4 also have eosinophil-attracting capabilities. MCP-3 was identified from cytokine-stimulated osteosarcoma cells by its ability to induce monocyte migration in vitro (31). MCP-3 is 15-fold more potent than MCP-2 and slightly less potent than RANTES as an eosinophil chemoattractant. In addition, MCP-3 can activate purified basophils, but with slightly less potency than MCP-1. Increased MCP-3 mRNA has been observed in biopsies from asthmatics and was predominantly located in the bronchial submucosa, with very low expression in the epithelium (16).

MCP-4 is also an eosinophil chemoattractant, as well as inducing histamine release from IL-3-primed basophils, with potency similar to MCP-3, and raises intracellular calcium levels in purified eosinophils. Evidence for the involvement of MCP-4 in allergic reactions in vivo derive from a study showing increased MCP-4 mRNA in bronchial biopsies from atopic and non-atopic patients, where MCP-4 was located throughout the bronchial epithelium and submucosa (16).

The remaining member of the MCP family, MCP-5, was originally cloned in the mouse. MCP-5 shows chemoattractant activity for monocytes, lymphocytes, and eosinophils and is up-regulated during a mouse model of allergic pulmonary inflammation (32). Moreover, antibody neutralization studies have shown that MCP-5 is involved in the trafficking of leukocytes through the lung interstitium (33). In the absence of MCP-5, cells are not retained in the lung interstitium but progress toward the airway lumen. Therefore, bronchial hyperresponsiveness (BHR) and mucus hypersecretion do not occur. Human MCP-5 has yet to be cloned, and it is thought that the human counterpart of MCP-5 is MCP-1.

D. Monocyte-Derived Chemokine (MDC)

MDC (CCL22) was originally described as a chemoattractant for monocytes, monocyte-derived dendritic cells, and natural killer cells (34), and is a functional ligand for CCR4 (35). Although the in vitro functions of MDC would imply that it plays a role in the inflammatory process in allergic asthma, there has been little study in patients as yet. One study has found that MDC was only weakly expressed in the bronchial epithelium of asthmatics, but the intensity was not significantly different from that of normal subjects (36).

E. Thymus and Activation-Regulated Chemokine (TARC)

TARC/CCL17 selectively attracts T cells (37) and signals via the receptor CCR4 (38). Moreover, TARC, like MDC, selectively attracts T cells of the T-helper 2 (Th2) Subtype (39). TARC expression has been demonstrated in the bronchial epithelium of asthmatics and normal subjects, with the asthmatics showing a more intense expression than the normal subjects (36). Neutralization of TARC during allergic inflammation in vivo attenuated ovalbumin (OVA)–induced airway eosinophilia, airway hyperreactivity, and diminished Th2 cytokine production (40).

The analyses described above have described the cellular distribution of a number of inflammatory chemokines in biopsies from patients with asthma (summarized in Tables 1 and 2). Immunohistochemical analysis of chemokine expression in the lung has also been undertaken in mouse models of allergic airway disease, and these studies have determined important facets of chemokine function. In models of disease it is possible to examine expression during a time course after allergen challenge. These studies have revealed an important feature of chemokine expression that could be key to understanding action(s) in vivo, i.e., spatial distribution. It is presumed that chemokines generate chemotactic gradients in vivo. The location, range, and distribution of these chemotactic gradients depend on the spatial location of the cell(s) source for the specific chemokine. The mapping of the chemotactic gradients and their pattern of expression will be essential to determine and ultimately understand the specific role of a given chemokine in the inflammatory disease process. As yet the majority of this work has been done in the mouse, although some studies have looked at human biopsies collected at two time points following segmental allergen challenge in humans (16).

VII. Evidence for the Functional Roles of Chemokines in Asthma

As described above, multiple chemokines and receptors are expressed during the allergic reaction, and while the extent of investigation has been limited in humans to expression analysis and direct injection of chemokine in vivo, functional analysis of chemokines and their receptors has been conducted in animal models of asthma. Mouse models of allergic airway disease (AAD) have been invaluable in attempts to dissect the roles that individual cells and molecules play in the development of different pathophysiologies associated with asthma. These models are specifically suited for study of chemokine function in vivo because (1) multiple leukocyte subpopulations are recruited to the lung in sequential fashion; (2) some of these populations are clearly regulatory in nature (e.g., Th2 cells), whereas others have an effector role (e.g., eosinophils) and the immunological/physiological functions of one or the other can be distinguished with different end-point assays; (3) the recruitment of leukocyte subsets to the lung can be monitored at different, distinct anatomical sites: perivascular, interstital, and in the airway lumen; (4) the anatomical location of these leukocyte subsets can be correlated with physiological end points that are essential for disease: airway hyperresponsiveness (AHR) and mucus hypersecretion. These models have been used to define the roles that chemokine–receptor interactions play in vivo to mediate the recruitment of specific leukocyte subtypes to the lung over time following allergen challenge. A summary of the findings of these studies is given in Table 3. Studies with neutralizing antibodies, genetically deficient mice, and small-molecule antagonists have revealed critical roles for eotaxin, RANTES, MCP-1, MCP-3, MCP-5, MDC, MIP-1α, SDF-1α, and TARC in eosinophilia and airway hyper-reactivity (33, 41–44). These studies have involved the blockage of a single chemokine at intervals in a number of different models of AAD. While there are limitations to these studies, they clearly show that chemokines play an important role in the disease process. Interestingly, they have shown that chemokines not only contribute to tissue inflammation by recruiting and activating leukocytes, but also mediate degranulation and cause mediator release from effector cells such as basophils, mast cells, neutrophils, and eosinophils.

VIII. Migration of Antigen-Specific Effector T Cells

T cells are critical mediators of the allergic inflammatory response, and as such they and their secreted products, such as IL-4, IL-5, and IL-13, are found in biopsies and BAL from patients. Moreover, in vivo depletion experiments in mice or the use of mice genetically deficient in T cells have shown that a functional CD4 population is critical for the development of allergic inflammation (45,46). The delivery of functional subsets of T cells to particular tissues or microenvironments is a tightly controlled process involving a complex series of molecules expressed by a variety of cell types. This is especially important for T cells, since effector T cells can be divided into distinct subsets based on their cytokine profiles and functional properties. Th1 cells characteristically produce IFN-γ and contribute to host defense against pathogens, whereas Th2 cells produce IL-4 and IL-5 and are associated with allergic reactions involving IgE, eosinophils, and basophils (47). Th2 cells and the cytokines they secrete are thought to be critically important for the development of injury during allergic reactions such as asthma. However, it is unclear, how or why the Th2 subset migrates to the lung. Several theories have been proposed to explain how T cells traffic to the lung during disease, implicating both chemokines and their receptors in the process. One purports operation of a lung lymphocyte homing pathway similar to that proposed for the skin (48,49) whereby selected populations of T cells express a specific set of molecules to enable them to navigate to a particular tissue. A recent study set out to examine the molecules expressed on lung T cells so as to identify a distinct lung homing pathway (50). Lung T cells

Table 3 In Vivo Function of Chemokines and Their Receptors During Active Immunization Models[a]

Chemokine	Treatment	Effect	Ref.
Eotaxin	Neutralizing antibodies	Decrease in eosinophil recruitment	33
	Neutralizing antibodies	Reduced Th2 recruitment	58
	Gene knockout	Partial reduction in eosinophil recruitment	115
	Gene knockout	No effect	116
MCP-1	Neutralizing antibodies	Reduction in AHR and lavage and tissue eosinophilia, inflammatory mediator release	33, 43, 44
MCP-3	Neutralizing antibody	Reduced lavage eosinophilia	117
MCP-5	Neutralizing antibodies	Reduction of tissue eosinophil recruitment and AHR	32, 38
RANTES	Neutralizing antibodies	Reduced eosinophilia	44
	Receptor antagonist	Reduction in tissue and lavage eosinophilia	33
MIP-1α	Neutralizing antibodies	Reduced eosinophilia	44
		Partial reduction in eosinophilia and AHR	33
MDC	Neutralizing antibodies	Reduction of tissue eosinophil recruitment and AHR	42
		Reduced Th2 recruitment	58
TARC	Neutralizing antibodies	Reduction of tissue eosinophil recruitment and AHR, decreased Th2 cytokine production	40
SDF-1α	Neutralizing antibodies	Reduction of tissue eosinophil recruitment and AHR	118
CCR1	Gene knockout	Decreased Th2 cytokines, airway remodeling	119
CCR2	Gene knockout	Reduced airway hyperreactivity and BAL histamine	43
		No effect	120
CCR4	Gene knockout	No effect	121
CCR8	Gene knockout	Decreased eosinophilia and serum IL-5	59
IL-8R	Gene knockout	Increased B cell recruitment, serum IgE, decreased AHR	122
CXCR4	Neutralizing antibodies	Reduction of tissue eosinophil recruitment and AHR	118

[a]The table summarizes the results of various investigators in abrogating chemokine ligand or receptor function by genetically deficient mice or the use of neutralizing antibodies or receptor antagonists. The treatment column signifies the method by which particular chemokines were blocked. The effect column denoted the resulting change in phenotype after blockage. For further details of each experiment, please see individual references.

were found to express a pattern of chemokine receptors distinct from gut- or skin-homing T cells, indicating that a separate lung homing population exists. However, molecules that specifically identify this population have not yet been described.

The other theory rests on the recent observation that chemokine receptor expression appears to be tightly regulated on effector T cells. T-helper cells express a restricted panel of receptors for chemokines and migrate differentially in response to the chemokines that bind to these receptors (51,52). Eotaxin and TARC/MDC are among the chemokines that seem to attract selectively Th2 but not Th1 cells (51,52). Eotaxin binds CCR3 with high affinity and fidelity (12,53), whereas MDC interacts specifically with CCR4 (35). The attraction of these Th2 cells by eotaxin may represent a mechanism by which an allergen-driven reaction escalates with the production of IL-4 and IL-5, both of which are necessary for the differentiation and activation of eosinophils. Similarly, CCR4 has been identified on Th2 cells (52,54), and its ligands MDC and TARC have been shown to attract Th2 cells in preference to Th1 cells (42,52,54,55). CCR8 is selectively expressed on Th2 cells (56), particularly after activation of the T-cell receptor (57).

The role of the CCR3/eotaxin or CCR4/MDC axes in attracting effector Th2 cells has been investigated during an in vivo inflammatory processes. A mouse model of AAD based on the adoptive transfer of polarized effector Th cells was used to determine the functional importance of these chemokine receptor/ligand axes in mediating the recruitment of antigen-specific Th2 cells in vivo (58). Tracking of the transferred Th2 cells after repeated antigen challenge has established that both CCR3/eotaxin and CCR4/MDC axes contribute to the recruitment of Th2 cells to the lung, demonstrating the in vivo relevance of the expression of these receptors on Th2 cells (58). This finding emphasizes the relevance of previous in vitro results and demonstrates for the first time in vivo that CCR3 and CCR4 are more than markers of Th2 cells but have a critical pathophysiological significance in the development of AAD (as determined by their impact in BHR and eosinophilia).

The findings from these studies also reinforce the idea that chemokine receptors and their ligands function in a coordinated cooperative manner. The CCR3/eotaxin pathway was found to be critical in the acute stages of a response after initial challenge, however, repeated antigen challenge resulted in an increased frequency of CCR4 expressing Th2 cells. Consequently, the CCR4/MDC pathway ultimately dominates in the recruitment of antigen-specific Th2 cells. Based on these findings it was proposed that the CCR4/MDC axis is primarily responsible for the long-term recruitment of antigen-specific Th2 cells to target organs, such as airways, during chronic inflammatory responses in which there is repeated exposure to allergen. Of course, this view does not exclude the critical relevance that the early recruitment of Th2 cells by CCR3/eotaxin might have for the overall development of the allergic inflammatory response.

The receptor for I-309/CCL1, CCR8, is also selectively expressed on Th2 cells, indicating that this receptor may also be important in recruitment of Th2 cells to the lung. A recent study using mice genetically deficient in CCR8 demonstrates that CCR8 is important in the recruitment of eosinophils to the lung (59). However, the importance of this axis in asthmatic patients has not yet been investigated. Moreover, it remains to be seen whether allergen challenge induces the recruitment of effector lymphocytes following up-regulation of chemokines that interact with particular receptors on Th2 cells, or whether the expression of a district set of molecules guides particular populations of lymphocytes specifically to the lung.

IX. Role of Chemokines in the Polarization of the Allergic Response

In addition to the initiation and maintenance of leukocyte accumulation, CC chemokine members may have the capacity to drive the inflammatory reaction by augmenting or directionally differentiating T lymphocytes toward a Th1- or Th2-type response. In particular, MCP-1 may drive undifferentiated in vitro T-cell populations toward an IL-4-producing Th2-type cell, while MIP-1α appears to promote the development of a Th1-type response by enhancing IFN-γ secretion and decreasing Il-4 production (60). Additional evidence of the role of MCP-1 in controlling Th2 differentiation comes from a study showing that mice deficient in MCP-1 are unable to mount Th2 responses (61). Lymph node cells from immunized MCP-1$^{-/-}$ mice synthesize extremely low levels of IL-4, IL-5, and IL-10, but normal levels of IL-2 and IFN-γ. Consequently, these mice are not able to accomplish the normal immunoglobulin subclass switch that is characteristic of Th2 responses. This influence on Th2 polarization is likely to have far-reaching effects on disease pathogenesis. As outlined above, MCP-1 is expressed in the lung during asthma, and blockage in mouse models has profound effects on lung and lavage cellularity and AHR (33). These wide-ranging effects indicate that in ths situation MCP-1 is acting as more than just a monocyte chemoattractant. It is likely that MCP-1 has an important role in driving the asthmatic response, perhaps as early as during the primary sensitization phases.

X. Coordination of Chemokine Responses

In vitro characterization of chemokine functions suggests that there is redundancy within the family since many chemokines have overlapping actions and promiscuous receptor usage. Furthermore, expression studies in humans and animal models have determined that multiple chemokines are expressed in the lung in asthma. This might imply that some of the chemokines detected by expression analysis are redundant during the allergic response. However, detailed study of animal models of airway inflammation has shown that the production of these chemokines in vivo is organized and occurs in a coordinated manner. Detailed examination of murine models of pulmonary allergic inflammation have shown that leukocyte recruitment and development of AHR involves the action of both eosinophilic (eotaxin, RANTES, MCP-5, and MIP-1α) and noneosinophilic chemokines (MCP-1, MCP-3, MDC) (33,41,42). This indicates the absence of redundancy because these chemokines seem to exert a critical role at different stages and on different pathways of the development of AAD.

MCP-1 in particular has been shown to have an important role in the early stages of the response to allergen. Neutralization of MCP-1 during the sensitization and challenge phases of an allergen model affects recruitment of lymphocytes, monocytes, and eosinophils, as well as development of AHR (33). This effect may be attributable to the ability of MCP-1 to induce mast cell activation and LTC$_4$ release in the airway, both of which directly contribute to AHR (33,43).

The recruitment of eosinophils is also mediated in a coordinated fashion. A number of CC chemokines are able to mediate the migration of eosinophils, including the eotaxins, RANTES, MIP-1α, MCP-3, and MCP-4. Mouse studies have indicated that neutraliztion of either eotaxin or RANTES elicits a decrease in eosinophil recruitment to the lungs and airways, with a concomitant decrease in AHR (33). However, in the same model blockage of MIP-1α had little effect. In contrast, other models have shown that blockage of MIP-1α has a significant effect on eosinophil recruitment (44). Although the exact contribution of individual chemokines varies according to the particular allergy model used, it is clear that chemokines function in a tightly controlled fashion, with particular chemokines operating at key stages of the response.

XI. Synergy with Other Inflammatory Mediators

During an immune response, the ability to recruit and activate leukocytes is dependent on the local production of a particular chemokine and the cellular expression of the appropriate receptor. As described above, there are a number of chemokines postulated to have a role in the allergic response. Although it appears that common pathways, such as NKκB- and AP-1-induced promoter activation, mediate chemokine production, it is becoming increasingly clear that chemokines are differentially regulated by specific cytokines. Eotaxin, MCP-1, MDC, and MCP-4 are all up-regulated by IL-4 and/or IL-13, presumably by a STAT6-dependent pathway (62–64). This is supported by studies in which adoptive transfer of wild-type OVA-specific Th2 cells into STAT6-deficient mice led to an absence of chemokine production and of eosinophilic airway inflammation normally observed in wild-type recipient mice. Similarly, production of MDC, a Th2-selective chemokine, seems to be regulated by T-cell cytokines. Th2-derived cytokines, such as IL4 and IL-3, induce MDC production by monocytes, whereas the Th1-derived cytokine IFN-γ inhibits production (52,55). This suggests that an MDC-based amplification circuit of Th2 responses is in operation. Moreover, it is an example of how cytokines and chemokines interact to regulate the immune response.

XII. Chemotaxis Versus Chemokinesis

The process by which cells move along an increasing gradient of chemokine is known as *chemotaxis* and is particular because it allows for the directed, selective recruitment of cells. In direct contrast to this is a process called *chemokinesis*, whereby cells move in a nondirectional manner in response to an inflammatory stimulus. For example, eosinophil migration in response to chemokines (eotaxin-1 and 2, RANTES, MIP-1α, and MCP-3), lipid mediators (PAF, LTB$_4$), and low-molecular-weight chemoattractants (anaphylatoxin C5a and bacterial-derived peptide fMLP) is chemotactic. In this case, the specific receptor profile expressed on the cell surface of the eosinophil dictates which chemoattractants regulate movement and to what extent migration can be induced. In direct contrast, the eosinophil-specific cytokines (IL-5, IL-3, and GM-CSF), signaling through receptors of the cytokine superfamily, appear to prime eosinophil responses to chemoattractants (65). Molecules that prime cells for movement increase a cell's responsiveness to extracellular stimuli, possibly by promoting receptor aggregation and the colocalization of downstream signaling mediators, inducing receptor activation and possibly phosphorylation on subsequent stimulation of the same pathway. In terms of eosinophil migration, priming results in an increase in chemokinetic or nondirectional movement that is distinguishable in vitro from classical chemotactic migration.

Although there are a number of mediators that synergize with chemoattractants, the best characterized, and perhaps most important in the context of development of an allergic response, is the unique relationship between IL-5 and eotaxin-1. In vitro eotaxin-1 has been shown to induce the chemotaxis of mature guinea pig eosinophils, whereas IL-5 only promotes chemokinesis (66). Similar observations have been made with IL-5 and eotaxin in chemotaxis assays on isolated human peripheral eosinophils (67,68).

The specific role of IL-5 and eotaxin-1 in the regulation of eosinophil trafficking has initiated investigation in to the mechanisms of cooperation between these two molecules. Under basal conditions eosinophils normally reside in the bone marrow and tissues. In response to specific stimuli (inflammatory or parasitic), increased numbers of eosinophils migrate to the site of inflammation. Investigation of eosinophil trafficking in animal models has revealed that

IL-5 and eotaxin-1 cooperate to perform fundamental roles under basal conditions and during allergy to regulate recruitment of eosinophils to specific sites (66,69,70). Eotaxin-1 is constitutively expressed in a number of tissues; however, allergen challenge in sensitized animals or individuals leads to an early increase in production and recruitment of eosinophils (10,13,71). This eosinophilia is thought to occur in response to the secretion of eotaxin-1 from pulmonary endothelial and epithelial cells, which has been observed in a variety of animal models and in asthmatic patients (11,13,46,72). Other chemokines interacting with CCR3, such as RANTES, MIP-1α, and MCP-3, may potentiate eosinophil migration through the tissues. However, IL-5 released from mast cells and T cells in the late-phase response provides the key signal for eosinophil mobilization from the bone marrow and amplifies the chemoattractant potential of chemokines in the tissue. In particular, it is this "priming" of eosinophils by IL-5 that amplifies intracellular signaling systems coupled to chemokine receptors and thus potentiates tissue eosinophilia (69,70). IL-5 and eotaxin may also cooperate to regulate eosinophil homing and tissue accumultion by regulating adhesion pathways used by eosinophils (73). The chemotactic and chemokinetic activities of eotaxin and IL-5 clearly underlie the potential of these mediators to elicit, and cooperatively enhance, eosinophil migration. The cross-talk between IL-5 and eotaxin signaling pathway appears to play a key role in the selective recruitment and homing of eosinophils to the lung during an allergic response.

XIII. Regulation of Chemokine Responses

A prominent feature of the chemokine family is the fact that many chemokines are promiscuous and bind to multiple receptors. Moreover, many chemokines have overlapping functions. This begs the question, how are responses regulated? As outlined above, chemokines exert their effects through interaction with G-protein-coupled receptors on the cell surface. Sophisticated mechanisms exist at multiple levels (both extracellular and intracellular) to regulate cellular responses through these types of receptors. It is thought that some of these control processes serve to increase the specificity and selectivity of responses within the chemokine family.

Treatment with a chemoattractant can render a cell less responsive to subsequent stimulation by the same agonist—a process termed *homologous desensitization* (74). Treatment with some chemokines can also render the cell less responsive to a subsequent treatment with agonists that bind different receptors, a process that can be mediated by heterologous receptor desensitization (74), heterologous receptor sequestration (75), or, potentially, inhibition of downstream machinery. Both homologous and heterologous cross-talk between agonists and their receptors are potential mechanisms by which leukocyte migration can be controlled regulated.

A complex network of molecules function intracellularly to induce signaling through receptors, thus inserting further control and regulatory mechanisms for those receptors. Chemokine receptors are coupled to heterotrimeric G proteins, which consist of α, β, and γ subunits. Four families of G subunits can be distinguished based on their function and amino acid sequence homology, and are termed G_s, G_i, G_q, and G_{12}. In vitro studies suggest that G_i family members are essential for mediating chemoattractant responses (76–78). In order to function, G subunits must switch between an inactive GDP-bound and an active GTP-bound conformation. Essential elements in this GDP/GTP cycling are positive regulators that accelerate the nucleotide exchange on G and negative regulators that increase the intrinsic GTPase activity of G. GTPase-activating proteins have only been recognized relatively recently for heterotrimeric G proteins. Evidence suggests that a group of proteins with a common domain, the RGS (for regulator of *G* protein signaling) domain, can control aspects of G-protein-stimulated signaling pathways (79–82). Therefore, RGS proteins enhance the endogenous GTPase activity of G proteins, thus decreasing the half-life of the active GTP-bound state and limiting the duration of $G\alpha_i$ signaling. At least 19 mammalian RGS members have been identified. Many RGS members have been shown to bind $G\alpha_i$ proteins and activate the $G\alpha_i$ subunit's intrinsic GTPase activity in in vitro biochemical assays.

The highly homologous RGS domain is a region of about 120 amino acids, thought to confer the GAP activity of the protein by stabilizing the GTP-to-GDP transition state of G subunits. Most RGS proteins are relatively small, consisting of 200 amino acids, but an increasing number of larger RGS proteins have been described that contain additional functional domains, such as a PDZ domain in RGS12, a Dbl homology domain in p115RhoGEF, and a B-raf homology domain in RGS14 (83). Studies on the specificity of RGS molecules for different G proteins to date have indicated that human RGS1, RGS3, RGS4, and RGS16 predominantly interact with G_i subunits, RGS2 with G_q, RGSZ1 with G_z, and p115RhoGEF with $G_{12/13}$. However, these relationships may not be rigid, as some studies have indicated that RGS1 and RGS3 can also inhibit signaling via G_q-coupled receptors (84–86), while RGS2 may antagonize some G_i-coupled receptors (81). Evidence is accumulating that the specificity of RGS proteins can also be regulated through interaction with the GPCRs themselves (84,87,88), but further work is needed to understand how individual RGS proteins regulate individual GPCRs. Since RGS proteins regulate GPCR function it was postulated that they might also regulate cellular migratory and proadhesive responses to chemoattractants. At first it was difficult to predict whether RGS proteins would stimulate or inhibit chemotaxis and adhesion responses. However, it has since been demonstrated that RGS1, RGS3, and RGS4 modulate the ability of motile lymphoid cells to migrate along a chemoattractant gradient, presumably by decreasing the half-life of the activated G protein (78). These results suggest that the duration of the $G\alpha_i$ active state is a major determinant of the chemotactic response that requires coordination and integration of multiple downstream responses over a prolonged period. In contrast, RGS2 was unable to modulate migration to any chemoattractant in the same system (78). RGS1, RGS3, and RGS4 significantly inhibited rapid, chemoattractant-triggered adhesion as well, though to a lesser extent than chemotaxis. Similarly, RGS1 and an isoform of RGS3 were found to be effective inhibitors of chemotaxis toward the lymphoid tissue chemokines stromal cell–derived factor-1, B-lymphocyte chemoattractant, and EBV-induced molecule-1 ligand chemokine, whereas RGS2 had a limited effect on the same chemokines (89). This suggests that antigen-mediated changes in RGS molecule expression are part of the mechanism by which antigen receptor signaling regulates B-cell migration lymphoid tissues. The regulated expression of RGS molecules, in conjunction with Gα_i specificities, regulatory interactions, and subcellular localization of RGS proteins, may help control leukocyte migratory responses to chemoattractants, thus regulating the microenvironmental trafficking of leukocytes in vivo.

The next step in the intracellular signaling process comes after G proteins have dissociated into their Gα and Gβ subunits. Gβ subunits are able to activate the membrane-associated enzyme phospholipase Cβ2(PLC), which in turn cleaves phosphatidylinositol 4,5-bisphosphate (PIP$_2$) to form the intracellular second messengers phosphatidylinositol 1,4,5-trisphosphate (IP$_3$) and diacylglycerol (DAG). IP$_3$ mobilizes intracellular stored calcium whereas DAG acts in conjunction with calcium to activate various isoforms of protein kinase C (PKC). The activation of PKC and various calcium-sensitive protein kinases catalyzes protein phosphorylation, which activates a series of coordinated signaling events that ultimately result in cellular responses (90–93). There is increasing evidence that chemokine receptors can also activate several different intracellular effectors downstream of G$_i$ coupling, including the low molecular weight proteins Rho and Ras (94,91), phospholipase A$_2$, phosphatidylinositol 3-kinase (95), tyrosine kinase (96–98), and the MAP kinase pathway (99).

After activation, chemokine receptors become either partially or totally desensitized to repeated stimulation with the same or other agonists. This process is thought to involve phosphorylation of serine and threonine residues at the C tail of the receptor by G-protein-coupled receptor kinases and receptor sequestration by internalization. Desensitization may be critical for maintaining the capacity of the cell to sense a chemoattractant gradient (92).

XIV. Chemokines and Their Receptors as Novel Therapeutic Agents

One of the hallmark features of the asthmatic reaction is the influx of a range of inflammatory cells to the lung parenchyma and airways. The most common approach to resolving, or at least ameliorating, this recruitment is to suppress the inflammatory response. Traditionally this has been accomplished by administration of corticosteroids, cyclosporin A, and similar anti-inflammatory agents. However, these agents are broad acting, whereas chemokine antagonists offer the possibility of more specific inhibition with fewer side effects. The success of small-molecule inhibitors of GPCRs in the treatment of various other diseases has led the pharmaceutical and biotechnology industries to investigate the production of small-molecule inhibitors of chemokine receptors. As such chemokine antagonists are being hailed as the new generation of anti-inflammatory agents. There is compelling evidence for this to be the case, since there is a large body of evidence showing that blockage of chemokines suppresses inflammatory diseases in a variety of animal models. Moreover, many viruses have been shown to use internally expressed chemokine antagonists to subvert immune responses.

A. Small-Molecule Antagonists

This theoretical strategy has been put into practice with some success in the development of antagonists for CCR5 and CXCR4 in view of the critical role of these receptors in HIV infection (100–102). Targeting of chemokine receptors to suppress cell recruitment to the lung is an area of intense investigation for novel asthma therapy. In particular, receptors expressed on eosinophils have been targeted. CCR3 is an obvious choice since it is expressed on eosinophils, but also Th2 cells—both of which are critical in the development of the asthmatic response (12,51,53). A range of chemokines interact with CCR3—mainly eotaxin, but also RANTES, MCP-4, and MCP-3—all of which have been documented to be expressed in asthma. Signaling through CCR1 and CCR3 has also been blocked in vitro using a single compound UCB35625 (103). However, no in vivo data are available. Another area of investigation is the suppression of Th2 responses since this population of effector cells is though to be responsible for the initial development and subsequent escalation of the allergic response. Receptors on Th2 cells include CCR3, CCR4, and CCR8. To date there are no compounds that selectively target chemokine receptors, but these receptors are the subject of intense investigation.

B. Modified Chemokines

Discovery and development of pharmaceutical antagonists is a long and expensive process. Consequently, other strategies are being pursued. Modified chemokines and N-terminal peptides can be engineered to allow them to retain binding specificity and affinity to a receptor while blocking intracellular signaling and therefore function. Several examples of which have been described in the literature. A modified version of RANTES, whereby an additional methionine residue was added to the N terminus (104), was used in an in vivo mouse model of allergic pulmonary disease and was found to decrease both cellular inflammation and AHR (33). Similarly, another antagonist was formulated by addition of an aminooxypentane residue at the N terminus of RANTES (AOP-RANTES) and has been shown to inhibit HIV-1 infectivity in macrophages and lymphocytes (100). Another CCR3 antagonist, termed CKβ7, has been generated by an amino-terminal alanine-methionine swap of macrophage inflammatory protein-4 (MIP-4) (105). Whereas Met-RANTES inhibits eosinophil effector function through antagonizing CCR1 and CCR3, CKβ7 specifically antagonizes CCR3. CKβ7 is a more potent CCR3 antagonist than Met-RANTES and prevents signaling through CCR3 at concentrations of 1 nM. However, the success of modified chemokines or N-terminal peptides as antagonists depends mostly on their capacity to fully occupy the chemokine receptor/s at nanomolar concentrations, competing with the natural ligand's binding and thus blocking signaling. One of the advantages of using a modified ligand is that most of the receptors used by that ligand can be blocked, or partially blocked, by a single antagonist (106,107).

C. Viral Antagonists

Another potential source of chemokine antagonists comes from the observation that many viruses use chemokines antagonists to subvert immune responses (108). Chemokine homologues, such as vMIP-II, were probably pirated by viruses for broad antagonistic activity. VMIP-II is encoded by Kaposi's sarcoma herpes virus HHV8 (109,110). This viral chemokine antagonizes many of the Th1-associated receptors, such as CCR1, CCR2, and CCR5, but stimulates Th2-associated receptors, such as CCR3 and CCR8 (111). Other viruses use membrane-expressed chemokine receptor homologues, such as US28, a protein encoded by cytomegalovirus, to soak up chemokines to suppress host responses (112). A noteworthy feature of most viral chemokines or chemokine-binding proteins is their broad chemokine or receptor binding capabilities, which suggests that viruses need to circumvent chemokine redundancy for effective immune subversion.

D. Neutralizing Antibodies

Another strategy to modify chemokine function is by the generation of specific monoclonal antibodies against chemokines or their receptors. A range of in vivo studies with mouse models of allergic disease have demonstrated the benefits of blocking ligands (33), reviewed by (6); however, the range of chemokine functions, particularly those in lymphocyte homeostasis, suggests that targeting receptors may be a more effective therapeutic prospect. A neutralizing monoclonal antibody against CCR3 blocks chemotaxis and calcium flux induced by all CCR3 ligands in human eosinophils in vitro (113). Moreover, a neutralizing monoclonal anti-CCR3 antibody was shown to inhibit eosinophil recruitment to the skin in an in vivo guinea pig model (114). However, the effect of this antibody on allergic pulmonary inflammation has yet to be determined.

XV. Conclusion

The discovery and continued characterization of the chemokine family of ligands and receptors has contributed to a greater understanding of the recruitment of inflammatory cells to the lung during allergic asthma. The particular feature of this family that makes these molecules especially attractive therapeutic targets is their specificity. Unlike the pleiotropic effects of cytokines, chemokines target-specific leukocyte subtypes. Thus, an agent designed to target a particular chemokine–receptor interaction would be expected to have a physiologically limited effect, with a reduced set of side effects. The challenge in the future is to design specific and selective antagonists for a new generation of therapeutic agents.

References

1. Lawrence MB, Springer TA. Leukocytes roll on a selectin at physiologic flow rates: distinction from and prerequisite for adhesion through integrins. Cell 1991; 65:859–873.
2. Tanaka Y, Adams DH, Shaw S. Proteoglycans on endothelial cells present adhesion-inducing cytokines to leukocytes. Immunol Today 1993; 14:111–115.
3. Springer TA. Traffic signals for lymphocyte recirculation and leukocyte emigration: the multistep paradigm. Cell 1994; 76:301–314.
4. Pan Y, Lloyd C, Zhou H, Dolich S, Deeds J, Gonzalo JA. Neurotactin, a membrane-anchored chemokine upregulated in brain inflammation. Nature 1997; 387:611–617.
5. Bazan JF, Bacon KB, Hardiman G, Wang W, Greaves DR, Zlotnik A. A new class of membrane-bound chemokine with a CX_3C motif. Nature 1997; 385:640–644.
6. Homey B, Zlotnik A. Chemokines in allergy. Curr Opin Immunol 1999; 11:626–634.
7. Watson B. In: Akinstall S, ed. The G-protein linked receptor facts book. London: Academic Press, 1994.
8. Murdoch C, Finn A. Chemokine receptors and their role in inflammation and infectious diseases. Blood 2000; 95:3032–3043.
9. Jose PJ, Adcock IM, Griffiths-Johnson DA, Berkman N, Wells TNC, Williams TJ. Eotaxin: Cloning of an eosinophil chemoattractant cytokine and increased mRNA expression in allergen-challenged guinea-pig lungs. Biochem Biophys Res Commun 1994; 205:788–794.
10. Gonzalo J-A, Jia G-Q, Aguirre V, Friend D, Cocyle AJ, Jenkins NA, Lin GS, Katz H, Lichtman A, Copeland N, Kopf M, Gutierrez-Ramos JC. Mouse eotaxin expression parallels eosinophil accumulation during lung allergic

inflammation but it is not restricted to a Th2-type response. Immunity 1996; 4:1–14.

11. Rothenberg ME, Luster AD, Leder P. Murine eotaxin: An eosinophil chemo-attractant inducible in endothelial cells and in interleukin 4-induced tumor suppression. Proc Natl Acad Sci USA 1995; 92:8960–8964.

12. Ponath PD, Qin S, Post TW, Wang J, Wu L, Gerard NP, Newman W, Gerard C, Mackay CR. Molecular cloning and characterization of a human eotaxin receptor expressed selectively on eosinophils. J Exp Med 1996; 183:2437–2448.

13. Lamkhioued B, Renzi PM, Younes A, Garcia-Zepeda EA, Allakhverdi Z, Ghaffar O. Increased expression of eotaxin in bronchoalveolar lavage and airways of asthmatics contributes to the chemotaxis of eosinophils to the site of inflammation. J Immunol 1997; 159:4593–4601.

14. Brown JR, Kleimberg J, Marini M, Sun G, Bellini A, Mattoli S. Kinetics of eotaxin expression and its relationship to eosinophil accumulation and activation in bronchial biopsies and bronchoalveolar lavage (BAL) of asthmatic patients after allergen inhalation. Clin Exp Immunol 1998; 114:137–146.

15. Ying S, Robinson DS, Meng Q, Barata LT, McEuen AR, Buckley MG, Walls AF, Askenase PW, Kay AB. C-C chemokines in allergen-induced late-phase cutaneous responses in atopic subjects: association of eotaxin with early 6-hour eosinophils, and of eotaxin-2 and monocyte chemoattractant protein-4 with the later 24-hour tissue eosinophilia, and relationship to basophils and other C-C chemokines (monocyte chemoattractant protein-3 and RANTES). J Immunol 1999; 163:3976–3984.

16. Ying S, Meng Q, Zeibecoglou K, Robinson DS, Macfarlane A, Humbert M, Kay AB. Eosinophil chemotactic chemokines (eotaxin, eotaxin-2, RANTES, monocyte chemoattractant protein-3 (MCP-3), and (MCP-4), and C-C chemokine receptor 3 expression in bronchial biopsies from atopic and nonatopic (Intrinsic) asthmatics. J Immunol 1999; 163:6321–6329.

17. Nakamura H, Weiss ST, Israel E, Luster AD, Drazen JM, Lilly CM. Eotaxin and impaired lung function in asthma. Am J Respir Crit Care Med 1999; 160:1952–1956.

18. Teran LM. CCL chemokines and asthma. Immunol Today 2000; 21:235–242.

19. Ying S, Robinson DS, Meng Q, Rottman J, Kennedy R, Ringler DJ, Mackay CR, Daugherty BL, Springer MS, Durham SR, Williams TJ, Kay AB. Enhanced expression of eotaxin and CCR3 mRNA and protein in atopic asthma. Association with airway hyperresponsiveness and predominant co-localization of eotaxin mRNA to bronchial epithelial and endothelial cells. Eur J Immunol 1997; 27:3507–3516.

20. Mattoli S, Stacey MA, Sun G, Bellini A, Marini M. Eotaxin expression and eosinophilic inflammation in asthma. Biochem Biophys Res Commun 1997; 236:299–301.

21. Patel VP, Kreider BL, Li Y, Li H, Leung K, Salcedo T, Nardelli B, Pippalla V, Gentz S, Thotakura R, Parmelee D, Gentz R, Garotta G. Molecular and functional characterization of two novel human C-C chemokines as inhibitors of two distinct classes of myeloid progenitors. J Exp Med 1997; 185:1163–1172.

22. White JR, Imburgia C, Dul E, Appelbaum E, O'Donnell K, O'Shannessy DJ, O'Shannessy DJ, Brawner M, Fornwald J, Adamou J, Elshourbagy NA, Kaiser K, Foley JJ, Schmidt DB, Johanson K, Macphee C, Moores K, McNulty D, Scott GF, Schleimer RP, Sarau HM. Cloning and functional characterization of a novel human CC chemokine that binds to the CCR3 receptor and activates human eosinophils. J Leukoc Biol 1997; 62:667–675.

23. Forssmann U, Uguccioni M, Loetscher P, Dahinden CA, Langen H, Thelen M, Baggiolini M. Eotaxin-2, a novel CC chemokine that is selective for the chemokine receptor CCR3, and acts like eotaxin on human eosinophil and basophil leukocyes. J Exp Med 1997; 185:2171–2176.

24. Jahnsen FL, Haye R, Gran E, Brandtzaeg P, Johansen FE. Glucocorticosteroids inhibit mRNA expression for eotaxin, eotaxin-2, and monocyte-chemotactic protein-4 in human airway inflammation with eosinophilia. J Immunol 1999; 163:1545–1551.

25. Shinkai A, Yoshisue H, Koike M, Shoji E, Nakagawa S, Saito A, Takeda T, Imabeppu S, Kato Y, Hanai N, Anazawa H, Kuga T, Nishi T. A novel human CC chemokine, eotaxin-3, which is expressed in IL-4-stimulated vascular endothelial cells, exhibits potent activity toward eosinophils. J Immunol 1999; 163:1602–1610.

26. Kitaura M, Suzuki N, Imai T, Takagi S, Suzuki R, Nakajima T, Hirai K, Nomiyama H, Yoshie O. Molecular cloning of a novel human CC chemokine (eotaxin-3) that is a functional ligand of CC chemokine receptor 3. J Biol Chem 1999; 274:27975–27980.

27. Kameyoshi Y, Dorschner A, Mallet AI, Christophers E, Schröder J-M. Cytokine RANTES released by thrombin-stimulated platelets is a potent attractant for human eosinophils. J Exp Med 1992; 176:587–592.

28. Teran LM, Noso N, Carroll M, Davies DE, Holgate S, Schroder J-M. Eosinophil recruitment following allergen challenge is associated with the release of the chemokine RANTES into asthmatic airways. J Immunol 1996; 157:1806–1812.

29. Holgate ST, Bodey KS, Janezic A, Frew AJ, Kaplan AP, Teran LM. Release of RANTES, MIP-1 alpha, and MCP-1 into asthmatic airways following endobronchial allergen challenge. Am J Respir Crit Care Med 1997; 156:1377–1383.

30. Teran LM, Park HS, Djukanovic R, Roberts K, Holgate S. Cultured nasal polyps from nonatopic and atopic patients release RANTES spontaneously and after stimulation with phytohemagglutinin. J Allergy Clin Immunol 1997; 100:499–504.

31. Van Damme J, Proost P, Lenaerts J-P, Opdenakker G. Structural and functional identification of two human, tumor-derived monocyte chemotactic proteins (MCP-2 and MCP-3) belonging to the chemokine family. J Exp Med 1992; 176:59–65.

32. Jia GQ, Gonzalo JA, Lloyd C, Kremer L, Lu L, Martinez-A C, Wershil BK, Gutierrez-Ramos JC. Distinct expression and function of the novel mouse chemokine monocyte chemotactic protein-5 in lung allergic inflammation. J Exp Med 1996; 184:1939–1951.

33. Gonzalo JA, Lloyd CM, Wen D, Albar JP, Wells TN, Proudfoot A, Martinez-A C, Dorf M, Bjerke T, Coyle AJ, Gutierrez-Ramos JC. The co-ordinated action of CC chemokines in the lung orchestrates allergic inflammation and airways hyperresponsiveness. J Exp Med 1998; 188:157–167.

34. Godiska R, Chantry D, Raport CJ, Sozzani S, Allavena P, Leviten D, Mantovani A, Gray PW. Human macophage-derived chemokine (MDC), a novel chemo-attractant for monocytes, monocyte-derived dendritic cells, and natural killer cells. J Exp Med 1997; 185:1595–1604.

35. Imai T, Chantry D, Raport CJ, Wood CL, Nishimura M, Godiska R, Yoshie O, Gray PW. Macrophage-derived chemokine is a functional ligand for the CC chemokine receptor 4. J Biol Chem 1998; 273:1764–1768.

36. Sekiya T, Miyamasu M, Imanishi M, Yamada H, Nakajima T, Yamaguchi M, Fujisawa T, Pawankar R, Sano Y, Ohta K, Ishii A, Morita Y, Yamamoto K, Matsushima K, Yoshie O, Hirai K. Inducible expression of a Th2-type CC chemokine thymus- and activation-regulated chemokine by human bronchial epithelial cells. J Immunol 2000; 165:2205–2213.

37. Imai T, Yoshida T, Baba M, Nishimura M, Kakizaki M, Yoshie O. Molecular cloning of a novel T cell-directed CC chemokine expressed in thymus by signal sequence trap using Epstein-Barr virus vector. J Biol Chem 1996; 271:21514–21521.

38. Imai T, Baba M, Nishimura M, Kakizaki M, Takagi S, Yoshie O. The T cell–directed CC chemokine TARC is a highly specific biological ligand for CC chemokine receptor 4. J Biol Chem 1997; 272:15036–15042.

39. Imai T, Nagira M, Takagi S, Kakizaki M, Nishimura M, Wang J, Gray PW, Matsushima K, Yoshie O. Selective recruitment of CCR4-bearing Th2 cells toward antigen-presenting cells by the CC chemokines thymus and activation-regulated chemokine and macrophage-derived chemokine. Int Immunol 1999; 11:81–88.

40. Kawasaki S, Takizawa H, Yoneyama H, Nakayama T, Fujisawa R, Izumizaki M, Imai T, Yoshie O, Homma I, Yamamoto K, Matsushima K. Intervention of thymus and activation-regulated chemokine attenuates the development of allergic airway inflammation and hyperresponsiveness in mice. J Immunol 2001; 166:2055–2062.

41. Stafford S, Li H, Forsythe PA, Ryan M, Bravo R, Alam R. Monocyte chema-tactic protein-3 (MCP-3)/fibroblast-induced cytokine (FIC) in eosinophilic inflammation of the airways and the inhibitory effects of an anti-MCP-3/FIC antibody. J Immunol 1997; 158:4953–4960.

42. Gonzalo JA, Pan Y, Lloyd CM, Jia GQ, Yu G, Dussault B, Powers CA, Proudfoot AE, Coyle AJ, Gearing D, Gutierrez-Ramos JC. Mouse monocyte–derived chemokine is involved in airway hyperreactivity and lung inflammation. J Immunol 1999; 163:403–411.

43. Campbell EM, Charo IF, Kunkel SL, Strieter RM, Boring L, Gosling J, Lukacs NW. Monocyte chemoattractant protein-1 mediates cockroach allergen-induced bronchial hyperreactivity in normal but not CCR2-/-mice: the role of mast cells. J Immunol 1999; 163:2160–2167.

44. Lukacs NW, Strieter RM, Warmington K, Lincoln P, Chensue SW, Kunkel SL. Differential recruitment of leukocyte populations and alteration of airway hyperreactivity by C-C family chemokines in allergic airway inflammation. J Immunol 1997; 158:4398–4404.

45. Gavett SH, Chen X, Finkelman F, Wills-Karp M. Depletion of murine CD4+ T lymphocytes prevents antigen-induced airway hyperreactivity and pulmonary eosinophilia. Am J Respir Cell Mol Biol 1994; 10:587–593.

46. Gonzalo JA, Lloyd CM, Kremer L, Finger E, Martinez-A C, Siegelman MH, Cybulsky M, Gutierrez-Ramos JC. Eosinophil recruitment to the lung in a murine model of allergic inflammation. The role of T cells, chemokines and adhesion receptors. J Clin Invest 1996; 98:2332–2345.

47. Mosmann TR, Coffman RL. Th1 and Th2 cells: Different patterns of lymphokine secretion lead to different functional properties. Ann Rev Immunol 1989; 7: 145–173.

48. Campbell JJ, Haraldsen G, Pan J, Rottman J, Qin S, Ponath P, Andrew DP, Warnke R, Ruffing N, Kassam N, Wu L, Butcher EC. The chemokine receptor CCR4 in vascular recognition by cutaneous but not intestinal memory T cells. Nature 1999; 400:776–780.

49. Zabel BA, Agace WW, Campbell JJ, Heath HM, Parent D, Roberts AI, Ebert EC, Kassam N, Qin S, Zovko M, LaRosa GJ, Yang LL, Soler D, Butcher EC, Ponath PD, Parker CM, Andrew DP. Human G protein-coupled receptor GPR-9-6/CC chemokine receptor 9 is selectively expressed on intestinal homing T lymphocytes, mucosal lymphocytes, and thymocytes and is required for thymus-expressed chemokine-mediated chemotaxis. J Exp Med 1999; 190:1241–1256.

50. Campbell JJ, Brightling CE, Symon FA, Qin S, Murphy KE, Hodge M, Andrew DP, Wu L, Butcher EC, Wardlaw AJ. Expression of chemokine receptors by lung T cells from normal and asthmatic subjects. J Immunol 2001; 166: 2842–2848.

51. Sallusto F, Mackay CR, Lanzavecchia A. Selective expression of the eotaxin receptor CCR3 by human T helper 2 cells. Science 1997; 277:2005–2007.

52. Bonecchi R, Bianchi G, Bordignon PP, D'Ambrosio D, Lang R, Borsatti A, Sozzani S, Allavena P, Gray PA, Mantovani A, Sinigaglia F. Differential expression of chemokine receptors and chemotactic responsiveness of type 1 T helper cells (Th1s) and Th2s. J Exp Med 1998; 187:129–134.

53. Daugherty BL, Siciliano SJ, DeMartino J, Malkowitz L, Sirontino A, Springer MS. Cloning, expression and characterization of the human eosinophil eotaxin receptor. J Exp Med 1996; 183:2349–2354.

54. Sallusto F, Lenig D, Mackay CR, Lanzavecchia A. Flexible programs of chemokine receptor expression on human polarised T helper 1 and 2 lymphocytes. J Exp Med 1998; 187:875–883.

55. Andrew DP, Chang MS, McNinch J, Wathen ST, Rihanek M, Tseng J, Spellberg JP, Elias CG 3rd. STCP-1 (MDC) CC chemokine acts specifically on chronically activated Th2 lymphocytes and is produced by monocytes on stimulation with Th2 cytokines IL-4 and IL-13. J Immunol 1998; 161:5027–5038.

56. Zingoni A, Soto H, Hedrick JA, Stoppacciaro A, Storlazzi CT, Sinigaglia F, D'Ambrosio D, O'Garra A, Robinson D, Rocchi M, Santoni A, Zlotnik A, Napolitano M. The chemokine receptor CCR8 is preferentially expressed in Th2 but not Th1 cells. J Immunol 1998; 161:547–551.

57. D'Ambrosio D, Iellem A, Bonecchi R, Mazzeo D, Sozzani S, Mantovani A, Sinigaglia F. Selective up-regulation of chemokine receptors CCR4 and CCR8 upon activation of polarized human type 2 Th cells. J Immunol 1998; 161:5111–5115.

58. Lloyd CM, Delaney T, Nguyen T, Tian J, Martinez-A C, Coyle AJ, Gutierrez-Ramos JC. CC chemokine receptor (CCR)3/Eotaxin is followed by CCR4/

monocyte-derived chemokine in mediating pulmonary T helper lymphocyte type 2 recruitment after serial antigen challenge in vivo. J Exp Med 2000; 191:265–273.

59. Chensue SW, Lukacs NW, Yang TY, Shang X, Frait KA, Kunkel SL, Kung T, Wiekowski MT, Hedrick JA, Cook DN, Zingoni A, Narula SK, Zlotnik A, Barrat FJ, O'Garra A, Napolitano M, Lira SA. Aberrant in vivo t helper type 2 cell response and impaired eosinophil recruitment in cc chemokine receptor 8 knockout mice. J Exp Med 2001; 193:573–584.

60. Karpus WJ, Lukacs NW, Kennedy KJ, Smith WS, Hurst SD, Barrett TA. Differential CC chemokine-induced enhancement of T helper cell cytokine production. J Immunol 1997; 158:4129–4136.

61. Gu L, Tseng S, Horner RM, Tam C, Loda M, Rollins BJ. Control of TH2 polarization by the chemokine monocyte chemoattractant protein-1. Nature 2000; 404:407–411.

62. Goebeler M, Schnarr B, Toksoy A, Kunz M, Brocker EB, Duschl A, Gillitzer R. Interleukin-13 selectively induces monocyte chemoattractant protein-1 synthesis and secretion by human endothelial cells. Involvement of IL-4R alpha and Stat6 phosphorylation. Immunology 1997; 91:450–457.

63. Pype JL, Dupont LJ, Menten P, Van Coillie E, Opdenakker G, Van Damme J, Chung KF, Demedts MG, Verleden GM. Expression of monocyte chemotactic protein (MCP)-1, MCP-2, and MCP-3 by human airway smooth-muscle cells. Modulation by corticosteroids and T-helper 2 cytokines. Am J Respir Cell Mol Biol 1999; 21:528–536.

64. Zhang S, Lukacs NW, Lawless VA, Kunkel SL, Kaplan MH. Cutting edge: differential expression of chemokines in Th1 and Th2 cells is dependent on Stat6 but not Stat4. J Immunol 2000; 165:10–14.

65. Sanderson CJ. Interleukin-5, eosinophils, and disease. Blood 1992; 79:3101–3109.

66. Palframan RT, Collins PD, Severs NJ, Rothery S, Williams TJ, Rankin SM. Mechanisms of acute eosinophil mobilization from the bone marrow stimulated by interleukin 5: the role of specific adhesion molecules and phosphatidylinositol 3-kinase. J Exp Med 1998; 188:1621–1632.

67. Schweizer RC, van Kessel-Welmers BA, Warringa RA, Maikoe T, Raaijmakers JA, Lammers JW, Koenderman L. Mechanisms involved in eosinophil migration. Platelet-activating factor-induced chemotaxis and interleukin-5-induced chemokinesis are mediated by different signals. J Leuk Biol 1996; 59:347–356.

68. Shahabuddin S, Ponath P, Schleimer RP. Migration of eosinophils across endothelial cell monolayers: interactions among IL-5, endothelial-activating cytokines, and C-C chemokines. J Immunol 2000; 164:3847–3854.

69. Collins PD, Marleau S, Griffiths-Johnson DA, Jose PJ, Williams TJ. Cooperation between interleukin-5 and the chemokine eotaxin to induce eosinophil accumulation in vivo. J Exp Med 1995; 182:1169–1174.

70. Mould AW, Matthaei Ki, Young IG, Foster PS. Relationship between interleukin-5 and eotaxin in regulating blood and tissue eosinophilia in mice. J Clin Invest 1997; 99:1064–1071.

71. Humbles AA, Conroy DM, Marleau S, Rankin SM, Palframan RT, Proudfoot AEI, Wells TN, Li D, Jeffery PK, Griffiths-Johnson DA, Williams TJ, Jose PJ. Kinetics of eotaxin generation and its relationship to eosinophil accumulation in

allergic airways disease: analysis in a guinea pig model in vivo. J Exp Med 1997; 186:601–612.

72. Cook EB, Stahl JL, Lilly CM, Haley KJ, Sanchez H, Luster AD, Graziano FM, Rothenberg ME. Epithelial cells are a major cellular source of the chemokine eotaxin in the guinea pig lung. Allergy Asthma Proc 1998; 19:15–22.

73. Palframan RT, Collins PD, Williams TJ, Rankin SM. Eotaxin induces a rapid release of eosinophils and their progenitors from the bone marrow. Blood 1998; 91:2240–2248.

74. Freedman NJ, Lefkowitz RJ. Desensitization of G protein–coupled receptors. Recent Prog Horm Res 1996; 51:319–351.

75. Sabroe I, Williams TJ, Hebert CA, Collins PD. Chemoattractant cross-desensitisation of the human neutrophil interleukin-8 receptor involves receptor internalisation and differential receptor subtype regulation. J Immunol 1997; 158:1361–1369.

76. Arai H, Tsou Cl, Charo IF. Chemotaxis in a lymphocyte cell line transfected with C-C chemokine receptor 2B: evidence that directed migration is mediated by betagamma dimers released by activation of Galphai-coupled receptors. Proc Natl Acad Sci USA 1997; 94:14495–14499.

77. Arai H, Charo IF. Differential regulation of G-protein-mediated signaling by chemokine receptors. J Biol Chem 1996; 271:21814–21819.

78. Bowman EP, Campbell JJ, Druey KM, Scheschonka A, Kehrl JH, Butcher EC. Regulation of chemotactic and proadhesive responses to chemoattractant receptors by RGS (regulator of G-protein signaling) family members. J Biol Chem 1998; 273:28040–28048.

79. De Vries L, Mousli M, Wurmser A, Farquhar MG. GAIP, a protein that specifically interacts with the trimeric G protein G alpha i3, is a member of a protein family with a highly conserved core domain. Proc Natl Acad Sci USA 1995; 92:11916–11920.

80. Koelle MR, Horvitz HR. EGL-10 regulates G protein signaling in the *C. elegans* nervous system and shares a conserved domain with many mammalian proteins. Cell 1996; 84:115–125.

81. Druey KM, Blumer KJ, Kang VH, Kehrl JH. Inhibition of G-protein-mediated MAP kinase activation by a new mammalian gene family. Nature 1996; 379:742–746.

82. Dohlman HG, Thorner J. RGS proteins and signaling by heterotrimeric G proteins. J Biol Chem 1997; 272:3871–3874.

83. De Vries L, Gist FM. RGS proteins: more than just GAPs for heterotrimeric G proteins. Trends Cell Biol 1999; 9:138–144.

84. Xu X, Zeng W, Popov S, Berman DM, Davignon I, Yu K, Yowe D, Offermanns S, Muallem S, Wilkie TM. RGS proteins determine signaling specificity of Gq-coupled receptors. J Biol Chem 1999; 274:3549–3556.

85. Dulin NO, Sorokin A, Reed E, Elliott S, Kehrl JH, Dunn MJ. RGS3 inhibits G protein-mediated signaling via translocation to the membrane and binding to Galpha11. Mol Cell Biol 1999; 19:714–723.

86. Neill JD, Duck LW, Sellers JC, Musgrove LC, Scheschonka A, Druey KM, Kehrl JH. Potential role for a regulator of G protein signaling (RGS3) in gonadotropin-

releasing hormone (GnRH) stimulated desensitization. Endocrinology 1997; 138:843–846.

87. Snow BE, Hall RA, Krumins AM, Brothers GM, Bouchard D, Brothers CA, Chung S, Mangion J, Gilman AG, Lefkowitz RJ, Siderovski DP. GTPase activating specificity of RGS12 and binding specificity of an alternatively spliced PDZ (PSD-95/Dlg/ZO-1) domain. J Biol Chem 1998; 273:17749–17755.

88. Zeng W, Xu X, Popov S, Mukhopadhyay S, Chidiac P, Swistok J, Danho W, Yagaloff KA, Fisher SL, Ross EM, Muallem S, Wilkie TM. The N-terminal domain of RGS4 confers receptor-selective inhibition of G protein signaling. J Biol Chem 1998; 273:34687–34690.

89. Reif K, Cyster JG. RGS molecule expression in murine B lymphocytes and ability to down-regulate chemotaxis to lymphoid chemokines. J Immunol 2000; 164:4720–4729.

90. Wu D, LaRosa GJ, Simon MI. G protein-coupled signal transduction pathways for interleukin-8. Science 1993; 261:101–103.

91. Bokoch GM. Chemoattractant signaling and leukocyte activation. Blood 1995; 86:1649–1660.

92. Murphy PM. Chemokine receptors: structure, function and role in microbial pathogenesis. Cyt Growth Factor Rev 1996; 7:47–64.

93. Kuang Y, Wu Y, Jiang H, Wu D. Selective G protein coupling by C-C chemokine receptors. J Biol Chem 1996; 271:3975–3978.

94. Bacon KB, Szabo MC, Yssel H, Bolen JB, Schall TJ. RANTES induces tyrosine kinase activity of stably complexed p125FAK and ZAP-70 in human T cells. J Exp Med 1996; 184:873–882.

95. Turner SJ, Domin J, Waterfield MD, Ward SG, Westwick J. The CC chemokine monocyte chemotactic peptide-1 activates both the class I p85/p110 phosphatidylinositol 3-kinase and the class II PI3K-C2alpha. J Biol Chem 1998; 25987–25995.

96. Huang R, Lian JP, Robinson D, Badwey JA. Neutrophils stimulated with a variety of chemoattractants exhibit rapid activation of p21-activated kinases (Paks): separate signals are required for activation and inactivation of paks. Mol Cell Biol 1998; 18:7130–7138.

97. Mellado M, Rodriguez-Frade JM, Aragay A, del Real G, Martin AM, Vila-Coro AJ, Serrano A, Mayor F Jr, Martinez-A C. The chemokine monocyte chemotactic protein 1 triggers Janus kinase 2 activation and tyrosine phosphorylation of the CCR2B receptor. J Immunol 1998; 161:805–813.

98. Ganju RK, Dutt P, Wu L, Newman W, Avraham H, Avraham S, Groopman JE. Beta-chemokine receptor CCR5 signals via the novel tyrosine kinase RAFTK. Blood 1998; 91:791–797.

99. Kampen GT, Stafford S, Adachi T, Jinquan T, Quan S, Grant JA, Skov PS, Poulsen LK, Alam R. Eotaxin induces degranulation and chemotaxis of eosinophils through the activation of ERK2 and p38 mitogen-activated protein kinases. Blood 2000; 95:1911–1917.

100. Simmons G, Clapham PR, Picard L, Offord RE, Rosenkilde MM, Schwartz TW, Buser R, Wells TN, Proudfoot AE. Potent inhibition of HIV-1 infectivity in macrophage and lymphocytes by a novel CCR5 antagonist. Science 1997; 276:276–279.

101. Baba M, Nishimura O, Kanzaki N, Okamoto M, Sawada H, Iizawa Y, Shiraishi M, Aramaki Y, Okonogi K, Ogawa Y, Meguro K, Fujino M. A small-molecule, nonpeptide CCR5 antagonist with highly potent and selective anti-HIV-1 activity. Proc Natl Acad Sci USA 1999; 96:5698–5703.

102. Howard OM, Korte T, Tarasova NI, Grimm M, Turpin JA, Rice WG, Michejda CJ, Blumenthal R, Oppenheim JJ. Small molecule inhibitor of HIV-1 cell fusion blocks chemokine receptor-mediated function. J Leukoc Biol 1998; 64:6–13.

103. Sabroe I, Peck MJ, Van Keulen BJ, Jorritsma A, Simmons G, Clapham PR, Williams TJ, Pease JE. A small molecule antagonist of the chemokine receptors CCR1 and CCR3: Potent inhibition of eosinophil function and CCR3-mediated HIV-1 entry. J Biol Chem 2000; 275:25985–25992.

104. Proudfoot AE, Power CA, Hoogewerf AJ, Montjovent MO, Borlat F, Offord RE, Wells TN. Extension of recombinant human RANTES by the retention of the initiating methionine produces a potent antagonist. J Biol Chem 1996; 271:2599–2603.

105. Nibbs RJ, Salcedo TW, Campbell JD, Yao XT, Li Y, Nardelli B, Olsen HS, Morris TS, Proudfoot AE, Patel VP, Graham GJ. C-C chemokine receptor 3 antagonism by the beta-chemokine macrophage inflammatory protein 4, a property strongly enhanced by an amino-terminal alanine-methionine swap. J Immunol 2000; 164(3):1488–1497.

106. Elsner J, Petering H, Hochstetter R, Kimmig D, Wells TN, Kapp A, Proudfoot AE. The CC chemokine antagonist Met-RANTES inhibits eosinophil effector functions through the chemokine receptors CCR1 and CCR3. Eur J Immunol 1997; 27:2892–2898.

107. Elsner J, Mack M, Bruhl H, Dulkys Y, Kimmig D, Simmons G, Clapham PR, Schlondorff D, Kapp A, Wells TN, Proudfoot AE. Differential activation of CC chemokine receptors by AOP-RANTES. J Biol Chem 2000; 275:7787–7794.

108. Alcami A, Koszinowski UH. Viral mechanisms of immune evasion. Mol Med Today 2000; 6:365–372.

109. Kledal TN, Rosenkilde MM, Coulin F, Simmons G, Johnsen AH, Alouani S, Power CA, Luttichau HR, Gerstoft J, Clapham PR, Clark-Lewis I, Wells TN, Schwartz TW. A broad-spectrum chemokine antagonist encoded by Kaposi's sarcoma–associated herpesvirus. Science 1997; 277:1656–1659.

110. 3: Boshoff C, Endo Y, Collins PD, Takeuchi Y, Reeves JD, Schweickart VL, Siani MA, Sasaki T, Williams TJ, Gray PW, Moore PS, Chang Y, Weiss RA. Angiogenic and HIV-inhibitory functions of KSHV-encoded chemokines. Science 1997; 278:290–294.

111. Sozzani S, Allavena P, Vecchi A, Van Damme J, Mantovani A. Chemokine receptors: interaction with HIV-1 and viral-encoded chemokines. Pharm Acta Helv 2000; 74:305–312.

112. Gao JL, Murphy PM. Human cytomegalovirus open reading frame US28 encodes a functional beta chemokine receptor. J Biol Chem 1994; 269:28539–28542.

113. Health H, Qin S, Rao P, Wu L, LaRosa G, Kassam N, Ponath PD, Mackay CR. Chemokine receptor usage by human eosinophils. The importance of CCR3 demonstrated using an antagonistic monoclonal antibody. J Clin Invest 1997; 99:178–184.

114. Sabroe I, Conroy DM, Gerard NP, Li Y, Collins PD, Post TW, Jose PJ, Williams TJ, Gerard CJ, Ponath PD. Cloning and characterisation of the guinea pig eosinophil eotaxin receptor, CCR3: blockade using a monoclonal antibody in vivo. J Immunol 1998; 161:6139–6147.

115. Rothenberg ME, MacLean JA, Pearlman E, Luster AD, Leder P. Targeted disruption of the chemokine eotaxin partially reduces antigen-induced tissue eosinophilia. J Exp Med 1997; 185:785–790.

116. Yang Y, Loy J, Ryseck RP, Carrasco D, Bravo R. Antigen-induced eosinophilic lung inflammation develops in mice deficient in chemokine eotaxin. Blood 1998; 92:3912–3923.

117. Stafford S, Li H, Forsythe PA, Ryan M, Bravo R, Alam R. Monocyte chemotactic protein-3 (MCP-3)/fibroblast-induced cytokine (FIC) in eosinophilic inflammation of the airways and the inhibitory effects of an anti-MCP-3/FIC antibody. J Immunol 1997; 158:4953–4960.

118. Gonzalo JA, Lloyd CM, Peled A, Delaney T, Coyle AJ, Gutierrez-Ramos JC. Critical involvement of the chemotactic axis CXCR4/stromal cell-derived factor-1 alpha in the inflammatory component of allergic airway disease. J Immunol 2000; 165:499–508.

119. Blease K, Mehrad B, Standiford TJ, Lukacs NW, Kunkel SL, Chensue SW, Lu B, Gerard CJ, Hogaboam CM. Airway remodeling is absent in CCR1-/- mice during chronic fungal allergic airway disease. J Immunol 2000; 165:1564–1572.

120. MacLean JA, De Sanctis GT, Ackerman KG, Drazen JM, Sauty A, DeHaan E, Green FH, Charo IF, Luster AD. CC chemokine receptor-2 is not essential for the development of antigen-induced pulmonary eosinophilia and airway hyperresponsiveness. J Immunol 2000; 165:6568–6575.

121. Chvatchko Y, Hoogewerf AJ, Meyer A, Alouani S, Juillard P, Buser R, Conquet F, Proudfoot AE, Wells TN, Power CA. A key role for CC chemokine receptor 4 in lipopolysaccharide-induced endotoxic shock. J Exp Med 2000; 191:1755–1764.

122. De Sanctis GT, MacLean JA, Qin S, Wolyniec WW, Grasemann H, Yandava CN, Jiao A, Noonan T, Stein-Streilein J, Green FH, Drazen JM. Interleukin-8 receptor modulates IgE production and B-cell expansion and trafficking in allergen-induced pulmonary inflammation. J Clin Invest 1999; 103:507–515.

17

Cytokine Regulation of Bronchial Hyperresponsiveness

JOHAN C. KIPS and ROMAIN A. PAUWELS

Ghent University Hospital
Ghent, Belgium

I. Introduction

Bronchial hyperresponsiveness (BHR) is a cardinal feature of altered airway behavior in asthma. It describes the increased twitchiness of the airways, which results in a bronchoconstrictor response to a variety of stimuli at a level of intensity that in normal individuals is insufficient to affect airway caliber. The two main determinants of BHR are hypersensitivity and hyperreactivity of the airways (1,2). Hypersensitivity (or deviation supersensitivity) is reflected by a leftward shift of the dose–response curve to a bronchoconstrictor agonist. This is most likely caused by an increased accessibility of the agonist to its receptor site in the airway wall. Hyperreactivity (or nondeviation supersensitivity) describes the exaggerated maximal airway narrowing in asthmatics and is characterized by an increase or even loss of a plateau on the dose–response curve to bronchoconstrictor agonists (3). Clinically, hyperreactivity is more important than hypersensitivity because enhanced airway narrowing can lead to airway closure resulting in death by asphyxia. The precise mechanisms that underlie airway hyperreactivity remain to be fully established. Different hypotheses have highlighted the impact of an increase in airway wall thickness, loss of parenchymal elastic recoil on contracting airway smooth muscle, and increased smooth muscle contractility on this phenomenon (4–6) (Fig. 1). The development of structural airway changes, so-called airway remodeling, is thought to largely contribute to this phenomenon through alterations in the composition of the extracellular matrix (ECM) and smooth muscle hypertrophy (7).

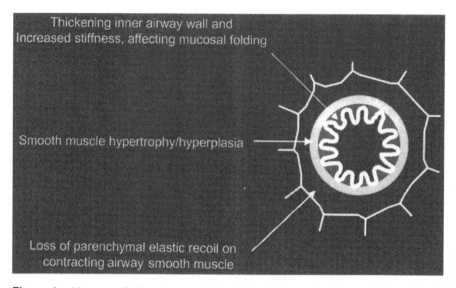

Figure 1 Airway wall changes postulated to contribute to airway hyperreactivity.

    How exactly each of the cytokines present in asthmatic airways reg-
ulates BHR also is unclear. Compared with normal individuals, asthmatic
airways contain increased amounts of a multitude of cytokines, which can
grossly be grouped into T-helper 2 (Th2), proinflammatory, and fibrogenic
cytokines, as well as chemokines. In addition, reduced levels of immumo-
dulatory molecules, such as interleukin-12 (IL-12) or interferon-γ (IFN-γ),
have been reported (8) (Fig. 2). At present, the potential contribution of
these various groups is deduced from descriptive data in humans, coupled to
a more functional analysis in in vivo animal models. An obvious limitation of
this approach has been the lack of an animal model that fully reflects all
features of asthma. Most of these models display a short-lived, relatively
small increase in airway responsiveness. In addition, the morphological
alterations are usually limited to acute inflammatory changes. However,
attempts are now increasingly undertaken to develop in vivo animal models
that display features of airway remodeling and a more persistent increase in
airway responsiveness, thus mimicking more closely human asthma (9).
Together with the increased availability of specific cytokine antagonists for
human use, it can be anticipated that this will lead to better insight into the
cytokine regulation of BHR. This, in turn, will probably result in novel
therapeutic strategies.
    In this chapter, rather than attempting to cover all cytokines we have
tried to focus on a few that have been highlighted as potential therapeutic
targets (Table 1).

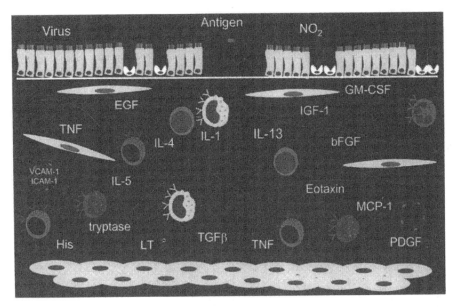

Figure 2 Schematic representation of the cytokine network in asthmatic airways.

II. Th2-Like Cytokines

Th2 CD4$^+$ T cells are currently considered to largely orchestrate the chronic mucosal inflammation underlying asthma (10). Within the range of cytokines produced by Th2 cells, IL-4, IL-13, IL-5, and IL-9 have attracted considerable interest to date.

A. IL-4/IL-13

IL-4 has a broad range of biological activities. In general terms, it can be described as the main cytokine involved in the pathogenesis of allergic responses, at the same time down-regulating acute inflammatory changes. Additional effects that seem of particular importance for asthma include stimulation of mucus-producing cells and fibroblasts, thus also implicating IL-4 in the pathogenesis of airway remodeling (11–13). Inhalation of recombinant human IL-4 has been confirmed to induce airway eosinophilia and to cause some increase in the degree of BHR in atopic asthmatics (14). In addition, bronchial biopsies have confirmed increased expression of IL-4 and the IL-4 receptor α chain (IL-4Rα), both at the protein and the mRNA level, in the airway mucosa of atopic and even nonatopic asthmatics, when compared with nonasthmatic controls (15–18). Polymorphisms of the IL-4 and IL-4Rα chain have also been related to asthma severity. In particular, the IL-4-589T allele, which has been

Table 1 Summary of Asthma-Related Cytokines

Main cellular source	Major effects
Th2 cytokines	
IL-4 Th2 cells, MC, Eo	Differentiation/proliferation Th2 cells Inhibition of development of Th1 cells
IL-4/IL-13	Isotype switching of B cells from IgG to IgE synthesis Up-regulation FcεRII and MHC Class II Ag expression on antigen-presenting cells Up-regulation endothelial VCAM-1 expression Down-regulation endothelial ICAM-1 expression Down-regulation production of proinflammatory cytokines (TNF-α, IL-1β) and chemokines (RANTES, IL-8) Promoting growth of human basophils and eosinophils Chemotaxis and activation of fibroblasts Stimulation of mucus production
IL-5 Th2 cells, Mc, Eo	Proliferation, differentiation, maturation, activation of eosinophils Enhanced eosinophil survival Responsiveness of eosinophils to homing signals Eosinophil chemoattraction at higher concentration Enhanced mediator release human basophils
IL-9 Th2 cells, Mc, Eo	Stimulation of T-cell proliferation Growth and increased survival of mast cells Increased IgE production by B lymphocytes and up-regulated expression of the α chain of the FcεR$_I$ Enhanced IL-5 receptor expression, differentiation and survival of eosinophils

Cytokine	Source cells	Functions
Proinflammatory cytokines TNF-α IL-1-β	CD4 cells, MC, Eo Macro, epithelial, smooth muscle cells	Induction of IL-8 production by neutrophils Induction of CC chemokine production by epithelial cells Maturation and migration of dendritic cells Up-regulation of endothelial adhesion molecules Increased production cytokines, chemokines, and growth factors Activation inflammatory cells and release of inflammatory mediators Increased expression of inducible NO synthase Stimulation fibroblast and airway smooth muscle proliferation Increased production of ECM proteins and MMP
Immunomodulatory cytokines IL-10	CD4 cells, monocytes macrophage, MC	Suppression proinflammatory cytokines production and up-regulation IL-1Ra synthesis Inhibition of MHC class II expression on APC Inhibition of IFN-γ and IL-2 production by TH1 cells Inhibition of IL-4 and IL-5 production by Th2 cells Inhibition of eosinophil survival and IL-4-induced IgE synthesis Growth costimulation of mast cells Inhibition of smooth muscle cell proliferation Reduction collagen and MMP synthesis
IFN-γ	Th1, CD8, NK cells	Inhibition of Th2 cell activation Inhibition of IL-4 induced IgE and IgG$_4$ synthesis by B cells Prevention of antigen-induced eosinophil recruitment Up-regulation adhesion molecules, release proinflammatory cytokines

(Continued)

Table 1 Continued

Main cellular source	Major effects
IL-12	DC, B cells, monocytes, macrophages	Enhanced Th1 cell development, inhibition expansion Th2 cells
		Stimulation of IFNγ production from NK and T cells
		Stimulation of IL-10 production from mononuclear cells
IL-18	Monocytes	Activation of NK cells and monocytes
		Induction of IL-13 and eotaxin production
		Coadministered with IL-12: induction IFN-γ synthesis, inhibition of IL-4-dependent IgE synthesis and up-regulation IL-12R expression

associated with increased IL-4 gene expression, was found to be a risk factor for life-threatening asthma (19). As for IL-4, increased expression of IL-13 mRNA and protein has been demonstrated in asthmatic airways (20–22). Both cytokines have very similar biological activities. This is reflected in the structure of their receptors. IL-4R is a heterodimer, consisting of the IL-4 binding IL-4Rα chain and a second chain that is either the γc chain, shared in common with the receptor for IL-2, IL-7, IL-9, and IL-15, or the IL-13Rα chain (23,24). IL-13R consists of the IL-13Rα1 or α2 chain, which binds IL-13, and again the IL-4Rα chain (25). The signal transduction pathway in common to the IL-4 and IL-13 receptor involves the intracytoplasmatic domain of both chains and is largely signal transducer and activator of transcription-6 (STAT-6) dependent. IL-4 can bind to both receptors through the IL-4Rα chain; IL-13 binds only to its own receptor. At the exception of T cells which do not carry functional IL-13 receptors, most cell types respond similarly to IL-4 and IL-13, indicating that they carry either IL-13R or both (26). Of note is that under certain experimental conditions, IL-4Rα-independent STAT6 activation by IL-13 has been shown to occur (27).

Because of this large degree of redundancy, it is difficult to establish with certainty the exact role of IL-4, relative to IL-13 in allergen-induced airway changes, but it would appear that both are functionally active. In vivo animal models illustrate that IL-4, but not IL-13, is essential for the development of antigen-induced eosinophil influx into the airways, IgE production, and increased airway responsiveness (28–31). The crucial role of IL-4 lies in its effect on Th2 cell development, rather than in IgE synthesis and subsequent mast cell degranulation, which in contrast to T cells has been shown not to play a major role in the induction of allergen-induced BHR (29,32–37). However, despite its important role in the initial Th2 cell development during primary sensitization, it would appear that IL-4 alone is insufficient to cause all allergen-induced airway changes (38,39) and that during secondary antigen exposure in sensitized animals, IL-13 release is functionally far more important (23,40). This concept is again illustrated in in vivo animal models. Neutralizing anti-IL-4 antibodies, administered during primary antigen sensitization, inhibit Th2 cell development (29). However, when given during secondary antigen presentation in sensitized animals, anti-IL-4 is far less effective in reducing Th2 cell cytokine production, eosinophil influx, and BHR, whereas anti-IL-4R antibodies maintain their therapeutic effect (29,38). This confirms in vitro data showing that once T cells have been committed to a Th2 phenotype, they become IL-4 independent (41). At the same time, this suggests that during secondary antigen exposure IL-13 plays a more important role than IL-4. In line with these observations, neutralizing endogenously released IL-13 with an IL-13Rα2 Fc fusion protein during secondary antigen exposure largely inhibits characteristics of asthma in murine models (30,42). Increasing evidence also implicates IL-13 in the pathogenesis of airway remodeling, which as already indicated is thought to contribute substantially to the pathogenesis of BHR.

Although both IL-4 and IL-13 activate fibroblast in vitro, transgene mice over-expressing IL-13 but not those overexpressing IL-4 develop airway fibrosis (39,43,44). Similarly, neutralization of IL-13 was shown to largely reverse the structural airway changes induced by chronic exposure to *Aspergillus* extract in CBA/J mice (45). Finally, the recent in vitro observation that IL-13, in contrast to IL-4, interferes with β_2-agonist-induced reduction in cell stiffness suggests that IL-13 might also have direct effects on airway smooth muscle behavior (46).

These observations have important therapeutic implications, as this leads to the assumption that interfering with the common pathway between IL-4 and IL-13, namely, IL-4Rα activation or STAT6 induction, might be of greater therapeutic benefit than antagonizing either cytokine alone. One of the approaches which has been developed in this respect consists of developing mutant IL-4 proteins that bind to the IL-4Rα chain without inducing signal transduction, thus acting as competitive antagonists to wild type IL-4 and IL-13 (47). Examples of mutant human IL-4 include IL-4.Y124D in which tyrosine in position 124 has been replaced by aspartic acid or the double mutant R121D/Y124D (Bay 19-996), which, in addition, includes substitution of arginine at position 121 by aspartic acid (48,49). Administration of this latter compound to sensitized primates prior to secondary allergen exposure inhibits the development of airway hyperresponsiveness and inflammation (50). Similarly, R121D/Y124D was shown in a hu-PBL-SCID model to inhibit the increase in airway responsiveness induced by exposure to aerosolized house dust mite allergen (51) (Fig. 3).

Another approach is to block the signal transduction pathway. Recent data indicate that this can be achieved through various mechanisms, including administration of SOCS-1 (suppressor of cytokine signaling-1) or decoy oligonucleotides, directed against STAT6 (52,53).

B. IL-5

The eosinophil is considered a key effector cell in the pathogenesis of allergic inflammation and the associated increase in BHR. Despite possible redundancy with other cytokines, such as IL-3 and granulocyte-macrophage colony-stimulating factor (GM-CSF), IL-5 seems to be the primary cytokine involved in vivo in the production, differentiation, maturation, and activation of eosinophils (54). Inhalation of IL-5 has been shown to increase the percentage of eosinophils in induced sputum and to augment airway hyperresponsiveness in asthma (55). Expression of IL-5 at mRNA and protein levels is increased in the mucosa of asthmatic airways (56,57). The functional role of IL-5 has been illustrated in animal models, showing that ovalbumin sensitization and exposure in IL-5$^{-/-}$ mice does not cause BHR, as opposed to that in wild-type mice (58). In subsequent studies it was shown that passive transfer of IL-4-secreting CD4$^+$ T cells from ovalbumin-sensitized wild-type mice to nonsensitized IL-5$^{-/-}$ mice led to airway eosinophilia and an increase in airway responsiveness when these

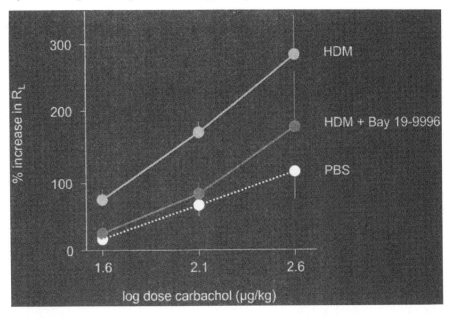

Figure 3 Effect of Bay 19-9996 on house dust mite allergen-induced airway reactivity in hu-PBL-SCID mice. (Adapted from Ref. 51.)

animals were exposed to aerosolized ovalbumin (59). Similarly, reconstituting IL-5 or IL-5 production, but not IgE, in IL-4$^{-/-}$ mice restored all the allergen-induced airway changes (60). This supports the concept that IL-4 and IL-5, possibly in combination with IL-13, are sequentially involved in the pathogenesis of allergic airway changes. IL-5 can affect airway responsiveness either directly, by influencing airway smooth muscle contractility (61), or indirectly through eosinophil recruitment (62). Eosinophils contain not only a wide range of proinflammatory and bronchoconstrictor agonists, but also a variety of profibrogenic cytokines and growth factors implicating these cells in the pathogenesis of airway remodeling (Fig. 4). Biopsy studies in human asthma relate increased expression of transforming growth factor-β (TGF-β) and IL-11 to the degree of subepithelial fibrosis (63,64). Both cytokines have colocalized predominantly to eosinophils. Antagonizing IL-5, therefore, could prove of substantial therapeutic benefit, especially as it would seem that the effect of IL-5 in humans is mainly focused on various aspects of eosinophil function, thus avoiding profound interference with the overall immune system. To date, the development of human anti-IL-5 antagonists has mainly focused on anti-human IL-5 monoclonal antibodies. Two single-dose trials in humans have been presented. SB240563 administered at a dose of 10 mg/kg in 8 subjects with mild allergic asthma was well tolerated and profoundly reduced circulating eosinophil counts for up to 16 weeks, but did not significantly inhibit the antigen-induced early or late asthmatic response, or the degree of airway

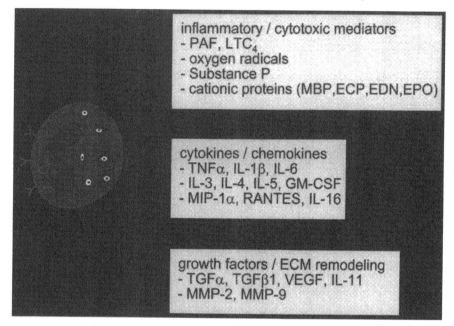

Figure 4   Eosinophil and related mediators and cytokines.

responsiveness (65). The second study was primarily a safety assessment in patients with severe asthma, treated with oral or high doses of inhaled steroids. A single dose of 1 mg/kg SCH55700 induced a similar long-lasting reduction in circulating blood eosinophil counts and was also well tolerated. However, no sustained difference on baseline FEV_1 was noted between 12 actively and 8 placebo-treated patients (66). The negative results of both studies would seem to question the importance of the IL-5/eosinophil axis in the pathogenesis of asthma, thus adding to previous animal studies that dissociate airway eosinophilia from airway responsiveness (67–69) or observations in humans that failed to correlate the degree of BHR to eosinophil numbers in biopsies or sputum from patients with mild asthma (70,71). However, before dismissing the role of the eosinophil in asthma, a few points need to be further considered. Eosinophils are predominantly tissue-dwelling cells. It cannot be excluded that chemotactic stimuli within the airways are sufficiently strong to maintain large number of eosinophils within the mucosa, despite the reduction in circulating eosinophil counts. SB240563 also significantly reduced sputum eosinophil counts (65). However, to what extent this correlates with depletion of tissue eosinophils remains to be fully established. In addition, in view of the possible role of the eosinophil on airway remodeling, a far more prolonged eosinophil clearance from the airway mucosa might be required to influence the clinical characteristics of the disease. Finally, it needs to be borne in mind that, within asthma, subgroups are likely to exist that might not all be eosinophil driven. Both above-mentioned studies were conducted in a limited number of patients who were not selected for eosinophils in blood or sputum. Larger trials that take into account these various points are required to further evaluate the role of IL-5 and the eosinophil in the pathogenesis of asthma, and BHR in particular.

C. IL-9

IL-9 is mainly derived from Th2 cells albeit that, as for the previously mentioned Th2 cytokines, other cellular sources have also been identified, including mast cells and eosinophils (72,73). IL-9 production by T cells is stimulated by IL-2, IL-10, IL-1, and TGF-β and inhibited by IFN-γ and IL-12. In vitro data indicate that, among other features, IL-9 stimulates activation and growth of T cells, supports the growth and increases the survival of mast cells, enhances the production of IgE from B cells, and induces CC chemokine production by epithelial cells. The potential role of IL-9 in asthma is further supported by the observation that lung specific overexpression in transgenic mice induces BHR, in conjunction with morphological changes that bear similarities to asthma (74). Human biopsy studies show increased expression of IL-9 in bronchial tissue from asthmatics (75). A correlation was found between IL-9 mRNA expression and methacholine responsiveness. In addition, genetic linkage analysis studies demonstrate an association between the IL-9 locus and BHR (76). The functional contribution relative to other Th2 cytokines remains to be further addressed.

III. Chemokines

Recruitment of inflammatory cells into the airway mucosa requires, in conjunction with the immunoregulatory activity of Th2 cells, expression of adhesion molecules on vascular endothelium and chemokine activity. An abundance of chemokines and chemokine receptors has been identified. Chemokines have been divided into C, CC, CXC, and CX3C based on the number and position of cysteine residues within their amino acid sequence. The overall biological activity of the different chemokines within each structurally related group is largely similar. The CXC or α-chemokines principally attract neutrophils and have therefore mainly been related to acute inflammatory processes. To date, investigation into the role of chemokines in allergic inflammation has focused predominantly on the CC or β-chemokine family, as they express chemotactic activity toward eosinophils as well as dendritic cells, T lymphocytes, basophils, and monocytes (77). The precise functional role of each chemokine within this group remains to be fully explored. A sequential role for different chemokines in the antigen-induced eosinophil recruitment and induction of BHR has been suggested (78,79). Of particular interest is the observation that the CCR3 receptor expression is limited to eosinophils, basophils, and Th2 cells. Several chemokines bind to the CCR3 receptor, including RANTES (regulated upon activation, normal T-cell expressed and secreted), MCP-3, MCP-4, and the CCR3-specific ligand eotaxin. Increased expression of eotaxin and the CCR3 receptor have been described in the bronchial mucosa from asthmatics (80). Eotaxin expression was shown to correlate with the degree of BHR. In addition, plasma eotaxin levels have been associated with impaired lung function in a large cohort of asthmatics (81). These various observations have raised interest in the CCR3 receptor as a potential therapeutic target (82). Blockage of the CCR3 receptor, either with monoclonal antibodies or with modified CC chemokines, such as methionylated (Met)-RANTES, or amino-oxypentane (AOP)-RANTES, have proven to reduce antigen-induced hyperresponsiveness in an in vivo animal model (79,83).

IV. Proinflammatory Cytokines

Another group of cytokines that could profoundly regulate BHR in asthma are the proinflammatory cytokines IL-1β and tumor necrosis factor-α (TNF-α) (84). The pleiotropic activities of TNF-α include proinflammatory effects, such as leukocyte recruitment through up-regulation of adhesion molecules on vascular endothelial cells and induction of chemokine synthesis (85). In addition, TNF-α and IL-1β might also play a central role in the remodeling process (86). TNF-α has been reported to increase the transcription of genes encoding for growth factors, such as platelet-derived growth factor (PDGF) or heparin-binding epithelial growth factor (HB-EGF), and to up-regulate expression of epithelial growth factor receptor (EGF-R) (87–89). The importance of the EGF system in the pathogenesis of remodeling has been highlighted (90). TNF-α also has the potential to stimulate the proliferation of smooth muscle cells and fibroblasts and to increase the production of ECM proteins, including collagen and tenascin, as well as matrix metalloproteinases (91–97). Moreover, by augmenting Gα protein expression, TNF-α has also been shown to increase smooth muscle tone and to enhance the carbachol-induced inhibition of adenylcyclase (98).

In view of this wide range of biological activities, it is not surprising that TNF-α can cause BHR as has been demonstrated in both animals and humans (99–101). Furthermore, elevated levels of TNF-α have been detected in sputum, bronchoalveolar lavage (BAL) fluids and biopsies from asthmatics (102–105). Genetic analysis also link TNFα to characteristics of asthma, as an association has been described between −308 TNF-α promotor polymorphism and the degree of BHR (106–108). Allele 2 of the −308 TNF-α polymorphism is characterized by increased releasability of TNF-α in response to various stimuli. Specific TNF antagonists have been developed (109). Their potential in asthma remains to be evaluated.

V. Immunomodulating Cytokines

An important aspect that must be borne in mind when evaluating the contribution of individual cytokines to the pathogenesis of BHR is that they act within a network. Cytokines that have the potential to counteract the effect of the above-mentioned Th2 and proinflammatory cytokines and might therefore be of therapeutic benefit include IFN-γ, IL-10, IL-12, and IL-18 (Fig. 5).

A. IL-10

IL-10 is a pleiotropic cytokine that has the potential to down-regulate both Th1 and Th2 cell–driven inflammatory processes (110). Of interest is that IL-10 might also have a beneficial effect on airway remodeling, as it has been shown to reduce collagen type I synthesis and vascular smooth muscle proliferation (111,112). However, the exact functional role of IL-10 at present remains unclear. Whether the expression of IL-10 is changed in asthma is uncertain, as in some studies reduced but in another study increased BAL levels were found (113–115). In animal models, exogenous administration of IL-10 during secondary antigen presentation reduces airway eosinophilia (116,117), whereas airway eosinophilia and total serum IgE are increased in

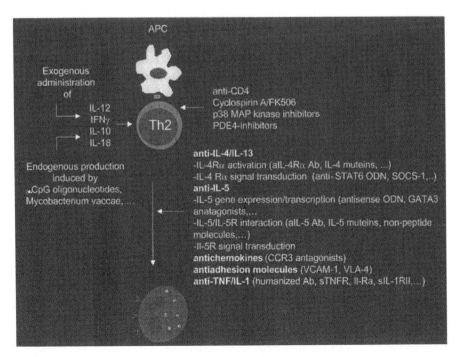

Figure 5 Possible anticytokine strategies in asthma.

sensitized IL-10 knockout mice (116–119). However, the effects of IL-10 on airway responsiveness are somewhat more contradictory. In some studies endogenous production of IL-10 was shown to dampen airway responsiveness (119), whereas other studies have shown that IL-10 enhances the allergen-induced increase in airway responsiveness, despite the reduction in eosinophil recruitment (117,120).

B. IL-12, IL-18, IFN-γ

IFN-γ has also been shown to prevent development of antigen-induced airway eosinophilia and hyperresponsiveness in in vivo animal models (121–123). Similarly, IFN-γ $R^{-/-}$ mice develop a prolonged airway eosinophilia in response to allergen (124). To date, however, exogenous administration of IFN-γ at tolerable doses in humans has proven disappointing. Nebulized IFN-γ was reported not to influence baseline FEV_1 in mild asthma, nor did subcutaneous administration of IFN-γ offer any improvement in steroid-dependent asthmatics (125,126).

IL-12 is produced by antigen-presenting cells and has been identified as a necessary growth factor for Th1 cell development during primary antigen presentation (127). In vivo animal models have confirmed that exogenous administration of IL-12 during the primary sensitization process suppresses antigen-induced Th2 cell development, favoring Th1 cell differentiation (128,129). More interesting from a therapeutic perspective is that even when only administered during secondary antigen exposure in sensitized animals, IL-12 retains the capacity to inhibit allergen-induced eosinophilia and airway hyperresponsiveness (128). The precise mechanisms underlying this effect are largely unknown. Fully committed Th2 cells have been shown to lose their IL-12 responsiveness (130). Therefore, reversal of a Th2 toward a Th1 phenotype at this stage is unlikely. IL-12 is also known to induce the production of IFN-γ and to down-regulate IL-5 synthesis, possibly through endogenous release of IL-10 (131,132). However, it has been shown that IL-12 retains its immunomodulatory effect in IFN-γ$R^{-/-}$ or IL-10$R^{-/-}$ mice (133,134). Therefore, the exact mechanisms of these IL-12-mediated effects need to be further established. Studies in humans indicate that IL-12 expression is reduced in bronchial biopsies from asthmatics individuals (21). However, whether exogenous administration of IL-12 will prove a therapeutic option at present is unclear. Cancer studies have revealed that treatment with IL-12 carries significant toxicity, limiting the dose that can be given (135). A recent allergen challenge study in mild asthma indicated that, despite substantially reducing circulating eosinophil counts, IL-12 did not influence the early or late asthmatic response (136). In addition, although IL-12 was given systemically in incremental doses, as is advocated to reduce toxicity, side effects still occurred. These included the development of a flu-like syndrome, increases in serum hepatic transaminases, and cardiac arrhythmias.

Alternative strategies that avoid the systemic toxicity but at the same time further enhance the local immunomodulatory effect of IL-12 are currently being explored. One of the possibilities consists of combining low doses of IL-12 to other cytokines. Interesting in this respect is the apparent synergistic activity with IL-18. IL-18 is mainly secreted by macrophages and was initially described as IFN-γ releasing factor (137). The absence of endogenous IL-18 enhances antigen-induced airway eosinophilia (138). However, the effect of exogenous IL-18 seems to depend on the circumstances of administration. It has been shown that when given alone IL-18 enhances antigen-induced recruitment of eosinophils into the airways of sensitized animals, possibly through induction of IL-13 and eotaxin synthesis (139,140). On the other hand, when given together with IL-12, Il-18 acts synergistically to induce IFN-γ production, inhibit IL-4-dependent IgE synthesis, and prevent antigen-induced BHR (141).

Another potential strategy consists of inducing the endogenous production of these immunomodulatory cytokines. Due to their paracrine activity, release within the mucosa might result in a far more pronounced effect yet have few side effects. A possible inducer that is being explored includes attenuated mycobacteria. Administration of *Mycobacterium vaccae* was reported to attenuate the allergen-induced late asthmatic response in atopic individuals (142). However, repeated low-dose administration in house dust mite allergic subjects with moderate to severe asthma revealed ineffective (143).

Another possibility is the administration of oligodeoxynucleotides (ODNs) containing unmethylated CpG motifs. These are potent immunomodulators that were initially thought to reverse a Th2 to a Th1 cell phenotype (144). Subsequent studies have shown that although they cannot fully redirect neonatally triggered Th2 cell development (145), they have an overall effect that counteracts Th2 stimulation. This includes release of IL-10, IL-12, IL-18, TNF-α, and IFN-α + IFN-β from mononuclear cells and IFN-γ from natural killer cells (146–152). As a result, when given prior to secondary antigen exposure, CpG ODNs inhibit antigen-induced BHR in in vivo animal models (153). Systemic administration, especially at higher doses, again results in toxicity (154,155). However, when given in lower doses together with antigen intratracheally, thus potentially avoiding systemic effects, the protective effect persists (156,157). Of particular interest from a therapeutic perspective is the observation from animal models that CpG-containing constructs not only prevent but may even reverse already established allergen-induced airway inflammation and hyperresponsiveness (158). This characteristic seems of particular interest for the development of novel forms of antigen-specific immunotherapy. Reversal of antigen-induced BHR has been confirmed by vaccination with an allergen cDNA containing plasmid. To be fully effective, however, fusion of the plasmid to IL-18 cDNA was required (159). These possible avenues to novel treatment modalities are currently being explored.

VI. Conclusion

It is clear that a wide range of cytokines known to be present in asthmatic airways have the potential to influence the degree of BHR. The functional role of each individual cytokine is largely determined by the presence of other components of the cytokine network that underlies asthma. Influencing this network either by antagonizing Th2 or proinflammatory cytokines or enhancing the effect of counteracting cytokines such as IL-12 or IL-18 remains an interesting therapeutic target for asthma.

References

1. Woolcock AJ, Salome CM, Yan K. The shape of the dose-response curve to histamine in asthmatic and normal subjects. Am Rev Respir Dis 1984; 130(1):71–75.
2. Sterk PJ, Bel EH. The shape of the dose-response curve to inhaled bronchoconstrictor agents in asthma and in chronic obstructive pulmonary disease. Am Rev Respir Dis 1991; 143(6):1433–1437.
3. Moreno RH, Hogg JC, Paré PD. Mechanics of airway narrowing. Am Rev Respir Dis 1986; 133:1171–1180.
4. Lambert RK, Wiggs BR, Kuwano K, Hogg JC, Pare PD. Functional significance of increased airway smooth muscle in asthma and COPD. J Appl Physiol 1993; 74(6):2771–2781.
5. Macklem PT. A theoretical analysis of the effect of airway smooth muscle load on airway narrowing. Am J Respir Crit Care Med 1996; 153(1):83–89.
6. Schmidt D, Rabe KF. Immune mechanisms of smooth muscle hyperreactivity in asthma. J Allergy Clin Immunol 2000; 105(4):673–682.
7. Kips JC, Pauwels RA. Airway wall remodelling: does it occur and what does it mean? Clin Exp Allergy 1999; 29(11):1457–1466.
8. Chung KF, Barnes PJ. Cytokines in asthma. Thorax 1999; 54(9):825–857.
9. Kips JC, Palmans E, Vanacker N, Pauwels RA. Is there an animal model of airway remodeling? In: Howarth PH, Wilson JW, Bousquet J, Rak S, Pauwels RA, eds. Airway Remodeling. (Lung Biology in Health and Disease, Vol 155). New York: Marcel Dekker, 2001:261–270.
10. Bousquet J, Jeffery PK, Busse WW, Johnson M, Vignola AM. Asthma. From bronchoconstriction to airways inflammation and remodeling. Am J Respir Crit Care Med 2000; 161(5):1720–1745.
11. Dabbagh K, Takeyama K, Lee HM, Ueki IF, Lausier JA, Nadel JA. IL-4 induces mucin gene expression and goblet cell metaplasia in vitro and in vivo. J Immunol 1999; 162(10):6233–6237.
12. Trautmann A, Krohne G, Brocker EB, Klein CE. Human mast cells augment fibroblast proliferation by heterotypic cell-cell adhesion and action of IL-4. J Immunol 1998; 160(10):5053–5057.
13. Doucet C, Brouty-Boyé D, Pottin-Clemenceau C, Canonica GW, Jasmin C, Azzarone B. Interleukin (IL) 4 and IL-13 act on human lung fibroblasts. J Clin Invest 1998; 101:2129–2139.

14. Shi HZ, Deng JM, Xu H, Nong ZX, Xiao CQ, Liu ZM et al. Effect of inhaled interleukin-4 on airway hyperreactivity in asthmatics. Am J Respir Crit Care Med 1998; 157(6 Pt 1):1818–1821.

15. Humbert M, Durham SR, Ying S, Kimmitt P, Barkans J, Assoufi B et al. IL-4 and IL-5 mRNA and protein in bronchial biopsies from patients with atopic and nonatopic asthma: evidence against "intrinsic" asthma being a distinct immunopathologic entity. Am J Respir Crit Care Med 1996; 154(5):1497–1504.

16. Ying S, Humbert M, Barkans J, Corrigan CJ, Pfister R, Menz G et al. Expression of IL-4 and IL-5 mRNA and protein product by CD4+ and CD8+ T cells, eosinophils, and mast cells in bronchial biopsies obtained from atopic and nonatopic (intrinsic) asthmatics. J Immunol 1997; 158(7):3539–3544.

17. Bradding P, Roberts JA, Britten KM, Montefort S, Djukanovic R, Mueller R et al. Interleukin-4, -5, and -6 and tumor necrosis factor-alpha in normal and asthmatic airways: evidence for the human mast cell as a source of these cytokines. Am J Respir Cell Mol Biol 1994; 10(5):471–480.

18. Kotsimbos TC, Ghaffar O, Minshall EM, Humbert M, Durham SR, Pfister R et al. Expression of the IL-4 receptor alpha-subunit is increased in bronchial biopsy specimens from atopic and nonatopic asthmatic subjects. J Allergy Clin Immunol 1998; 102(5):859–866.

19. Sandford AJ, Chagani T, Zhu S, Weir TD, Bai TR, Spinelli JJ et al. Polymorphisms in the IL4, IL4RA, and FCERIB genes and asthma severity. J Allergy Clin Immunol 2000; 106(1 Pt 1):135–140.

20. Humbert M, Durham SR, Kimmitt P, Powell N, Assoufi B, Pfister R et al. Elevated expression of messenger ribonucleic acid encoding IL-13 in the bronchial mucosa of atopic and nonatopic subjects with asthma. J Allergy Clin Immunol 1997; 99(5):657–665.

21. Naseer T, Minshall EM, Leung DY, Laberge S, Ernst P, Martin RJ et al. Expression of IL-12 and IL-13 mRNA in asthma and their modulation in response to steroid therapy. Am J Respir Crit Care Med 1997; 155(3):845–851.

22. Huang SK, Xiao HQ, Kleine-Tebbe J, Paciotti G, Marsh DG, Lichtenstein LM et al. IL-13 expression at the sites of allergen challenge in patients with asthma. J Immunol 1995; 155(5):2688–2694.

23. de Vries JE. The role of IL-13 and its receptor in allergy and inflammatory responses. J Allergy Clin Immunol 1998; 102(2):165–169.

24. Nelms K, Keegan AD, Zamorano J, Ryan JJ, Paul WE. The IL-4 receptor: signaling mechanisms and biologic functions. Anu Rev Immunol 1999; 17:701–738.

25. Callard RE, Matthews DJ, Hibbert L. IL-4 and IL-13 receptors: are they one and the same? Immunol Today 1996; 17(3):108–110.

26. Graber P, Gretener D, Herren S, Aubry JP, Elson G, Poudrier J et al. The distribution of IL-13 receptor alpha1 expression on B cells, T cells and monocytes and its regulation by IL-13 and IL-4. Eur J Immunol 1998; 28(12):4286–4298.

27. Mattes J, Yang M, Siqueira A, Clark K, MacKenzie J, McKenzie AN et al. IL-13 induces airways hyperreactivity independently of the IL-4R alpha chain in the allergic lung. J Immunol 2001; 167(3):1683–1692.

28. Brusselle GG, Kips JC, Tavernier JH, van der Heyden JG, Cuvelier CA, Pauwels RA et al. Attenuation of allergic airway inflammation in IL-4 deficient mice. Clin Exp Allergy 1994; 24(1):73–80.

29. Coyle AJ, Le Gros G, Bertrand C, Tsuyuki S, Heusser CH, Kopf M et al. Interleukin-4 is required for the induction of lung Th2 mucosal immunity. Am J Respir Cell Mol Biol 1995; 13(1):54–59.
30. Grunig G, Warnock M, Wakil AE, Venkayya R, Brombacher F, Rennick DM et al. Requirement for IL-13 independently of IL-4 in experimental asthma. Science 1998; 282(5397):2261–2263.
31. Webb DC, McKenzie AN, Koskinen AM, Yang M, Mattes J, Foster PS. Integrated signals between IL-13, IL-4, and IL-5 regulate airways hyperreactivity. J Immunol 2000; 165(1):108–113.
32. Brusselle G, Kips J, Joos G, Bluethmann H, Pauwels R. Allergen-induced airway inflammation and bronchial responsiveness in wild-type and interleukin-4-deficient mice. Am J Respir Cell Mol Biol 1995; 12(3):254–259.
33. Mehlhop PD, van de Rijn M, Goldberg AB, Brewer JP, Kurup VP, Martin TR et al. Allergen-induced bronchial hyperreactivity and eosinophilic inflammation occur in the absence of IgE in a mouse model of asthma. Proc Natl Acad Sci USA 1997; 94(4):1344–1349.
34. Takeda K, Hamelmann E, Joetham A, Shultz LD, Larsen GL, Irvin CG et al. Development of eosinophilic airway inflammation and airway hyperresponsiveness in mast cell-deficient mice. J Exp Med 1997; 186:54–59.
35. Li XM, Schofield BH, Wang QF, Kim KH, Huang SK. Induction of pulmonary allergic responses by antigen-specific Th2 cells. J Immunol 1998; 160(3):1378–1384.
36. Hogan SP, Matthaei KI, Young JM, Koskinen A, Young IG, Foster PS. A novel T cell–regulated mechanism modulating allergen-induced airways hyperreactivity in BALB/c mice independently of IL-4 and IL-5. J Immunol 1998; 161(3):1501–1509.
37. Cohn L, Tepper JS, Bottomly K. IL-4-independent induction of airway hyperresponsiveness by Th2, but not Th1, cells. J Immunol 1998; 161(8):3813–3816.
38. Gavett SH, O'Hearn DJ, Karp CL, Patel EA, Schofield BH, Finkelman FD et al. Interleukin-4 receptor blockade prevents airway responses induced by antigen challenge in mice. Am J Physiol 1997; 272(2 Pt 1):L253–L261.
39. Rankin JA, Picarella DE, Geba GP, Temann UA, Prasad B, DiCosmo B et al. Phenotypic and physiologic characterization of transgenic mice expressing interleukin 4 in the lung: lymphocytic and eosinophilic inflammation without airway hyperreactivity. Proc Natl Acad Sci USA 1996; 93(15):7821–7825.
40. McKenzie GJ, Fallon PG, Emson CL, Grencis RK, McKenzie AN. Simultaneous disruption of interleukin (IL)-4 and IL-13 defines individual roles in T helper cell type 2-mediated responses. J Exp Med 1999; 189(10):1565–1572.
41. Huang H, Hu-Li J, Chen H, Ben-Sasson SZ, Paul WE. IL-4 and IL-13 production in differentiated T helper type 2 cells is not IL-4 dependent. J Immunol 1997; 159(8):3731–3738.
42. Wills-Karp M, Luyimbazi J, Xu X, Schofield B, Neben TY, Karp CL et al. Interleukin-13: central mediator of allergic asthma. Science 1998; 282(5397): 2258–2261.
43. Zhu Z, Homer RJ, Wang Z, Chen Q, Geba GP, Wang J et al. Pulmonary expression of interleukin-13 causes inflammation, muscus hypersecretion, subepithelial fibrosis, physiologic abnormalities, and eotaxin production. J Clin Invest 1999; 103(6):779–788.

44. Fallon PG, Richardson EJ, McKenzie GJ, McKenzie AN. Schistosome infection of transgenic mice defines distinct and contrasting pathogenic roles for IL-4 and IL-13: IL-13 is a profibrotic agent. J Immunol 2000; 164(5): 2585–2591.

45. Blease K, Jakubzick C, Westwick J, Lukacs N, Kunkel SL, Hogaboam CM. Therapeutic effect of IL-13 immunoneutralization during chronic experimental fungal asthma. J Immunol 2001; 166(8):5219–5224.

46. Laporte JC, Moore PE, Baraldo S, Jouvin MH, Church TL, Schwartzman IN et al. Direct effects of interleukin-13 on signaling pathways for physiological responses in cultured human airway smooth muscle cells. Am J Respir Crit Care Med 2001; 164(1):141–148.

47. Tomkinson A, Duez C, Cieslewicz G, Pratt JC, Joetham A, Shanafelt MC et al. A murine IL-4 receptor antagonist that inhibits IL-4- and IL-13-induced responses prevents antigen-induced airway eosinophilia and airway hyperresponsiveness. J Immunol 2001; 166(9):5792–5800.

48. Aversa G, Punnonen J, Cocks BG, de Waal Malefyt R, Vega FJ, Zurawski SM et al. An interleukin 4 (IL-4) mutant protein inhibits both IL-4 or IL-13-induced human immunoglobulin G4 (IgG4) and IgE synthesis and B cell proliferation: support for a common component shared by IL-4 and IL-13 receptors. J Exp Med 1993; 178(6):2213–2218.

49. Tony HP, Shen BJ, Reusch P, Sebald W. Design of human interleukin-4 antagonists inhibiting interleukin-4-dependent and interleukin-13-dependent responses in T-cells and B-cells with high efficiency. Eur J Biochem 1994; 225(2):659–665.

50. Harris P, Lindell D, Fitch N, Gundel R. The IL-4 receptor antagonist (Bay 16-9996) reverses airway hyperresponsiveness in a primate model of asthma. Am J Respir Crit Care Med 1999;159, A230.

51. Tournoy KG, Kips JC, Pauwels RA. The allergen-induced airway hyperresponsiveness in a human-mouse chimera model of asthma is T cell and IL-4 and IL-5 dependent. J Immunol 2001; 166:6982–6991.

52. Losman JA, Chen XP, Hilton D, Rothman P. Cutting edge: SOCS-1 is a potent inhibitor of IL-4 signal transduction. J Immunol 1999; 162(7):3770–3774.

53. Wang LH, Yang XY, Kirken RA, Resau JH, Farrar WL. Targeted disruption of stat6 DNA binding activity by an oligonucleotide decoy blocks IL-4-driven T(H)2 cell response. Blood 2000; 95(4):1249–1257.

54. Tavernier J, Plaetinck G, Guisez Y, Van der Heyden J, Kips J, Peleman R et al. The role of IL-5 in the production and function of eosinophils. In: Whetton AD, Gordon JR, eds. Cell Biochemistry vol. 7 Hematopoietic cell growth factors and their receptors. New York: Plenum Press, 2000:321–361.

55. Shi HZ, Xiao CQ, Zhong D, Qin SM, Liu Y, Liang GR et al. Effect of inhaled interleukin-5 on airway hyperreactivity and eosinophilia in asthmatics. Am J Respir Crit Care Med 1998; 157(1):204–209.

56. Hamid Q, Azzawi M, Ying S, Moqbel R, Wardlaw AJ, Corrigan CJ et al. Expression of mRNA for interleukin-5 in mucosal bronchial biopsies from asthma. J Clin Invest 1991; 87(5):1541–1546.

57. Robinson DS, Ying S, Bentley AM, Meng Q, North J, Durham SR et al. Relationships among numbers of bronchoalveolar lavage cells expressing

messenger ribonucleic acid for cytokines, asthma symptoms, and airway methacholine responsiveness in atopic asthma. J Allergy Clin Immunol 1993; 92(3):397–403.

58. Foster PS, Hogan SP, Ramsay AJ, Matthaei KI, Young IG. Interleukin 5 deficiency abolishes eosinophilia, airways hyperreactivity, and lung damage in a mouse asthma model. J Exp Med 1996; 183(1):195–201.

59. Hogan SP, Koskinen A, Matthaei KI, Young IG, Foster PS. Interleukin-5-producing CD4+ T Cells play a pivotal role in aeroallergen-induced eosinophila, bronchial hyperreactivity, and lung damage in mice. Am J Respir Crit Care Med 1998; 157(1):210–218.

60. Hamelmann E, Takeda K, Haczku A, Cieslewicz G, Shultz L, Hamid Q et al. Interleukin (IL)-5 but not immunoglobulin E reconstitutes airway inflammation and airway hyperresponsiveness in IL-4-deficient mice. Am J Respir Cell Mol Biol 2000; 23(3):327–334.

61. Hakonarson H, Maskeri N, Carter C, Grunstein MM. Regulation of TH1- and TH2-type cytokine expression and action in atopic asthmatic sensitized airway smooth muscle. J Clin Invest 1999; 103(7):1077–1087.

62. Trifilieff A, Fujitani Y, Coyle AJ, Kopf M, Bertrand C. IL-5 deficiency abolishes aspects of airway remodelling in a murine model of lung inflammation. Clin Exp Allergy 2001; 31(6):934–942.

63. Minshall EM, Leung DYM, Martin RJ, Song YL, Cameron L, Ernst P et al. Eosinophil-associated TGF-betal mRNA expression and airways fibrosis in bronchial asthma. Am J Respir Cell Mol Biol 1997; 17:326–333.

64. Minshall E, Chakir J, Laviolette M, Molet S, Zhu Z, Olivenstein R et al. IL-11 expression is increased in severe asthma: association with epithelial cells and eosinophils. J Allergy Clin Immunol 2000; 105(2 Pt 1):232–238.

65. Leckie MJ, ten Brinke A, Khan J, Diamant Z, O'Connor B, Walls CM et al. Effects of an IL-5 blocking monoclonal antibody on eosinophils, airway hyperresponsiveness, and the late asthmatic response. Lancet 2000; 356: 2144–2148.

66. Kips J, O'connor BJ, Langley SJ, Woodcock AJ, Kerstjens HAM, Postma DS et al. Results of a phase I trial with SCH55700 a humanized anti-IL-5 antibody, in severe persistent asthma. Am J Respir Crit Care Med 2000; 161, A505.

67. Kips JC, Cuvelier CA, Pauwels RA, Effect of acute and chronic antigen inhalation on airway morphology and responsiveness in actively sensitized rats. Am Rev Respir Dis 1992; 145(6):1306–1310.

68. Tournoy KG, Kips JC, Schou C, Pauwels RA. Airway eosinophilia is not a requirement for allergen-induced airway hyperresponsiveness. Clin Exp Allergy 2000; 30(1):79–85.

69. Coyle AJ, Kohler G, Tsuyuki S, Brombacher F, Kopf M. Eosinophils are not required to induce airway hyperresponsiveness after nematode infection. Eur J Immunol 1998; 28(9):2640–2647.

70. Djukanovic R, Wilson JW, Britten KM, Wilson SJ, Walls AF, Roche WR et al. Quantitation of mast cells and eosinophils in the bronchial mucosa of symptomatic atopic asthmatics and healthy control subjects using immunohistochemistry. Am Rev Respir Dis 1990; 142(4):863–871.

71. Rosi E, Ronchi MC, Grazzini M, Duranti R, Scano G. Sputum analysis, bronchial hyperresponsiveness, and airway function in asthma: results of a factor analysis. J Allergy Clin Immunol 1999; 103(2 Pt 1):232–237.

72. Soussi-Gounni A, Kontolemos M, Hamid Q. Role of IL-9 in the pathophysiology of allergic diseases. J Allergy Clin Immunol 2001; 107(4):575–582.

73. Gounni AS, Nutku E, Koussih L, Aris F, Louahed J, Levitt RC et al. IL-9 expression by human eosinophils: regulation by IL-1beta and TNF-alpha. J. Allergy Clin Immunol 2000; 106(3):460–466.

74. Temann UA, Geba GP, Rankin JA, Flavell RA. Expression of interleukin 9 in the lungs of transgenic mice causes airway inflammation, mast cell hyperplasia, and bronchial hyperresponsiveness. J Exp Med 1998; 188(7):1307–1320.

75. Shimbara A, Christodoulopoulos P, Soussi-Gounni A, Olivenstein R, Nakamura Y, Levitt RC et al. IL-9 and its receptor in allergic and nonallergic lung disease: increased expression in asthma J Allergy Clin Immunol 2000; 105(1 Pt 1):108–115.

76. Nicolaides NC, Holroyd KJ, Ewart SL, Eleff SM, Kiser MB, Dragwa CR et al. Interleukin 9: a candidate gene for asthma. Proc Natl Acad Sci USA 1997; 94(24):13175–13180.

77. Baggiolini M. Chemokines and leukocyte traffic. Nature 1998; 392(6676):565–568.

78. Campbell EM, Kunkel SL, Strieter RM, Lukacs NW. Temporal role of chemokines in a murine model of cockroach allergen-induced airway hyperreactivity and eosinophilia. J Immunol 1998; 161(12):7047–7053.

79. Gonzalo JA, Lloyd CM, Wen D, Albar JP, Wells TN, Proudfoot A et al. The coordinated action of CC chemokines in the lung orchestrates allergic inflammation and airway hyperresponsiveness. J Exp Med 1998; 188(1):157–167.

80. Ying S, Robinson DS, Meng Q, Rottman J, Kennedy R, Ringler DJ et al. Enhanced expression of eotaxin and CCR3 mRNA and protein in atopic asthma. Association with airway hyperresponsiveness and predominant co-localization of eotaxin mRNA to bronchial epithelial and endothelial cells. Eur J Immunol 1997; 27(12):3507–3516.

81. Nakamura H, Weiss ST, Israel E, Luster AD, Drazen JM, Lilly CM. Eotaxin and impaired lung function in asthma. Am J Respir Crit Care Med 1999; 160(6):1952–1956.

82. Nibbs RJ, Salcedo TW, Campbell JD, Yao XT, Li Y, Nardelli B et al. C-C chemokine receptor 3 antagonism by the beta-chemokine macrophage inflammatory protein 4, a property strongly enhanced by an amino-terminal alanine-methionine swap. J Immunol 2000; 164(3):1488–1497.

83. Elsner J, Petering H, Hochstetter R, Kimmig D, Wells TN, Kapp A et al. The CC chemokine antagonist Met-RANTES inhibits eosinophil effector functions through the chemokine receptors CCR1 and CCR3. Eur J Immunol 1997; 27(11):2892–2898.

84. Kips J, Pauwels R. Proinflammatory cytokines. In: Barnes PJ, Grunstein MM, Leff AR, Woolley A, eds. Asthma, vol I. Philadelphia: Lippincott–Raven, 1997:653.

85. Hirata N, Kohrogi H, Iwagoe H, Goto E, Hamamoto J, Fujii K et al. Allergen exposure induces the expression of endothelial adhesion molecules in passively

sensitized human bronchus: time course and the role of cytokines. Am J Respir Cell Mod Biol 1998; 18(1):12–20.

86. Schwingshackl A, Duszyk M, Brown N, Moqbel R. Human eosinophils release matrix metalloproteinase-9 on stimulation with TNF-alpha. J Allergy Clin Immunol 1999; 104(5):983–989.

87. Kume N, Gimbrone MA. Lysophosphatidylcholine transcriptionally induces growth factor gene expression in cultured human endothelial cells. J Clin Invest 1994; 93(2):907–911.

88. Yoshizumi M, Kourembanas S, Temizer DH, Cambria RP, Quertermous T, Lee ME. Tumor necrosis factor increases transcription of the heparin-binding epidermal growth factor-like growth factor gene in vascular endothelial cells. J Biol Chem 1992; 267(14):9467–9469.

89. Takeyama K, Dabbagh K, Lee HM, Agusti C, Lausier JA, Ueki IF et al. Epidermal growth factor system regulates mucin production in airways. Proc Natl Acad Sci USA 1999; 96(6):3081–3086.

90. Holgate ST, Davies DE, Lackie PM, Wilson SJ, Puddicombe SM, Lordan JL. Epithelial-mesenchymal interactions in the pathogenesis of asthma. J Allergy Clin Immunol 2000; 105(2 Pt 1):193–204.

91. Chou DH, Lee W, McCulloch CA. TNF-alpha inactivation of collagen receptors: implications for fibroblast function and fibrosis. J Immunol 1996; 156(11): 4354–4362.

92. Gordon JR, Galli SJ. Promotion of mouse fibroblast collagen gene expression by mast cells stimulated via the Fc epsilon RI. Role for mast cell-derived transforming growth factor beta and turmor necrosis factor alpha. J Exp Med 1994; 180(6):2027–2037.

93. Rogalsky V, Todorov G, Den T, Ohnuma T. Increase in protein kinase C activity is associated with human fibroblast growth inhibition. FEBS Lett 1992; 304(2–3): 153–156.

94. Amrani Y, Panettieri RA, Frossard N, Bronner C. Activation of the TNF alpha-p55 receptor induces myocyte proliferation and modulates agonist-evoked calcium transients in cultured human tracheal smooth muscle cells. Am J Respir Cell Mol Biol 1996; 15(1):55–63.

95. Stewart AG, Tomlinson PR, Fernandes DJ, Wilson JW, Harris T. Tumor necrosis factor-alpha modulates mitogenic responses of human cultured airway smooth muscle. Am J Respir Cell Mol Biol 1995; 12:110–119.

96. Yang CM, Luo SF, Wang CC, Chiu CT, Chien CS, Lin CC et al. Tumour necrosis factor-alpha-and interleukin-1beta-stimulated cell proliferation through activation of mitogen-activated protein kinase in canine tracheal smooth muscle cells. Br J Pharmacol 2000; 130(4):891–899.

97. Panettieri RA, Lazaar AL, Pure E, Albelda SM. Activation of cAMP-dependent pathways in human airway smooth muscle cells inhibits TNF-alpha-induced ICAM-1 and VCAM-1 expression and T lymphocyte adhesion. J Immunol 1995; 154(5):2358–2365.

98. Hotta K, Emala CW, Hirshman CA. TNF-alpha upregulates Gialpha and Gqalpha protein expression and function in human airway smooth muscle cells. Am J Physiol 1999; 276(3 Pt 1):L405–L411.

99. Kips JC, Tavernier J, Pauwels RA. Tumor necrosis factor causes bronchial hyperresponsiveness in rats. Am Rev Respir Dis 1992; 145(2 Pt 1):332–336.

100. Wheeler AP, Jesmok G, Brigham KL. Tumor necrosis factor's effects on lung mechanics, gas exchange, and airway reactivity in sheep. J Appl Physiol 1990; 68(6):2542–2549.

101. Thomas PS, Yates DH, Barnes PJ. Tumor necrosis factor-alpha increases airway responsiveness and sputum neutrophilia in normal human subjects. Am J Respir Crit Care Med 1995; 152(1):76–80.

102. Broide DH, Lotz M, Cuomo AJ, Coburn DA, Federman EC, Wasserman SI. Cytokines in symptomatic asthma airways. J Allergy Clin Immunol 1992; 89(5):958–967.

103. Keatings VM, Barnes PJ. Granulocyte activation markers in induced sputum: comparison between chronic obstructive pulmonary disease, asthma, and normal subjects. Am J Respir Crit Care Med 1997; 155(2):449–453.

104. Keatings VM, Collins PD, Scott DM, Barnes PJ. Differences in interleukin-8 and tumor necrosis factor-alpha in induced sputum from patients with chronic obstructive pulmonary disease or asthma. Am J Respir Crit Care Med 1996; 153(2):530–534.

105. Ackerman V, Marini M, Vittori E, Bellini A, Vassali G, Mattoli S. Detection of cytokines and their cell sources in bronchial biopsy specimens from asthmatic patients. Relationship to atopic status, symptoms, and level of airway hyper-responsiveness. Chest 1994; 105(3):687–696.

106. Li Kam Wa TC, Mansur AH, Britton J, Williams G, Pavord I, Richards K et al. Association between – 308 tumour necrosis factor promoter polymorphism and bronchial hyperreactivity in asthma. Clin Exp Allergy 1999; 29(9):1204–1208.

107. Chagani T, Pare PD, Zhu S, Weir TD, Bai TR, Behbehani NA et al. Prevalence of tumor necrosis factor-alpha and angiotensin coverting enzyme polymorphisms in mild/moderate and fatel/near-fatel asthma. Am J Respir Crit Care Med 1999; 160(1):278–282.

108. Albuquerque RV, Hayden CM, Palmer LJ, Laing IA, Rye PJ, Gibson NA et al. Association of polymorphisms within the tumour necrosis factor (TNF) genes and childhood asthma. Clin Exp Allergy 1998; 28(5):578–584.

109. Luong BT, Chong BS, Lowder DM. Treatment options for rheumatoid arthritis: celecoxib, leflunomide, etanercept, and infliximab. Ann Pharmacother 2000; 34(6):743–760.

110. Koulis A, Robinson DS. The anti-inflammatory effects of interleukin-10 in allergic disease. Clin Exp Allergy 2000; 30(6):747–750.

111. Selzman CH, McIntyre RCJ, Shames BD, Whitehill TA, Banerjee A, Harken AH. Interleukin-10 inhibits human vascular smooth muscle proliferation. J Mol Cell Cardiol 1998; 30(4):889–896.

112. Reitamo S, Remitz A, Tamai K, Uitto J. Interleukin-10 modulates type I collagen and matrix metalloprotease gene expression in cultured human skin fibroblasts. J Clin Invest 1994; 94(6):2489–2492.

113. Borish L, Aarons A, Rumbyrt J, Cvietusa P, Negri J, Wenzel S. Interleukin-10 regulation in normal subjects and patients with asthma. J Allergy Clin Immunol 1996; 97(6):1288–1296.

114. John M, Lim S, Seybold J, Jose P, Robichaud A, O'Connor B et al. Inhaled corticosteroids increase interleukin-10 but reduce macrophage inflammatory protein-1alpha, granulocyte-macrophage colony-stimulating factor, and interferon-gamma release from alveolar macrophages in asthma. Am J Respir Crit Care Med 1998; 157(1):256–262.

115. Robinson DS, Tsicopoulos A, Meng Q, Durham S, Kay AB, Hamid Q. Increased interleukin-10 messenger RNA expression in atopic allergy and asthma. Am J Respir Cell Mol Biol 1996; 14(2):113–117.

116. Quinn TJ, Taylor S, Wohlford-Lenane CL, Schwartz DA. IL-10 reduces grain dust–induced airway inflammation and airway hyperreactivity. J Appl Physiol 2000; 88(1):173–179.

117. van Scott MR, Justice JP, Bradfield JF, Enright E, Sigounas A, Sur S. IL-10 reduces Th2 cytokine production and eosinophilia but augments airway reactivity in allergic mice. Am J Physiol Lung Cell Mol Physiol 2000; 278(4):L667–L674.

118. Zuany-Amorim C, Haile S, Leduc D, Dumarey C, Huerre M, Vargaftig BB et al. Interleukin-10 inhibits antigen-induced cellular recruitment into the airways of sensitized mice. J Clin Invest 1995; 95(6):2644–2651.

119. Tourney KG, Kips JC, Pauwels RA. Endogenous interleukin-10 suppresses allergen-induced airway inflammation and nonspecific airway responsiveness. Clin Exp Allergy 2000; 30(6):775–783.

120. Makela MJ, Kanehiro A, Borish L, Dakhama A, Loader J, Joetham A et al. IL-10 is necessary for the expression of airway hyperresponsiveness but not pulmonary inflammation after allergic sensitization. Proc Natl Acad Sci USA 2000; 97(11):6007–6012.

121. Li XM, Chopra RK, Chou TY, Schofield BH, Wills-Karp M, Huang SK. Mucosal IFN-gamma gene transfer inhibits pulmonary allergic responses in mice. J Immunol 1996; 157(8):3216–3219.

122. Lack G, Bradley KL, Hamelmann E, Renz H, Loader J, Leung DY et al. Nebulized IFN-gamma inhibits the development of secondary allergic responses in mice. J Immunol 1996; 157(4):1432–1439.

123. Iwamoto I, Nakajima H, Endo H, Yoshida S. Interferon gamma regulates antigen-induced eosinophil recruitment into the mouse airways by inhibiting the infiltration of CD4+ T cells. J Exp Med 1993; 177(2):573–576.

124. Coyle AJ, Tsuyuki S, Bertrand C, Huang S, Aguet M, Alkan SS et al. Mice lacking the IFN-gamma receptor have impaired ability to resolve a lung eosinophilic inflammatory response associated with a prolonged capacity of T cells to exhibit a Th2 cytokine profile. J Immunol 1996; 156(8):2680–2685.

125. Boguniewicz M, Martin RJ, Martin D, Gibson U, Celniker A, Williams M et al. The effects of nebulized recombinant interferon-gamma in asthmatic airways. J Allergy Clin Immunol 1995; 95(1 Pt 1):133–135.

126. Boguniewicz M, Schneider LC, Milgrom H, Newell D, Kelly N, Tam P et al. Treatment of steroid-dependent asthma with recombinant interferon-gamma. Clin Exp Allergy 1993; 23(9):785–790.

127. Rissoan MC, Soumelis V, Kadowaki N, Grouard G, Briere F, de Waal Malefyt R et al. Reciprocal control of T helper cell and dendritic cell differentiation. Science 1999; 283(5405):1183–1186.

128. Kips JC, Brusselle GJ, Joos GF, Peleman RA, Tavernier JH, Devos RR et al. Interleukin-12 inhibits antigen-induced airway hyperresponsiveness in mice. Am J Respir Crit Care Med 1996; 153(2):535–539.

129. Gavett SH, O'Hearn DJ, Li X, Huang SK, Finkelman FD, Wills-Karp M. Interleukin 12 inhibits antigen-induced airway hyperresponsiveness, inflammation, and Th2 cytokine expression in mice. J Exp Med 1995; 182(5):1527–1536.

130. Szabo SJ, Jacobson NG, Dighe AS, Gubler U, Murphy KM. Developmental commitment to the Th2 lineage by extinction of IL-12 signaling. Immunity 1995; 2(6):665–675.

131. Lee Y, Fu C, Chiang B. Administration of interleukin-12 exerts a therapeutic instead of a long-term preventive effect on mite Der p I allergen-induced animal model of airway inflammation. Immunology 1999; 97(2):232–240.

132. Wang ZE, Zheng S, Corry DB, Dalton DK, Seder RA, Reiner SL et al. Interferon gamma-independent effects of interleukin 12 administered during acute or established infection due to Leishmania major. Proc Natl Acad Sci USA 1994; 91(26):12932–12936.

133. Brusselle GG, Kips JC, Peleman RA, Joos GF, Devos RR, Tavernier JH et al. Role of IFN-gamma in the inhibition of the allergic airway inflammation caused by IL-12. Am J Respir Cell Mol Biol 1997; 17(6):767–771.

134. Tournoy KG, Kips JC, Pauwels RA. The counterbalancing effect of Th2-driven allergic airway inflammation by IL-12 does not require IL-10. J Allergy Clin Immunol 2001;107:483–491.

135. Leonard JP, Sherman ML, Fisher GL, Buchanan LJ, Larsen G, Atkins MB et al. Effects of single-dose interleukin-12 exposure on interleukin-12-associated toxicity and interferon-gamma production. Blood 1997; 90(7):2541–2548.

136. Bryan SA, O'Connor B, Matti S, Leckie MJ, Kanabar V, Khan J et al. Effects of recombinant human IL-12 on eosinophils, airway hyperresponsiveness and the late asthma response. Lancet 2000; 356, 2149–2153.

137. Okamura H, Tsutsi H, Komatsu T, Yutsudo M, Hakura A, Tanimoto T et al. Cloning of a new cytokine that induces IFN-gamma production by T cells. Nature 1995; 378(6552):88–91.

138. Kodama T, Matsuyama T, Kuribayashi K, Nishioka Y, Sugita M, Akira S et al. IL-18 deficiency selectively enhances allergen-induced eosinophilia in mice. J Allergy Clin Immunol 2000; 105(1 Pt 1): 45–53.

139. Wild JS, Sigounas A, Sur N, Siddiqui MS, Alam R, Kurimoto M et al. IFN-gamma-inducing factor (IL-18) increases allergic sensitization, serum IgE, Th2 cytokines, and airway eosinophilia in a mouse model of allergic asthma. J Immunol 2000; 164(5):2701–2710.

140. Kumano K, Nakao A, Nakajima H, Hayashi F, Kurimoto M, Okamura H et al. Interleukin-18 enhances antigen-induced eosinophil recruitment into the mouse airways. Am J Respir Crit Care Med 1999; 160(3):873–878.

141. Hofstra CL, Van A, I, Hofman G, Kool M, Nijkamp FP, Van Oosterhout AJ. Prevention of Th2-like cell responses by coadministration of IL-12 and IL-18 is associated with inhibition of antigen-induced airway hyperresponsiveness, eosinophilia, and serum IgE levels. J Immunol 1998; 161(9):5054–5060.

142. Camporota L, Corkhill A, Long H, Lau LC, Tukwell N, Lordan J et al. Effects of intradermal injection of SRL-172 (Killed Mycobacterium vaccae suspension) on

allergen-induced airway responses and IL-5 generation by PBMC in asthma. Am J Respir Crit Care Med 2000; 161:A477.

143. Shirtcliffe PM, Easthope SE, Cheng S, Weatherall M, Tan PL, Le Gros G et al. The effect of delipidated deglycolipidated (DDMV) and heat-killed Mycobacterium vaccae in asthma. Am J Respir Crit Care Med 2001; 163(6):1410–1414.

144. Chu RS, Targoni OS, Krieg AM, Lehmann PV, Harding CV. CpG oligodeoxynucleotides act as adjuvants that switch on T helper 1 (TH1) immunity. J Exp Med 1997; 186(10):1623–1631.

145. Kovarik J, Bozzotti P, Love-Human L, Pihlgren M, Davis HL, Lambert PH et al. CpG oligodeoxynucleotides can circumvent the Th2 polarization of neonatal responses to vaccines but may fail to fully redirect Th2 responses established by neonatal priming. J Immunol 1999; 162(3):1611–1617.

146. Krieg AM, Yi AK, Matson S, Waldschmidt TJ, Bishop GA, Teasdale R et al. CpG motifs in bacterial DNA trigger direct B-cell activation. Nature 1995; 374(6522):546–549.

147. Cowdery JS, Chace JH, Yi AK, Krieg AM. Bacterial DNA induces NK cells to produce IFN-gamma in vivo and increases the toxicity of lipopolysaccharides. J Immunol 1996; 156(12):4570–4575.

148. Klinman DM, Yi AK, Beaucage SL, Conover J, Krieg AM. CpG motifs present in bacteria DNA rapidly induce lymphocytes tos secrete interleukin 6, interleukin 12, and interferon gamma. Proc Natl Acad Sci USA 1996; 93(7):2879–2883.

149. Iho S, Yamamoto T, Takahashi T, Yamamoto S. Oligodeoxynucleotides containing palindrome sequences with internal 5'-CpG-3' act directly on human NK and activated T cells to induce IFN-gamma production in vitro. J Immunol 1999; 163(7):3642–3652.

150. Sato Y, Roman M, Tighe H, Lee D, Corr M, Nguyen MD et al. Immunostimulatory DNA sequences necessary for effective intradermal gene immunization. Science 1996; 273(5273):352–354.

151. Roman M, Matrin-Orozco E, Goodman JS, Nguyen MD, Sato Y, Ronaghy A et al. Immunostimulatory DNA sequences function as T helper-1-promoting adjuvants. Nat Med 1997; 3(8):849–854.

152. Chu RS, Askew D, Noss EH, Tobian A, Krieg AM, Harding CV. CpG oligodeoxynucleotides down-regulate macrophage class II MHC antigen processing. J Immunol 1999; 163(3):1188–1194.

153. Kline JN, Waldschmidt TJ, Businga TR, Lemish JE, Weinstock JV, Thorne PS et al. Modulation of airway inflammation by CpG oligodeoxynucleotides in a murine model of asthma. J Immunol 1998; 160(6):2555–2559.

154. Sparwasser T, Miethke T, Lipford G, Borschert K, Hacker H, Heeg K et al. Bacterial DNA causes septic shock. Nature 1997; 386(6623):336–337.

155. Sparwasser T, Miethke T, Lipford G, Erdmann A, Hacker H, Heeg K et al. Macrophages sense pathogens via DNA motifs: induction of tumor necrosis factor-alpha-mediated shock. Eur J Immunol 1997; 27(7):1671–1679.

156. Broide D, Schwarze J, Tighe H, Gifford T, Nguyen MD, Malek S et al. Immunostimulatory DNA sequences inhibit IL-5, eosinophilic inflammation, and airway hyperresponsiveness in mice. J Immunol 1998; 161(12):7054–7062.

157. Shirota H, Sano K, Kikuchi T, Tamura G, Shirato K. Regulation of T-helper type 2 cell and airway eosinophilia by transmucosal coadministration of antigen and

oligodeoxynucleotides containing CpG motifs. Am J Respir Cell Mol Biol 2000; 22(2):176–182.

158. Serebrisky D, Teper AA, Huang CK, Lee SY, Zhang TF, Schofield BH et al. CpG oligodeoxynucleotides can reverse Th2-associated allergic airway responses and alter the B7.1/B7.2 expression in a murine model of asthma. J Immunol 2000; 165(10):5906–5912.

159. Maecker HT, Hansen G, Walter DM, DeKruyff RH, Levy S, Umetsu DT. Vaccination with allergen-IL-18 fusion DNA protects against, and reverses established, airway hyperreactivity in a murine asthma model. J Immunol 2001; 166(2):959–965.

18

Immunological Functions of Inflammatory Mediators

DOMENICO SPINA and
CLIVE PAGE
Sackler Institute of Pulmonary
   Pharmacology
King's College London
London, England

ZUZANA DIAMANT
Erasmus University Medical Centre
Rotterdam, The Netherlands

ANTHONY P. SAMPSON
University of Southampton
   School of Medicine
Southampton General Hospital
Southampton, England

I. Introduction

Asthma is characterized by a complex inflammatory response involving resident (e.g., mast cells, macrophages, nerves), recruited (e.g., lymphocytes, eosinophils, monocytes), and structural cells (e.g., epithelium, airway smooth muscle, fibroblast). These cells can synthesize and secrete a vast number of mediators that may contribute to bronchoconstriction, submucosal gland secretion, vasodilation, bronchial wall edema, recruitment of inflammatory cells, airway remodeling, and bronchial hyperresponsiveness (BHR) observed in asthma. The role of individual mediators in the context of asthma has been greatly facilitated by the discovery of highly potent and selective mediator antagonists.

Given the complex nature of the pathophysiology of asthma and the vast array of potential mediators that are released and thought to contribute to this process, it is perhaps not surprising that few single mediator antagonists have been successfully developed for the treatment of asthma, perhaps with one exception to date (1). However, it is clear that many new candidate mediators continue to be investigated for their potential role in asthma and will be the subject of this chapter. However, for historical purposes, the current state of play of more traditional mediators will also be addressed and in general only studies performed in humans will be considered. For a more detailed review of the many potential mediators thought to play a role in asthma, one should consult a recently published review on this subject (2).

II. Histamine

Histamine is the classical mediator that has been extensively studied in the context of allergy and asthma. Histamine is stored in granules within mast cells and basophils and can be released under immunological conditions following the cross-linking of antigen to high-affinity IgE receptors present on the surface of mast cells and basophils or by nonimmunological stimuli (e.g., compound 48/80, calcium ionophore, substance P, and hypo-osmolar solutions). Histamine concentrations are elevated in bronchoalveolar lavage (BAL) fluid of asymptomatic mild asthmatics (3) and following antigen challenge (4,5). The acute bronchoconstriction observed following antigen challenge is attenuated by selective H_1 receptor antagonists (6). These studies confirm that the acute release of histamine following an allergic or nonallergic insult may lead to bronchoconstriction.

A. Histamine Receptors

Three histamine receptors have thus far been cloned in humans: H_1 (7), H_2 (8), and H_3 receptors (9). The signaling pathways of these cloned receptors result in the activation of phosphoinositide hydrolysis, stimulation, and inhibition of adenylyl cyclase, respectively. The H_3 receptor is abundantly expressed in the central nervous system, and while the levels of expression in the periphery were below the level of detection, it is clear that these receptors are located on peripheral nerve terminals in the lung (10). More recently a fourth histamine receptor has been cloned with 29%, 31%, and 58% sequence homology to H_1, H_2, and H_3 receptors, respectively (11–14). This novel receptor appears to be expressed in cells of the immune system, including T cells, dendritic cells, monocytes, mast cells, neutrophils, and eosinophils.

B. Effects of Histamine Relevant to Asthma

Histamine released in the airway induces bronchoconstriction via an H_1 receptor–dependent mechanism, but also has the potential to increase vascular permeability (15), vasodilation (16), and stimulate submucosal gland secretion (17), or thought to be mediated following activation of H_2 receptors. There is evidence that histamine may also stimulate sensitized afferent nerves. Thus, following viral infection, the bronchoconstriction to inhaled histamine is attenuated by muscarinic blockade, suggesting the reflex activation of cholinergic nerves (18). In vitro evidence supports the notion that stimulation of H_3 receptors on prejunctional cholinergic nerve terminals attenuates the release of acetylcholine in human bronchial preparations (10).

With regard to inflammatory cells, histamine has been shown to activate eosiniphils but the receptor subtype involved could not be clearly defined (19), and whether this is mediated via the newly described H_4 receptor subtype is not yet clear. However, there is considerable evidence that histamine can regulate the function of immune cells via a H_2 receptor–dependent mechanism. Thus, while histamine alone has no effect on cytokine release from human peripheral monocytes, it increased the gene expression and production of interleukin-10 (IL-10) from monocytes stimulated with lipopolysaccharide (LPS) by an H_2 receptor–dependent mechanism (20,21). Together these studies would support the view that histamine could potentially play a suppressive role in down-regulating TH2-mediated responses secondary to the stimulation of IL-10 production from antigen-presenting cells (APCs), as IL-10 is thought to play an important role in modulation of TH2-mediated inflammatory responses (22).

On the other hand, some evidence suggests that histamine may be proin-flammatory, possibly by altering the balance between Th1- and Th2-like cyto-kine release from lymphocytes. Thus, histamine inhibited the production of IL-12 from human monocytes stimulated with LPS (20,23). This inhibition of IL-12 production was mediated via activation of H_2 receptors on monocytes and not secondary to elevated levels of IL-10 (20,23). Similarly, histamine was shown to inhibit interferon-γ(IFN-γ) secretion while up-regulating IL-5 production following activation of T-cell clones derived from BAL fluid in asthmatic subjects (24). Similarly, histamine inhibited IFN-γ production from Th1 cells and IL-4 from Th0 clones (25) and inhibited IFN-γ production from murine splenocytes (26), consistent with the demonstration of the ability of histamine to inhibit IFN-γ gene expression stimulated by LPS in human peri-pheral blood mononuclear cells (27). In contrast, a recent study has shown that peripheral blood mononuclear cells produce an increase in IL-18 and IFN-γ in response to histamine via a H_2 receptor–dependent mechanism (28). Alter-natively, histamine may contribute toward the inflammatory process by stimulating the production of IL-16 from airway epithelial cells, a potent che-moattractant for T lymphocytes (29). Taken together, these studies suggest that histamine might also contribute to perpetuation of the inflammatory response via an H_2 receptor–dependent mechanism.

C. Role of Histamine Receptor Antagonists in Asthma

H_1 receptor antagonists are widely used in the treatment of allergic diseases where the release of histamine is thought to play an important role in the symptoms associated with hay fever, urticaria, and mild asthma (6). However, it is clear that a number of H_1 receptor antagonists, including cetirizine, terfena-dine, ebastine, oxatimide, loratidine, and ketotifen, demonstrate anti-inflam-matory activity unrelated to H_1 receptor blockade. For example, cetirizine inhibits fMet-Leu-Phe (FMLP)–and platelet-activating factor (PAF)–induced chemotaxis of eosinophils (30,31), and superoxide generation by eosinophils (31); inhibits FMLP-, leukotriene $B_4(LTB_4)$–induced chemotaxis of lymphocytes and monocytes (32), and inhibited eosinophil survival in vitro (33). Similarly, oxatimide inhibited antigen-induced degranulation of human lung mast cells and basophils in vitro (34), and ketotifen has been shown to inhibit PAF-induced eosinophilia in vivo (35). The mechanism by which these drugs inhibit inflammatory cell function is unclear but may be related to stabilization of cell membranes and interference with intracellular calcium mobilization.

A number of clinical studies have reported that cetirizine can attenuate the wheal-and-flare response following intradermal injection of antigen while having no effect on the late cutaneous response or the attendant eosinophilia and deposition of eosinophil cationic protein (ECP) (36,37). Similarly, 3-week treatment with cetirizine failed to attenuate early-and late-phase response; however, the effect of cetirizine on BHR following antigen challenge is controversial (38,39). Nonetheless, 15-day treatment with cetirizine significantly reduced the expression of intracellular adhesion molecule-1(ICAM-1) and eosinophil number in scrapings from nasal mucosa in children sensitive to house dust mite (40). Following 26 weeks of treatment, cetirizine has also been shown to reduce a number of clinical symptoms in patients with perennial asthma (41) and suggest that these drugs appear to be more effective in mild forms of allergic disease. Moreover, 18-month treatment with cetirizine in young children (18–24 months) with atopic dermatitis reduced the likelihood of asthma developing (42).

III. Lipid Mediators

A. Prostanoids

Eicosanoids are derivatives of arachidonic acid (AA), a 20-carbon polyunsaturated fatty acid (eicosatetra-5,8,11,14-enoic acid; $20:4\omega6$), usually esterified in membrane phospholipids at the *sn*-2 position (43). For eicosanoid synthesis, release of AA from membrane phospholipids occurs by the calcium-dependent action of phospholipase A_2 (PL A_2) or by the sequential action of PLC and a diglyceride lipase (44,45). Arachidonic acid can be converted by enzymes of the cyclooxygenase pathway, COX-1 and COX-2 isoenzymes, followed by a number of synthases and isomerases resulting in the release of prostaglandin D_2 (PGD_2), $PGF_{2\alpha}$, PGE_2, prostacyclin (PGI_2), or thromboxane A_2 (TXA_2).

COX1 is constitutively expressed in a number of cells, including mast cells and airway epithelium (46). In contrast, various proinflammatory cytokines stimulate the induction of COX2 in human airway epithelium (47) and smooth muscle (48) in culture and suggest that, during inflammation, COX2 expression may be augmented. However, immunohistochemical examination of bronchial biopsies from subjects with mild to severe asthma revealed the presence of both COX1 and COX2 in airway epithelium, in the absence of a preferential increase in COX2 expression (49).

Prostanoid Receptors

Eight prostanoid receptors have thus far been cloned from different genes that are characteristic of G-protein-coupled receptors, including EP(1-4), DP, FP, IP, and TP based on their selectivity for the prostanoids PGE_2, PGD_2, $PGF_{2\alpha}$, PGI_2, and TXA_2, respectively (50,51). Stimulation of these receptors leads to the activation of adenylyl cyclase (EP_2, EP_4, DP, TP, IP), inhibition of adenylyl cyclase (EP_3, TP), and activation of phosphoinositide hydrolysis/calcium mobilization (EP_1, EP_3, FP, IP, and TP)(50,51).

Effects of Prostanoid Relevant to Asthma

Immediately following acute antigen challenge of asthmatic subjects, increased levels of $PGF_{2\alpha}$, PGD_2, and TXB_2 are detected in BAL fluid (3,52,53) most likely derived from the activation of mast cells, although potential other sources of these prostanoids include macrophages and airway epithelium. Nonsteroidal anti-inflammatory drugs (NSAIDs) have a modest inhibitory action against the acute bronchoconstriction to allergen (54,55) and suggest that other mediators contribute to a significantly greater extent than prostanoids to the acute bronchoconstriction following allergen challenge. However, several studies have reported that NSAIDs can inhibit the late response to allergen (55–57).

When inhaled, prostanoids like PGD_2, $PGF_{2\alpha}$, and TXA_2 induce bronchoconstriction (58–60) but, more interestingly, increase airway responsiveness to spasmogens unrelated to alterations in airway caliber (61,62) and suggest that prostanoids may play a greater role in modulating airway responsiveness. Indeed, the increase in airway responsiveness following antigen challenge is attenuated following inhalation of NSAIDs in some asthmatic subjects (54,55). The role of PGD_2 in the allergic inflammatory response has been further investigated in DP receptor knockout mice. It appears that this prostanoid has an important role in the development of a Th2 phenotype as evidenced by an impairment of Th2 cytokine secretion, reduction in lymphocyte and consequently eosinophil recruitment to the airways following antigen challenge of immunized mice compared with wild-type controls (63). However, it appears that the role of this prostanoid in the context of airway inflammation is more complex as highlighted by the findings of augmented allergic responses in PGH_1 and PGH_2 synthase knockout mice (64), possibly a consequence of prostanoids that may exert negative feedback regulation of the inflammatory process (65).

The profiles of prostanoids formed by COX1 and COX2 are similar, although the role of PGE_2 in the context of airway inflammation is complex. Thus, PGE_2 relaxes human airway smooth muscle (66), inhibits the proliferation of human airway smooth muscle (48), and induced bronchodilation when inhaled by asthmatic subjects (67). Similarly, PGE_2 inhibits the development of the late asthmatic response that is unrelated to functional antagonism of airway smooth muscle contraction (67,68). Furthermore, PGE_2 attenuates the attendant increase in sputum eosinophilia following allergen challenge

(68), suggesting that this prostanoid may have anti-inflammatory properties. It is unclear whether this is related to suppression of eosinophil recruitment to the airways, but the fact that this response can be observed within minutes after administration of PGE_2 (65) suggests that such an inhibitory effect could therefore be a consequence of a reduction in adhesion molecule expression, thereby inhibiting eosinophil adhesion to epithelial surfaces (69). This clinical evidence in support of an inhibitory effect of PGE_2 on the inflammatory response is also consistent with experimental evidence in murine models. Thus, treatment with indomethacin augmented the recruitment of eosinophils to the airways following antigen challenge that was associated with elevated levels of IL-5 and IL-13 in a murine model of allergic inflammation (70). Similarly, PGH_1 and PGH_2 synthase–deficient mice were also characterized by enhanced allergic responses (64). The mechanism by which PGE_2 down-regulates the inflammatory response is unclear but might be due to suppression of the production of proinflammatory cysteinyl leukotrienes (71), although it remains to be established how cysteinyl leukotrienes up-regulate Th2 cytokine production. The potential beneficial effect of PGE_2 on airway inflammation in asthma might explain in part why NSAIDs can induce exacerbation of asthma in aspirin-sensitive asthmatic subjects. The acute administration of PGE_2 prior to allergen challenge of asthmatic subjects was shown to suppress the increase in mast cell–derived PGD_2 and cysteinyl leukotrienes in BAL fluid (65). This is entirely consistent with the observation that aspirin can increase the levels of leukotrienes while reducing the levels of PGE_2 in BAL fluid of asthmatic subjects (72).

In contrast, other studies have shown that PGE_2 may have proinflammatory properties. Hence, PGE_2 induces cough in healthy and asthmatic subjects (73), and in some subjects NSAIDs can partially attenuate the late asthmatic response (55). Furthermore, PGE_2 has the potential to promote Th2 cell development and allergic inflammation by virtue of its ability to down-regulate IFN-γ and IL-12 production from T lymphocytes and monocytes, respectively (74–76).

The potential anti- and proinflammatory properties of PGE_2 may reflect activation of different prostanoid receptor subtypes on different cells. Thus, bronchodilation appears to be mediated by EP_2 receptors in mice (77), while $EP_{2/4}$ but not EP_3 receptors are implicated in the secretion of the proinflammatory cytokine, IL-6 from human airway epithelial cells (78), and the sensitization of afferent nerves appears to involve EP_{3C} and EP_4 receptors (79,80).

Role of COX Inhibitors and Receptor Antagonists in Asthma

The nonselective inhibition of the synthesis of anti- and proinflammatory prostanoids following administration of NSAIDs perhaps explains why this class of drug has mixed therapeutic activity in asthma. Other therapeutic strategies include the development of selective prostanoid receptor antagonists and enzyme inhibitors. Some of these drugs have been investigated for their potential use in the management of asthma. The TXA_2 antagonist Bay U3405 produced a modest decrease in airway responsiveness to methacholine following 2-week treatment in asthmatics (81) but was ineffective against bronchoconstriction induced by bradykinin following a single oral administration of this drug (82). Similarly, the TXA_2 antagonist GR32191 was ineffective against methacholine responsiveness in adult asthmatics following 3 weeks of treatment (83). These studies suggest that TXA_2 antagonists alone are unlikely to suppress baseline airway hyperresponsiveness (AHR) in asthmatics.

The TXA_2 synthase inhibitor ozagrel (OKY-046) reduced cough sensitivity to capsaicin (84) and bronchoconstriction to acetaldehyde in asthmatic subjects (85), indicating a possible role for TXA_2 in sensitization of afferent nerves. This is entirely consistent with the lack of effect of 1-week treatment with UK-38,485 on airways responsiveness to methacholine (86), which elicits bronchoconstriction predominantly via a nonneuronal mechanism of action (87). Similarly, while acute treatment with CGS 13080 attenuated the acute bronchoconstrictor response to antigen, the late asthmatic response and attendant BHR was not inhibited (88).

B. Cysteinyl Leukotrienes

In addition to prostaglandins and thromboxane, other eicosanoids can be synthesized from arachidonic acid and are thought to be involved in the pathogenesis of asthma. Cysteinyl leukotrienes (cysLTs) are an example.

5-Lipoxygenase Pathway

Arachidonic acid can be converted by various lipoxygenases into mono-, di-, and trihydroxylated derivatives such as lipoxins, hydroxyeicosatetraenoic acids(HETEs), and LTs (89). LTs are not stored inside the cell but generated de novo upon cell activation. Following activation, LT synthesis is initiated by 5-lipoxygenase (5-LO), a 78-kD hydrophilic enzyme (90,91). 5-LO is translocated to the nuclear membrane, where it receives AA donated by an integral membrane protein termed 5-LO-activating protein (FLAP) (92), allowing for the transformation of AA into 5-hydroperoxyeicosatetraenoic acid (5-HPETE) (93). 5-HPETE may degrade nonenzymatically into the weak neutrophil chemotaxin 5-HETE, or be further transformed by 5-LO to the unstable epoxide LTA_4 (94). 5-LO is the target of one class of LT-modifying drugs, the 5-LO inhibitors, exemplified by zileuton (A-64077; Zyflo) (95). 5-LO inhibitors compete with AA at the 5-LO active site and block the synthesis of LTA_4, and consequently both the formation of LTB_4 and cysLTs (96). Recently, variants of the 5-LO promoter genotype have been reported in asthmatic patients. This may account for differences between the so-called responders and nonresponders to drugs modifying the 5-LO pathway (1,97). The activity of 5-LO in intact cells requires Ca^{2+} and ATP (91) and the provision of AA by the 18-kD membrane protein FLAP, which is located in the nuclear envelope (98–101). Cellular activation leads to the translocation of PLA_2 and 5-LO from the cytoplasm to the nuclear envelope (101–103), where AA is transferred to FLAP and then donated to 5-LO (104). This process is blocked by the second class of leukotrieno-modifying drugs, the FLAP inhibitors, including MK-886, MK-0591, Bay X1005, and Bay Y1015, which bind to FLAP and prevent its donating AA to 5-LO (105,106). In this manner, the synthesis of LTs may be inhibited.

Synthesis of Leukotrienes

Depending on the cell type, LTA_4 can be metabolized either into LTB_4 by LTA_4 hydrolase or into cysLTs (LTC_4, LTD_4, and LTE_4) by LTC_4 synthase. Upon stimulation, neutrophils, monocytes, and macrophages predominantly release LTB_4 (107–110). This is accomplished by LTA_4 hydrolase, a 68- to 71-kD cytosolic zinc-containing epoxide hydrolase with a high degree of substrate specificity (111), possessing additional activity as an arginine aminopeptidase (112,113). LTB_4 ($5S,12R$-dihydroxy-6,8,11,14-ETE) is a potent chemoattractant for neutrophils and other leukocytes, acting at specific surface (BLT) receptors on target cells. The BLT receptor has been cloned in HL-60 cells and shown to be a 352-amino-acid G-protein-linked receptor, activation of which leads to a rise in intracellular Ca^{2+} and chemotaxis (114). LTB_4 instilled into the human airway induces airway neutrophilia, as has been shown in a BAL study (115). However inhaled LTB_4 did not cause bronchoconstriction or alter airway responsiveness either in nonasthmatic individuals or in patients with asthma (116). In one study in asthmatic subjects, a specific BLT receptor antagonist (LY 293111) did not affect allergen-induced airway responses, despite a reduction in neutrophil counts in the BAL fluid (117). In conclusion, there is little coherent evidence that LTB_4 plays an important role in the pathophysiology of asthma (118). However, BLT receptor antagonists may find clinical application in the treatment of patients with chronic obstructive pulmonary disease (COPD) (119).

Alternatively, LTA_4 can be conjugated with glutathione at the C-6 position by LTC_4 synthase, producing LTC_4, the first of the LTs implicated in asthma. This occurs mainly in eosinophils, but also in basophils, monocytes, and mast cells (120–122). LTC_4 is released from the cell by a specific export carrier (123) and may be converted by γ-glutamyl transpeptidase and dipeptidase activities in lung tissue and in plasma into LTD_4 and LTE_4, respectively (124–126). Degradation of the cysLTs occurs by ω oxidation followed by successive cycles of β oxidation in the liver (127), although a fixed proportion of intravenous or inhaled ^3H-LTC_4 (about 5%) is excreted as LTE_4 in the urine (128). Consequently, urinary LTE_4 concentrations are used as a marker of whole-body production of cysLTs, and hence as a measure of bioactivity of LT synthesis inhibitors (LTSIs) in vivo.

In bronchial biopsies of patients with aspirin-sensitive asthma (ASA) who have constitutively high baseline cysLT production, an enhanced target organ sensitivity to cysLTs, and an overall good clinical response to LTRAs, the prevalence of eosinophils expressing LTC_4 synthase is fourfold higher than in those from patients with aspirin-tolerant asthma, and 19-fold more prevalent than in bronchial biopsies of nonasthmatics (129). A variant allele for LTC_4 synthase (A-444C) has been described (130). The variant A/C and C/C genotypes are found in high frequency (75%) in ASA patients (130) and in other chronic severe asthmatics (56%) in comparison with normals (32%) (130,131). In nonasthmatics, the presence of variant genotypes was not associated with increased urinary levels of LTE_4 at baseline, but following in vitro activation of eosinophils cysLT synthesis was threefold higher in subjects with the variant genotypes compared with the wild-type genotype (131). In severe asthmatics with the variant genotypes, increases in baseline FEV_1 were observed following 2 weeks of oral treatment with zafirlukast, whereas lung function did not improve in the wild-type genotypes (131). This study suggests that irrespective of aspirin sensitivity the C_{-444} variant genotypes of LTC_4 synthase are associated with a predisposition to higher cysLT synthesis, and that in patients with severe persistent asthma the variant genotypes may be markers of an LT-dependent form of asthma with a potentially good clinical response to LT modulators (131).

Leukotriene Receptors

The leukotrienes C_4, D_4, and E_4 comprise the "slow-reacting substance of anaphylaxis" (SRS-A), first described as bronchoconstrictor activity more than 60 years ago by Kellaway and Trethewie in guinea pigs (132), and some 10 years later confirmed by Brocklehurst and colleagues who demonstrated the presence of similar bronchoactive substances in human airways in vitro (133). Although separate receptors for LTC_4 and LTD_4 have been identified in guinea pig lungs, in human airways all cysLTs appear to act at the same receptors (134,135) termed $cysLT_1$ and $cysLT_2$ receptors. Both cysLT receptors have been recently cloned in humans, and expression studies demonstrated high concentrations of the $cysLT_1$ receptors in several tissue, including airway smooth muscle and inflammatory leukocytes (136). Moreover, the $cysLT_2$ receptor has been predominantly found in alveolar macrophages, but also in airway smooth muscle, peripheral inflammatory leukocytes, and some other organs as well (137).

The third major group of anti-LT drugs comprises the cysLT receptor antagonists (LTRAs) (138), which specifically block the $cysLT_1$ receptor on airway smooth muscle and other lung tissues. These compounds include zafirlukast (ICI-204,219; Accolate), montelukast (MK-0476; Singulair), and pranlukast (ONO-1078 = SB205,312 = Ultair). At present, only one LTRA (Bay U9773, not registered) has been shown to block both the $cysLT_1$ and the $cysLT_2$ receptor. The $cysLT_2$ receptor is suspected of mediating some of the vascular effects of cysLTs within human airways (137,139), although additional research is required to elucidate this mechanism.

Leukotriene-Releasing Cells

The LT profile generated in response to immunological and nonimmuno-logical stimuli varies among cell types. The potential of intact cells to produce LTs de novo depends on their coexpression of 5-LO and FLAP (100), whereas the subsequent synthesis of LTB_4 and/or cysLTs depends on the expression of the terminal enzymes LTA_4 hydrolase and LTC_4 synthase. Some cells express both enzymes, whereas others predominantly or exclusively express only one. Neutrophils preferentially secrete LTB_4, while eosinophils preferentially generate LTC_4 (107,120). Similarly, human lung mast cells and basophils preferentially secrete cysLTs (121,122). Monocytes are capable of producing both LTB_4 and smaller amounts of cysLTs (109), with an increased capacity for synthesis of LTB_4 as they differentiate into alveolar macrophages (110). In contrast to myeloid cells, the capacity of lymphocytes to generate LTs is contentious. Early reports on T lymphocytes generating LTs (140) have been disputed (141). Lymphoblastoid B-cell lines and human tonsillar B cells have low levels of 5-LO and FLAP activity (142,143). In addition, a range of lymphocyte cell lines, tonsillar B cells, and peripheral T cell have LTA_4 hydrolase activity (144), suggesting that LTB_4 may be formed by T or B lymphocytes (145). However, lymphocytes appear to lack LTC_4 synthase and thus do not generate cysLTs.

Regulation of the 5-Lipoxygenase Pathway

The human gene for 5-LO has been localized to chromosome 10 (146). Although the 5-LO gene promoter contains recognition sequences for the Sp1 and AP-2 transcription factors, it lacks the TATA and CCAAT sequences expected in an inducible gene (147). Alternatively, the 5-LO gene promoter contains a recognition sequence for the NF-κB transcription factor, which is associated with cytokines and adhesion molecules, suggesting that 5-LO products can be coregulated with other proinflammatory mediators. The gene for FLAP has been localized to chromosome 13, and in contrast to 5-LO, the FLAP promoter has TATA sequences and other features characteristic of a highly inducible gene (148). Its promoter also has a glucocorticoid response element (GRE), suggesting that FLAP expression may be regulated by glucocorticosteroids. Curiously, in human neutrophils, dexamethasone increases the expression of FLAP (149), and consequently up-regulates the activity of the 5-LO pathway, although a reduction might have been expected. Furthermore, both LTA_4 hydrolase and LTC_4 synthase cDNAs have been cloned (150). Intriguingly, the LTC_4 synthase gene localizes to human chromosome 5q35 (151), close to the loci of genes coding for IL-3, IL-4, IL-5, IL-6, IL-9, IL-13, and other eosinophil- and mast cell–regulating molecules implicated in asthma. In human neutrophils, granulocyte-macrophage colony-stimulating factor (GM-CSF) can induce the expression of 5-LO and FLAP, causing an increased LTB_4 synthesis (152). This mechanism accounts for the enhanced LTB_4-producing capacity occurring when monocytes differentiate into alveolar macrophages (102). In eosinophils, IL-5 and IL-3 promote the sequential expression of 5-LO, FLAP, and LTC_4 synthase in eosinophils differentiating from $CD34^+$ cord blood precursor cells, inducing an increase in cysLT synthesis (153). In mature human eosinophils, IL-5 also promotes the expression of FLAP but not of 5-LO (154). In murine mast cells, IL-3 promotes the expression of 5-LO, FLAP, and LTC_4 synthase (155), and in the human mast cell line HMC-1, stem cell factor increases 5-LO expression and activity (156). In conclusion, the cytokine microenvironment in asthmatic airways not only promotes influx of eosinophils and activation of mast cells, but also determines their capacity for eicosanoids synthesis toward cysLT production.

Effects of cysLTs Relevant to Asthma

Airway Smooth Muscle Spasm

Several studies confirmed that the cysLTs are potent bronchoconstrictors in both nonasthmatic and asthmatic subjects, with LTC_4 and LTD_4 being more than 1000-fold more potent than histamine and producing contractions lasting 2–8 times longer than those induced by histamine (157–162). LTD_4 is the most potent cysLT, whereas LTE_4 is less potent but produces the most sustained contractions. CysLTs contract human airway smooth muscle via stimulation of the $cysLT_1$ receptors and, according to indirect evidence in humans, possibly by secondary release of neuropeptides as well (163).

Inhaled LTC_4 and LTD_4 are more potent bronchoconstrictors in the airways of patients with asthma compared to nonasthmatic subjects, which is consistent with the presence of BHR in asthma. However, the degree of BHR is les than that seen with other agonists: asthmatic subjects respond to methacholine at a 55-fold lower concentration than nonasthmatic individuals, but respond to LTC_4 at a one-fourth and LTD_4 at one-eleventh of the concentration required in nonasthmatics (160,164). This could be due to production of endogenous cysLTs in asthmatics airways, inducing down-regulation of the $CysLT_1$ receptors, and thus a reduced response to exogenous cysLTs (165). Interestingly, asthmatic airways appear to be uniquely hyperresponsive to LTE_4, being 14-, 15-, 6-, 9-, and 219-fold more responsive to histamine, methacholine, LTC_4, LTD_4, and LTE_4, respectively, compared with airways of nonasthmatics (166). A possible explanation for these findings may be a differential expression of the cysLT receptor subtypes in nonasthmatic and asthmatic subjects, but this awaits further investigation.

Vascular Leakage and Formation of Mucosal Edema

The principal vascular effect of cysLTs is a direct action on the permeability of postcapillary venules (167). CysLTs are 2–3 times more potent than histamine in causing plasma extravasation in guinea pig trachea in vivo, an effect that was blocked by FPL-55712, an early specific LTRA (168). Furthermore, the allergen-induced increase in plasma extravasation in the airways of guinea pigs was blocked by the LTRA pranlukast, showing the involvement of endogenous cysLTs in this response (169).

Mucus Hypersecretion

Although plugging of the small airways by mucus is a common post mortem finding in status asthmaticus, excessive mucus secretion may also occur within the airways of patients with moderate persistent asthma. CysLTs affect mucus secretion directly via stimulating effects on goblet cells and submucosal glandular cells (170,171), and indirectly via the activation of airway nerves, inducing reflex secretion from submucosal glands (172). Following inhalation of cysLTs, expectoration of mucus is a common finding in both asthmatic and nonasthmatic individuals. In human studies in vivo, mucociliary transport in the asthmatic airways is diminished by inhaled allergen; this response was restored by the LTRA FPL-55712 (173). Hence, evidence has been provided that endogenous cysLTs are involved in mucus hypersecretion following allergen stimulation. The contribution of persistent overproduction of cysLTs inducing mucus hypersecretion to impaired lung function in asthma has not yet been clarified.

Effects on Inflammatory Cells

Several lipoxygenase derived mediators are potent chemotaxins for eosinophils but also cause nonspecific chemoattraction of other cell types, especially neutrophils (174–176). However, eosinophils that have been specifically primed by IL-5, may be selectively recruited by such a chemotaxin (177). In the last decade, it has been demonstrated that cysLTs are both potent and specific chemotaxins for eosinophils. In vitro, subnanomolar concentrations of LTD_4 chemoattract human eosinophils, whereas much higher concentrations were needed to cause chemotaxis of neutrophils (176). This response was blocked by the LTRA pobilukast (SKF 104,353) (176). In guinea pigs, inhalation of a single dose of LTC_4 or LTD_4 (but not LTB_4) has been shown to induce a dose-related eosinophil infiltration of the airways, persisting for up to 4 weeks (178,179). This inflammatory response was inhibited by the LTRAs MK-571 and pranlukast, and by an antibody to IL-5 (178,179). In ovalbumin-sensitized guinea-pigs, antigen inhalation has been shown to induce a four-fold eosinophil infiltrate of the bronchial submucosa at 12 h postchallenge. Furthermore, it appeared that this response was induced by endogenous cysLT release, as it was specifically blocked by the LTRA MK-571, but not by H_1 or H_2 receptor antagonists or by a COX inhibitor (180). In the same manner, the antigen-induced increases in AHR and in BAL eosinophil counts are blocked by the LTRA ICI 198,615 in cynomolgus monkeys (181). In another study in sheep, the rises in BAL eosinophils and in AHR following antigen challenge were blocked by the 5-LO inhibitor zileuton (A-64077) (182). Similarly, in 5-LO gene–disrupted mice, most of the rise in airway eosinophils, and the entire rise in allergen-induced AHR, occurring in the wild-type mice following allergen appeared to be absent (71).

Although these findings indicate that 5-LO products are the predominant factors in allergen-induced airway eosinophilia in these animal models, with IL-5 playing a minor role, it is not yet clear whether cysLTs and IL-5 act independently or synergistically to elicit the response.

In patients with mild to moderate persistent asthma who were treated with on-demand β_2 agonists only, inhalation of LTE_4 has been shown to cause eosinophilia in bronchial biopsies 4 h after inhalation (183). Similarly, LTD_4 induced eosinophils in sputum of asthmatics at the same time point following inhalation (184). In a recent study in asthmatics, LTs prolonged eosinophil survival by inhibiting the apoptosis of these inflammatory cells. This effect was reversed by LT modulators including an LTRA (pobilukast), a 5-LO inhibitor (BWA4C), and a FLAP antagonist (MK-886) (185). Furthermore, following segmental allergen challenge of asthmatic subjects, the induced rise in eosinophils in the BAL was significantly reduced by pretreatment with the 5-LO inhibitor zileuton and by the LTRA zafirlukast, 24 and 48 h post-allergen, respectively (186,187). Likewise, long-term administration of the LTRAs pranlukast and montelukast significantly reduced eosinophils in bronchial biopsies and induced sputum and peripheral blood of patients with moderate persistent asthma who were not treated with corticosteroids (188,189).

Effects on Nerves

In guinea pig airways, LTD_4-induced bronchoconstriction and plasma exudation have been shown to be partly mediated by tachykinin release, suggesting that LTD_4 can release neuropeptides from sensory nerves in this animal model (190,191). The neutral endopeptidase (NEP) inhibitor thiorphan, when given by inhalation, increased the maximal bronchoconstrictor response to inhaled LTD_4 in nonasthmatic subjects. These findings suggest that at least a part of the proinflammatory response to inhaled LTD_4 in human airways is caused by endogenous tachykinin release (192). Intervention studies with nontoxic and specific neurokinin receptor antagonists for human use are needed to investigate whether cysLTs exert their bronchoactive effects by secondary release of tachykinins.

Airway Remodeling

In patients with longstanding asthma, there are structural changes within the airways, including an increase in total airway smooth muscle (ASM) mass (193). In rats, the enhanced airway responsiveness following allergen exposure is caused by an increase in airway smooth muscle mass (194). Both these increases were blocked by the LTRAs MK-571 and pranlukast (194,195), suggesting a role of cysLTs in both phenomena. Additional evidence for a role of cysLTs in airway remodeling has been provided by two in vitro studies. In the first study, LTD_4 potentiated rabbit ASM proliferation to the mitogen insulin-like growth factor (IGF) (196). In another study, LTD_4 potentiated the effect of epidermal growth factor (EGF) on human ASM proliferation that was blocked by pranlukast (197). Additional studies in asthma in vivo are needed to confirm a role of cysLTs in the pathophysiology of airway remodeling in asthma.

Bronchial Hyperresponsiveness

BHR to various stimuli is a hallmark of asthma. CysLTs cause increases in airway responsiveness to other mediators. In nonasthmatic individuals, inhalation of a single bronchoconstrictor dose of LTD_4 increases airway responsiveness to methacholine twofold, with the maximal increase at 7 days and persisting for up to 14 days (198). In asthmatic subjects, inhaled cysLTs induce a three- to four-fold BHR to histamine, with the effect of a single dose of LTE_4 lasting up to a week (199). The mechanisms underlying BHR in allergic asthma are not fully understood, but a number of factors may be involved. Evidence suggests that BHR may be due to subthreshold airway narrowing caused by persistent overproduction of cysLTs by activated mast cells and/or eosinophils, which would increase resting ASM tone and promote airway edema (168) and mucus plugging (172). Moreover, the resting tone of human bronchi has been reduced by a specific LTSI (AA-861) and by an LTRA (MCI-286), but not by specific blockade of prostaglandin, thromboxane, histamine, or muscarinic cholinergic activity (200), suggesting that cysLTs play a pivotal role in regulating basal airway tone. In mice, targeted disruption of the 5-LO gene completely abolished development of BHR following antigen challenge that occurs in the 5-LO wild-type mouse (71). Evidence that cysLTs are involved in the pathophysiology of BHR in asthma has been provided by a few studies. In two allergen challenge studies in asthma, pretreatment with the LTRAs zafirlukast and pranlukast has been shown to reduce the allergen-induced BHR to histamine at 6 h and to methacholine at 24 postallergen, respectively (201,202). In another study in asthmatics, the protective effect of a single dose of the 5-LO inhibitor zileuton against BHR to cold, dry air in susceptible asthmatics lasted for up to 10 days (203). In another study in patients with mild to moderate persistent asthma who were not using maintenance therapy with glucocorticosteroids, treatment with pranlukast for 4 weeks resulted in a clinically significant reduction in AHR to methacholine (188). This effect was accompanied by significant reductions in symptoms and inflammatory cells in bronchial biopsies.

Role of Leukotriene Modulators in Asthma

In the last two decades, a growing number of studies in humans have been performed to investigate the effects of LT modulation on clinical asthma. From these studies it has now become clear that LT synthesis inhibitors (5-LO inhibitors and FLAP antagonists) and LT receptor antagonists (LTRAs) have similar clinical activity. These drugs can reduce bronchoconstriction and exhibit modest antieosinophilic activity (53,204–207). In various bronchoprovocation studies in asthmatics, these drugs have been shown to protect against challenges with exercise, cold, dry air, allergen, and aspirin (208). In studies in chronic asthma of differing severity, improvements have been reported in clinical symptoms, asthma exacerbation rates, lung function parameters, AHR, and peripheral and airway eosinophilia (208,209). Most of these effects became even more prominent when LT modulators were administered in combination with inhaled corticosteroids (207,210). Future studies should indicate the long-term effects of these compounds on various chronic sequelae of asthma, including airway remodeling.

C. Other Lipid Mediators

Several other lipid mediators, including HPETE, mono- and di-HETE and lipoxins are metabolic products of the mammalian 12- or 15-lipoxygenase enzyme. These enzymes catalyze the insertion of molecular oxygen at carbon 12 and 15 of arachidonic acid, respectively, and have been implicated as potential mediators of airway inflammation (89).

12-LO

The 12-LO enzyme was initially described in platelets (211,212) but is also found in monocytes, endothelial cells, vascular smooth muscle cells (213), and human skin (214). Furthermore, an additional 12-LO enzyme has recently been discovered that catalyzes the formation of $(12R)$-H(P)ETE in the skin (215) and tonsillar epithelial cells (216). 12-LO products have a number of biological actions include stimulating the production of collagenase from rat fibroblast (217), increasing monocyte adhesion to vascular endothelium (213), and stimulating mucus secretion (218).

15-LO

The 15-LO enzyme is found in a variety of cells and represents a major metabolic pathway for the conversion of AA in airway epithelial cells (219–222), eosinophils (223–225), macrophages (109,226), endothelial cells (227), monocytes (228), and dendritic cells (225). A second 15-LO enzyme has also been cloned and found to be expressed in the lung (229). The expression of 15-LO can be increased by Th2 cytokines including IL-4 and IL-13 as demonstrated in airway epithelial cells (230–232), dendritic cells (225), and monocytes (228,233,234) by a STAT6-dependent pathway (235), suggesting that 15-LO activity may be increased during an inflammatory episode in the lung, particularly as this response is characterized by the activation of Th2-dependent pathways (see cytokines).

The release of 15-LO products from the lung has been documented in a number of studies. Thus, generation of large quantities of 15-HETE is observed following antigen challenge of human lung form asthmatic subjects in vitro

(236) and following bronchial allergen challenge in vivo (52). Furthermore, pollutants such as ozone can stimulate the release of 15-HETE from human tracheal epithelial cells in culture (237). While the constitutive expression of 15-LO in the epithelium does not appear to be increased in asthma, there was an increase in the number of 15-LO-positive cells infiltrating the airways of these subjects and found to be localized, but not exclusively, to eosinophils (238). Similarly, the expression of 15-LO was increased in macrophages found in sputum samples taken from asthmatic compared with controls and this was associated with significantly greater levels of 15-HETE recovered from sputum samples in asthmatic patients (239). Together these studies demonstrate that 15-LO activity is up-regulated in asthma releasing significant quantities of 15-LO products within the airways.

The biological effect of 15-LO products has also been investigated. Thus, mono- and di-HETES are chemotactic for neutrophils (240–242) and eosinophils (243,244). Furthermore, 15-HETE is a potent stimulus for mucus secretion in humans (218), stimulates LTC_4 release from mastocytoma cells (245), inhibits cyclooxygenase activity (246), and may act as endogenous ligands for the peroxisome proliferator–activated receptor (PPAR-γ) (247). 15-HPETE has been shown to induce a slowly developing contraction of human airway smooth muscle in vitro (222) which may, in part, be secondary to metabolism of 15-HPETE to lipoxins (248,249) or following activation of PKC (250).

In the context of airway responsiveness, there is a paucity of data concerning the effect of 15-LO products on this response. 15-HETE has been shown to reduce airway responsiveness to histamine but prolonged the acute bronchospasm to inhaled antigen in asthmatic subjects (251,252). As mentioned previously, 15-LO catalyzes the insertion of molecular oxygen to the C-15 position of AA, which leads to the formation of the 15-HPETE. However, since this is a short-lived product, much of our understanding of the function of the 15-LO pathway stems from studies examining the biology of mono- and di-HETEs whereas there is a paucity of data concerning the biology of 15-HPETE. It is therefore of considerable interest that, like 8R,15S-diHETE (253), 15-HPETE (254) can increase the responsivity of painful stimuli by modulating afferent C-fiber activity and is therefore implicated as a potential hyperalgesia-inducing agent. In a similar context, the local instillation of 15-HPETE into the airways increased airway responsiveness to histamine in rabbits, which was not mimicked by the reduced product, 15-HETE, suggesting this was a specific effect related to 15-HPETE (255). This increase in BHR induced by 15-HPETE was associated with a cellular infiltrate that mainly consisted of neutrophils; however, it is unlikely that this cell accounted for the changes in airway responsivity, since 15-HETE during promotion of the recruitment of neutrophils to the airways did not induce BHR. Similarly, in a murine model of allergic inflammation, BHR and not the pulmonary recruitment of inflammatory cells was inhibited in 12/15-LO knockout mice (256).

The mechanism of the BHR appeared to be mediated via the activation of capsaicin-sensitive afferent nerves since this response was abrogated in animals chemically treated with capsaicin, a treatment modality that is often used to impair afferent nerve activity (255). The implication of these findings is that, as in the skin, 15-HPETE may alter afferent activity in the airways, promoting neural reflexes to spasmogenic agonists like histamine and thereby contributing to BHR in this model. The molecular target for 15-HPETE on airway sensory nerves has not been elucidated; however, it has recently been shown that products of the 12/15-LO pathway, including 15-HPETE, can increase the open probability of cloned and native vanilloid receptors (257). This is of considerable interest as this receptor has been implicated as a molecular integrator for hyperalgesia in a variety of pain models (258,259). It is plausible, therefore, that the close anatomical proximity between 15-LO expressed in the respiratory epithelium and afferent nerves that innervate this structure would provide the link between local inflammatory insult to the airways, sensitization of afferent nerves, and ultimately development of BHR. This argument is particularly persuasive in view of the findings that 15-LO activity and/or expression can be upregulated by inflammatory cytokines, thereby achieving high local concentrations in the airway wall.

Lipoxins

Lipoxins(LX) are trihydroxytetranene metabolites formed by the chemical insertion of molecular oxygen into C-15 and C-5 of AA via the corresponding LO enzyme, of which there are two major isomers (LXA_4 and LXB_4). These mediators are formed in the lung and are elevated in various pathological conditions, including asthma (226,260). LTA_4 has no effect on baseline lung function but appears to attenuate bronchoconstriction induced by LTC_4, possibly by acting as a receptor antagonist (261). Furthermore, a number of cellular studies demonstrate that LXs possess anti-inflammatory activity. Thus, LXA_4 inhibits human neutrophil (262) and eosinophil chemotaxis (263), and this mediator can suppress the recruitment of eosinophils to sites of inflammation (264). The notion that LXA_4 may serve as an endogenous anti-inflammatory agent is intriguing and might explain why some asthmatic subjects are aspirin intolerant as these individuals appear to have a reduced capacity to generate this substance (265).

IV. Peptide Mediators

A number of peptide mediators, including bradykinin, sensory neuropeptides (substance P, neurokinin A), and endothelin, are released in the lung and have a wide range of pharmacological activity. A number of studies in humans have shown that these mediators may contribute to various aspects of the inflammatory response in asthma.

A. Bradykinin

The kinins, bradykinin and lysylbradykinin, are synthesized from high (plasma) and low (tissue) molecular weight precursors (the kininogens, respectively) by the action of serine proteases (the kininogenases) (266). Bradykinin and lysylbradykinin are converted by carboxypeptidase M and N, respectively, to desArg^9-bradykinin and desArg^{10}-lysylbradykinin, respectively, following removal of the C-terminal arginine residue. Bradykinin has a short plasma half-life and is terminated by the action of angiotensin-converting enzyme (ACE) present in the endothelium and airway epithelium (267,268). Bradykinin produced in the airway wall is also terminated by neutral endopeptidase (NEP) present in the epithelium and airway smooth muscle. Kininogenase activity has been detected in BAL fluid in asymptomatic asthmatic subjects (269), and both kininogenase activity and kinin levels were increased following antigen challenge (270). Whether this reflects both an increase in kinin production and a reduction in the activity of degradative enzymes present in the lung is not clear. However, it was of interest that the level of immunoreactivity to ACE protein the epithelium was significantly diminished in biopsies from asthmatic subjects not receiving anti-inflammatory treatment (268).

Bradykinin Receptors

Human B_1 and B_2 receptors have been cloned and are characteristic of G-protein-coupled receptors linked to PLC (271,272). Both bradykinin and lysylbradykinin are equieffective at B_2 receptors, whereas desArg^{10}-bradykinin and desArg^{10}-lysylbradykinin are inactive. In contrast, the carboxypeptidase metabolites appear to be more potent that their parent peptides on the B_1 receptor. In the airways, B_2 receptors are present on various cells, including vascular endothelium, airway smooth muscle, submucosal glands, nerves, and airway epithelium (273). B_2 receptors are constitutively expressed on most cell types whereas expression of B_1 receptors can be induced by a variety of inflammatory cytokines including IL-1β (274). Another interesting feature of B_2 receptors is their susceptibility to desensitization compared with the inducible B_1 receptor and suggests that the B_1 receptor may play a greater role during an inflammatory response (274,275).

Effects of Bradykinin Relevant to Asthma

When inhaled, bradykinin produces modest if any bronchoconstriction in healthy subjects but is a potent bronchoconstrictor agonist in asthmatic subjects (276). It appears that this effect is mediated by B_2 receptors as desArg^9-bradykinin, which is selective for B_1 receptors, was without effect (277). However, the fact that desArg^9-bradykinin is at least two orders of magnitude less active than desArg^{10}-lysylbradykinin against the human B_1 receptor suggests that the latter is more likely to be the endogenous activator of this receptor

(272,275). Hence, the role of B_1 receptors in the physiological response to bradykinin in the airways remains an open question. Recently, it has been confirmed that, unlike bradykinin, desArg[10]-lysylbradykinin does not elicit bronchoconstriction in asthmatic subjects or evoke cough, thereby conclusively demonstrating no role for B_1 receptors in this response (278). These findings are also consistent with studies of human isolated bronchial preparations showing that contractile responses to bradykinin is antagonized by the B_2-selective antagonist icatibant (279,280).

The mechanism of bronchoconstriction induced by bradykinin has also been investigated and shown to involve a neuronal reflex (276). It does not appear to be secondary to the release of histamine from airway mast cells (277) or to the generation of COX products including TXA_2 (82,276,277), although in one study it was reported that inhaled lysine-aspirin attenuated bronchoconstrictor responses to bradykinin (281). Interestingly, bronchoconstriction to inhaled bradykinin was augmented following ingestion of the nitric oxide synthase inhibitor N^G-Nitro-L-Arginine, suggesting that nitric oxide functionally antagonizes this response in asthmatic subjects (282). Bradykinin stimulates a subpopulation of afferent nerves, C-fibers (283), and mediates the release of sensory neuropeptides from these nerves (284). Studies in the upper respiratory tract provide convincing evidence that bradykinin can stimulate sensory nerves, resulting in glandular secretion and vascular permeability (278,285–287). Similarly, bradykinin can also induce cough in healthy and asthmatic subjects (73). Clinical studies also suggest that bradykinin induces bronchoconstriction via activation of afferent nerves and subsequent reflex bronchoconstriction. The antiallergic agents sodium cromoglycate and nedocromil sodium inhibit bronchoconstriction to bradykinin, and these agents have been demonstrated to alter afferent nerve activity in animals (288,289). The up-regulation of this neural pathway during inflammation might explain the observation that the increase in airway responsiveness to bradykinin following antigen challenge is greater than that observed with methacholine and, moreover, persists for several days thereafter (290). Furthermore, airway responsiveness to bradykinin but not methacholine correlated with the number of eosinophils in BAL fluid, bronchial biopsies, and sputum (291,292). It remains to be established what role, if any, B_1 receptors play in this regard, but this seems less likely in view of an absence of effect of desArg[10]-lysylbradykinin on bronchomotor tone in vivo (278). The possibility that cytokines released into the airways amplify bradykinin responsiveness downstream of the B_2 receptor remains a distinct possibility to explain the increased airway responsiveness observed in this peptide (293).

In the context of modulation of inflammatory cell function, a variety of studies have demonstrated, using isolated human cell populations, that bradykinin can augment the function of neutrophils, monocytes, macrophages, and fibroblasts by activation of B_1 and B_2 receptors expressed on these cells (293). In the context of allergic inflammation, the role of bradykinin in eosinophil recruitment to sites of inflammation is not a consistent finding (294,295). However, there is considerable evidence showing that bradykinin can stimulate the release of a variety of cytokines and chemokines that are chemoattractant for neutrophils and monocytes from a number of cells, including macrophages (296), bronchial epithelial cells (297), and fibroblasts (298). Thus, bradykinin generated locally the lung during an inflammatory insult may contribute to the recruitment of neutrophils and monocytes to the lung. Similarly, the expression of B_1 receptors on $CD3^+$ T lymphocytes has been documented, activation of which produces antimigratory effects (299). However, the expression of kinin receptors and their function on Th2 lymphocytes remains to be established.

Role of Bradykinin Antagonists in Asthma

The effect of bradykinin receptor antagonists in respiratory disease is only beginning to be explored. A 4-week treatment with the B_2-selective antagonist icatibant (HOE 140) was shown to provide small improvement in various clinical indices (300), whereas acute intranasal treatment with icatibant prior to allergen exposure abolished nasal hyperresponsiveness in subjects with seasonal rhinitis (287).

B. Sensory Neuropeptides

In mammals, the preprotachykinin-I (PPT-I) gene encodes substance P and neurokinin A (NKA) whereas PPT-II encodes neurokinin B (NKB) (301–304). Alternate splicing of the PPT-I gene results in formation of three mRNAs designated α-, β-, and γ-PPT. Posttranslational processing of α-, β- and γ-PPT mRNA yields substance P and, from the two latter forms of mRNA, NKA. Furthermore, neuropeptide K and neuropeptide-γ are (N-terminally) extended forms of NKA produced by β- and γ-PPT mRNA respectively, whereas NKA (3–10) is produced from β- and γ-PPT mRNA. α and β-Calcitonin gene–related peptide (α-CGRP and β-CGRP) are products of two distinct calcitonin genes (305,306), and expression of mRNA for all of these sensory neuropeptides has been demonstrated in primary afferent neurons (307–309).

More recently, studies employing retrograde techniques have revealed that almost all afferent nerves guinea pig trachea arise from cell bodies within the nodose ganglion; however, most of the nerves that contain neuropeptides have cell bodies that arise from the jugular ganglion (310). This latter finding is consistent with an earlier observation that vagal section above, but not below, the nodose ganglion resulted in significant loss in substance P-like immunoreactivity in the guinea pig (311). In human studies, neuropeptides including substance P, CGRP, NKA, neuropeptide Y, and vasointestinal polypeptide (VIP) have been detected in the lung. Immunohistochemical techniques reveal that fibers containing substance P and NKA are sparsely distributed within the bronchial epithelium, around blood vessels, bronchial smooth muscle, and local tracheobronchial ganglia (312–316). It has even been suggested there is an absence of substance P-like immunoreactivity in the lung, despite demonstrable substance P in other tissues (317). However, it is unlikely that substance P is absent from this organ because substantial amounts have been extracted from human lung using a high-performance liquid chromatography (NPLC) technique (318). Various factors, including tissue processing, staining, age of subject, and type of subject studied can be important in influencing the detection of neuropeptides human lung. More recently, it has been proposed that neuropeptides like NKA have a role in human lung development as there was evidence of NKA immunoreactivity in nerve fibers and NK_2 receptor protein on airway smooth muscle in samples with gestational age greater than 12 weeks (316). The activation of these receptors with an NK_2 receptor agonist or capsaicin resulted in contraction of airway smooth muscle.

Neuropeptide Receptors

Three distinct types of tachykinin receptors exist in humans based on cloning and expression studies (319–322) and evidence from the comparison of tachykinin agonist potency in various tissues across different animal species, including human (323,324). The rank order of potency of mammalian tachykinins is as follows: substance P > NKA > NKBS for NK_1 receptors; NKA > NKB > substance P for NK_2 receptors; and NKB > NKA > substance P for NK_3 receptors. The tachykinin receptors are characteristic of G-protein-coupled receptors, activation of which can lead to both stimulation of phosphoinositide production and elevation of cyclic AMP (325).

Autoradiographic studies have detected binding sites for substance P over airway smooth muscle in the rabbit (326). However, little, if any, binding for substance P was detected over airway smooth muscle in humans (327,328), even though binding sites for substance P have been reported in one study of human airway smooth muscle (329). Whether methodological differences can account for these discrepancies is unclear but would seem unlikely, given that substance P binding sites were clearly detected in the microvasculature and submucosal glands of human (327,328). A more likely explanation is that functional NK_1 receptor may have a more peripheral distribution. Thus, studies have revealed that tachykinins contract human isolated airways via NK_2 receptors (316, 330,331) although in small-diameter airways (approximately 1 mm), contractile responses to substance P are mediated via an NK_1-dependent mechanism (332,333). The contractile response mediated by NK_1 receptors appears to be lower than that achieved following activation of airway smooth muscle NK_2 receptors but nonetheless is associated with elevations in phosphatidylinositol-3 (IP_3) and interestingly appears to be indirect and secondary to the release of cyclooxygenase products (332,333).

Other studies have documented possible changes in neurokinin receptor expression in respiratory disease. An increase in mRNA transcripts for NK_1 (334) and NK_2 (335) receptors was demonstrated in lung tissue from asthmatic as opposed to nonasthmatic subjects. In accordance with these findings, there is evidence of increased expression of NK_1 receptor protein the epithelium and, to a lesser extent, submucosal tissue from asthmatic as opposed to nonasthmatic subjects (315). In another study, both NK_1 and NK_2 receptor protein was detected in human airways localized to airway smooth muscle, glandular tissue, and vascular endothelium, whereas NK_1 receptors were occasionally found localized to nerves. In contrast, NK_2 receptors were found localized to macrophages, T lymphocytes, and mast cells (336). The level of expression did not differ among subjects who smoked in comparison with healthy controls.

Effects of Neuropeptide Relevant to Asthma

There are various reports indicating that neuropeptide levels within the lung may be altered in asthmatic airways. For instance, it has been claimed that substance P–containing nerves are more abundant in airway submucosa obtained at autopsy from asthmatics as than healthy individuals (337), although this observation was not confirmed in other studies (315,338,339). However, it was of interest to note that substance P-like immunoreactivity was increased within the epithelium that might have implications for regulation of epithelial cell function (315). Using HPLC, a reduction in substance P-like immunoreactivity was observed in lungs of individuals who died of asthma or who were undergoing thoracotomy, compared with age-matched nondiseased subjects (318). Similar changes have been reported in other diseases. In rheumatoid arthritis, there appears to be a loss of substance P- and CGRP-like immunocreactivity in sensory nerves in synovial tissue (340), whereas individuals with idiopathic cough who have increased sensitivity to capsaicin have increased levels of CGRP and, to a lesser extent, substance P immunoreactivity in nerves bronchial biopsies as compared with healthy subjects (341). These differences in levels of tachykinin immunoreactivity observed in inflamed airways might reflect turnover of neuropeptides secondary to activation of afferent nerves and provides circumstantial evidence for the release of sensory neuropeptides in asthma. This view is consistent with the detection of increased substance P-like immunoreactivity in BAL fluid in atopic asthmatics as compared with healthy individuals (342). Furthermore, concentrations of substance P-like immunoreactivity in BAL fluid was further increased in atopic asthmatics who had experienced an acute reaction to inhaled allergen (342). Elevated levels of substance P-like immunoreactivity have also been detected in the sputum of patients with asthma or chronic bronchitis patients as compared with healthy individuals following hypertonic saline inhalation (343). These findings are complimented by the observation that chronic treatment with capsaicin reduced symptoms and vascular reactivity in patients with severe chronic nonallergic rhinitis (344), suggesting that sensory neuropeptides are involved in the increased responsiveness of the upper respiratory tract.

Both substance P and NKA contract human bronchi (345,346), but the vanilloid receptor agonist capsaicin elicits only a modest contractile response and is at least two to three orders of magnitude less potent than in guinea pig (346–348). Capsaicin can also mediate an inhibitory response that is not dependent on the release of sensory neuropeptides (348), thereby potentially masking the excitatory action of this substance in these in vitro studies. To date, no study has convincingly demonstrated contractile responses in human airway tissue that are secondary to release of sensory neuropeptides from excitatory nonadrenergic noncholinergic (eNANC) nerves (346,349). Interestingly, a recent study has shown that capsaicin can induce contraction of airway smooth muscle in isolated perfused human fetal lung that was secondary to the release of NKA (316), suggesting that regulation of airway smooth muscle tone by neuropeptides is more important during development of the lung and less so in the adult.

Intravenous (350,351) or aerosolized (352) substance P produced marginal changes in lung function in healthy individuals, whereas NKA produced a small bronchoconstrictor response (351). In contrast, these substances elicit more consistent bronchoconstriction in asthmatic subjects (353). This might reflect the increased expression of neurokinin receptors observed in lung tissue in asthma (334,335). Alternatively, alterations in the pathways that degrade neuropeptides the lung might contribute to this increased responsivity to sensory neuropeptides in asthma.

Histochemical, immunohistochemical, and biochemical studies have revealed that neutral endopeptidase is found in the lung of guinea pigs (354,355) and humans (267) localized predominantly to the epithelium and is responsible for the degradation of tackykinins (224). Bronchoconstriction to inhaled NKA in healthy individuals was augmented by prior inhalation of the neutral endopeptidase inhibitor thiorphan, which may explain the propensity of asthmatics to bronchoconstrict in response to inhaled NKA (352,356). However, the neutral endopeptidase inhibitors thiorphan (357) and phosphoramidon (358) augmented the bronchoconstrictor response to NKA in mild asthmatics to a similar degree to that observed in healthy individuals (357). It seems likely, therefore, that asthmatics are intrinsically more responsive to NKA as a manifestation of the mechanism that determines differential responsivity between asthmatic and healthy subjects for other indirect-acting stimuli. Anticholinergic drugs have a modest inhibitory effect on the bronchoconstrictor responses to both substance P (359) and NKA (360) in asthmatics, suggesting that sensory neuropeptides may also stimulate parasympathetic neural pathways.

There is considerable evidence to support the notion that sensory neuropeptides released within the airway wall may play an important immunomodulatory role and thereby regulate the function of a number of inflammatory cells (361,362). Thus, neuropeptides, including substance P, are potent stimuli for the degranulation (363,364) and migration of human eosinophils (365);

proliferation and chemotaxis of human fibroblasts (366); chemotaxis of human immature dendritic cells, albeit at high concentrations (367); adhesion of neutrophils to a fibroblast monolayer and migration across a lung fibroblast barrier (368); adhesion of human neutrophils to epithelial cells in a synergistic manner with LPS (369); superoxide production from human monocytes (370); monocyte chemotaxis (371); TNF-α and IL-1β production from human monocytes (372,373); chemotaxis of human CD3$^+$ T lymphocyte (371); activation (374) and proliferation of T lymphocytes (375). Similarly, NKA was demonstrated to stimulate the migration of human bronchial epithelial cells in culture (376). Further evidence also support a role for substance P and NK$_1$ receptors in the recruitment of inflammatory cells to sites of inflammation. Thus, studies using human dermal microvascular cells reveal that substance P can stimulate the expression of adhesion molecules VCAM-1 and ICAM-1 secondary to elevation of intracellular calcium and following activation of the transcription factors NF-κB and NF-AT, respectively (377).

While a number of studies have suggested that the effect of neuropeptides on inflammatory cells might be mediated by a nonneurokinin receptor (378,379), it is also clear that neurokinin receptors exist on these cells that are functionally coupled to intracellular pathways whose activation leads to the pharmacological effects of exogenously administered substance P in many of the studies outlined above. Functional studies support a role for NK$_1$ receptors in mediating the pharmacological actions of exogenously administered substance P on inflammatory cell function. Thus, superoxide release from human macrophages (370), chemotaxis of monocytes and T lymphocytes (371), TNF-α secretion from human monocytes (373), and migration of neutrophils through a fibroblast barrier (368) was antagonized by NK$_1$-selective antagonists. Furthermore, using reverse-transcription polymerase chain reaction (RT-PCR), NK$_1$ mRNA was detected in human monocytes and lymphocytes from peripheral blood (380–382) and macrophages from sputum (383). Most studies investigating the role of tachykinin receptors in modulating inflammatory cell function utilize peripheral blood. However, it appears that the level of NK$_1$ receptor expression may be increased in cells derived from mucosal tissue (382,383), suggesting that factors which regulate the transmigration and/or differentiation of cells into tissue compartments may also be a signal for neurokinin receptor expression. This might have important functional consequences in disease states were neurokinin receptor expression may be increased (334,335). Thus, superoxide radical production was significantly greater in monocytes from individuals with interstitial lung disease than in that from healthy subjects (370).

Interestingly, it appears that while the principle site of synthesis for neuropeptides like substance P is neuronal, more recently it has been shown that substance P appears to be expressed in a number of inflammatory cells, including eosinophils (384), endothelial cells (385), monocytes (380), macrophages (383), and lymphocytes (381). The implication of these novel findings is that neuropeptides might act in an autocrine or paracrine fashion to influence inflammatory cell function.

While the majority of experimental evidence supports the view that NK_1 receptors are distributed in inflammatory cells in humans, recent observations indicate the presence of NK_2 receptor protein in a variety of inflammatory cells, including macrophages, mast cells and T lymphocytes (336). This is consistent with evidence supporting a functional role for NK_2 receptors on mononuclear cells (370,371) and fibroblasts (366). While an absence of NK_2 receptor protein in the epithelium has been shown in adult lung (336), there is evidence of localization of this receptor, albeit to a small population of epithelial cells in the developing lung (316), consistent with the demonstration of functional receptors on human bronchial epithelial cells in culture (376). Whether disease status or methodological differences can account for this lack of evidence of NK_2 receptor protein on epithelial cells in some studies is unclear at present. However, disease status may be an important factor as shown by the apparent discrepancy with regard to the level of epithelial NK_1 receptor protein expression in different respiratory conditions (315,336).

Role of Neurokinin Receptor Antagonists in Asthma

With the availability of neurokinin antagonists, a number of studies have begun to explore the role of sensory neuropeptides in asthma. The nonselective NK_1 and NK_2 antagonist FK-224 has been reported to inhibit (386) or be marginally effective against (387) bradykinin-induced bronchoconstriction and ineffective against NKA induced bronchoconstriction in asthmatics (388). The latter outcome brings into question the utility of this antagonist to evaluate the role of neuropeptides in asthma. However, selective NK_2 antagonist SR48968 attenuated NKA-induced bronchoconstriction in asthma (389) but was without effect against bronchoconstriction elicited by adenosine (390), suggesting that NK_2 receptors are not obligatory for the maintenance of BHR in asthma. On the other hand, the NK_1 receptor antagonist FK-888 improved the recovery from exercise-induced airway narrowing in asthmatics (391), whereas the NK_1-selective antagonist CP99994 was without effect on hypertonic saline–induced bronchoconstriction and cough in asthmatic subjects (392).

C. Endothelin

Endothelins (ETs) were originally discovered as potent vasoconstrictor peptides, and a wide range of studies have shown that these peptide mediators exhibit activity in the airways and may have a role in the pathophysiology of asthma (393). There are three ET peptides each encoded by three distinct genes (394). ET-1 is formed as a proteolytic product from the precursor peptide, pre-proET-1, via an intermediary product, big-ET-1. The conversion of big-ET-1 to ET-1 occurs via the action of endothelin-converting enzyme (ECE). The expression of mRNA for the ETs and ECE has been documented in human bronchial epithelial cells (395), which can be up-regulated by a variety of proinflammatory cytokines (396,397). There also resides within the epithelium neutral endopeptidase, which is known to degrade ET (398). Thus, the epithelium and other cell types the lung, including macrophages, neuroendocrine cells, vascular smooth muscle cells, and endothelial cells, may serve as a potential source for ETs and thereby play a role in airway inflammation (393,399).

Endothelin Receptors

A least two receptor subtypes (ET_A and ET_B) have been found for the ETs characteristic of G-protein-coupled receptors. ET-1 and ET-2 are selective for ET_A receptors compared with ET-3, whereas all three ETs bind to ET_B with high affinity (399). Autoradiographic studies have documented the presence of ET_B receptors in airway smooth muscle of healthy (400) and asthmatic subjects (401), with no obvious difference in distribution and/or density.

Effects of Endothelin Relevant to Asthma

Elevated levels of ET have been detected in BAL fluid from asthmatic subjects not taking glucocorticosteroid therapy (402) and consistent with an increase in the expression of immunoreactive ET in epithelium from biopsies taken from asthmatic subjects (403,404). However, acute bronchoconstriction to allergen inhalation (405) or hypertonic saline (406) does not appear to be associated with the release of ET-1. This is perhaps not surprising as this mediator is not stored and requires de novo synthesis, which might be expected to occur several hours following acute challenge. ET-1 is a potent bronchoconstrictor agonist in asthmatic subjects but has no effect in healthy subjects (407).

Although it is clear that ET induces significant bronchospasm in asthmatic subjects, the role of this mediator in promoting the inflammatory response has received scant attention. A recent study has shown that acute exposure with ET did not result in the accumulation of inflammatory cells to the airways as reflected by cell numbers enumerated in sputum. Furthermore, there was no increase in sputum levels of TNF-α, IL-1β, or albumin, suggesting a lack of proinflammatory activity (408). However, in the absence of a positive control it remains to be established whether ET has proinflammatory activity in asthma.

ET is a potent contractile agonist of human airway smooth muscle (400,409) and augments cholinergic nerve–mediated responses in human airways in vitro (410), both effects mediated via the activation of ET_B receptors. Furthermore, while ET did not stimulate the proliferation of human airway smooth muscle, this agonist augmented the proliferative response to EGF via an ET_A receptor–dependent manner (411). A similar finding has been observed regarding human bronchial fibroblasts, where ET required costimulatory signals from other growth factors increase DNA synthesis and collagen production from these cells (412). This latter finding might offer an explanation of why ET alone failed to elicit an inflammatory response in asthmatic subjects (408) and may require cooperation from other inflammatory mediators.

A number of in vitro studies have documented the capacity of ET to stimulate cellular activity in humans. Thus, ET stimulates the secretion of various cytokines, including IL-1β, TNF-α, and IL-6, from human macrophages (413) and monocytes (414); increases expression of adhesion molecules on vascular endothelial cells (415,416); and induces neutrophil aggregation (417), migration (418), and chemotaxis of monocytes (419). Animal studies have shown that ET can stimulate the recruitment of $CD4^+$ and $CD8^+$ T lymphocytes to sites of inflammation by an ET_A receptor–dependent mechanism (420). Similarly, mice overexpressing the ET-1 gene were characterized by an increase in the number of $CD4^+$ T lymphocytes recruited to the lung (421). Furthermore, eosinophilic recruitment to the lung in various inflammatory models appears to involve ET as reflected by the ability of ET receptor antagonists to inhibit the recruitment of eosinophils to sites of inflammation (422,423). The mechanism by which ET promotes eosinophil recruitment to the airways remains to be established but could involve up-regulation of adhesion molecules on vascular endothelium (415,416,424). Similarly, by stimulating TNF-α and IL-1β production from resident lung cells, ET may indirectly induce chemotaxis via CC chemokine production from airway epithelium (425). Alternatively, modulation of lymphocyte recruitment or alterations in Th2 cytokine generation from these cells in response to endothelin could promote eosinophil recruitment to the airways (420,421,423).

A number of studies have employed transgenic and knockout models to further address the role of ET in the lung. Mice that overexpress the gene for ET-1 were characterized by a pulmonary fibrosis with increased deposition of extracellular matrix protein located in perivascular and peribronchial regions (421). Interestingly, there was an absence of airway smooth muscle proliferation, which is consistent with in vitro studies demonstrating the requirement of costimulatory signals to stimulate airway smooth muscle proliferation (411). Mice heterozygous for the ET-1 mutant allele and characterized by significantly lower levels of ET-1 in plasma and lung appear to be more responsive to the bronchoconstrictor action of methacholine yet are normally responsive to serotonin (426). The mechanism of this effect does not appear to be related to alterations in airway wall structure (427) but might be related to an impairment in the production of nitric oxide by virtue of the decreased levels of ET in this model (426). The effect of ET antagonists on clinical asthma awaits documentation in humans.

V. Nitric Oxide

It is two decades since the discovery that the endothelium released a soluble factor that relaxed vascular smooth muscle (428), coined endothelium-derived relaxing factor, later identified as nitric oxide (NO) (429,430). NO is derived from the amino acid L-arginine by the enzyme nitric oxide synthase (NOS), of which exist the calcium-dependent, constitutive, endothelial isoform eNOS (or NOS3) and the neural (central and peripheral) isoform nNOS (or NOS1). These isoforms are also expressed in tissue other than their original designation. Thus, nNOS is also present in human bronchial epithelium (431). A third isoform is only expressed following an inflammatory insult (iNOS or NOS2), is less dependent on calcium for activation, and produces significant quantities of NO. This latter isoform is thought to play a role in pathophysiological situations.

A. Nitric Oxide Synthesis

In the lung, NOS3 is localized to endothelial cells in the bronchial circulation and within the epithelium (432), whereas NOS1 is predominantly localized to cholinergic nerves (433). In asthmatic airways, NOS2 is predominantly found in the airway epithelium (434,435) and inflammatory cells, notably macrophages, neutrophils, and eosinophils (435). Clinical studies have detected the presence of NO in exhaled airway of asthmatic subjects (436), which is increased during the late asthmatic response (437), supporting the view that during airway inflammation the expression of NOS2 is increased.

B. Effects of NO Relevant to Asthma

The functional consequences of NO in the airways has been investigated in a number of studies. In human airways it appears that NO is the neurotransmitter that mediates the nonadrenergic noncholinergic inhibitory response (438) and is consistent with the localization of NOS immunoreactivity to cholinergic nerves (439). NO is a potent vasodilator of the pulmonary circulation (440), and may either inhibit (441) or promote (442) plasma protein extravasation in the airways. The latter action is dependent on the expression of NOS2. These studies suggest that NO generated from NOS1 and NOS3 may play a protective role in the lung. Indeed, NOS inhibitors augment bronchoconstriction to inhaled bradykinin in asthmatic subjects (282) and increased nasal reactivity to both histamine and bradykinin in normal subjects (443).

It has recently been proposed that NO may promote the development of the atopic state by suppressing the function of Th1 lymphocytes, which act as a braking mechanism to the development of Th2-mediated responses (i.e., atopy) (444). However, human T lymphocytes of either Th1 or Th2 phenotype are susceptible to inhibition by NO, suggesting that there is no preferential downregulation of Th1 cell function (445). Similarly, other studies also support the view that NO may play a protective role during inflammation. Thus, NO has been shown to inhibit cytokine and chemokine production from human alveolar macrophages stimulated with LPS (446) that may be secondary to suppression of the activation of the proinflammatory transcription factor NF-κB (447). Similarly, NO was shown to inhibit NF-κB activity and release of the CC chemokine MCP-1 from human endothelial cells (448). Nitric oxide also inhibited the expression of VCAM-1 expression induced by TNF-α on human saphenous vein endothelial cells in culture, via increased expression of IκBα, an inhibitor of NF-κB (449). While NO has been shown to attenuate histamine release from human basophils in vitro (450), it is less likely that NO modulates mast cell function in vivo, as the NOS inhibitor L-nitroarginine methyl ester (L-NAME) failed to exacerbate acute bronchoconstriction to inhaled allergen in asthmatic subjects (451). In contrast to these findings, some studies support a role for NO as a proinflammatory mediator. Thus, NO donors promote activation of NF-κB in human peripheral blood lymphocytes (452), and NO has been implicated in promoting survival of human eosinophil via disruption of Fas receptor–mediated cell death (453,454).

Animal studies have documented increased NOS2 expression at various times following antigen challenge in immunized rodents (455–460). However, under different circumstances, airway inflammation can be induced in the absence of up-regulation of NOS2 expression the lung (461), perhaps reflecting differences in the intensity of the inflammatory response induced in these models. Inhibition of NOS activity with the use of inhibitors also highlights the role of different NOS isoforms in the pulmonary recruitment of eosinophils in these models. Thus, nonselective NOS inhibitors significantly reduced the recruitment of eosinophils to the lung following antigen challenge (461,462). However, the relative contribution of different NOS isoforms in these models is suggested by the findings that relatively selective NOS2 inhibitors either were ineffective (461) or suppressed (459,460,463) eosinophil recruitment to the lung. A potential mechanism by which NO facilitates eosinophil recruitment may be linked to increased CC chemokine expression in these models (463).

Further studies in mice with a gene disruption for the various NOS isoforms have also yielded conflicting outcomes. Thus, eosinophil recruitment following antigen challenge is either attenuated (457) or unaffected (458) following disruption of the NOS2 gene. Moreover, targeted disruption of the NOS1 and NOS3 genes was without effect on eosinophil recruitment (458), which seems at odds with the NOS inhibitor data outlined earlier. This discrepancy might relate to functional redundancy with respect to the different NOS isoforms for the recruitment of eosinophils to the lung or, more likely, that NO is not obligatory for eosinophil recruitment. Indeed, depending on the model employed, an anti-inflammatory role can be documented for NO. Thus, eosinophil recruitment was exacerbated in allergic mice following treatment with L-NAME, implicating NO as having an anti-inflammatory role in this model (464). While the mechanism by which NO may promote or inhibit eosinophil recruitment to the airways in these models is not clear, this was associated with a suppression (463) or augmentation (464) of CC chemokine expression, respectively.

In both knockout studies outlined above, BHR to methacholine following antigen challenge was not significantly altered in the absence of NOS2, thereby ruling out an obligatory role for NO generated during an inflammatory insult on airway lung mechanics. Interestingly, there was a discrepancy between the degree of baseline airway responsivity to methacholine in nonimmunized mice that probably reflected the different methods used to measure respiratory lung mechanics in these models (457,458). However, in contrast to these knockout studies, one study has reported a potential role for NO generated by NOS2 for the induction of BHR when it was demonstrated that treatment with a selective NOS2 inhibitor abolished the increase in airway responsiveness to methacholine following antigen challenge (460).

Under different experimental conditions it appears that NO may have a beneficial role and prevent the development of AHR (464). This might be due to the actions of NO produced from consitutively expressed NOS, which produces discreet amounts of NO compared with the inducible isoform, thereby acting as an endogenous suppressor of airway reactivity. It appears that NOS1 and, to a lesser extent, NOS3 are important determinans of baseline bronchial reactivity to spasmogenic agonists (458,465), although the mechanism is unclear. NOS3 appears to suppress neural responses to cholinergic stimulation in the mouse (466), and in ET-1 knockout mice the increase in baseline airways responsiveness to methacholine was attributed to a loss of NO in these mice (426).

C. NOS Inhibitors in Asthma

The NOS inhibitor L-NAME failed to attenuate the early and late asthmatic response following antigen challenge in asthmatic subjects (451). The level of expired NO was significantly decreased following treatment with L-NAME, which probably reflects inhibition of NOS1 and NOS3, since there was a lack of increase in expired NO during the late asthmatic response (8–10 h) in the placebo arm. This suggests that NOS2 expression was not increased during this time period and therefore makes interpretation of the data difficult. However, 21 h after allergen challenge there was a significant increase in expired NO that was not evident in the L-NAME-treated group, possibly reflecting an increase in NOS2 expression. Whether the development of more selective NOS2 inhibitors will prove of greater benefit in asthma requires further investigation. The lack of effect of L-NAME on AHR might be related to the removal of a protective endogenous dilator from the airways (282,443) or loss of a negative-feedback regulator which tends to suppress the allergic inflammatory (467).

VI. Conclusion

It is clear that there are a plethora of mediators too numerous to cover in one chapter that can modulate and influence inflammatory cell function. What is particularly striking is the sheer complexity of signaling that occurs during an inflammatory insult, and it is perhaps not surprising that single-mediator antagonists have proven inadequate in the management of diseases like asthma. The potential for interaction and synergism between different mediators upon inflammatory and immune cell function highlights the need for an integrative approach to fully comprehend the role of different mediators in the regulation of cellular function in airway disease.

References

1. Drazen JM, Israel E, O'Byrne PM. Treatment of asthma with drugs modifying the leukotriene pathway. N Engl J Med 1999; 340:197–206.
2. Barnes PJ, Fan CK, Page CP. Inflammatory mediators of asthma: an update. Pharmacol Rev 1998; 50:515–596.
3. Liu MC, Bleecker ER, Lichtenstein LM, Kagey-Sobotka A, Niv Y, McLemore TL, Permutt S, Proud D, Hubbard WC. Evidence for elevated levels of histamine, prostaglandin D2, and other bronchoconstriction prostaglandins in the airways of subjects with mild asthma. Am Rev Respir Dis 1990; 142:126–132.
4. Wenzel SE, Fowler AA, III, Schwartz LB. Activation of pulmonary mast cells by bronchoalveolar allergen challenge. In vivo release of histamine and tryptase in atopic subjects with and without asthma. Am Rev Respir Dis 1988; 137:1002–1008.
5. Liu MC, Hubbard WC, Proud D, Stealey BA, Galli SJ, Kagey-Sobotka A, Bleecker ER, Lichtenstein LM. Immediate and late inflammatory responses to ragweed antigen challenge of the peripheral airways in allergic asthmatics: cellular, mediator, and permeability changes. Am Rev Respir Dis 1991; 144:51–58.
6. Holgate ST, Finnerty JP. Antihistamines in asthma. J Allergy Clin Immunol 1989; 83:537–547.
7. De Backer MD, Gommeren W, Moereels H, Nobels G, Van Gompel P, Leysen JE, Luyten WH. Genomic cloning, heterologous expression and pharmacological characterization of a human histamine H1 receptor. Biochem Biophys Res Commun 1993; 197:1601–1608.
8. Gantz I, Munzert G, Tashiro T, Schaffer M, Wang L, DelValle J, Yamada T. Molecular cloning of the human histamine H2 receptor. Biochem Biophys Res Commun 1991; 178:1386–1392.
9. Lovenberg TW, Roland BL, Wilson SJ, Jiang X, Pyati J, Huvar A, Jackson MR, Erlander MG. Cloning and functional expression of the human histamine H3 receptor. Mol Pharmacol 1999; 55:1101–1107.
10. Ichinose M, Stretton CD, Schwartz JC, Barnes PJ. Histamine H3-receptors inhibit cholinergic neurotransmission in guinea-pig airways. Br J Pharmacol 1989; 97:13–15.
11. Oda T, Morikawa N, Saito Y, Masuho Y, Matsumoto S. Molecular cloning and characterization of a novel type of histamine receptor preferentially expressed in leukocytes. J Biol Chem 2000; 275:36781–36786.
12. Morse KL, Behan J, Laz TM, West RE, Greenfeder SA, Anthes JC, Umland S, Wan Y, Hipkin RW, Gonsiorek W, Shin N, Gustafson EL, Qiao X, Wang S, Hedrick JA, Greene J, Bayne M, Monsma FJ. Cloning and characterization of a novel human histamine receptor. J Pharmacol Exp Ther 2001; 296:1058–1066.

13. Liu C, Ma X, Jiang X, Wilson SJ, Hofstra CL, Blevitt J, Pyati J, Li X, Chai W, Carruthers N, Lovenberg TW. Cloning and pharmacological characterization of a fourth histamine receptor (H(4)) expressed in bone marrow. Mol Pharmacol 2001; 59:420–426.

14. Zhu Y, Michalovich D, Wu H, Tan KB, Dytko GM, Mannan IJ, Boyce R, Alston J, Tierney LA, Li X, Herrity NC, Vawter L, Sarau HM, Ames RS, Davenport CM, Hieble JP, Wilson S, Bergsma DJ, Fitzgerald LR. Cloning, expression, and pharmacological characterization of a novel human histamine receptor. Mol Pharmacol 2001; 59:434–441.

15. Braude S, Royston D, Coe C, Barnes PJ. Histamine increases lung permeability by an H2-receptor mechanism. Lancet 1984; 2:372–374.

16. Kaliner M, Sigler R, Summers R, Shelhamer JH. Effects of infused histamine: Analysis of the effects of H-1 and H-2 histamine receptor antagonists on cardiovascular and pulmonary responses. J Allergy Clin Immunol 1981; 68:365–371.

17. Shelhamer JH, Marom Z, Kaliner M. Immunologic and neuropharmacologic stimulation of mucous glycoprotein release from human airways in vitro. J Clin Invest 1980; 66:1400–1408.

18. Empey DW, Laitinen LA, Jacobs L, Gold WM, Nadel JA. Mechanisms of bronchial hyperreactivity in normal subjects after upper respiratory tract infection. Am Rev Respir Dis 1976; 113:131–139.

19. Raible DG, Lenahan T, Fayvilevich Y, Kosinski R, Schulman ES. Pharmacologic characterization of a novel histamine receptor on human eosinophils. Am J Respir Crit Care Med 1994; 149:1506–1511.

20. Elenkov IJ, Webster E, Papanicolaou DA, Fleisher TA, Chrousos GP, Wilder RL. Histamine potently suppresses human IL-12 and stimulates IL-10 production via H2 receptors. J Immunol 1998; 161:2586–2593.

21. Sirois J, Menard G, Moses AS, Bissonnette EY. Importance of histamine in the cytokine network in the lung through H2 and H3 receptors: stimulation of IL-10 production. J Immunol 2000; 164:2964–2970.

22. Pretolani M. Interleukin-10: an anti-inflammatory cytokine with therapeutic potential. Clin Exp Allergy 1999; 29:1164–1171.

23. van der Pouw Kraan TC, Snijders A, Boeije LC, de Groot ER, Alewijnse AE, Leurs R, Aarden LA. Histamine inhibits the production of interleukin-12 through interaction with H2 receptors. J Clin Invest 1998; 102:1866–1873.

24. Krouwels FH, Hol BEA, Lutter R, Bruinier B, Bast A, Jansen HM, Out TA. Histamine affects interleukin-4, interleukin-5, and interferon-gamma production by human T cell clones from the airways and blood. Am J Respir Cell Mol Biol 1998; 18:721–730.

25. Lagier B, Lebel B, Bousquet J, Pene J. Different modulation by histamine of IL-4 and interferon-gamma (IFN-gamma) release according to the phenotype of human Th0, Th1 and Th2 clones. Clin Exp Immunol 1997; 108:545–551.

26. Osna N, Elliott K, Khan MM. Regulation of interleukin-10 secretion by histamine in TH2 cells and splenocytes. Int Immunopharmacol 2001; 1:85–96.

27. Horvath BV, Szalai C, Mandi Y, Laszlo V, Radvany Z, Darvas Z, Falus A. Histamine and histamine-receptor antagonists modify gene expression and biosynthesis of interferon gamma in peripheral human blood mononuclear cells and in CD19-depleted cell subsets. Immunol Lett 1999; 70:95–99.

28. Kohka H, Nishibori M, Iwagaki H, Nakaya N, Yoshino T, Kobashi K, Saeki K, Tanaka N, Akagi T. Histamine is a potent inducer of IL-18 and IFN-gamma in human peripheral blood mononuclear cells. J Immunol 2000; 164:6640–6646.

29. Mashikian MV, Tarpy RE, Saukkonen JJ, Lim KG, Fine GD, Cruikshank WW, Center DM. Identification of IL-16 as the lymphocyte chemotactic activity in the bronchoalveolar lavage fluid of histamine-challenged asthmatic patients. J Allergy Clin Immunol 1998; 101:786–792.

30. Charlesworth EN, Kagey Sobotka A, Norman PS, Lichtenstein LM. Effect of cetirizine on mast cell-mediator release and cellular traffic during the cutaneous late-phase reaction. J Allergy Clin Immunol 1989; 83:905–912.

31. Okada C, Eda R, Miyagawa H, Sugiyama H, Hopp RJ, Bewtra AK, Townley RG. Effect of cetirizine on human eosinophil superoxide generation, eosinophil chemotaxis and eosinophil peroxidase in vitro. Int Arch Allergy Immunol 1994; 103:384–390.

32. Jinquan T, Reimert CM, Deleuran B, Zachariae C, Simonsen C, Thestrup Pedersen K. Cetirizine inhibits the in vitro and ex vivo chemotactic response of T lymphocytes and monocytes. J Allergy Clin Immunol 1995; 95:979–986.

33. Sedgwick JB, Busse WW. Inhibitory effect of cetirizine on cytokine-enhanced in vitro eosinophil survival. Ann Allergy Asthma Immunol 1997; 78:581–585.

34. Patella V, de Crescenzo G, Marino O, Spadaro G, Genovese A, Marone G. Oxatomide inhibits the release of proinflammatory mediators from human basophils and mast cells. Int Arch Allergy Immunol 1996; 111:23–29.

35. Arnoux B, Denjean A, Page CP, Nolibe D, Morley J, Benveniste J. Accumulation of platelets and eosinophils in baboon lung after PAF-acether challenge. Inhibition by ketotifen. Am Rev Respir Dis 1988; 137:855–860.

36. Atkins PC, Zweiman B, Moskovitz A, von Allmen C, Ciliberti M. Cellular inflammatory responses and mediator release during early developing late-phase allergic cutaneous inflammatory responses: effects of cetirizine. J Allergy Clin Immunol 1997; 99:806–811.

37. Zweiman B, Atkins PC, Moskovitz A, von Allmen C, Ciliberti M, Grossman S. Cellular inflammatory responses during immediate, developing, and established late-phase allergic cutaneous reactions: effects of cetirizine. J Allergy Clin Immunol 1997; 100:341–347.

38. de Bruin Weller MS, Rijssenbeek Nouwens LH, de Monchy JG. Lack of effect of cetirizine on early and late asthmatic response after allergen challenge. J Allergy Clin Immunol 1994; 94:231–239.

39. Bentley AM, Walker S, Hanotte F, De Vos C, Durham SR. A comparison of the effects of oral cetirizine and inhaled beclomethasone on early and late asthmatic responses to allergen and the associated increase in airways hyperresponsiveness. Clin Exp Allergy 1996; 26:909–917.

40. Fasce L, Ciprandi G, Pronzato C, Cozzani S, Tosca MA, Grimaldi I, Canonica GW. Cetirizine reduces ICAM-I on epithelial cells during nasal minimal persistent inflammation in asymptomatic children with mite-allergic asthma. Int Arch Allergy Immunol 1996; 109:272–276.

41. Aaronson DW. Evaluation of cetirizine in patients with allergic rhinitis and perennial asthma. Ann Allergy Asthma Immunol 1996; 76:440–446.

42. Simons FER. Prospective, long-term safety evaluation of the H1-receptor antagonist cetirizine in very young children with atopic dermatitis. J Allergy Clin Immunol 1999; 104:433–440.

43. Stossel TP, Mason RJ, Smith AL. Lipid peroxidation by human blood phagocytes. J Clin Invest 1974; 54:638–645.

44. Gallela G, Medini L, Stragliotto E, Stefanini P, Rise P, Tremoli E, Galli C. In human monocytes interleukin-1 stimulates a phospholipase C active on phosphatidylcholine and inactive on phosphatidylinositol. Biochem Pharmacol 1992; 44:715–720.

45. Samuelsson B. Leukotrienes: mediators of immediate hypersensitivity reactions and inflammation. Science 1983; 220:568–575.

46. Mitchell JA, Larkin S, Williams TJ. Cyclooxygenase-2: regulation and relevance in inflammation. Biochem Pharmacol 1995; 50:1535–1542.

47. Mitchell JA, Belvisi MG, Akarasereenont P, Robbins RA, Kwon O-J, Croxtall J, Barnes PJ, Vane JR. Induction of cyclo-oxygenase-2 by cytokines in human pulmonary epithelial cells: regulation by dexamethasone. Br J Pharmacol 1994; 113:1008–1014.

48. Johnson SR, Knox AJ. Synthetic functions of airway smooth muscle in asthma. Trends Pharmacol Sci 1997; 18:288–292.

49. Demoly P, Jaffuel D, Lequeux N, Weksler B, Creminon C, Michel F, Godard P, Bousquet J. Prostaglandin H synthase 1 and 2 immunoreactivities in the bronchial mucosa of asthmatics. Am J Respir Crit Care Med 1997; 155:670–675.

50. Narumiya S, Sugimoto Y, Ushikubi F. Prostanoid receptors: structures, properties, and functions. Physiol Rev 1999; 79:1193–1226.

51. Sugimoto Y, Narumiya S, Ichikawa A. Distribution and function of prostanoid receptors: studies from knockout mice. Prop Lipid Res 2000; 39:289–314.

52. Murray JJ, Tonnel AB, Brash AR, Roberts JL, Gasset P, Workman R, Capron A, Coates JA. Release of prostaglandin D2 into human airways during acute allergen challenge. N Engl J Med 1986; 315:800–804.

53. Dworski R, Fitzgerald GA, Oates JA, Sheller JR. Effect of oral prednisone on airway inflammatory mediators in atopic asthma. Am J Respir Crit Care Med 1994; 149:953–959.

54. Sestini P, Refini RM, Pieroni MG, Vaghi A, Robuschi M, Bianco S. Protective effect of inhaled lysine acetylsalicylate on allergen-induced early and late asthmatic reactions. J Allergy Clin Immunol 1997; 100:71–77.

55. Sestini P, Refini RM, Pieroni MG, Vaghi A, Robuschi M, Bianco S. Different effects of inhaled aspirin-like drugs on allergen-induced early and late asthmatic responses. Am J Respir Crit Care Med 1999; 159:1228–1233.

56. Fairfax AJ, Hanson JM, Morley J. The late reaction following bronchial provocation with house dust mite allergen. Dependence on arachidonic acid metabolism. Clin Exp Immunol 1983; 52:393–398.

57. Joubert JR, Shephard E, Mouton W, Van Zyl L, Viljoen I. Non-steroid anti-inflammatory drugs in asthma: dangerous or useful therapy? Allergy 1985; 40:202–207.

58. Hardy CC, Robinson C, Tattersfield AE, Holgate ST. The bronchoconstrictor effect of inhaled prostaglandin D2 in normal and asthmatic men. N Engl J Med 1984; 311:209–213.

59. Fish JE, Jameson LS, Albright A, Norman PS. Modulation of the bronchomotor effects of chemical mediators by prostaglandin F(2alpha) in asthmatic subjects. Am Rev Respir Dis 1984; 130:571–574.

60. Saroea HG, Inman MD, O'Byrne PM. U46619-induced bronchoconstriction in asthmatic subjects is mediated by acetylcholine release. Am J Respir Crit Care Med 1995; 151:321–324.

61. Heaton RW, Henderson AF, Dunlop LS, Costello JF. The influence of pretreatment with prostaglandin F(2alpha) on bronchial sensitivity to inhaled histamine and methacholine in normal subjects. Br J Dis Chest 1984; 78:168–173.

62. Fuller RW, Dixon CMS, Dollery CT, Barnes PJ. Prostaglandin D2 potentiates airway responsiveness to histamine and methacholine. Am Rev Respir Dis 1986; 133:252–254.

63. Matsuoka T, Hirata M, Tanaka H, Takahashi Y, Murata T, Kabashima K, Sugimoto Y, Kobayashi T, Ushikubi F, Aze Y, Eguchi N, Urade Y, Yoshida N, Kimura K, Mizoguchi A, Honda Y, Nagai H, Narumiya S. Prostaglandin D2 as a mediator of allergic asthma. Science 2000; 287:2013–2017.

64. Gavett SH, Madison SL, Chulada PC, Scarborough PE, Qu W, Boyle JE, Tiano HF, Lee CA, Langenbach R, Roggli VL, Zeldin DC. Allergic lung responses are increased in prostaglandin H synthase-deficient mice. J Clin Invest 1999; 104:721–732.

65. Hartert TV, Dworski RT, Mellen BG, Oates JA, Murray JJ, Sheller JR, Prostaglandin E(2) decreases allergen-stimulated release of prostaglandin D(2) in airways of subjects with asthma. Am J Respir Crit Care Med 2000; 162:637–640.

66. Knight DA, Stewart GA, Thompson PJ. Prostaglandin E2, but not prostacyclin inhibits histamine-induced contraction of human bronchial smooth muscle. Eur J Pharmacol 1995; 272:13–19.

67. Pavord ID, Wong CS, Williams J, Tattersfield AE. Effect of inhaled prostaglandin E2 on allergen-induced asthma. Am Rev Respir Dis 1993; 148:87–90.

68. Gauvreau GM, Watson RM, O'Byrne PM. Protective effects on inhaled PGE2 on allergen-induced airway responses and airway inflammation. Am J Respir Crit Care Med 1999; 159:31–36.

69. Noguchi K, Iwasaki K, Endo H, Kondo H, Shitashige M, Ishikawa I. Prostaglandins E2 and I2 downregulate tumor necrosis factor alpha-induced intercellular adhesion molecule-1 expression in human oral gingival epithelial cells. Oral Microbiol Immunol 2000; 15:299–304.

70. Peebles RSJ, Dworski R, Collins RD, Jarzecka K, Mitchell DB, Graham BS, Sheller JR. Cyclooxygenase inhibition increases interleukin 5 and interleukin 13 production and airway hyperresponsiveness in allergic mice. Am J Respir Crit Care Med 2000; 162:676–681.

71. Irvin CG, Tu YP, Sheller JR, Frunk CD. 5-Lipoxygenase products are necessary for ovalbumin-induced airway responsiveness in mice. Am J Physiol 1997; 272:L1053–L1058.

72. Szczeklik A, Sladek K, Dworski R, Nizankowska E, Soja J, Sheller J, Oates J. Bronchial aspirin challenges causes specific eicosanoid response in aspirin-sensitive asthmatics. Am J Respir Crit Care Med 1996; 154:1608–1614.

73. Choudry NB, Fuller RW, Pride NB. Sensitivity of the human cough reflex: Effect of inflammatory mediators prostaglandin E2, bradykinin, and histamine. Am Rev Respir Dis 1989; 140:137–141.

74. Betz M, Fox BS. Prostaglandin E2 inhibits production of Th1 lymphokines but not of Th2 lymphokines. J Immunol 1991; 146:108–113.

75. Snijdewint FG, Kalinski P, Wierenga EA, Bos JD, Kapsenberg ML. Prostaglandin E2 differentially modulates cytokine secretion profiles of human T helper lymphocytes. J Immunol 1993; 150:5321–5329.

76. van der Pouw Kraan TC, Boeije LC, Smeenk RJ, Wijdenes J, Aarden LA. Prostaglandin-E2 is a potent inhibitor of human interleukin 12 production. J Exp Med 1995; 181:775–779.

77. Sheller JR, Mitchell D, Meyrick B, Oates J, Breyer R. EP(2) receptor mediates bronchodilation by PGE(2) in mice. J Appl Physiol 2000; 88:2214–2218.

78. Tavakoli S, Cowan MJ, Benfield T, Logun C, Shelhamer JH. Prostaglandin E(2)-induced interleukin-6 release by a human airway epithelial cell line. Am J Physiol Lung Cell Mol Physiol 2001; 280:L127–L133.

79. Southall MD, Vasko MR. Prostaglandin receptor subtypes, EP3C and EP4, mediate the prostaglandin E2–induced cAMP production and sensitization of sensory neurons. J Biol Chem 2001; 276:16083–16091.

80. Minami T, Nakano H, Kobayashi T, Sugimoto Y, Ushikubi F, Ichikawa A, Narumiya S, Ito S. Characterization of EP receptor subtypes responsible for prostaglandin E(2)–induced pain responses by use of EP(1) and EP(3) receptor knockout mice. Br J Pharmacol 2001; 133:438–444.

81. Aizawa H, Shigyo M, Nogami H, Hirose T, Hara N. BAY u3405, a thromboxane A2 antagonist, reduces bronchial hyperresponsiveness in asthmatics. Chest 1996; 109:338–342.

82. Rajakulasingam K, Johnston SL, Ducey J, Ritter W, Howarth PH, Holgate ST. Effect of thromboxane A2-receptor antagonist on bradykinin-induced bronchoconstriction in asthma. J Appl Physiol 1996; 80:1973–1977.

83. Stenton SC, Young CA, Harris A, Palmer JB, Hendrick DJ, Walters EH. The effect of GR32191 (a thromboxane receptor antagonist) on airway responsiveness in asthma. Pulmon Pharmacol 1992; 5:199–202.

84. Fujimura M, Kamio Y, Kasahara K, Bando T, Hashimoto T, Matsuda T. Prostanoids and cough response to capsaicin in asthma and chronic bronchitis. Eur Respir J 1995; 8:1499–1505.

85. Myou S, Fujimura M, Nishi K, Ohka T, Masuda T. Inhibitory effect of a selective thromboxane synthetase inhibitor, OKY-046, on acetaldehyde-induced bronchoconstriction in asthmatic patients. Chest 1994; 106:1414–1418.

86. Gardiner PV, Young CL, Holmes K, Hendrick DJ, Walters EH. Lack of short-term effect of the thromboxane synthetase inhibitor UK-38,485 on airway reactivity to methacholine in asthmatic subjects. Eur Respir J 1993; 6:1027–1030.

87. Vidruk EH, Hahn HL, Nadel JA, Sampson SR. Mechanisms by which histamine stimulates rapidly adapting receptors in dog lungs. J Appl Physiol 1977; 43:397–402.

88. Manning PJ, Stevens WH, Cockcroft DW, O'Byrne PM. The role of thromboxane in allergen-induced asthmatic responses. Eur Respir J 1991; 4:667–672.

89. Samuelsson B, Dahlen SE, Lindgren JA, Rouzer CA, Serhan CN. Leukotrienes and lipoxins: structures, biosynthesis, and biological effects. Science 1987; 237:1171–1176.

90. Dixon RA, Jones RE, Diehl RE, Bennett CD, Kargman S, Rouzer CA. Cloning of the cDNA for human 5-lipoxygenase. Proc Natl Acad Sci USA 1988; 85:416–420.

91. Rouzer CA, Bennett CD, Diehl RE, Jones RE, Kargman S, Rands E, Dixon RA. Cloning and expression of human leukocyte 5-lipoxygenase. Adv Prostaglandin Thromboxane Leukot Res 1989; 19:474–477.

92. Evans JF, Leville C, Mancini JA, Prasit P, Therien M, Zamboni R, Gauthier JY, Fortin R, Charleson P, MacIntyre DE. 5-Lipoxygenase-activating protein is the target of a quinoline class of leukotriene synthesis inhibitors. Mol Pharmacol 1991; 40:22–27.

93. Samuelsson B, Haeggstrom JZ, Wetterholm A. Leukotriene biosynthesis. Ann N Y Acad Sci 1991; 629:89–99.

94. Rouzer CA, Matsumoto T, Samuelsson B. Single protein from human leukocytes possesses 5-lipoxygenase and leukotriene A4 synthase activities. Proc Natl Acad Sci USA 1986; 83:857–861.

95. McGill KA, Busse WW. Zileuton. Lancet 1996; 348:519–524.

96. Bell RL, Young PR, Albert D, Lanni C, Summers JB, Brooks DW, Rubin P, Carter GW. The discovery and development of zileuton: an orally active 5-lipoxygenase inhibitor. Int J Immunopharmacol 1992; 14:505–510.

97. In KH, Asano K, Beier D, Grobholz J, Finn PW, Silverman EK, Silverman ES, Collins T, Fischer AR, Keith TP, Serino K, Kim SW, De Sanctis GT, Yandava C, Pillari A, Rubin P, Kemp J, Israel E, Busse W, Ledford D, Murray JJ, Segal A, Tinkleman D, Drazen JM. Naturally occurring mutations in the human 5-lipoxygenase gene promoter that modify transcription factor binding and reporter gene transcription. J Clin Invest 1997; 99:1130–1137.

98. Dixon RA, Diehl RE, Opas E, Rands E, Vickers PJ, Evans JF, Gillard JW, Miller DK. Requirement of a 5-lipoxygenase-activating protein for leukotriene synthesis. Nature 1990; 343:282–284.

99. Miller DK, Gillard JW, Vickers PJ, Sadowski S, Leveille C, Mancini JA, Charleson P, Dixon RA, Ford-Hutchinson AW, Fortin R. Identification and isolation of a membrane protein necessary for leukotriene production. Nature 1990; 343:278–281.

100. Reid GK, Kargman S, Vickers PJ, Mancini JA, Leveille C, Ethier D, Miller DK, Gillard JW, Dixon RA, Evans JF. Correlation between expression of 5-lipoxygenase-activating protein, 5-Lipoxygenase, and cellular leukotriene synthesis. J Biol Chem 1990; 265:19818–19823.

101. Woods JW, Evans JF, Ethier D, Scott S, Vickers PJ, Hearn L, Heibein JA, Charleson S, Singer II. 5-Lipoxygenase and 5-lipoxygenase-activating protein are localized in the nuclear envelope of activated human leukocytes. J Exp Med 1993; 178:1935–1946.

102. Pueringer RJ, Bahns CC, Monick MM, Hunninghake GW. A23187 stimulates translocation of 5-lipoxygenase from cytosol to membrane in human alveolar macrophages. Am J Physiol 1992; 262:L454–L458.

103. Peters-Golden M, McNish RW. Redistribution of 5-lipoxygenase and cytosolic phospholipase A2 to the nuclear fraction upon macrophage activation. Biochem Biophys Res Commun 1993; 196:147–153.

104. Abramovitz M, Wong E, Cox ME, Richardson CD, Li C, Vickers PJ. 5-Lipoxygenase-activating protein stimulates the utilization of arachidonic acid by 5-lipoxygenase. Eur J Biochem 1993; 215:105–111.

105. Ford-Hutchinson AW. FLAP: a novel drug target for inhibiting the synthesis of leukotrienes. Trends Pharmacol Sci 1991; 12:68–70.

106. Mancini JA, Prasit P, Coppolino MG, Charleson P, Leger S, Evans JF, Gillard JW, Vickers PJ. 5-Lipoxygenase-activating protein is the target of a novel hybrid of two classes of leukotriene biosynthesis inhibitors. Mol Pharmacol 1992; 41:267–272.

107. Sun FF, McGuire JC. Metabolism of arachidonic acid by human neutrophils. Characterization of the enzymatic reactions that lead to the synthesis of leukotriene B4. Biochim Biophys Acta 1984; 794:56–64.

108. Sala A, Bolla M, Zarini S, Muller-Peddinghaus R, Folco G. Release of leukotriene A4 versus leukotriene B4 from human polymorphonuclear leukocytes. J Biol Chem 1996; 271:17944–17948.

109. Bigby TD, Holtzman MJ. Enhanced 5-lipoxygenase activity in lung macrophages compared to monocytes from normal subjects. J Immunol 1987; 138:1546–1550.

110. Damon M, Chavis C, Godard P, Michel FB, Crastes DP. Purification and mass spectrometry identification of leukotriene D4 synthesized by human alveolar macrophages. Biochem Biophys Res Commun 1983; 111:518–524.

111. Samuelsson B, Funk CD. Enzymes involved in the biosynthesis of leukotriene B4. J Biol Chem 1989; 264:19469–19472.

112. Orning L, Gierse JK, Fitzpatrick FA. The bifunctional enzyme leukotriene-A4 hydrolase is an arginine aminopeptidase of high efficiency and specificity. J Biol Chem 1994; 269:11269–11273.

113. Orning L, Gierse J, Duffin K, Bild G, Krivi G, Fitzpatrick FA. Mechanism-based inactivation of leukotriene A4 hydrolase/aminopeptidase by leukotriene A4. Mass spectrometric and kinetic characterization. J Biol Chem 1992; 267: 22733–22739.

114. Yokomizo T, Izumi T, Chang K, Takuwa Y, Shimizu T. A G-protein-coupled receptor for leukotriene B4 that mediates chemotaxis. Nature 1997; 387:620–624.

115. Martin TR, Pistorese BP, Chi EY, Goodman RB, Matthay MA. Effects of leukotriene B4 in the human lung. Recruitment of neutrophils into the alveolar spaces without a change in protein permeability. J Clin Invest 1989; 84:1609–1619.

116. Sampson SE, Costello JF, Sampson AP. The effect of inhaled leukotriene B4 in normal and in asthmatic subjects. Am J Respir Crit Care Med 1997; 155:1789–1792.

117. Evans DJ, Barnes PJ, Spaethe SM, van Alstyne EL, Mitchell MI, O'Connor BJ. Effect of a leukotriene B4 receptor antagonist, LY293111, on allergen induced responses in asthma. Thorax 1996; 51:1178–1184.

118. Christie PE, Barnes NC. Leukotriene B4 and asthma. Thorax 1996; 51: 1171–1173.

119. Evans RB. Comparative results of leukotriene modifiers in COPD and asthma. Am J Respir Crit Care Med 1998; 157:A413.

120. Weller PF, Lee CW, Foster DW, Corey EJ, Austen KF, Lewis RA. Generation and metabolism of 5-lipoxygenase pathway leukotrienes by human eosinophils: predominant production of leukotriene C4. Proc Natl Acad Sci USA 1983; 80:7626–7630.

121. MacGlashan DWJ, Peters SP, Warner J, Lichtenstein LM. Characteristics of human basophil sulfidopeptide leukotriene release: releasability defined as the ability of the basophil to respond to dimeric cross-links. J Immunol 1986; 136:2231–2239.

122. Peters SP, MacGlashan DWJ, Schleimer RP, Hayes EC, Adkinson NFJ, Lichtenstein LM. The pharmacologic modulation of the release of arachidonic acid metabolites from purified human lung mast cells. Am Rev Respir Dis 1985; 132:367–373.

123. Lam BK, Xu K, Atkins MB, Austen KF. Leukotriene C4 uses a probenecid-sensitive export carrier that does not recognize leukotriene B4. Proc Natl Acad Sci USA 1992; 89:11598–11602.

124. Snyder DW, Aharony D, Dobson P, Tsai BS, Krell RD. Pharmacological and biochemical evidence for metabolism of peptide leukotrienes by guinea-pig airway smooth muscle in vitro. J Pharmacol Exp Ther 1984; 231:224–229.

125. Koller M, Konig W, Brom J, Bremm KD, Schonfeld W, Knoller J. Functional characteristics of leukotriene C4- and D4-metabolizing enzymes (gamma-glutamyl transpeptidase, dipeptidase) within human plasma. Biochim Biophys Acta 1985; 836:56–62.

126. Conroy DM, Piper PJ. Metabolism and generation of cysteinyl-containing leukotrienes by human airway preparations. Ann N Y Acad Sci 1991; 629:455–457.

127. Keppler D, Huber M, Hagmann W, Ball HA, Guhlmann A, Kastner S. Metabolism and analysis of endogenous cysteinyl leukotrienes. Ann N Y Acad Sci 1988; 524:68–74.

128. Maltby NH, Taylor GW, Ritter JM, Moore K, Fuller RW, Dollery CT. Leukotriene C4 elimination and metabolism in man. J Allergy Clin Immunol 1990; 85:3–9.

129. Cowburn AS, Sladek K, Soja J, Adamek L, Nizankowska E, Szczeklik A, Lam BK, Penrose JF, Austen FK, Holgate ST, Sampson AP. Overexpression of leukotriene C4 synthase in bronchial biopsies from patients with aspirin-intolerant asthma. J Clin Invest 1998; 101:834–846.

130. Sanak M, Simon HU, Szczeklik A. Leukotriene C4 synthase promoter polymorphism and risk of aspirin-induced asthma. Lancet 1997; 350:1599–1600.

131. Sampson AP, Siddiqui S, Buchanan D, Howarth PH, Holgate ST, Holloway JW, Sayers I. Variant LTC(4) synthase allele modifies cysteinyl leukotriene synthesis in eosinophils and predicts clinical response to zafirlukast. Thorax 2000; 55 Suppl 2:S28–S31.

132. Kellaway CH, Trethewie WR. The liberation of a slow reacting smooth muscle-stimulating substance in anaphylaxis. Q J Exp Physiol 1940; 30:121–145.

133. Brocklehurst WE. The release of histamine and formation of slow-reacting substance (SRS-A) during anaphylactic shock. J Physiol 1960; 151:416–435.

134. Buckner CK, Krell RD, Laravuso RB, Coursin DB, Bernstein PR, Will JA. Pharmacological evidence that human intralobar airways do not contain different receptors that mediate contractions to leukotriene C4 and leukotriene D4. J Pharmacol Exp Ther 1986; 237:558–562.

135. Gorenne I, Norel X, Brink C. Cysteinyl leukotriene receptors in the human lung: what's new? Trends Pharmacol Sci 1996; 17:342–345.

136. Lynch KR, O'Neill GP, Liu Q, Im D-S, Sawyer N, Metters KM, Coulombe N, Abramovitz M, Figueroa DJ, Zeng Z, Connolly BM, Bai C, Austin CP, Chateauneuf A, Stocco R, Greig GM, Kargman S, Hooks SB, Hosfield E, Williams Jr DL, Ford-Hutchinson AW, Caskey CT, Evans JF. Characterization of the human cysteinyl leukotriene CysLT$_1$ receptor. Nature 1999; 399:789–793.

137. Heise CE, O'Dowd BF, Figueroa DJ, Sawyer N, Nguyen T, Im DS, Stocco R, Bellefeuille JN, Abramovitz M, Cheng R, Williams DLJ, Zeng Z, Liu Q, Ma L, Clements MK, Coulombe N, Liu Y, Austin CP, George SR, O'Neill GP, Metters KM, Lynch KR, Evans JF. Characterization of the human cysteinyl leukotriene 2 receptor. J Biol Chem 2000; 275:30531–30536.

138. Holgate ST, Bradding P, Sampson AP. Leukotriene antagonists and synthesis inhibitors: new directions in asthma therapy. J Allergy Clin Immunol 1996; 98:1–13.

139. Gardiner PJ, Abram TS, Tudhope SR, Cuthbert NJ, Norman P, Brink C. Leukotriene receptors and their selective antagonists. Adv Prostaglandin Thromboxane Leukot Res 1994; 22:49–61.

140. Atluru D, Lianos EA, Goodwin JS. Arachidonic acid inhibits 5-lipoxygenase in human T cells. Biochem Biophys Res Commun 1986; 135:670–676.

141. Goldyne ME, Rea L. Stimulated T cell and natural killer (NK) cell lines fail to synthesize leukotriene B4. Prostaglandins 1987; 34:783–795.

142. Jakobsson PJ, Odlander B, Steinhilber D, Rosen A, Claesson HE. Human B lymphocytes possess 5-lipoxygenase activity and convert arachidonic acid to leukotriene B4. Biochem Biophys Res Commun 1991; 178:302–308.

143. Jakobsson PJ, Steinhilber D, Odlander B, Radmark O, Claesson HE, Samuelsson B. On the expression and regulation of 5-lipoxygenase in human lymphocytes. Proc Natl Acad Sci USA 1992; 89:3521–3525.

144. Odlander B, Jakobsson PJ, Rosen A, Claesson HE. Human B and T lymphocytes convert leukotriene A4 into leukotriene B4. Biochem Biophys Res Commun 1988; 153:203–208.

145. Samuelsson B, Claesson HE. Leukotriene B4: biosynthesis and role in lymphocytes. Adv Prostaglandin Thromboxane Leukot Res 1990; 20:1–13.

146. Funk CD, Hoshiko S, Matsumoto T, RadMark O, Samuelsson B. Characterization of the human 5-lipoxygenase gene. Proc Natl Acad Sci USA 1989; 86:2587–2591.

147. Hoshiko S, Radmark O, Samuelsson B. Characterization of the human 5-lipoxygenase promoter. Proc Natl Acad Sci USA 1990; 87:9073–9077.

148. Kennedy BP, Diehl RE, Boie Y, Adam M, Dixon RA. Gene characterization and promoter analysis of the human 5-lipoxygenase-activating protein (FLAP). J Biol Chem 1991; 266:8511–8516.

149. Pouliot M, McDonald PP, Borgeat P, McColl SR. Granulocyte/macrophage colony-stimulating factor stimulates the expression of the 5-lipoxygenase-

activating protein (FLAP) in human neutrophils. J Exp Med 1994; 179:1225–1232.

150. Mancini JA, Evans JF. Cloning and characterization of the human leukotriene A4 hydrolase gene. Eur J Biochem 1995; 231:65–71.

151. Penrose JF, Spector J, Baldasaro M, Xu K, Boyce J, Arm JP, Austen KF, Lam BK. Molecular cloning of the gene for human leukotriene C4 synthase. Organization, nucleotide sequence, and chromosomal localization to 5q35. J Biol Chem 1996; 271:11356–11361.

152. McDonald PP, Pouliot M, Borgeat P, McColl SR. Induction by chemokines of lipid mediator synthesis in granulocyte-macrophage colony-stimulating factor-treated human neutrophils. J Immunol 1993; 151:6399–6409.

153. Boyce JA, Lam BK, Penrose JF, Friend DS, Parsons S, Owen WF, Austen KF. Expression of LTC4 synthase during the development of eosinophils in vitro from cord blood progenitors. Blood 1996; 88:4338–4347.

154. Cowburn AS, Holgate ST, Sampson AP. IL-5 increases expression of 5-lipoxygenase-activating protein and translocates 5-lipoxygenase to the nucleus in human blood eosinophils. J Immunol 1999; 163:456–465.

155. Murakami M, Austen KF, Bingham CO, Friend DS, Penrose JF, Arm JP. Interleukin-3 regulates development of the 5-lipoxygenase/leukotriene C4 synthase pathway in mouse mast cells. J Biol Chem 1995; 270:22653–22656.

156. Macchia L, Hamberg M, Kumlin M, Butterfield JH, Haeggstrom JZ. Arachidonic acid metabolism in the human mast cell line HMC-1: 5-lipoxygenase gene expression and biosynthesis of thromboxane. Biochim Biophys Acta 1995; 1257:58–74.

157. Weiss JW, Drazen JM, Coles N, McFadden ERJ, Weller PF, Corey EJ, Lewis RA, Austen KF. Bronchoconstrictor effects of leukotriene C in humans. Science 1982; 216:196–198.

158. Holroyde MC, Altounyan RE, Cole M, Dixon M, Elliott EV. Bronchoconstriction produced in man by leukotrienes C and D. Lancet 1981; 2:17–18.

159. Weiss JW, Drazen JM, McFadden ERJ, Weller P, Corey EJ, Lewis RA, Austen KF. Airway constriction in normal humans produced by inhalation of leukotriene D. Potency, time course, and effect of aspirin therapy. JAMA 1983; 249:2814–2817.

160. Griffin M, Weiss JW, Leitch AG, McFadden ERJ, Corey EJ, Austen KF, Drazen JM. Effects of leukotriene D on the airways in asthma. N Engl J Med 1983; 308:436–439.

161. Davidson AB, Lee TH, Scanlon PD, Solway J, McFadden ERJ, Ingram RHJ, Corey EJ, Austen KF, Drazen JM. Bronchoconstrictor effects of leukotriene E4 in normal and asthmatic subjects. Am Rev Respir Dis 1987; 135:333–337.

162. Barnes NC, Piper PJ, Costello JF. Comparative effects of inhaled leukotriene C4, leukotriene D4, and histamine in normal human subjects. Thorax 1984; 39:500–504.

163. Gardiner PJ, Cuthbert NJ. Characterisation of the leukotriene receptor(s) on human isolated lung strips. Agents Actions Suppl 1988; 23:121–128.

164. Bisgaard H, Groth S, Dirksen H. Leukotriene D4 induces bronchoconstriction in man. Allergy 1983; 38:441–443.

165. O'Byrne PM. Leukotrienes, airway hyperresponsiveness, and asthma. Ann NY Acad Sci 1988; 524:282–288.

166. Arm JP, O'Hickey SP, Hawksworth RJ, Fong CY, Crea AE, Spur BW, Lee TH. Asthmatic airways have a disproportionate hyperresponsiveness to LTE4, as compared with normal airways, but not to LTC4, LTD4, methacholine, and histamine. Am Rev Respir Dis 1990; 142:1112–1118.

167. Joris I, Majno G, Corey EJ, Lewis RA. The mechanism of vascular leakage induced by leukotriene E4. Endothelial contraction. Am J Pathol 1987; 126:19–24.

168. Woodward DF, Weichman BM, Gill CA, Wasserman MA. The effect of synthetic leukotrienes on tracheal microvascular permeability. Prostaglandins 1983; 25:131–142.

169. Obata T, Kobayashi T, Okada Y, Nakagawa N, Terawaki T, Aishita H. Effect of a peptide leukotriene antagonist, ONO-1078 on antigen-induced airway microvascular leakage in actively sensitized guinea pigs. Life Sci 1992; 51:1577–1583.

170. Hoffstein ST, Malo PE, Bugelski P, Wheeldon EB. Leukotriene D4 (LTD4) induces mucus secretion from goblet cells in the guinea pig respiratory epithelium. Exp Lung Res 1990; 16:711–725.

171. Goswami SK, Ohashi M, Stathas P, Marom ZM. Platelet-activating factor stimulates secretion of respiratory glycoconjugate from human airways in culture. J Allergy Clin Immunol 1989; 84:726–734.

172. Marom Z, Shelhamer JH, Back MK, Morton DR, Kaliner M. Slow-reacting substances, leukotrienes C4 and D4, increase the release of mucus from human airways in vitro. Am Rev Respir Dis 1982; 126:449–451.

173. Ahmed T, Greenblatt DW, Birch S, Marchette B, Wanner A. Abnormal mucociliary transport in allergic patients with antigen-induced bronchospasm: role of slow reacting substance of anaphylaxis. Am Rev Respir Dis 1981; 124:110–114.

174. Ford-Hutchinson AW, Bray MA, Doig MV, Shipley ME, Smith MJ. Leukotriene B, a potent chemokinetic and aggregating substance released from polymorphonuclear leukocytes. Nature 1980; 286:264–265.

175. Spada CS, Nieves AL, Krauss AH, Woodward DF. Comparison of leukotriene B4 and D4 effects on human eosinophil and neutrophil motility in vitro. J Leukoc Biol 1994; 55:183–191.

176. Page CP. The contribution of platelet-activating factor to allergen-induced eosinophil infiltration and bronchial hyperresponsiveness. Lipids 1991; 26:1280–1282.

177. Sehmi R, Wardlaw AJ, Cromwell O, Kurihara K, Waltmann P, Kay AB. Interleukin-5 selectively enhances the chemotactic response of eosinophils obtained from normal but not eosinophilic subjects. Blood 1992; 79:2952–2959.

178. Chan CC, McKee K, Tagari P, Chee P, Ford-Hutchinson A. Eosinophil-eicosanoid interactions: inhibition of eosinophil chemotaxis in vivo by a LTD4-receptor antagonist. Eur J Pharmacol 1990; 191:273–280.

179. Underwood DC, Osborn RR, Newsholme SJ, Torphy TJ, Hay DWP. Persistent airway eosinophilia after leukotriene (LT) D4 administration in the guinea pig: modulation by the LTD4 receptor antagonist, pranlukast, or an interleukin-5 monoclonal antibody. Am J Respir Crit Care Med 1996; 154:850–857.

180. Foster A, Chan CC. Peptide leukotriene involvement in pulmonary eosinophil migration upon antigen challenge in the actively sensitized guinea pig. Int Arch Allergy Appl Immunol 1991; 96:279–284.

181. Turner CR, Smith WB, Andresen CJ, Swindell AC, Watson JW. Leukotriene D4 receptor antagonism reduces airway hyperresponsiveness in monkeys. Pulm Pharmacol 1994; 7:49–58.

182. Abraham WM, Ahmed A, Cortes A, Sielczak MW, Hinz W, Bouska J, Lanni C, Bell RL. The 5-lipoxygenase inhibitor zileuton blocks antigen-induced late airway responses, inflammation and airway hyperresponsiveness in allergic sheep. Eur J Pharmacol 1992; 217:119–126.

183. Laitinen LA, Laitinen A, Haahtela T, Vilkka V, Spur BW, Lee TH. Leukotriene E4 and granulocytic infiltration into asthmatic airways. Lancet 1993; 341: 989–990.

184. Diamant Z, Hiltermann JT, Van Rensen EL, Callenbach PM, Veselic, Van d, V, Sont JK, Sterk PJ. The effect of inhaled leukotriene D4 and methacholine on sputum cell differentials in asthma. Am J Respir Crit Care Med 1997; 155:1247–1253.

185. Lee E, Robertson T, Smith J, Kilfeather S. Leukotriene receptor antagonists and synthesis inhibitors reverse survival in eosinophils of asthmatic individuals. Am J Respir Crit Care Med 2000; 161:1881–1886.

186. Kane GC, Pollice M, Kim CJ, Cohn J, Dworski RT, Murray JJ, Sheller JR, Fish JE, Peters SP. A controlled trial of the effect of the 5-lipoxygenase inhibitor, zileuton, on lung inflammation produced by segmental antigen challenge in human beings. J Allergy Clin Immunol 1996; 97:646–654.

187. Calhoun WJ, Lavins BJ, Minkwitz MC, Evans R, Gleich GJ, Cohn J. Effect of zafirlukast (Accolate) on cellular mediators of inflammation: bronchoalveolar lavage fluid findings after segmental antigen challenge. Am J Respir Crit Care Med 1998; 157:1381–1389.

188. Nakamura Y, Hoshino M, Sim JJ, Ishii K, Hosaka K, Sakamoto T. Effect of the leukotriene receptor antagonist pranlukast on cellular infiltration in the bronchial mucosa of patients with asthma. Thorax 1998; 53:835–841.

189. Pizzichini E, Leff JA, Reiss TF, Hendeles L, Boulet LP, Wei LX, Efthimiadis AE, Zhang J, Hargreave FE. Montelukast reduces airway eosinophilic inflammation in asthma: a randomized, controlled trial. Eur Respir J 1999; 14:12–18.

190. Martins MA, Shore SA, Drazen JM. Release of tachykinins by histamine, methacholine, PAF, LTD4, and substance P from guinea pig lungs. Am J Physiol 1991; 261:L449–L455.

191. Ishikawa J, Ichinose M, Miura M, Kageyama N, Yamauchi H, Tomaki M, Sasaki Y, Shirato K. Involvement of endogenous tachykinins in LTD4-induced airway responses. Eur Respir J 1996; 9:486–492.

192. Diamant Z, Timmers MC, Van d, V, Booms P, Sont JK, Sterk PJ. Effect of an inhaled neutral endopeptidase inhibitor, thiorphan, on airway responsiveness to leukotriene D4 in normal and asthmatic subjects. Eur Respir J 1994; 7:459–466.

193. Ebina M, Takahashi T, Chiba T, Motomiya M. Cellular hypertrophy and hyperplasia of airway smooth muscles underlying bronchial asthma. A 3-D morphometric study. Am Rev Respir Dis 1993; 148:720–726.

194. Wang CG, Du T, Xu LJ, Martin JG. Role of leukotriene D4 in allergen-induced increases in airway smooth muscle in the rat. Am Rev Respir Dis 1993; 148:413–417.

195. Salmon M, Walsh DA, Koto H, Barnes PJ, Chung KF. Repeated allergen exposure of sensitized Brown-Norway rats induces airway cell DNA synthesis and remodelling. Eur Respir J 1999; 14:633–641.

196. Cohen P, Noveral JP, Bhala A, Nunn SE, Herrick DJ, Grunstein MM. Leukotriene D4 facilitates airway smooth muscle cell proliferation via modulation of the IGF axis. Am J Physiol 1995; 269:L151–L157.

197. Panettieri RA, Tan EM, Ciocca V, Luttmann MA, Leonard TB, Hay DW. Effects of LTD4 on human airway smooth muscle cell proliferation, matrix expression, and contraction in vitro: differential sensitivity to cysteinyl leukotriene receptor antagonistis. Am J Respir Cell Mol Biol 1998; 19:453–461.

198. Kaye MG, Smith LJ. Effects of inhaled leukotriene D4 and platelet-activating factor on airway reactivity in normal subjects. Am Rev Respir Dis 1990; 141: 993–997.

199. Arm JP, Spur BW, Lee TH. The effects of inhaled leukotriene E4 on the airway responsiveness to histamine in subjects with asthma and normal subjects. J Allergy Clin Immunol 1988; 82:654–660.

200. Kohno S, Tsuzuike N, Yamamura H, Nabe T, Horiba M, Ohata K. Important role of peptide leukotrienes (p-LTs) in the resting tonus of isolated human bronchi. Jpn J Pharmacol 1993; 62:351–355.

201. Taylor IK, O'Shaughnessy KM, Fuller RW, Dollery CT. Effect of cysteinyl-leukotriene receptor antagonist ICI 204.219 on allergen-induced bronchoconstriction and airway hyperreactivity in atopic subjects [see comments]. Lancet 1991; 337:690–694.

202. Hamilton A, Faiferman I, Stober P, Watson RM, O'Byrne PM. Pranlukast, a cysteinyl leukotriene receptor antagonist, attenuates allergen-induced early- and late-phase bronchoconstriction and airway hyperresponsiveness in asthmatic subjects. J Allergy Clin Immunol 1998; 102:177–183.

203. Dekhuijzen PNR, Bootsma GP, Wielders PLML, Van den Berg LRM, Festen J, van Herwaarden CLA. Effects of single-dose zileuton on bronchial hyperresponsiveness in asthmatic patients with inhaled corticosteroids. Eur Respir J 1997; 10:2749–2753.

204. Hui KP, Taylor IK, Taylor GW, Rubin P, Kesterson J, Barnes NC, Barnes PJ. Effect of a 5-lipoxygenase inhibitor on leukotriene generation and airway responses after allergen challenge in asthmatic patients. Thorax 1991; 46: 184–189.

205. Gaddy JN, Margolskee DJ, Bush RK, Williams VC, Busse WW. Bronchondilation with a potent and selective leukotriene D4 (LTD4) receptor antagonist (MK-571) in patients with asthma. Am Rev Respir Dis 1992; 146:358–363.

206. Lammers JW, Van Daele P, Van den Elshout FM, Decramer M, Buntinx A, De L, I, Friedman B. Bronchodilator properties of an inhaled leukotriene D4 antagonist (verlukast—MK-0679) in asthmatic patients. Pulm Pharmacol 1992; 5:121–125.

207. Laviolette M, Malmstrom K, Lu S, Chervinsky P, Puject JC, Peszek I, Zhang J, Reiss TF. Montelukast added to inhaled beclomethasone in treatment of asthma.

Montelukast/Beclomethasone Additivity Group. Am J Respir Crit Care Med 1999; 160:1862–1868.

208. Diamant Z, Sampson AP. Leukotriene modulators. In: Yeadon M, Diamant Z, New and Exploratory Therapeutic Agents for Asthma. New York: Marcel Dekker, 2000:285–328.

209. Diamant Z, Grootendorst DC, Veselic-Charvat M, Timmers MC, De Smet M, Leff JA, Seidenberg BC, Zwinderman AH, Peszek I, Sterk PJ. The effect of montelukast (MK-0476), a cysteinyl leukotriene receptor antagonist, on allergen-induced airway responses and sputum cell counts in asthma. Clin Exp Allergy 1999; 29:42–51.

210. Virchow J, Prasse A, Naya I, Summerton L, Harris A. Zafirlukast improves asthma control in patients receiving high-dose inhaled corticosteroids. Am J Respir Crit Care Med 2000; 162:578–585.

211. Hamberg M, Samuelsson B. Prostaglandin endoperoxides. Novel transformations of arachidonic acid in human platelets. Proc Natl Acad Sci USA 1974: 71:3400–3404.

212. Nugteren DH. Arachidonate lipoxygenase in blood platelets. Biochim Biophys Acta 1975; 380:299–307.

213. Patricia MK, Kim JA, Harper CM, Shih PT, Berliner JA, Natarajan R, Nadler JL, Hedrick CC. Lipoxygenase products increase monocyte adhesion to human aortic endothelial cells. Arterioscler Thromb Vasc Biol 1999; 19:2615–2622.

214. Hussain H, Shornick LP, Shannon VR, Wilson JD, Funk CD, Pentland AP, Holtzman MJ. Epidermis contains platelet-type 12-lipoxygenase that is over-expressed in germinal layer keratinocytes in psoriasis. Am J Physiol 1994; 266:C243–C253.

215. Boeglin WE, Kim RB, Brash AR. A 12R-lipoxygenase in human skin: mechanistic evidence, molecular cloning, and expression. Proc Natl Acad Sci USA 1998; 95:6744–6749.

216. Schneider C, Keeney DS, Boeglin WE, Brash AR. Detection and cellular localization of 12R-lipoxygenase in human tonsils. Arch Biochem Biophys 2001; 386:268–274.

217. Mariani TJ, Sandefur S, Roby JD, Pierce RA. Collagenase-3 induction in rat lung fibroblasts requires the combined effects of tumor necrosis factor-alpha and 12-lipoxygenase metabolites: a model of macrophage-induced, fibroblast-driven extracellular matrix remodeling during inflammatory lung injury. Mol Biol Cell 1998; 9:1411–1424.

218. Marom Z, Shelhamer JH, Sun F, Kaliner M. Human airway monohydroxyeicosatetraenoic acid generation and mucus release. J Clin Invest 1983; 72:122–127.

219. Hunter JA, Finkbeiner WE, Nadel JA, Goetzl EJ, Holtzman MJ. Predominant generation of 15-lipoxygenase metabolites of arachidonic acid by epithelial cells from human trachea. Proc Natl Acad Sci USA 1985; 82:4633–4637.

220. Henke D, Danilowicz RM, Curtis JF, Boucher RC, Eling TE. Metabolism of arachidonic acid by human nasal and bronchial epithelial cells. Arch Biochem Biophys 1988; 267:426–436.

221. Nadel JA, Conrad DJ, Ueki IF, Schuster A, Sigal E. Immunocytochemical localization of arachidonate 15-lipoxygenase in erythrocytes, leukocytes, and airway cells. J Clin Invest 1991; 87:1139–1145.

222. Salari H, Schellenberg RR. Stimulation of human airway epithelial cells by platelet activating factor (PAF) and arachidonic acid produces 15-hydroxy-eicosatetraenoic acid (15-HETE) capable of contracting bronchial smooth muscle. Pulm Pharmacol 1991; 4:1–7.

223. Turk J, Maas RL, Brash AR, Roberts LJ, Oates JA. Arachidonic acid 15-lipoxygenase products from human eosinophils. J Biol Chem 1982; 257: 7068–7076.

224. Nadel JA. Neutral endopeptidase modulates neurogenic inflammation. Eur Respir J 1991; 4:745–754.

225. Spanbroek R, Hildner M, Kohler A, Muller A, Zintl F, Kuhn H, Radmark O, Samuelsson B, Habenicht AJ. IL-4 determines eicosanoid formation in dendritic cells by down-regulation of 5-lipoxygenase and up-regulaion of 15-lipoxygenase 1 expression. Proc Natl Acad Sci USA 2001; 98:5152–5157.

226. Levy BD, Romano M, Chapman HA, Reilly JJ, Drazen J, Serhan CN. Human alveolar macrophages have 15-lipoxygenase and generate 15(S)-hydroxy-5,8,11-cis-13-trans-eicosatetraenoic acid and lipoxins. J Clin Invest 1993; 92:1572–1579.

227. Hopkins NK, Oglesby TD, Bundy GL, Gorman RR. Biosynthesis and metabolism of 15-hydroperoxy-5,8,11,13-eicosatetraenoic acid by human umbilical vein endothelial cells. J Biol Chem 1984; 259:14048–14053.

228. Conrad DJ, Kuhn H, Mulkins M, Highland E, Sigal E. Specific inflammatory cytokines regulate the expression of human monocyte 15-lipoxygenase. Proc Natl Acad Sci USA 1992; 89:217–221.

229. Brash AR, Boeglin WE, Chang MS. Discovery of a second 15S-lipoxygenase in humans. Proc Natl Acad Sci USA 1997; 94:6148–6152.

230. Brinckmann R, Topp MS, Zalan I, Heydeck D, Ludwig P, Kuhn H, Berdel WE, Habenicht JR. Regulation of 15-lipoxygenase expression in lung epithelial cells by interleukin-4 Biochem J 1996; 318 (Pt 1):305–312.

231. Jayawickreme SP, Gray T, Nettesheim P, Eling T. Regulation of 15-lipoxygenase expression and mucus secretion by IL-4 in human bronchial epithelial cells. Am J Physiol 1999; 276:L596–L603.

232. Profita M, Vignola AM, Sala A, Mirabella A, Siena L, Pace E, Folco G, Bonsignore G. Interleukin-4 enhances 15-lipoxygenase activity and incorporation of 15(S)-HETE into cellular phospholipids in cultured pulmonary epithelial cells. Am J Respir Cell Mol Biol 1999; 20:61–68.

233. Sigal E, Sloane DL, Conrad DJ. Human 15-lipoxygenase: induction by interleukin-4 and insights into positional specificity. J Lipid Mediat 1993; 6:75–88.

234. Nassar GM, Morrow JD, Roberts LJ, Lakkis FG, Badr KF. Induction of 15-lipoxygenase by interleukin-13 in human blood monocytes. J Biol Chem 1994; 269:27631–27634.

235. Conrad DJ, Lu M. Regulation of human 12/15-lipoxygenase by Stat6-dependent transcription Am J Respir Cell Mol Biol 2000; 22:226–234.

236. Dahlen SE, Hansson G, Hedqvist P, Bjorck T, Granstrom E, Dahlen B. Allergen challenge of lung tissue from asthmatics elicits bronchial contraction that correlates with the release of leukotrienes C4, D4, and E4. Proc Natl Acad Sci USA 1983; 80:1772–1716.

237. Alpert SE, Walenga RW. Ozone exposure of human tracheal epithelial cells inactivates cyclooxygenase and increases 15-HETE production. Am J Physiol 1995; 269:L734–L743.

238. Bradding P, Redington AE, Djukanovic R, Conrad DJ, Holgate ST. 15-lipoxy-genase immunoreactivity in normal and in asthmatic airways. Am J Respir Crit Care Med 1995; 151:1201–1204.

239. Profita M, Sala A, Riccobono L, Paterno A, Mirabella A, Bonanno A, Guerrera D, Pace E, Bonsignore G, Bousquet J, Vignola AM. 15-Lipoxygenase expression and 15(S)-hydroxyeicoisatetraenoic acid release and reincorporation in induced sputum of asthmatic subjects. J Allergy Clin Immunol 2000; 105:711–716.

240. Shak S, Perez HD, Goldstein IM. A novel dioxygenation product of arachidonic acid possesses potent chemotactic activity for human polymorphonuclear leuko-cytes. J Biol Chem 1983; 258:14948–14953.

241. Johnson HG, McNee ML, Sun FF. 15-Hydroxyeicosatetraenoic acid is a potent inflammatory mediator and agonist of canine tracheal mucus secretion. Am Rev Respir Dis 1985; 131:917–922.

242. Kirsch CM, Sigal E, Djokic TD, Graf PD, Nadel JA. An in vivo chemotaxis assay in the dog trachea: evidence for chemotactic activity of 8,15-diHETE. J Appl Physiol 1988; 64:1792–1795.

243. Morita E, Schroder JM, Christophers E. Production of 15-hydroxyeicosa-tetraenoic acid by purified human eosinophils and neutrophils. Scand J Immunol 1990; 32:497–502.

244. Schewenk U, Morita E, Engel R, Schroder JM. Identification of 5-oxo-15-hydroxy-6,8,11,13-eicosatetraenoic acid as a novel and potent human eosi-nophil chemotactic eicosanoid. J Biol Chem 1992; 267:12482–12488.

245. Goetzl EJ, Phillips MJ, Gold WM. Stimulus specificity of the generation of leukotrienes by dog mastocytoma cells. J Exp Med 1983; 158:731–737.

246. Setty BN, Stuart MJ. 15-Hydroxy-5,8,11,13-eicosatetraenoic acid inhibits human vascular cyclooxygenase. Potential role in diabetic vascular disease. J Clin Invest 1986; 77:202–211.

247. Huang JT, Welch JS, Ricote M, Binder CJ, Willson TM, Kelly C, Witztum JL, Funk CD, Conrad D, Glass CK. Interleukin-4-dependent production of PPAR-gamma ligands in macrophages by 12/15-lipoxygenase. Nature 1999; 400:378–382.

248. Dahlen SE, Raud J, Serhan CN, Bjork J, Samuelsson B. Biological activities of lipoxin A include lung strip contraction and dilation of arterioles in vivo. Acta Physiol Scand 1987; 130:643–647.

249. Meini S, Evangelista S, Geppetti P, Szallasi A, Blumberg PM, Manzini S. Pharmacologic and neurochemical evidence for the activation of capsaicin-sensitive sensory nerves by lipoxin A4 in guinea pig bronchus. Am Rev Respir Dis 1992; 146:930–934.

250. Hansson A, Serhan CN, Haeggstrom J, Ingelman-Sundberg M, Samuelsson B. Activation of protein kinase C by lipoxin A and other eicosanoids. Intracellular action of oxygenation products of arachidonic acid. Biochem Biophys Res Commun 1986; 134:1215–1222.

251. Lai CK, Polosa R, Holgate ST. Effect of 15-(s)-hydroxyeicosatetraenoic acid on allergen-induced asthmatic responses. Am Rev Respir Dis 1990; 141:1423–1427.

252. Lai CK, Phillips GD, Jenkins JR, Holgate ST. The effect of inhaled 15-(s)-hydroxyeicosatetraenoic acid (15-HETE) on airway calibre and non-specific

responsiveness in normal and asthmatic human subjects. Eur Respir J 1990; 3:38–45.

253. White DM, Basbaum AI, Goetzl EJ, Levine JD. The 15-lipoxygenase product, 8R,15S-diHETE, stereospecifically sensitizes C-fiber mechanoheat nociceptors in hairy skin of rat. J Neurophysiol 1990; 63:966–970.

254. Adcock JJ, Garland LG. The contribution of sensory reflexes an "hyperalgesia" to airway hyperresponsiveness. In: Page CP, Gardner PJ, eds. Airway Hyper-responsiveness: Is It Really Important for Asthma? Oxford, UK: Blackwell Scientific, 1993:234–255.

255. Riccio MM, Matsumoto T, Adcock JJ, Douglas GJ, Spina D, Page CP. The effect of 15-HPETE on airway responsiveness and pulmonary cell recruitment in rabbits. Br J Pharmacol 1997; 122:249–256.

256. Luu BQ, Broide DH, Conard DJ, 12/15-lipoxygenase in murine model of allergen-induced airway inflammation. Am J Respir Crit Care Med 2001; 163:A433.

257. Hwang SW, Cho H, Kwak J, Lee SY, Kang CJ, Jung J, Cho S, Min KH, Suh YG, Kim D, Oh U. Direct activation of capsaicin receptors by products of lipoxygenases: endogenous capsaicin-like substances. Proc Natl Acad Sci USA 2000; 97:6155–6160.

258. Caterina MJ, Leffler A, Malmberg AB, Martin WJ, Trafton J, Peterson-Zeitz KR, Koltzenburg M, Basbaum AI, Julius D. Impaired nociception and pain sensation in mice lacking the capsaicin receptor. Science 2000; 288:306–313.

259. Davis JB, Gray J, Gunthorpe MJ, Hatcher JP, Davey PT, Overend P, Harries MH, Latcham J, Clapham C, Atkinson K, Hughes SA, Rance K, Grau E, Harper AJ, Pugh PL, Rogers DC, Bingham S, Randall A, Sheardown SA. Vanilloid receptor-1 is essential for inflammatory thermal hyperalgesia. Nature 2000; 405:183–187.

260. Lee TH, Crea AE, Gant V, Spur BW, Marrow BE, Nicolaou KC, Reardon E, Brezinski M, Serhan CN. Identification of lipoxin A4 and its relationship to the sulfidopeptide leukotrienes C4, D4, and E4 in the bronchoalveolar lavage fluids obtained from patients with selected pulmonary diseases. Am Rev Respir Dis 1990; 141:1453–1458.

261. Christie PE, Spur BW, Lee TH. The effects of lipoxin A4 on airway response in asthmatic subjects. Am Rev Respir Dis 1992; 145:1281–1284.

262. Lee TH, Lympany P, Crea AE, Spur BW. Inhibition of leukotriene B4-induced neutrophil migration by lipoxin A4: structure–function relationship. Biochem Biophys Res Commun 1991; 180:1416–1421.

263. Soyombo O, Spur BW, Lee TH. Effects of lipoxin A4 on chemotaxis and degranulation of human eosinophils stimulated by platelet-activating factor and N-formyl-L-methionyl-L-leucyl-L-phenylalanine. Allergy 1994; 49:230–234.

264. Bandeira-Melo C, Bozza PT, Diaz BL, Cordeiro RS, Jose PJ, Martins MA, Serhan CN. Cutting edge: lipoxin (LX) A4 and aspirin-triggered 15-epi-LXA4 block allergen-induced eosinophil trafficking. J Immunol 2000; 164: 2267–2271.

265. Sanak M, Levy BD, Clish CB, Chiang N, Gronert K, Mastalerz L, Serhan CN, Szczeklik A. Aspirin-tolerant asthmatics generate more lipoxins than aspirin-intolerant asthmatics. Eur Respir J 2000; 16:44–49.

266. Proud D. The kinin system in rhinitis and asthma. Clin Rev Allergy Immunol 1998; 16:351–364.

267. Johnson AR, Ashton J, Schulz WW, Erdos EG. Neutral metalloendopeptidase in human lung tissue and cultured cells. Am Rev Respir Dis 1985; 132:564–568.

268. Roisman GL, Danel CJ, Lacronique JG, Alhenc-Gelas F, Dusser DJ. Decreased expression of angiotensin-converting enzyme in the airway epithelium of asthmatic subject is associated with eosinophil inflammation. J Allergy Clin Immunol 1999; 104:402–410.

269. Christiansen SC, Proud D, Cochrane CG. Detection of tissue kallikrein in the bronchoalveolar lavage fluid of asthmatic subjects. J Clin Invest 1987; 79:188–197.

270. Christiansen SC, Proud D, Sarnoff RB, Juergens U, Cochrane CG, Zuraw BL. Elevation of tissue kallikrein and kinin in the airways of asthmatic subjects after endobronchial allergen challenge. Am Rev Respir Dis 1992; 145:900–905.

271. Hess JF, Borkowski JA, Young GS, Strader CD, Ransom RW. Cloning and pharmacological characterization of a human bradykinin (BK-2) receptor. Biochem Biophys Res Commun 1992; 184:260–268.

272. Menke JG, Borkowski JA, Bierilo KK, MacNeil T, Derrick AW, Schneck KA, Ransom RW, Strader CD, Linemeyer DL, Hess JF. Expression cloning of a human B1 bradykinin receptor. J Biol Chem 1994; 269:21583–21586.

273. Mak JCW, Barnes PJ. Autoradiographic visualization of bradykinin receptors in human and guinea pig lung. Eur J Pharmacol 1991; 194:37–43.

274. Ahluwalia A, Perretti M. B1 receptors as a new inflammatory target. Could this B the 1? Trends Pharmacol Sci 1999; 20:100–104.

275. Austin CE, Faussner A, Robinson HE, Chakravarty S, Kyle DJ, Bathon JM, Proud D. Stable expression of the human kinin B1 receptor in Chinese hamster ovary cells. Characterization of ligand binding and effector pathways. J Biol Chem 1997; 272:11420–11425.

276. Fuller RW, Dixon CM, Cuss FM, Barnes PJ. Bradykinin-induced bronchoconstriction in humans. Mode of action. Am Rev Respir Dis 1987; 135:176–180.

277. Polosa R, Holgate ST. Comparative airway response to inhale bradykinin, kallidin, and [des-Arg9]bradykinin in normal and asthmatic subjects. Am Rev Respir Dis 1990; 142:1367–1371.

278. Reynolds CJ, Togias A, Proud D. Airway neural responses to kinins: tachyphylaxis and role of receptor subtypes. Am J Respir Crit Care Med 1999; 159:431–438.

279. Molimard M, Martin CA, Naline E, Hirsch A, Advenier C. Contractile effects of bradykinin on the isolated human small bronchus. Am J Respir Crit Care Med 1994; 149:123–127.

280. Hulsmann AR, Raatgeep HR, Saxena PR, Kerrebijn KF, De Jongste JC. Bradykinin-induced contraction of human peripheral airways mediated by both bradykinin beta 2 and thromboxane prostanoid receptors. Am J Respir Crit Care Med 1994; 150:1012–1018.

281. Polosa R, Milazzo VL, Magri S, Pagano C, Paolino G, Santonocito G, Prosperini G, Crimi N. Activity of inhaled lysine acetylsalicylate (L-ASA) on bradykinin-induced bronchoconstriction in asthmatics: evidence of contribution of prostaglandins. Eur Respir J 1997; 10:866–871.

282. Ricciardolo FLM, Geppetti P, Mistretta A, Nadel JA, Sapienza MA, Bellofiore S, Di Maria GU. Randomised double-blind placebo-controlled study of the effect of inhibition of nitric oxide synthesis in bradykinin-induced asthma. Lancet 1996; 348:374–377.

283. Fox AJ, Barnes PJ, Urban L, Dray A. An in vitro study of the properties of single vagal afferents innervating guinea-pig airways. J Physiol Lond 1993; 469:21–35.

284. Saria A, Martling CR, Yan Z, Theodorsson Norheim E, Gamse R, Lundberg JM. Release of multiple tachykinins from capsaicin-sensitive sensory nerves in the lung by bradykinin, histamine, dimethylphenyl piperazinium, and vagal nerve stimulation. Am Rev Respir Dis 1988; 137:1330–1335.

285. Sanico AM, Philip G, Proud D, Naclerio RM, Togias A. Comparison of nasal mucosal responsiveness to neuronal stimulation in non-allergic and allergic rhinitis: effects of capsaicin nasal challenge. Clin Exp Allergy 1998; 28:92–100.

286. Sanico AM, Atsuta S, Proud D, Togias A. Plasma extravasation through neuronal stimulation in human nasal mucosa in the setting of allergic rhinitis. J Appl Physiol 1998; 84:537–543.

287. Turner P, Dear J, Scadding G, Foreman JC. Role of Kinins in seasonal allergic rhinitis: icatibant, a bradykinin B2 receptor antagonist the hyperresponsiveness and nasal eosinophilia induced by antigen. J Allergy Clin Immunol 2001; 107:105–113.

288. Dixon CM, Barnes PJ. Bradykinin-induced bronchoconstriction: inhibition by nedocromil sodium and sodium cromoglycate. Br J Clin Pharmacol 1989; 27:831–836.

289. Jackson DM, Norris AA, Eady RP. Nedocromil sodium and sensory nerves in the dog lung. Pulm Pharmacol 1989; 2:179–184.

290. Berman AR, Togias AG, Skloot G, Proud D. Allergen-induced hyperresponsiveness to bradykinin is more pronounced than that to methacholine. J Appl Physiol 1995; 78:1844–1852.

291. Roisman GL, Lacronique JG, Desmazes-Dufeu N, Carre C, Le Cae A, Dusser DJ, Airway responsiveness to bradykinin is related to eosinophilic inflammation in asthma. Am J Respir Crit Care Med 1996; 153:381–390.

292. Polosa R, Renaud L, Cacciola R, Prosperini G, Crimi N, Djukanovic R. Sputum eosinophilia is more closely associated with airway responsiveness to bradykinin than methacholine in asthma. Eur Respir J 1998; 12:551–556.

293. Bockmann S, Paegelow I. Kinins and kinin receptors: importance for the activation of leukocytes. J Leukoc Biol 2000; 68:587–592.

294. Farmer SG, Wilkins DE, Meeker SA, Seeds EA, Page CP. Effects of bradykinin receptor antagonists on antigen-induced respiratory distress, airway hyperresponsiveness and eosinophilia in guinea-pigs. Br J Pharmacol 1992; 107:653–659.

295. Woisin FE, Matsumoto T, Douglas GJ, Paul W, Whalley ET, Page CP. Effect of antagonists for NK(2) and B(2) receptors on antigen-induced airway responses in allergic rabbits. Pulm Pharmacol Ther 2000; 13:13–23.

296. Tiffany CW, Burch RM. Bradykinin stimulates tumor necrosis factor and interleukin-1 release from macrophages. FEBS Lett 1989; 247:189–192.

297. Koyama S, Rennard SI, Robbins RA. Bradykinin stimulates bronchial epithelial cells to release neutrophil and monocyte chemotactic activity. Am J Physiol 1995; 269:L38–L44.

298. Koyama S, Sato E, Numanami H, Kubo K, Nagai S, Izumi T. Bradykinin stimulates lung fibroblasts to release neutrophil and monocyte chemotactic activity. Am J Respir Cell Mol Biol 2000; 22:75–84.

299. Prat A, Weinrib L, Becher B, Poirier J, Duquette P, Couture R, Antel JP. Bradykinin B1 receptor expression and function on T lymphocytes in active multiple sclerosis. Neurology 1999; 53:2087–2092.

300. Akbary AM, Wirth KJ, Scholkens BA. Efficacy and tolerability of Icatibant (Hoe 140) in Patients with moderately severe chronic bronchial asthma. Immunopharmacology 1996; 33:238–242.

301. Nawa H, Hirose T, Takashima H, Inayama S, Nakanishi S. Nucleotide sequences of cloned cDNAs for two types of bovine brain substance P precursor. Nature 1983; 306:32–36.

302. Nawa H, Kotani H, Nakanishi S. Tissue-specific generation of two pre-protachykinin mRNAs from one gene by alternative RNA splicing. Nature 1984; 312:729–734.

303. Kotani H, Hoshimaru M, Nawa H, Nakanishi S. Structure and gene organization of bovine neuromedin K precursor. Proc Natl Acad Sci USA 1986; 83:7074–7078.

304. Krause JE, Chirgwin JM, Carter MS, Xu ZS, Hershey AD. Three rat pre-protachykinin mRNAs encode the neuropeptides substance P and neurokinin A. Proc Natl Acad Sci USA 1987; 84:881–885.

305. Amara SG, Jonas V, Rosenfeld MG, Ong ES, Evans RM. Alternative RNA processing in calcitonin gene expression generates mRNAs encoding different polypeptide products. Nature 1982; 298:240–244.

306. Amara SG, Arriza JL, Leff SE, Swanson LW, Evans RM, Rosenfeld MG. Expression in brain of a messenger RNA encoding a novel neuropeptide homologous to calcitonin gene-related peptide. Science 1985; 229:1094–1097.

307. Gibson SJ, Polak JM, Giaid A, Hamid QA, Kar S, Jones PM, Denny P, Legon S, Amara SG, Craig RK. Calcitonin gene-related peptide messenger RNA is expressed in sensory neurones of the dorsal root ganglia and also in spinal motoneurones in man and rat. Neurosci Lett 1988; 91:283–288.

308. Minami M, Kuraishi Y, Kawamura M, Yamaguchi T, Masu Y, Nakanishi S, Satoh M. Enhancement of preprotachykinin A gene expression by adjuvant-induced inflammation in the rat spinal cord: possible involvement of substance P–containing spinal neurons in nociception. Neurosci Lett 1989; 98:105–110.

309. Rethelyi M, Metz CB, Lund PK. Distribution of neurons expressing calcitonin gene-related peptide mRNAs in the brain stem, spinal cord and dorsal root ganglia of rat and guinea-pig. Neuroscience 1989; 29:225–239.

310. Kummer W, Fischer A, Kurkowski R, Heym C. The sensory and sympathetic innervation of guinea-pig lung and trachea as studied by retrograde neuronal tracing and double-labelling immunohistochemistry. Neuroscience 1992; 49: 715–737.

311. Lundberg JM, Brodin E, Saria A. Effects and distribution of vagal capsaicin-sensitive substance P neurons with special reference to the trachea and lungs. Acta Physiol Scand 1983; 119:243–252.

312. Lundberg JM, Hokfelt T, Martling CR, Saria A, Cuello C. Substance P–immunoreactive sensory nerves in the lower respiratory tract of various mammals including man. Cell Tissue Res 1984; 235:251–261.

313. Hislop AA, Wharton J, Allen KM, Polak JM, Haworth SG. Immunohisto-chemical localization of peptide-containing nerves in human airways: age-related changes. Am J Respir Cell Mol Biol 1990; 3:191–198.

314. Komatsu T, Yamamoto M, Shimokata K, Nagura H. Distribution of substance P–immunoreactive and calcitonin gene–related peptide-immunoreactive nerves in normal human lungs. Int Arch Allergy Appl Immunol 1991; 95:23–28.

315. Chu HW, Kraft M, Krause JE, Rex MD, Martin RJ. Substance P and its receptor neurokinin 1 expression in asthmatic airways. J Allergy Clin Immunol 2000; 106:713–722.

316. Haley KJ, Sunday ME, Osathanondh R, Du J, Vathanaprida C, Karpitsky VV, Krause JE, Lilly CM. Developmental expression of neurokinin A and functional neurokinin-2 receptors in lung. Am J Physiol Lung Cell Mol Physiol 2001; 280:L1348–L1358.

317. Laitinen LA, Laitinen A, Panula PA, Partanen M, Tervo K, Tervo T. Immu-nohistochemical demonstration of substance P in the lower respiratory tract of the rabbit and not of man. Thorax 1983; 38:531–536.

318. Lilly CM, Hall AE, Rodger IW, Kobzik L, Haley KJ, Drazen JM. Substance P–induced histamine release in tracheally perfused guinea pig lungs. J Appl Physiol 1995; 78:1234–1241.

319. Gerard NP, Eddy RLJ, Shows TB, Gerard C. The human neurokinin A (sub-stance K) receptor. Molecular cloning of the gene, chromosome localization, and isolation of cDNA from tracheal and gastric tissues. J Biol Chem 1990; 265:20455–20462.

320. Gerard NP, Garraway LA, Eddy RLJ, Shows TB, Iijima H, Paquet JL, Gerard C. Human substance P receptor (NK-1): organization of the gene, chromosome localization, and functional expression of cDNA clones. Biochemistry 1991; 30:10640–10646.

321. Huang RR, Cheung AH, Mazina KE, Strader CD, Fong TM. cDNA sequence and heterologous expression of the human neurokinin-3 receptor. Biochem Bio-phys Res Commun 1992; 184:966–972.

322. Buell G, Schulz MF, Arkinstall SJ, Maury K, Missotten M, Adami N, Talabot F, Kawashima E. Molecular characterisation, expression and location of human neurokinin-3 receptor. FEBS Lett 1992; 299:90–95.

323. Maggi CA. Tachykinins and calcitonin gene-related peptide (CGRP) as co-transmitters released from peripheral endings of sensory nerves. Prog Neurobiol 1995; 45:1–98.

324. Bertrand C, Geppetti P. Tachykinin and kinin receptor antagonists: thera-peutic perspectives in allergic airway disease. Trends Pharmacol Sci 1996; 17:255–259.

325. Nakajima H, Iwamoto I, Tomoe S, Matsumura R, Tomioka H, Takstsu K, Yoshida S, CD4+ T-lymphocytes and interleukin-5 mediate antigen-induced eosinophil infiltration into the mouse trachea. Am Rev Respir Dis 1992; 146:374–377.

326. Black J, Diment L, Armour C, Alouan L, Johnson P, Distribution of substance P receptors in rabbit airways, functional and autoradiographic studies. J Pharmacol Exp Ther 1990; 253:381–386.

327. Goldie RG. Receptors in asthmatic airways. Am Rev Respir Dis 1990; 141:S151–S156.

328. Walsh DA, Salmon M, Featherstone R, Wharton J, Church MK, Polak JM. Differences in the distribution and characteristics of tachykinin NK1 binding sites between human and guinea pig lung. Br J Pharmacol 1994; 113:1407–1415.

329. Carstairs JR, Barnes PJ. Autoradiographic mapping of substance P receptors in lung. Eur J Pharmacol 1986; 127:295–296.

330. Naline E, Devillier P, Drapeau G, Toty L, Bakdach H, Regoli D, Advenier C. Characterization of neurokinin effects and receptor selectivity in human isolated bronchi. Am Rev Respir Dis 1989; 140:679–686.

331. Advenier C, Naline E, Toty L, Bakdach H, Emonds A, Vilain P, Breliere JC, Le Fur G. Effects on the isolated human bronchus of SR 48968, a potent and selective nonpeptide antagonist of the neurokinin A (NK2) receptors. Am Rev Respir Dis 1992; 146:1177–1181.

332. Naline E, Molimard M, Regoli D, Emonds-Alt X, Bellamy JF, Advenier C. Evidence for functional tachykinin NK1 receptors on human isolated small bronchi. Am J Physiol 1996; 271:L763–L767.

333. Amadesi S, Moreau J, Tognetto M, Springer J, Trevisani M, Naline E, Advenier C, Fisher A, Vinci D, Mapp C, Miotto D, Cavallesco G, Geppetti P. NK1 receptor stimulation causes contraction and inositol phosphate increase in medium-size human isolated bronchi. Am J Respir Crit Care Med 2001; 163: 1206–1211.

334. Adcock IM, Peters M, Gelder C, Shirasaki H, Brown CR, Barnes PJ. Increased tachykinin receptor gene expression in asthmatic lung and its modulation by steroids. J Mol Endocrinol 1993; 11:1–7.

335. Bai TR, Zhou D, Weir T, Walker B, Hegele R, Hayashi S, McKay K, Bondy GP, Fong T. Substance P (NK1)- and neurokinin A (NK2)-receptor gene expression in inflammatory airway diseases. Am J Physiol 1995; 269:L309–L317.

336. Mapp CE, Miotto D, Braccioni F, Saetta M, Turato G, Maestrelli P, Krause JE, Karpitskiy V, Boyd N, Geppetti P, Fabbri LM. The distribution of neurokinin-1 and neurokinin-2 receptors in human central airways. Am J Respir Crit Care Med 2000; 161:207–215.

337. Ollerenshaw SL, Jarvis D, Sullivan CE, Woolcock AJ. Substance P immunoreactive nerves in airways from asthmatics and nonasthmatics. Eur Respir J 1991; 4:673–682.

338. Howarth PH, Djukanovic R, Wilson JW, Holgate ST, Springall DR, Polak JM. Mucosal nerves in endobronchial biopsies in asthma and non-asthma. Int Arch Allergy Appl Immunol 1991; 94:330–333.

339. Chanez P, Springall D, Vignola AM, Moradoghi-Hattvani A, Polak JM, Godard P, Bousquet J. Bronchial mucosal immunoreactivity of sensory neuropeptides in severe airway diseases. Am J Respir Crit Care Med 1998; 158:985–990.

340. Mapp PI, Kidd BL, Gibson SJ, Terry JM, Revell PA, Ibrahim NB, Blake DR, Polak JM. Substance P-, calcitonin gene-related peptide- and C-flanking peptide of neuropeptide Y–immunoreactive fibres are present in normal synovium but depleted in patients with rheumatoid arthritis. Neuroscience 1990; 37:143–153.

341. O'Connell F, Springall DR, Moradoghli-Haftvani A, Krausz T, Price D, Fuller RW, Polak JM, Pride NB. Abnormal intraepithelial airway nerves in persistent unexplained cough? Am J Respir Crit Care Med 1995; 152:2068–2075.

342. Nieber K, Baumgarten CR, Rathsack R, Furkert J, Oehme P, Kunkel G. Substance P and beta-endorphin-like immunoreactivity in lavage fluids of subjects with and without allergic asthma. J Allergy Clin Immunol 1992; 90:646–652.

343. Tomaki M, Ichinose M, Miura M, Hirayama Y, Yamauchi H, Nakajima N, Shirato K. Elevated substance P content in induced sputum from patients with asthma and patients with chronic bronchitis. Am J Respir Crit Care Med 1995; 151:613–617.

344. Lacroix JS, Buvelot JM, Polla BS, Lundberg JM. Improvement of symptoms of non-allergic chronic rhinitis by local treatment with capsaicin. Clin Exp Allergy 1991; 21:595–600.

345. Advenier C, Naline E, Drapeau G, Regoli D. Relative potencies of neurokinins in guinea-pig trachea an human bronchus. Eur J Pharmacol 1987; 139:133–137.

346. Lundberg JM, Martling CR, Saria A. Substance P and capsaicin-induced contraction of human bronchi. Acta Physiol Scand 1983; 119:49–53.

347. Honda I, Kohrogi H, Yamaguchi T, Ando M, Araki S, Enkephalinase inhibitor potentiates substance P- and capsicin-induced bronchial smooth muscle contractions in humans. Am Rev Respir Dis 1991; 143:1416–1418.

348. Chitano P, Di Blasi P, Lucchini RE, Calabro F, Saetta M, Maestrelli P, Fabbri LM, Mapp CE. The effects of toluene diisocyanate and of capsaicin on human bronchial smooth muscle in vitro. Eur J Pharmacol 1994; 270:167–173.

349. De Jongste JC, Mons H, Bonta IL, Kerrebijn KF. Nonneural components in the response of fresh human airways to electric field stimulation. J Appl Physiol 1987; 63:1558–1566.

350. Fuller RW, Maxwell DL, Dixon CM, McGregor GP, Barnes VF, Bloom SR, Barnes PJ. Effect of substance P on cardiovascular and respiratory function in subjects. J Appl Physiol 1987; 62:1473–1479.

351. Evans TW, Dixon CM, Clarke B, Conradson TB, Barnes PJ. Comparison of neurokinin A and substance P on cardiovascular and airway function in man. Br J Clin Pharmacol 1988; 25:273–275.

352. Joos G, Pauwels R, Van Der Straeten M. Effect of inhaled substance P and neurokinin A on the airways of normal and asthmatic subjects. Thorax 1987; 42:779–783.

353. Van Schoor J, Joos GF, Pauwels RA. Indirect bronchial hyperresponsiveness in asthma: mechanisms, pharmacology and implications for clinical research. Eur Respir J 2000; 16:514–533.

354. Djokic TD, Nadel JA, Dusser DJ, Sekizawa K, Graf PD, Borson DB. Inhibitors of neutral endopeptidase potentiate electrically and capsaicin-induced non-cholinergic contraction in guinea pig bronchi. J Pharmacol Exp Ther 1989; 248:7–11.

355. Kummer W, Fischer A. Tissue distribution of neutral endopeptidase 24.11 ("enkephalinase") activity in guinea pig trachea. Neuropeptides 1991; 18:181–186.

356. Cheung D, Bel EH, den Hartigh J, Dijkman JH, Sterk PJ. The effect of an inhaled neutral endopeptidase inhibitor, thiorphan, on airway responses to neurokinin A in normal humans in vivo. Am Rev Respir Dis 1992; 145:1275–1280.

357. Cheung D, Timmers MC, Zwinderman AH, den Hartigh J, Dijkman JH, Sterk PJ. Neutral endopeptidase activity and airway hyperresponsiveness to neurokinin A in asthmatic subjects in vivo. Am Rev Respir Dis 1993; 148:1467–1473.

358. Crimi N, Palermo F, Oliveri R, Polosa R, Magri S, Mistretta A. Inhibition of neutral endopeptidase potentiates bronchoconstriction induced by neurokinin A in asthmatic patients [see comments]. Clin Exp Allergy 1994; 24:115–120.

359. Crimi N, Palermo F, Oliveri R, Palermo B, Vancheri C, Polosa R, Mistretta A. Influence of antihistamine (astemizole) and anticholinergic drugs (ipratropium bromide) on bronchoconstriction induced by substance P. Ann Allergy 1990; 65:115–120.

360. Joos G, Pauwels R, Van Der Straeten M. The effect of oxitropium bromide on neurokinin A–induced bronchoconstriction in asthmatic subjects. Pulm Pharmacol 1988; 1:41–45.

361. Joos GF, Germonpre PR, Pauwels RA. Neural mechanisms in asthma. Clin Exp Allergy 2000; 30 Suppl 1:60–65.

362. Lambrecht BN. Immunologists getting nervous: neuropeptides, dendritic cells and T cell activation. Respir Res 2001; 2:133–138.

363. Kroegel C, Giembycz MA, Barnes PJ. Characterization of eosinophil cell activation by peptides. Differential effects of substance P, melittin, and FMET-Leu-Phe. J Immunol 1990; 145:2581–2587.

364. el-Shazly AE, Masuyama K, Ishikawa T. Mechanisms involved in activation of human eosinophil exocytosis by substance. P: an in vitro model of sensory neuroimmunomodulation. Immunol Invest 1997; 26:615–629.

365. Dunzendorfer S, Meierhofer C, Wiedermann CJ. Signaling in neuropeptide-induced migration of human eosinophils. J Leukoc Biol 1998; 64:828–834.

366. Harrison NK, Dawes KE, Kwon OJ, Barnes PJ, Laurent GJ, Chung KF. Effect of neuropeptides on human lung fibroblast proliferation and chemotaxis. Am J Physiol 1995; 268:L278–L283.

367. Dunzendorfer S, Kaser A, Meierhofer C, Tilg H, Wiedermann CJ. Cutting edge: peripheral neuropeptides attract immature and arrest mature blood-derived dendritic cells. J Immunol 2001; 166:2167–2172.

368. Kahler CM, Pischel A, Kaufmann G, Wiedermann CJ. Influence of neuropeptides on neutrophil adhesion and transmigration through a lung fibroblast barrier in vitro. Exp Lung Res 2001; 27:25–46.

369. Kuo HP, Lin HC, Hwang KH, Wang CH, Lu LC. Lipopolysaccharide enhances substance P–mediated neutrophil adherence to epithelial cells and cytokine release. Am J Respir Crit Care Med 2000; 162:1891–1897.

370. Brunelleschi S, Nicali R, Lavagno L, Viano I, Pozzi E, Gagliardi L, Ghio P, Albera C. Tachykinin activation of human monocytes from patients with interstitial lung disease, healthy smokers or healthy volunteers. Neuropeptides 2000; 34:45–50.

371. Hood VC, Cruwys SC, Urban L, Kidd BL. Differential role of neurokinin receptors in human lymphocyte and monocyte chemotaxis. Regul Pept 2000; 96:17–21.

372. Lotz M, Vaughan JH, Carson DA. Effect of neuropeptides on production of inflammatory cytokines by human monocytes. Science 1988; 241:1218–1221.

373. Ho WZ, Stavropoulos G, Lai JP, Hu BF, Magafa V, Anagnostides S, Douglas SD. Substance P C-terminal octapeptide analogues augment tumor necrosis factor–alpha release by human blood monocytes and macrophages. J Neuroimmunol 1998; 82:126–132.

374. Calvo CF, Chavanel G, Senik A. Substance P enhances IL-2 expression in activated human T cells. J Immunol 1992; 148:3498–3504.

375. Payan DG, Brewster DR, Goetzl EJ. Specific stimulation of human T lymphocytes by substance P. J Immunol 1983; 131:1613–1615.

376. Kim JS, Rabe KF, Magnussen H, Green JM, White SR. Migration and proliferation of guinea pig and human airway epithelial cells in response to tachykinins. Am J Physiol 1995; 269:L119–L126.

377. Quinlan KL, Naik SM, Cannon G, Armstrong CA, Bunnett NW, Ansel JC, Caughman SW. Substance P activates coincident NF-AT- and NF-kappa B–dependent adhesion molecule gene expression in microvascular endothelial cells through intracellular calcium mobilization. J Immunol 1999; 163: 5656–5665.

378. Kavelaars A, Broeke D, Jeurissen F, Kardux J, Meijer A, Franklin R, Gelfand EW, Heijnen CJ. Activation of human monocytes via a non-neurokinin substance P receptor that is coupled to Gi protein, calcium, phospholipase D, MAP kinase, and IL-6 production. J Immunol 1994; 153:3691–3699.

379. Jeurissen F, Kavelaars A, Korstjens M, Broeke D, Franklin RA, Gelfand EW, Heijnen CJ. Monocytes express a non-neurokinin substance P receptor that is functionally coupled to MAP kinase. J Immunol 1994; 152:2987–2994.

380. Ho WZ, Lai JP, Zhu XH, Uvaydova M, Douglas SD. Human monocytes and macrophages express substance P and neurokinin-1 receptor. J Immunol 1997; 159:5654–5660.

381. Lai JP, Douglas SD, Ho WZ. Human lymphocytes express substance P and its receptor. J Neuroimmunol 1998; 86:80–86.

382. Goode T, O'Connell J, Ho WZ, O'Sullivan GC, Collins JK, Douglas SD, Shanahan F. Differential expression of neurokinin-1 receptor by human mucosal and peripheral lymphoid cells. Clin Diagn Lab Immunol 2000; 7:371–376.

383. Germonpre PR, Bullock GR, Lambrecht BN, Van DV, V, Luyten WH, Joos GF, Pauwels RA. Presence of substance P and neurokinin 1 receptors in human sputum macrophages and U-937 cells. Eur Respir J 1999; 14:776–782.

384. Aliakbari J, Sreedharan SP, Turck CW, Goetzl EJ. Selective localization of vasoactive intestinal peptide and substance P in human eosinophils. Biochem Biophys Res Commun 1987; 148:1440–1445.

385. Linnik MD, Moskowitz MA. Identification of immunoreactive substance P in human and other mammalian endothelial cells. Peptides 1989; 10:957–962.

386. Ichinose M, Nakajima N, Takahashi T, Yamauchi H, Inoue H, Takishima T. Protection against bradykinin-induced bronchoconstriction in asthmatic patients by neurokinin receptor antagonist. Lancet 1992; 340:1248–1251.

387. Schmidt D, Jorres RA, Rabe KF, Magnussen H. Reproducibility of airway response to inhaled bradykinin and effect of neurokinin receptor antagonist FK-224 in asthmatic subjects. Eur J Clin Pharmacol 1996; 50:269–273.

388. Joos GF, Van Schoor J, Kips JC, Pauwels RA. The effect of inhaled FK224, a tachykinin NK-1 and NK-2 receptor antagonist, on neurokinin A-induced

bronchoconstriction in asthmatics. Am J Respir Crit Care Med 1996; 153:1781–1784.

389. Van Schoor J, Joos G, Chasson B, Brouard R, Pauwels R. The effect of the oral nonpeptide NK2 receptor antagonist SR48968 on neurokinin A–induced bronchoconstriction in asthmatics. Eur Respir J 1996; 9:289s.

390. Kraan J, Vink-Klooster H, Postma DS. The NK-2 receptor antagonist SR 48968C does not improve adenosine hyperresponsiveness and airway obstruction in allergic asthma. Clin Exp Allergy 2001; 31:274–278.

391. Ichinose M, Miura M, Yamauchi H, Kageyama N, Tomaki M, Oyake T, Ohuchi Y, Hida W, Miki H, Tamura G, Shirato K. A neurokinin 1-receptor antagonist improves exercise-induced airway narrowing in asthmatic patients. Am J Respir Crit Care Med 1996; 153:936–941.

392. Fahy JV, Wong HH, Geppetti P, Reis JM, Harris SC, Maclean DB, Nadel JA, Boushey HA. Effect of an NK1 receptor antagonist (CP-99,994) on hypertonic saline-induced bronchoconstriction and cough in male asthmatic subjects. Am J Respir Crit Care Med 1995; 152:879–884.

393. Hay DWP. Endothelin-1: an interesting peptide or an important mediator in pulmonary diseases? Pulm Pharmacol Ther 1998; 11:141–146.

394. Inoue A, Yanagisawa M, Takuwa Y, Mitsui Y, Kobayashi M, Masaki T. The human preproendothelin-1 gene. Complete nucleotide sequence and regulation of expression. Biol Chem 1989; 264:14954–14959.

395. Saleh D, Furukawa K, Tsao MS, Maghazachi A, Corin B, Yanagisawa M, Barnes PJ, Giaid A. Elevated expression of endothelin-1 and endothelin-converting enzyme-1 in idiopathic pulmonary fibrosis: possible involvement of proinflammatory cytokines. Am J Respir Cell Mol Biol 1997; 16:187–193.

396. Shima H, Yamanouchi M, Omori K, Sugiura M, Kawashima K, Sato T. Endothelin-1 production and endothelin converting enzyme expression by guinea pig airway epithelial cells. Biochem Mol Biol Int 1995; 37:1001–1010.

397. Endo T, Uchida Y, Matsumoto H, Suzuki N, Normura A, Hirata F, Hasegawa S. Regulation of endothelin-1 synthesis in cultured guinea pig airway epithelial cells by various cytokines. Biochem Biophys Res Commun 1992; 186:1594–1599.

398. Hay DWP. Guinea-pig tracheal epithelium and endothelium. Eur J Pharmacol 1989; 171:241–245.

399. Mullol J, Picado C. Endothelin in nasal mucosa: role in nasal function and inflammation. Clin Exp Allergy 2000; 30:172–177.

400. Knott PG, D'Aprile AC, Henry PJ, Hay DWP, Goldie RG. Receptors for endothelin-1 in asthmatic human peripheral lung. Br J Pharmacol 1995; 114:1–3.

401. Goldie RG, Henry PJ, Knott PG, Self GJ, Luttmann MA, Hay DWP. Endothelin-1 receptor density, distribution, and function in human isolated asthmatic airways. Am J Respir Crit Care Med 1995; 152:1653–1658.

402. Redington AE, Springall DR, Ghatei MA, Lau LCK, Bloom SR, Holgate ST, Polak JM, Howarth PH. Endothelin in bronchoalveolar lavage fluid and its relation to airflow obstruction in asthma. Am J Respir Crit Care Med 1995; 151:1034–1039.

403. Springall DR, Howarth PH, Counihan H, Djukanovic R, Holgate ST, Polak JM. Endothelin immunoreactivity of airway epithelium in asthmatic patients. Lancet 1991; 337:697–701.

404. Redington AE, Springall DR, Meng Q-H, Tuck AB, Holgate ST, Polak JM, Howarth PH. Immunoreactive endothelin in bronchial biopsy specimens: increased expression in asthma and modulation by corticosteroid therapy. J Allergy Clin Immunol 1997; 100:544–552.

405. Redington AE, Springall DR, Ghatei MA, Madden J, Bloom SR, Frew AJ, Polak JM, Holgate ST, Howarth PH. Airway endothelin levels in asthma: influence of endobronchial allergen challenge and maintenance corticosteroid therapy. Eur Respir J 1997; 10:1026–1032.

406. Makker HK, Springall DR, Redington AE, Ghatei MA, Bloom SR, Polak JM, Howarth PH, Holgate SR. Airway endothelin levels in asthma: influence of endobronchial hypertonic saline challenge. Clin Exp Allergy 1999; 29:241–247.

407. Chalmers GW, Little SA, Patel KR, Thomson NC. Endothelin-1-induced bronchoconstriction in asthma. Am J Respir Crit Care Med 1997; 156:382–388.

408. Chalmers GW, MacLeod KJ, Thomson LJ, Little SA, Patel KR, McSharry C, Thomson NC. Sputum cellular and cytokine responses to inhaled endothelin-1 in asthma. Clin Exp Allergy 1999; 29:1526–1531.

409. Henry PJ, Rigby PJ, Self GJ, Preuss JM, Goldie RG. Relationship between endothelin-1 binding site densities and constrictor activities in human and animal airway smooth muscle. Br J Pharmacol 1990; 100:786–792.

410. Fernandes LB, Henry PJ, Rigby PJ, Goldie RG. Endothelin(B) (ET(B)) receptor-activated potentiation of cholinergic nerve-mediated contraction in human bronchus. Br J Pharmacol 1996; 118:1873–1874.

411. Panettieri RA, Hall IP, Maki CS, Murray RK. α-Thrombin increases cystolic calcium and induces human airway smooth muscle cell proliferation. Am J Respir Cell Mol Biol 1995; 13:205–216.

412. Dube J, Chakir J, Dube C, Grimard Y, Laviolette M, Boulet LP. Synergistic action of endothelin (ET)-1 on the activation of bronchial fibroblast isolated from normal and asthmatic subjects. Int J Exp Pathol 2000; 81:429–437.

413. Chanez P, Vignola AM, Albat B, Springall DR, Polak JM, Godard P, Bousquet J. Involvement of endothelin in mononuclear phagocyte inflammation in asthma. J Allergy Clin Immunol 1996; 98:412–420.

414. Helset E, Sildnes T, Seljelid R, Konopski ZS. Endothelin-1 stimulates human monocytes in vitro to release TNF-α, IL-1β and IL-6. Mediators Inflamm 1993; 2:417–422.

415. McCarron RM, Wang L, Stanimirovic DB, Spatz M. Endothelin induction of adhesion molecule expression on human brain microvascular endothelial cells. Neurosci Lett 1993; 156:31–34.

416. Ishizuka T, Takamizawa-Matsumoto M, Suzuki K, Kurita A. Endothelin-1 enhances vascular cell adhesion molecule-1 expression in tumor necrosis factor alpha-stimulated vascular endothelial cells. Eur J Pharmacol 1999; 369:237–245.

417. Gomez-Garre D, Guerra M, Gonzalez E, Lopez-Farre A, Riesco A, Caramelo C, Escanero J, Egido J. Aggregation of human polymorphonuclear leukocytes by endothelin: role of platelet-activating factor. Eur J Pharmacol 1992; 224:167–172.

418. Elferink JG, de Koster BM. Endothelin-induced activation of nuetrophil migration. Biochem Pharmacol 1994; 48:865–871.

419. Achmad TH, Rao GS. Chemotaxis of human blood monocytes toward endothelin-1 and the influence of calcium blockers. Biochem Biophys Res Commun 1992; 189:994–1000.

420. Sampaio AL, Rae GA, Henriques MM. Role of endothelins on lymphocyte accumulation in allergic pleurisy. J Leukoc Biol 2000; 67:189–195.

421. Hocher B, Schwarz A, Fagan KA, Thone-Reineke C, El-Hag K, Kusserow H, Elitok S, Bauer C, Neumayer HH, Rodman DM, Theuring F. Pulmonary fibrosis and chronic lung inflammation in ET-1 transgenic mice. Am J Respir Cell Mol Biol 2000; 23:19–26.

422. Finsnes F, Skjonsberg OH, Tonnessen T, Naess O, Lyberg T, Christensen G. Endothelin production and effects of endothelin antagonism during experimental airway inflammation. Am J Respir Crit Care Med 1997; 155:1404–1412.

423. Fujitani Y, Trifilieff A, Tsuyuki S, Coyle AJ, Bertrand C. Endothelin receptor antagonists inhibit antigen-induced lung inflammation in mice. Am J Respir Crit Care Med 1997; 155:1890–1894.

424. Zouki C, Baron C, Fournier A, Filep JG. Endothelin-1 enhances neutrophil adhesion to human coronary artery endothelial cells: role of ET(A) receptors and platelet-activating factor. Br J Pharmacol 1999; 127:969–979.

425. Finsnes F, Lyberg T, Christensen G, Skjonsberg OH. Effect of endothelin antagonism on the production of cytokines in eosinophilic airway inflammation. Am J Physiol Lung Cell Mol Physiol 2001; 280:L659–L665.

426. Nagase T, Kurihara H, Kurihara Y, Aoki T, Fukuchi Y, Yazaki Y, Ouchi Y. Airway hyperresponsiveness to methacholine in mutant mice deficient in endothelin-1. Am J Respir Crit Care Med 1998; 157:560–564.

427. Nagase T, Kurihara H, Kurihara Y, Aoki-Nagase T, Nagai R, Ouchi Y. Disruption of ET-1 gene enhances pulmonary responses to methacholine via functional mechanism in knockout mice. J Appl Physiol 1999; 87:2020–2024.

428. Furchgott RF, Zawadzki JV. The obligatory role of endothelial cells in the relaxation of arterial smooth muscle by acetylcholine. Nature 1980, 5789–376.

429. Palmer RMJ, Ferrige AG, Monocada S. Nitric oxide release accounts for the biological activity of endothelium-derived relaxing factor. Nature 1987; 327:524–526.

430. Ignarro LJ, Byrns RE, Buga GM, Wood KS. Endothelium-derived relaxing factor from pulmonary artery and vein possesses pharmacologic and chemical properties identical to those of nitric oxide radical. Circ Res 1987; 61:866–879.

431. Kobzik L, Bredt DS, Lowenstein CJ, Drazen J, Gaston B, Sugarbaker D, Stamler JS. Nitric oxide synthase in human and rat lung: immunocytochemical and histochemical localization. Am J Respir Cell Mol Biol 1993; 9:371–377.

432. Shaul PW, North AJ, Wu LC, Wells LB, Brannon TS, Lau KS, Michel T, Margraf LR, Star RA. Endothelial nitric oxide synthase is expressed in cultured human bronchiolar epithelium. J Clin Invest 1994; 94:2231–2236.

433. Fischer A, Mundel P, Mayer B, Preissler U, Philippin B, Kummer W. Nitric oxide synthase in guinea pig lower airway innervation. Neurosci Lett 1993; 149:157–160.

434. Hamid Q, Springall DR, Riveros-Moreno V, Chanez P, Howarth P, Redington A, Bousquet J, Godard P, Holgate S, Polak JM. Induction of nitric oxide synthase in asthma. Lancet 1993; 342:1510–1513.

435. Saleh D, Ernst P, Lim S, Barnes PJ, Giaid A. Increased formation of the potent oxidant peroxynitrite in the airways of asthmatic patients is associated with

induction of nitric oxide synthase: effect of inhaled glucocorticoid. FASEB J 1998; 12:929–937.

436. Kharitonov SA, Yates D, Robbins RA, Logan-Sinclair R, Shinebourne EA, Barnes PJ. Increased nitric oxide in exhaled air of asthmatic patients. Lancet 1994; 343:133–135.

437. Kharitonov SA, O'Connor BJ, Evans DJ, Barnes PJ. Allergen-induced late asthmatic reactions are associated with elevation of exhaled nitric oxide. Am J Respir Crit Care Med 1995; 151:1894–1899.

438. Belvisi MG, Stretton CD, Miura M, Verleden GM, Tadjkarimi S, Yacoub MH, Barnes PJ. Inhibitory NANC nerves in human tracheal smooth muscle: a quest for the neurotransmitter. J Appl Physiol 1992; 73:2505–2510.

439. Ward JK, Belvisi MG, Springall DR, Abelli L, Tadjkarimi S, Yacoub HM, Barnes PJ. Human iNANC bronchodilatation and nitric oxide–immuno-reactive nerves are reduced in distal airways. Am J Respir Cell Mol Biol 1995; 13:175–184.

440. Higenbottam T. Lung disease and pulmonary endothelial nitric oxide. Exp Physiol 1995; 80:855–864.

441. Erjefalt JS, Erjefalt I, Sundler F, Persson CGA. Mucosal nitric oxide may toni-cally suppress airways plasma exudation. Am J Respir Crit Care Med 1994; 150:227–232.

442. Bernareggi M, Mitchell JA, Barnes PJ, Belvisi MG. Dual action of nitric oxide on airway plasma leakage. Am J Respir Crit Care Med 1997; 155:869–874.

443. Turner PJ, Maggs JR, Foreman JC. Induction by inhibitors of nitric oxide syn-thase of hyperresponsiveness in the human nasal airway. Br J Pharmacol 2000; 131:363–369.

444. Barnes PJ, Liew FY. Nitric oxide and asthmatic inflammation. Immunol Today 1995; 16:128–130.

445. Bauer H, Jung T, Tsikas D, Stichtenoth DO, Frolich JC, Neumann C. Nitric oxide inhibits the secretion of T-helper 1- and T-helper 2-associated cytokines in activated human T cells. Immunology 1997; 90:205–211.

446. Thomassen MJ, Buhrow LT, Connors MJ, Kaneko FT, Erzurum SC, Kavuru MS. Nitric oxide inhibits inflammatory cytokine production by human alveolar macrophages. Am J Respir Cell Mol Biol 1997; 17:279–283.

447. Raychaudhuri B, Dweik R, Connors MJ, Buhrow L, Malur A, Drazba J, Arroliga AC, Erzurum SC, Kavuru MS, Thomassen MJ. Nitric oxide blocks nuclear factor-kappaB activation in alveolar macrophages. Am J Respir Cell Mol Biol 1999; 21:311–316.

448. Zeiher AM, Fisslthaler B, Schray-Utz B, Busse R. Nitric oxide modulates the expression of monocyte chemoattractant protein 1 in cultured human endothelial cells. Circ Res 1995; 76:980–986.

449. Spiecker M, Peng HB, Liao JK. Inhibition of endothelial vascular cell adhesion molecule-1 expression by nitric oxide involves the induction and nuclear trans-location of IkappaBalpha. J Biol Chem 1997; 272:30969–30974.

450. Iikura M, Takaishi T, Hirai K, Yamada H, Iida M, Koshino T, Morita Y. Exogeneous nitric oxide regulates the degranulation of human basophils and rat peritoneal mast cells. Int Arch Allergy Immunol 1998; 115:129–136.

451. Taylor DA, McGrath JL, O'Connor BJ, Barnes PJ. Allergen-induced early and late asthmatic responses are not affected by inhibition of endogenous nitric oxide. Am J Respir Crit Care Med 1998; 158:99–106.

452. Lander HM, Sehajpal P, Levine DM, Novogrodsky A. Activation of human peripheral blood mononuclear cells by nitric oxide–generating compounds. J Immunol 1993; 150:1509–1516.

453. Beauvais F, Michel L, Dubertret L. The nitric oxide donors, azide and hydroxylamine, inhibit the programmed cell death of cytokine-deprived human eosinophils. FEBS Lett 1995; 361:229–232.

454. Hebestreit H, Dibbert B, Balatti I, Braun D, Schapowal A, Blaser K, Simon H-U. Disruption of Fas receptor signaling by nitric oxide in eosinophils. J Exp Med 1998; 187:415–425.

455. Yeadon M, Price R. Induction of calcium-independent nitrix oxide synthase by allergen challenge in sensitized rat lung in vivo. Br J Pharmacol 1995; 116:2545–2546.

456. Liu SF, Haddad EB, Adcock I, Salmon M, Koto H, Gilbey T, Barnes PJ, Chung KF. Inducible nitric oxide synthase after sensitization and allergen challenge of Brown Norway rat lung. Br J Pharmacol 1997; 121:1241–1246.

457. Xiong Y, Karupiah G, Hogan SP, Foster SP, Ramsay AJ. Inhibition of allergic airway inflammation in mice lacking nitric oxide synthase 2. J Immunol 1999; 162:445–452.

458. De Sanctis GT, MacLean JA, Hamada K, Mehta S, Scott JA, Jiao A, Yandava CN, Kobzik L, Wolyniec WW, Fabian AJ, Venugopal CS, Grasemann H, Huang PL, Drazen JM. Contribution of nitric oxide synthases 1, 2, and 3 to airway hyperresponsiveness and inflammation in a murine model of asthma. J Exp Med 1999; 189:1621–1630.

459. Iijima H, Duguet A, Eum SY, Hamid Q, Eidelman DH. Nitric oxide and protein nitration are eosinophil dependent in allergen-challenged mice. Am J Respir Crit Care Med 2001; 163:1233–1240.

460. Koarai A, Ichinose M, Sugiura H, Yamagata S, Hattori T, Shirato K. Allergic airway hyperresponsiveness and eosinophil infiltration is reduced by a selective iNOS inhibitor, 1400W, in mice. Pulm Pharmacol Ther 2000; 13:267–275.

461. Feder LS, Stelts D, Chapman RW, Manfra D, Crawley Y, Jones H, Minnicozzi M, Fernandez X, Paster T, Egan RW, Kreutner W, Kung TT. Role of nitric oxide on eosinophilic lung inflammation in allergic mice. Am J Respir Cell Mol Biol 1997; 17:436–442.

462. Ferreira HH, Bevilacqua E, Gagioti SM, De L, I, Zanardo RC, Teixeira CE, Sannomiya P, Antunes E, De Nucci G. Nitric oxide modulates eosinophil infiltration in antigen-induced airway inflammation in rats. Eur J Pharmacol 1998; 358:253–259.

463. Trifilieff A, Fujitani Y, Mentz F, Dugas B, Fuentes M, Bertrand C. Inducible nitric oxide synthase inhibitors suppress airway inflammation in mice through down-regulation of chemokine expression. J Immunol 2000; 165:1526–1533.

464. Blease K, Kunkel SL, Hogaboam CM. Acute inhibition of nitric oxide exacerbates airway hyperresponsiveness, eosinophilia and C-C chemokine generation in a murine model of fungal asthma. Inflamm Res 2000; 49:297–304.

465. De Sanctis G, Itoh A, Green F. T lymphocytes regulate genetically determined airway hyperresponsiveness in mice. Nature Med 1997; 3:460–462.
466. Kakuyama M, Ahluwalia A, Rodrigo J, Vallance P. Cholinergic contraction is altered in nNOS knockouts. Cooperative modulation of neural bronchoconstriction by nNOS and COX. Am J Respir Cirt Care Med 1999; 160:2072–2078.
467. Thomassen MJ, Raychaudhuri B, Dweik RA, Farver C, Buhrow L, Malur A, Connors MJ, Drazba J, Hammel J, Erzurum SC, Kavuru MS. Nitric oxide regulation of asthmatic airway inflammation with segmental allergen challenge. J Allergy Clin Immunol 1999; 104:1174–1182.

19

Virally Induced Eosinophilic Airway Inflammation

WIESLAWA OLSZEWSKA
and PETER J.M. OPENSHAW

National Heart and Lung Institute
Imperial College School of Medicine
London, England

I. Lung Eosinophilia

Eosinophils are polymorphonuclear leukocytes (PMNs) that originate from bone marrow and circulate via the blood. They home to mucosal sites in the respiratory, gastrointestinal and genitourinary tracts. The process of maturation and migration of eosinophils requires a number of cytokines and chemokines.

In the naive, clean, uninfected lung, epithelial cells and macrophages are the major resident mucosal cells. However, normal environmental exposure to inhaled particles and to infectious agents recruits a significant number of granulocytes (mostly PMNs) and lymphocytes to the epithelium. During infectious challenge, respiratory epithelial cells produce chemokines, which attract other cells to the site of infection. These include monocyte chemotactic protein-1 (MCP-1), MCP-3, macrophage inflammatory protein-1α (MIP-1α), and RANTES (1–3). The recruitment and activation of other cells, including eosinophils, is therefore determined an inflammatory response in the lung, either to hypersensitivity reactions or to infectious agents.

An eosinophilic pulmonary infiltrate is characteristic of a range of etiologically distinct diseases, some of which are also characterized by blood eosinophilia. These include:

1. Asthmatic or allergic pulmonary eosinophilia—particularly that associated with hypersensitivity to allergens or pathogens (*Aspergillus fumigatus*, *Candida albicans*, or *Pseudomonas aeruginosa*)

2. Löffler's syndrome—seen during the passage of the parasitic larvae (most often *Ascaris lumbricoides*) through the lung
3. Tropical pulmonary eosinophilia—often representing a hypersensitivity reaction to filarial infestation
4. Chronic idiopathic eosinophilic pneumonia
5. Drug-related eosinophilia—usually associated with aspirin, tetracycline, naproxen, nitrofurantoin, or imipramine administration
6. Polyarteritis nodosa and allergic granulomatosis (Churg-Strauss syndrome)—vasculitides characterized by the presence of activated and degranulating eosinophils

II. Respiratory Viral Infections

Respiratory infections are leading causes of mortality and morbidity as well as economic loss throughout the world (4). These infections occur at all ages but have the highest mortality rates among the very young, the very old, and the immunocompromised. It has been estimated that the incidence of acute respiratory infections in children of 0–59 months of age varies from 13 to 17 new episodes per 100 child-weeks and the fatality rate is in the range from 3% to 26% in hospitalized children (5). In developing countries, lower respiratory tract infections in children are most important causes of disability and death (6,7). The incidence of respiratory tract infections has increased globally in recent years, in part because of aging of the population (8).

In infancy, respiratory syncytial virus (RSV) is the main cause of viral pneumonia and bronchiolitis (9,10). Infants may be particularly susceptible because the lungs are still in the process of adapting to extrauterine life, the alveolae are still septating, the deadspace is relatively large, the ribs are flexible and horizontal (11), and the immune system is immature. All of these factors predispose to wheezing, dyspnea, sometimes hypoxia during infantile viral inflections.

Immunocompromised persons are at increased risk of developing severe respiratory illness due to respiratory viruses. Recent reports show that in 133 consecutive patients with bone marrow transplants who developed a viral respiratory infection, the mortality rate for RSV was 61%, for parainfluenza virus 39%, and for adenovirus 72% (12). In addition, patients who develop neutropenia after chemotherapy are at increased risk of common respiratory viral infections, particularly with RSV.

As described above, eosinophilic lung disease is well known in many parasitic, bacterial, and fungal infections. However, viral pulmonary eosinophilia is rare but has been described after infection with human rhinovirus (HRV) (13–15) parainfluenza-3 virus (PIV-3) (16,17), and pneumonia virus of mice (PVM) (18). HRVs cause the majority of common colds in older children and in adults, and are a frequent cause of asthma exacerbation. Patients subjected to bronchial mucosal biopsies during experimental infections with HRV serotype 16 show an increase in histamine responsiveness during the cold, accompanied by increases in submucosal lymphocytes and in epithelial eosinophils. In asthmatics, this local eosinophilia persisted into convalescence, but it resolved rapidly in normal volunteers (19). The evidence for a role of eosinophils in human RSV bronchiolitis is indirect. Eosinophil cationic protein (ECP) is significantly higher in children with RSV respiratory tract infection, and ECP levels correlate with severity of disease (20).

In experimental models, pulmonary eosinophilia has been most comprehensively investigated during RSV disease. After infection with RSV, human or murine cells produce RANTES, IL-8, and MIP-1α (1,2,21). In vivo, bronchial lavage (BAL) fluid from children with RSV infections contains higher RANTES levels than those from RSV-negative children (1). Similarly, lower respiratory tract secretions from mechanically ventilated patients with RSV bronchiolitis have raised levels of RANTES, MIP-1α, and ECP (an eosinophil degranulation product) (21). Since RANTES is a major chemoattractant for eosinophils, it maybe assumed that high levels of this chemokine in the lung may be predictive of pulmonary eosinophilic disease and that elevated ECP levels may indicate the recruitment of activated eosinophils. However, only rarely do RSV-infected children have increased numbers of eosinophils in the BAL fluid as assessed by conventional cell staining and light microscopy. In children in whom samples can be obtained (i.e., those with diseases of unusual severity), the BAL fluid shows an increase in mononuclear cells and PMNs (22).

Children admitted with viral bronchiolitis have an increased incidence of repeated wheezing in later childhood and are often diagnosed as asthmatic (23). This effect seems to continue up to the age of 11–13 years, but not beyond (24). It is not clear whether RSV bronchiolitis is causally linked to later recurrent childhood wheeze, but these are plausible mechanisms that would explain such an effect (25).

III. Vaccine-Enhanced RSV Disease in Humans

In the reports of formalin vaccine disease enhancement, there was only limited information regarding the nature of the augmented disease. Augmentation was practically confined to younger (mostly seronegative) vaccinees experiencing natural RSV infection in the first or second year after vaccination. In one study, infants and children between 2 months and 9 years of age were immunized with the vaccine, which was prepared by formalin inactivation and alum precipitation of whole RSV (FI-RSV). During primary RSV infection these children developed a severe form of airway inflammation, with up to 80% of them requiring hospitalization due to bronchitis, bronchiolitis, or pneumonia (26). In two fatal cases, intensive cellular infiltrates comprising mononuclear cells, eosinophils, and PMNs were found. RSV was recovered from lung tissue, and pure cultures of *Escherichia coli* or *Klebsiella* were grown in vitro. Blood eosinophilia was also described among vaccinees during subsequent RSV infection (27). Eosinophilic lung inflammation in children previously immunized with FI-RSV suggests an immune-mediated event initiated by the vaccine. Although it is to be hoped that this vaccine augmentation will never again be induced in human studies, there has been considerable progress in understanding RSV vaccine–induced immunopathology in animal models.

IV. Animal Models of RSV-Induced Lung Eosinophilia

Vaccine-enhanced RSV disease has been extensively investigated in animal models (28). Animals that are immunized with FI-RSV and subsequently challenged with RSV develop enhanced acute lung inflammation with eosinophil infiltration (29,30). We have shown that eosinophils increase in bone marrow by the first day after intranasal RSV challenge, followed by a substantial rise in BAL fluid and (interstitial lung) eosinophil infiltration from day 4 to 9. Interestingly, the number of eosinophils circulating in the blood is only slightly raised, showing that peripheral eosinophilia is not necessarily present when lung eosinophilia occurs (Fig. 1).

It was originally suggested that antigen–antibody immune complexes were responsible for enhanced RSV disease (31). These were thought to result from an excess of non-neutralizing antibody produced to epitopes changed by the process of formalin inactivation. However, the dominant role of CD4[+] T cells in enhanced lung pathology has been demonstrated by studies of the

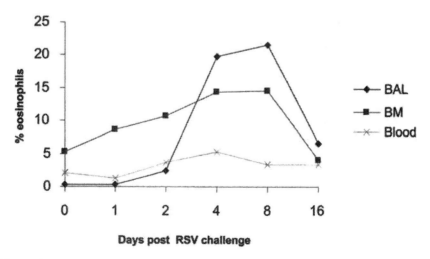

Figure 1

mouse model of RSV disease. Connors et al. showed that $CD4^+$ T cells are crucial to the immunopathogenesis of vaccine-augmented RSV disease and that RSV-specific antibodies (in the absence of $CD4^+$ and $CD8^+$ T cells) are not sufficient to mediate pulmonary histopathology (32). In other species, it is possible that FI-RSV induces interferon(IFN)-enhancing antibody and that this is important in disease augmentation.

Cytokines produced by $CD4^+$ T cells also play a crucial role in enhanced inflammation, particularly Th2-type cytokines (as demonstrated by abundant interleukin-5 (IL-5), IL-13, IL-10 mRNA and protein). In addition, there is marked reduction in the expression of IL-12 mRNA in FI-RSV-immunized mice (30). The same report demonstrated a correlation between eosinophil/macrophage ratio and the signal for IL-5 mRNA. There have also been reports of enhanced lung pathology due to class II–restricted CTL in FI-RSV-immunized mice. By contrast, primary RSV infection apparently results in an increase in the frequency of only class I–restricted CTL precursors (33). The role of CD8 T cells in viral eosinophilia is not clear. Although some have reported that CD8 cells can make type 2 cytokines (34) and that such cells have a role (35), others have not been able to confirm this finding or to demonstrate the presence of such cells either in vivo or in vitro.

It has been shown that two major surface glycoproteins, the fusion protein (F) and the attachment protein (G), demonstrate differential influence on the host immune system (28). In BALB/c mice, scarification with recombinant vaccinia virus (rVV) expressing F protein of RSV (rVV-F) prior to RSV infection results in hemorrhagic lung disease with efflux of PMNs (reminiscent of "shock lung"), whereas priming with rVV expressing G protein (rVV-G) produces enhanced disease characterized by eosinophilic influx. Lymphocytes obtained from BAL fluid of rVV-F- or rVV-M2-sensitized mice have enhanced numbers of activated $CD8^+$ T cells (which are class I restricted and cytolytic) and $CD4^+$ T cells that produce mainly type 1 cytokines in vitro or ex vivo. By contrast, rVV-G priming induces $CD4^+$ cells that produce type 2 cytokines, and activated CD8 T cells are not enhanced by priming. To further dissect factors responsible for pulmonary eosinophilia, the role of priming with different RSV proteins has been extensively investigated in inbred mice (Fig. 2).

Inbred strains are used because the defined and fixed genetic background allows detailed immunological dissection of pathogenic factors, and different strains may be used to reproduce the spectrum of diseases seen in outbred human populations. Most strains of mouse are susceptible to infection with human isolates of RSV, but only support limited viral replication. Indeed, it is sometimes impossible to cause severe life-threatening disease in non-immunized mice even using the highest titer of RSV available. This reflects the situation in humans, in whom only 2–3% develop disease of sufficient severity to cause hospital admission. Moreover, RSV induces histological changes that resemble human bronchiolitis. The strain specific effects are complex: $H-2^d$ mice (BALB/c, DBA/2n, B10.D2) show lung eosinophilia, but $H-2^k$ mice

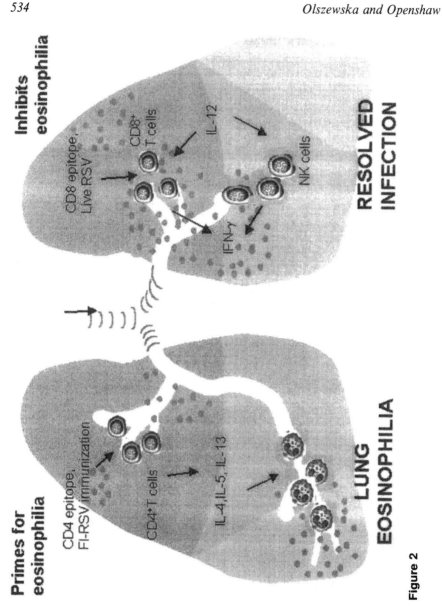

Figure 2

(CBA, C3H, B10.BR) do not. Among H-2^b strains, some are susceptible (i.e., BALB.B) but others resistant (C57BL/10) to the development of lung eosinophilia (36).

Cell transfer experiments confirm that injecting naive RSV-infected mice with CD4$^+$ and/or CD8$^+$ T cells fractionated from polyclonal RSV-specific T-cell lines produces disease enhancement similar to priming by scarification with rVV-G or rVV-F constructs. Mice receiving CD4$^+$ cells develop respiratory distress and lose up to 30% of their body weight, and an excessive number of eosinophils are present in BAL. On the other hand, CD8$^+$ T cells produce mild "shock lung" with PMNs and lung hemorrhage. The same study demonstrates that coinjecting CD8$^+$ cells can reduce the eosinophilogenic effects of CD4$^+$ cell transfer (37) and that both CD4 and CD8 T cells are antiviral in vivo (38). In support of these findings, Srikiatkhachorn and Braciale performed ingenious studies using a novel construct of rVV-G with M2 CD8$^+$ T-cell epitope inserted into it. Priming with this immunogen resulted in greatly reduced lung eosinophilia during the subsequent RSV challenge (39).

There are several explanations for the induction of eosinophilia in vivo after RSV infection in G-primed mice. G may lack relevant CD8$^+$ T-cell epitopes and therefore fail to generate CD8 cytotoxic (CTL) responses. Since CTLs are the major source of IFN-γ, absence of CTLs leads to deficient IFN-γ production and therefore to excess of helper T cells that default to type 2 cytokine production (38–40). These cytokines (IL-4 and IL-5) are expressed in BAL cells, peaking on day 4 after RSV challenge (41). It has recently been shown that the virus-specific T cells in the lung (but not in the spleen or in cultured cells) may have impaired function in terms of IFN-γ production (42). This would be additional factor favoring type 2 cytokine production by CD4 cells and therefore lung eosinophilia. Another possibility is that the ability of G to mimic the chemokine fractalkine (otherwise called neurotactin) and bind to CX3CR1, the fractalkine receptor (43). This may in some way cause selective recruitment of inflammatory cells, leading to a type 2–biased population of T cells. This topic is currently under investigation.

However, the secreted form of G and the route of immunization seem also to be important in determining the pattern of subsequent of lung pathology. Intraperitoneal administration of rVV-G does not lead to lung eosinophilia during subsequent RSV challenge (44), probably because of regional differences in antigen load or antigen presentation. In further studies, Bembridge et al. showed that gene gun delivery of a DNA vaccine encoding the F or G proteins primes for Th2 responses and that this could not be modulated by the co-delivery of plasmids encoding IL-2, IL-12, or IFN-γ (45). All animals produced IL-4 and IL-5 with very little IFN-γ, and BAL contained up to 7% of eosinophils. An eosinophilic response was not observed in mice immunized intraperitoneally with rVV expressing G protein although it was seen in animals scarified with the same antigen (44). The difference in pulmonary pathology observed between scarified or intraperitoneally or vaccinated mice was not reflected in a difference in cytokine production by splenocytes from vaccinated and challenged mice restimulated with RSV in vitro (44).

V. Modulating Lung Eosinophilia in Mice

A major advantage of the mouse model of RSV disease is that many depleting reagents, immunomodulators, knockouts, and cell surface markers are available for study. This has allowed the investigation of the role of specific cytokines and chemokines in normal and augmented disease. For example, it has been found that IL-12 down-regulates type 2 cytokine responses and lung eosinophilia in RSV-infected G-primed mice. The mechanism of this modulation is that IL-12 stimulates the production of IFN-γ by CTL and natural killer (NK) cells. Unfortunately, RSV-specific CTLs are also pathogenic alone (46) or in a situation where eosinophilia is reduced but disease severity is increased by IL-12 treatment (47).

Enhanced lung pathology seen after FI-RSV immunization can be lessened by treatment with neutralizing anti-IL-4 or anti-IL-10 antibodies (48). A more selective approach is to use depleting antibodies to T1/ST2, a surface receptor of the IL-1 receptor family, which defines a subset of Th2 cells. Anti-T1/ST2 treatment of RSV-infected mice primed with rVV-G reduces lung eosinophilia and disease severity, accompanied by a reduction in IL-5, tumor necrosis factor (TNF), and IFN-γ (but not IL-4) levels (49).

An alternative approach to disease modification is to eliminate proteins or fragments that are involved in augmented lung pathology. Thus, region 193–203 of G protein of RSV (identified as an epitope involved in the induction of pulmonary eosinophilia) was eliminated in altered recombinant G protein expressed in vaccinia virus. This construct was used for scarification prior to RSV infection and demonstrated that it is possible to induce protective immunity against RSV while avoiding eosinophilic response (50). Using a series of overlapping peptides, Tebbey et al. showed the dominant proliferative and cytokine responses to a peptide encompassing amino acids 184–198. Mice vaccinated with this peptide conjugated to keyhole limper hemocyanin showed marked pulmonary eosinophilia after challenge with live RSV. By contrast, mice immunized with the peptide 208–222 conjugate–induced IFN-γ-secreting spleen cells did not sensitise for pulmonary eosinophilia after challenge. In addition, they showed that some HLA A$_2$ human donors recognized peptide 184–198 (51).

VI. Role of Eosinophils in Viral Lung Disease

Although eosinophils are sometimes recruited to the lungs during viral infections, their role is not clear. It may simply be that virus-infected cells (epithelial cells and macrophages) produce various cytokines and chemokines, which generally attract other cells to the site of infection. The recruitment of eosinophils may be simply a bystander effect. Alternatively, it can be argued that eliciting an inappropriate Th2 response could be a survival advantage to a virus. Th1 responses have powerful antiviral effects, and Th2 responses may be more appropriate to helminthic infections and less potently antiviral (52).

The process of eosinophil maturation is highly dependent on IL-5 (53). It causes the bone marrow to release eosinophils into the circulation (54) and promotes their further maturation in peripheral tissues (55). In IL-5 knockout mice, airway eosinophilia does not develop unless IL-5 is administered (56,57).

It has been shown that eosinophils can specifically bind RSV and that eosinophils bind to cultured cells more avidly if they are RSV infected (58). As a result of eosinophil infection, increased production of superoxide has been demonstrated, as well as release of RANTES, MIP-1α, and other inflammatory mediators (3,59).

Human eosinophils are known to produce two different ribonucleases with antiviral activity against members of the Paramyxoviridae: eosinophil-derived neurotoxin (EDN) and ECP (60). Although many independent studies have found association between the production of these enzymes and the severity of RSV pulmonary disease (20,61,62), their role in host defense remains controversial and not fully understood. Investigations carried by Rosenberg and Domachowske demonstrated that eosinophils may mediate a direct, ribonuclease-dependent reduction in infectivity of RSV and that EDN can function alone as an independent antiviral agent mediating the destruction of extracellular virions (63). EDN and ECP may represent relatively unrecognized elements of innate antiviral host defenses (64).

Eosinophils can mediate antibody-dependent cell-mediated cytotoxicity due to expression of Fc receptors and ability to secrete lytic granules rich in mediators. When an infected target cell is bound by an eosinophil via the Fc receptor, the eosinophil releases the contents of cytoplasmic granules, which damage the target cell. The presence of complement receptor-1 on the surface of eosinophils provides another mechanism by which antibody-opsonized pathogens may be phagocytosed in the presence of C3b.

Along with having antiviral effects, eosinophils may clearly be harmful. They could contribute to the airway injury and obstruction (58) release superoxides, lysosomal hydrolase, and eosinophil-derived neurotoxin. Prolonged lung eosinophilia and high levels of ECP may be risk factors for the development of asthma.

VII. Infection History

The "hygiene hypothesis" suggests that normal exposure to environmental microbial agents prevent the development of asthma and atopy; it seems that infection history may also modify immune responses to RSV infection (65). In the mouse model of FI-RSV-enchanced disease, Waris and colleagues found that animals previously infected with RSV do not demonstrate augmented lung disease when they are immunized with FI-RSV vaccine before subsequent challenge (66). Responses were skewed toward Th1-type by priming with live RSV before FI-RSV vaccination, preventing enhanced disease. Similarly, prior infection with influenza virus prevent lung eosinophilia in the rVV-G sensitization model (67). Given the frequency of pathogen encounter during the first months and years of life (9), this phenomenon may be of great importance in explaining the age dependence of RSV disease.

VIII. Concluding Remarks

During viral infections of the lung, chemokines and cytokines are produced that may, under some circumstances, recruit eosinophils. Any mechanism that inhibits early IFN-γ production may skew immune response toward Th2 with cytokines (i.e., IL-4 and IL-5), which facilitate eosinophil migration and maturation at the site of infection. There is evidence that eosinophils can be both protective against viral infection and immunopathogenic. Understanding the role of eosinophils in viral lung diseases will help in the understanding of viral disorders, vaccinations strategies, and the relationship between viral infections and asthma.

References

1. Becker S, Reed W, Henderson FW, Noah TL. RSV infection of human airway epithelial cells causes production of the beta-chemokine RANTES. Am J Physiol 1997; 272:L512–L520.
2. Saito T, Deskin RW, Casola A, Haeberle H, Olszewska B, Ernst PB, Alam R, Ogra PL, Garofalo R. Respiratory syncytial virus induces selective production of the chemokine RANTES by upper airway epithelial cells. J Infect Dis 1997; 175:497–504.
3. Olszewska-Pazdrak PB, Casola A, Saito T, Alam R, Crowe SE, Mei F, Ogra PL, Garofalo RP. Cell-specific expression of RANTES, MCP-1, and MIP-1 alpha by lower airway epithelial cells and eosinophils infected with respiratory syncytial virus. J Virol 1998; 72:4756–4764.
4. Shann F. Pneumococcus and influenza. Lancet 1990; 335:898–901.
5. Selwyn BJ. The epidemiology of acute respiratory tract infection in young children: comparison of findings from several developing countries. Coordinated Data Group of BOSTID Researchers. Rev Infect Dis 1990; 12:S870–S888.
6. Pelletier DL, Frongillo EA, Schroeder DG, Habicht JP. The effects of malnutrition on child mortality in developing countries. Bull World Health Organ 1995; 73: 443–448.
7. Paxton LA, Redd SC, Steketee RW, Otieno JO, Nahlen B. An evaluation of clinical indicators for severe paediatirc illness. Bull World Health Organ 1996; 74:613–618.

8. Han LL, Alexander JP, Anderson LJ. Respiratory syncytial virus pneumonia among the elderly: an assessment of disease burden. J Infect Dis 1999; 179:25–30.

9. Denny FW, Jr. The clinical impact of human respiratory virus infections. Am J Respir Crit Care Med 1995; 152 (suppl).:S4–S12.

10. Hemming VG. Viral respiratory diseases in children: classification, etiology, epidemiology, and risk factors. J Pediatr 1994; 124:S13–S16.

11. Openshaw PJM, Edwards S, Helms P. Changes in rib cage geometry during childhood. Thorax 1984; 390:624–647.

12. Kaiser L, Couch RB, Galasso GJ, Glezen WP, Webster RG, Wright PF, Hayden FG. First International Symposium on Influenza and Other Respiratory Viruses: summary and overview: Kapalua, Maui, Hawaii, December 4–6, 1998. Antiviral Res 1999; 42:149–175.

13. Calhoun WJ, Dick EC, Schwartz LB, Busse WW. A common cold virus, rhinovirus 16, potentiates airway inflammation after segmental antigen bronchoprovocation in allergic subjects. J Clin Invest 1994; 94:2200–2208.

14. Gern JE, Vrtis R, Kelly EA, Dick EC, Busse WW. Rhinovirus produces non-specific activiation of lymphocytes through a monocyte-dependent mechanism. J Immunol 1996; 157:1605–1612.

15. Greiff, Andersson M, Andersson E, Linder M, Myint S, Svensson C, Persson CG. Experimental common cold increases mucosal output of eotaxin in atopic individuals. Allergy 1999; 54:1204–1208.

16. van Oosterhout AJ, van Ark I, Folkerts G, Van der Linde HJ, Savelkoul HF, Verheyen AK, Nijkamp FP. Antibody to interleukin-5 inhibits virus-induced airway hyperresponsiveness to histamine in guinea pigs. Am J Respir Crit Care Med 1995; 151:177–183.

17. Scheerens J, Folkerts G, Van-Der LH, Sterk PJ, Conroy DM, Williams TJ, Nijkamp FP. Eotaxin levels and eosinophils in guinea pig broncho-alveolar lavage fluid are increased at the onset of a viral respiratory infection. Clin Exp Allergy 1999; 29 (Suppl 2):74–77.

18. Domachowske JB, Bonville CA, Dyer KD, Easton AJ, Rosenberg HF. Pulmonary eosinophilia and production of MIP-1 alpha are prominent responses to infection with pneumonia virus of mice. Cell Immunol 2000; 200:98–104.

19. Fraenkel DJ, Bardin PG, Sanderson G, Lampe F, Johnston SL, Holgate ST. Lower airways inflammation during rhinovirus colds in normal and in asthmatic subjects. Am J Respir Crit Care Med 1995; 151:879–886.

20. Garofalo R, Kimpen JL, Welliver RC, Ogra PL. Eosinophil degranulation in the respiratory tract during naturally acquired respiratory syncytial virus infection. J Pediatr 1992; 120:28–32.

21. Harrison AM, Bonville CA, Rosenberg HF, Domachowske JB. Respiratory syncytical virus-induced chemokine expression in the lower airways: eosinophil recruitment and degranulation. Am J Respir Crit Care Med 1999; 159:1918–1924.

22. Everard ML, Milner AD. Testing of bronchoalveolar lavage for the laboratory diagnosis of respiratory syncytial virus infections. J Pediatr 1992; 121:168–169.

23. Sigurs N, Bjarnason R, Sigurbergsson F, Kjellman B, Bjorksten B. Asthma and immunoglobulin E antibodies after respiratory syncytial virus bronchiolitis: a prospective cohort study with matched controls. Pediatrics 1995; 95:500–505.

24. Stein RT, Sherrill D, Morgan WJ, Holberg CJ, Halonen M, Taussig LM, Wright AL, Martinez FD. Respiratory syncytial virus in early life and risk of wheeze and allergy by age 13 years. Lancet 1999; 354:541–545.

25. Openshaw PJM. Potential mechanisms causing delayed effects of respiratory syncytial virus infection. Am J Respir Crit Care Med 2001; 163:S10–S13.

26. Kim HW, Canchola JG, Brandt CD, Pyles G, Chanock RM, Jensen K, Parrott RH. Respiratory syncytial virus disease in infants despite prior administration of antigenic inactivated vaccine. Am J Epidemiol 1969; 89:422–434.

27. Chin J, Magoffin RL, Shearer LA, Schieble JH, Lennette EH. Field evaluation of a respiratory syncytial virsus vaccine and a trivalent parainfluenza virus vaccine in a pediatric population. Am J Epidemiol 1969; 89:449–463.

28. Openshaw PJM, Culley F, Olszewska W. Immunopathogenesis of vaccine-enhanced RSV disease. Vaccine 2001; 20:S27–S31.

29. Murphy BR, Sotnikov AV, Lawrence LA, Banks SM, Prince GA. Enhanced pulmonary histopathology is observed in cotton rats immunized with formalin-inactivated respiratory syncytial virus (RSV) or purified F glycoprotein and challenged with RSV 3-6 months after immunization. Vaccine 1990; 8:497–502.

30. Waris ME, Tsou C, Erdman DD, Zaki SR, Anderson LJ. Respiratory syncytial virus infection in BALB/c mice previously immunized with formalin-inactivated virus induces enhanced pulmonary inflammatory response with a predominant Th2-like cytokine pattern. J Virol 1996; 70:2852–2860.

31. Prince GA, Jenson AB, Hemming VG, Murphy BR, Walsh EE, Horswood RL, Chanock RM. Enhancement of respiratory syncytial virus pulmonary pathology in cotton rats by prior intramuscular inoclation of formalin-inactivated virus. J Virol 1986; 57:721–728.

32. Connors M, Kulkarni AB, Firestone CY, Holmes KL, Morse HC, Sotnikov AV, Murphy BR. Pulmonary histopathology induced by respiratory syncytial virus (RSV) challenge of formalin-inactivated RSV-immunized BALB/c mice is abrogated by depletion of CD4+T cells. J Virol 1992; 66:7444–7451.

33. Tripp RA, Anderson LJ. Cytotoxic T-lymphocyte precursor frequencies in BALB/c mice after acute respiratory syncytial virus (RSV) infection or immunization with a formalin-inactivated RSV vaccine. J Virol 1998; 72:8971–8975.

34. Coyle AJ, Erard F, Bertrand C, Walti S, Pircher H, Le Gros G. Virus-specific CD8+ cells can switch to interleukin 5 production and induce airway eosinophilia. J Exp Med 1995; 181:1229–1233.

35. Schwarze J, Makela M, Cieslewicz G, Dakhama A, Lahn M, Ikemura T, Joetham A, Gelfand EW. Transfer of the enhancing effect of respiratory syncytial virus infection on subsequent allergic airway sensitization by T lymphocytes. J Immunol 1999; 163:5729–5734.

36. Hussell T, Georgiou A, Sparer TE, Matthews S, Pala P, Openshaw PJM. Host genetic determinants of vaccine-induced eosinophilia during respiratory syncytial virus infection. J Immunol 1998; 161:6215–6222.

37. Alwan WH, Record FM, Openshaw PJM. CD4+ T cells clear virus but augment disease in mice infected with respiratory syncytial virus: comparison with the effects of CD8+ cells. Clin Exp Immunol 1992; 88:527–536.

38. Alwan WH, Kozlowska WJ, Openshaw PJM. Distinct types of lung disease caused by functional subsets of antiviral T cells. J Exp Med 1994; 179:81–89.

39. Srikiatkhachorn A, Braciale TJ. Virus specific CD8$^+$ T lymphocytes downregulate T helper cell type 2 cytokine secretion and pulmonary eosinophilia during experimental murine respiratory syncytial virus Infection. J Exp Med 1997; 186:421–432.

40. Hussell T, Baldwin CJ, O'Garra A, Openshaw PJM. CD8+ T-cells control Th2-driven pathology during pulmonary respiratory syncytial virus infection. Eur J Immunol 1997; 27:3341–3349.

41. Spender LC, Hussell T, Openshaw PJ. Abundant IFN-gamma production by local T cells in respiratory syncytial virus-induced eosinophilic lung disease. J Gen Virol 1998; 79:1751–1758.

42. Chang J, Srikiatkhachorn A, Braciale TJ. Visualization and characterization of respiratory syncytial virus F–specific CD8+ T cells during experimental virus infection. J Immunol 2001; 164:4254–4260.

43. Tripp RA, Jones LP, Haynes LM, Zheng H, Murphy PM, Anderson LJ. CX3C chemokine mimicry by respiratory syncytial virus G glycoprotein. Nat Immunol 2001; 2:732–738.

44. Bembridge GP, García-Beato R, Lopez JA, Melero JA, Taylor G. Subcellular site of expression and route of vaccination influence pulmonary eosinophilia following respiratory syncytial virus challenge in BALB/c mice sensitized to the attachment G protein. J Immunol 1998; 161:2473–2480.

45. Bembridge GP, Rodriguez N, Garcia-Beato R, Nicolson C, Melero JA, Taylor G. Respiratory syncytial virus infection of gene gun vaccinated mice induces Th2-driven pulmonary eosinophilia even in the absence of sensitization to the fusion (F) or attachment (G) protein. Vaccine 2000; 19:1038–1046.

46. Cannon MJ, Openshaw PJM, Anderson K, Wertz GW. Induction of virus-specific murine cytotoxic T cell responses by the G,M, 1A, and 1C gene products of respiratory syncytial virus. Virology 1988; submitted.

47. Hussell T, Openshaw PJM. IL-12 activated NK cells reduce lung eosinophilia to the attachment protein of respiratory syncytial virus but do not enhance the severity of illness after lung challenge in CD8 cell-immunodeficient conditions. J Immunol 2000; 165:7109–7115.

48. Connors M, Giese NA, Kulkarni AB, Firestone C-Y, Morse HC, III, Murphy BR. Enhanced pulmonary histopathology induced by respiratory syncytial virus (RSV) challenge of formalin-inactivated RSV-immunized BALB/c mice is abrogated by depletion of interleukin-4 (IL-4) and IL-10. J Virol 1994; 68:5321–5325.

49. Walzl G, Matthews S, Kendall S, Gutiérrez-Ramos JC, Coyle AJ, Openshaw PJM, Hussell T. Inhibition of T1/ST2 during respiratory syncytial virus infection prevents Th2- but not Th1-driven immunopathology. J Exp Med 2001; 193:785–792.

50. Sparer TE, Matthews S, Hussell T, Rae AJ, García-Barreno B, Melero JA, Openshaw PJ. Eliminating a region of respiratory syncytial virus attachment protein allows induction of protective immunity without vaccine-enhanced lung eosinophilia. J Exp Med 1998; 187:1921–1926.

51. Tebbey PW, Hagen M, Hancock GE. Atypical pulmonary eosinophilia is mediated by a specific amino acid sequence of the attachment (G) protein of respiratory syncytial virus. J Exp Med 1998; 188:1967–1972.

52. Openshaw PJ, O'Donnell DR. Asthma and the common cold: can viruses imitate worms? Thorax 1994; 49:101–103.

53. Dent LA, Strath M, Mellor AL, Sanderson CJ. Eosinophilia in transgenic mice expressing interleukin 5. J Exp Med 1990; 172:1425–1431.

54. Ying S, Robinson DS, Meng Q, Rottman J, Kennedy R, Ringler DJ, Mackay CR, Daugherty BL, Springer MS, Durham SR, Williams TJ, Kay AB. Enhanced expression of eotaxin and CCR3 mRNA and protein in atopic asthma: association with airway hyperresponsiveness and predominant co-localization of eotaxin mRNA to bronchial epithelial and endothelial cells. Eur J Immunol 1997; 27:3507–3516.

55. Cameron L, Christodoulopoulos P, Lavigne F, Nakamura Y, Eidelman D, McEuen A, Walls A, Tavernier J, Minshall E, Moqbel R, Hamid Q. Evidence for local eosinophil differentiation within allergic nasal mucosa: inhibition with soluble IL-5 receptor. J Immunol 2000; 164:1538–1545.

56. Foster PS, Hogan SP, Ramsay AJ, Matthaei KI, Young IG. Interleukin 5 deficiency abolishes eosinophilia, airways hyperreactivity, and lung damage in a mouse asthma model. J Exp Med 1996; 183:195–201.

57. Wang J, Palmer K, Lotvall J, Milan S, Lei XF, Matthaei KI, Gauldie J, Inman MD, Jordana M, Xing Z. Circulating, but not local lung, IL-5 is required for the development of antigen-induced airways eosinophilia. J Clin Invest 1998; 102:1132–1141.

58. Stark JM, Godding V, Sedgwick JB, Busse WW. Respiratory syncytial virus infection enhances neutrophil and eosinophil adhesion to cultured respiratory epithelial cells. Roles of CD18 and intercellular adhesion molecule-1. J Immunol 1996; 156:4774–4782.

59. Kimpen JL, Garofalo R, Welliver RC, Ogra PL. Activation of human eosinophils in vitro by respiratory syncytial virus. Pediatr Res 1992; 32:160–164.

60. Domachowske JB, Dyer KD, Adams AG, Rosenberg HF, Rosenberg. Eosinophil cationic protein/RNase 3 is another RNase A-family ribonuclease with direct antiviral activity. Nucl Acids Res 1998; 26:3358–3363.

61. Colocho Zelaya EA, Orvell C, Strannegard O. Eosinophil cationic protein in nasopharyngeal secretions and serum of infants infected with respiratory syncytial virus. Pediatr Allergy Immunol 1994; 5:100–106.

62. Oymar K, Elsayed S, Bjerknes R. Serum eosinophil cationic protein and interleukin-5 in children with bronchial asthma and acute bronchiolitis. Pediatr Allergy Immunol 1996; 7:180–186.

63. Domachowske JB, Dyer KD, Bonville CA, Rosenberg HF. Recombinant human eosinophil-derived neurotoxin/RNase 2 functions as an effective antiviral agent against respiratory syncytial virus. J Infect Dis 1998; 177:1458–1464.

64. Rosenberg HF, Domachowske JB. Eosinophils, ribonucleases and host defense: solving the puzzle. Immunol Res 1999; 20:261–274.

65. Pennycook A, Openshaw PJM, Hussell T. Partners in crime: co-infections in the developing world. Clin Exp Immunol 2000; 122:296–299.

66. Waris ME, Tsou C, Erdman DD, Day DB, Anderson LJ. Priming with live respiratory syncytial virus (RSV) prevents the enhanced pulmonary inflammatory response seen after RSV challenge in BALB/c mice immunized with formalin-inactivated RSV. J Virol 1997; 71:6935–6939.

67. Walzl G, Tafuro S, Moss PA, Openshaw PJM, Hussell T. Influenza virus lung infection protects from respiratory syncytial virus–induced immunopathology. J Exp Med 2000; 191:1317–1326.

20

Airway Remodeling as the Outcome of a Chronic Immune Response to Inhaled Allergen

ANTONIO M. VIGNOLA

University of Palermo
Palermo, Italy

JEAN BOUSQUET

Clinique des Maladies Respiratoires
INSERM U454
Montpellier, France

I. Introduction

"Remodel" is defined in the *Concise Oxford Dictionary* as "model again or differently, reconstruct." This is a critical aspect of wound repair in all organs representing a dynamic process which associates matrix production and degradation in reaction to an inflammatory insult (1) leading to a normal reconstruction process (model again) or a pathological one (model differently). Structural remodeling in airway diseases was initially proposed to describe changes induced in endothelial cells and extracellular matrix (ECM) by injury of the pulmonary circulation (2). It was then extended to many other pathological situations, including asthma (3,4).

The regeneration process in asthma follows the natural course of chronic inflammation and results in either tissue repair (a tightly regulated salutary biological response) or abnormal remodeling (an unregulated pathological process). This appears to be heterogeneous, leading, through a dynamic process of cell dedifferentiation, migration, differentiation, and maturation, to changes in connective tissue deposition (5). Although remodeling processes are almost invariably found in the airways of asthmatics, the extent of remodeling in asthma and its clinical consequences are still a matter of debate.

The links between allergen exposure in allergic asthmatics and remodeling is another important question that has not resolved yet. The airways are continuously exposed to several triggers, including allergens, pollutants, tobacco smoke, viruses, and bacteria. These agents are able to stimulate immune and inflammatory responses in the airways that can be sustained by the release of several factors, including chemokines and Th2-like cytokines.

II. Pathological Characteristics of Airway Remodeling

The airways in asthma display various structural alterations that can all contribute to airway remodeling and an overall increase in airway wall thickness. Not all features of remodeling are found in each asthmatic, but it appears that there are relatively few asthmatics without any pathological remodeling of the airways.

A. Extracellular Matrix

The ECM is a complex and dynamic meshwork influencing many cell biological functions, such as development, migration, and proliferation (6,7). The ECM also plays an essential supporting structural role that differs somewhat in the three physiological zones of the lung (8): the proximal, conducting airways and vasculature, the distal gas-exchanging respiratory zone (alveoli), and the intervening transitional zone (respiratory bronchioles). The ECM both allows some mobility to regulate airway and vascular diameter and is an essential stabilizer for preventing airway collapse during expiration. The macromolecules that constitute the EMC are secreted locally and consist of fibrous protein (fibronectin and laminin) embedded in a hydrated polysaccharide gel containing several glycosaminoglycans including hyaluronic acid (HA). ECM can be divided into two categories: the basement membrane and the interstitial matrix.

Thickening of the Reticular Basement Membrane
(i.e., Lamina Reticularis)

The basement membrane of surface epithelium is composed of several layers: the basal lamina (referred to as the "true" basement membrane) and the *lamina reticularis*. The basal lamina is of normal thickness in asthma. However, thickening of the *lamina reticularis* is a typical feature of the asthmatic bronchus, occurring early in the disease process. It consists of a plexiform deposition of immunoglobulins and/or collagen I and III and fibronectin (9), but apparently not of laminin (10). These proteins are likely produced by activated myofibroblasts (11) leading to a so-called pseudofibrosis of the airways. In some studies, the thickening could not be related to the severity, duration, or etiology of asthma (5,12–15), whereas a correlation with the severity of the disease has been observed in another study (16). Patients with rhinitis also present subepithelial fibrosis of the bronchi with a deposition of type I and III collagen and fibronectin (17). However, these features are less marked than in asthma.

Interstitial Matrix

Remodeling processes of the interstitial matrix are less well documented than the thickening of the reticular basement membrane. Several ECM abnormalities have been observed in asthmatics.

Most asthmatics present an *abnormal elastic fiber network* with fibers appearing fragmented (18,19) and hypertrophied as a result of the increased amount of collagen and myofibroblast matrix deposition occurring during the exaggerated elastic fiber deposition (20).

Hyaluronic acid levels have been found to be increased in the bronchoalveolar lavage (BAL) fluid of asthmatics (21). Moreover, there was a significant correlation between HA levels and the severity of asthma or the level of extracellular protein, suggesting a common activation of cells releasing these compounds.

Proteoglycans are complex macromolecules that consist of a protein core and one or more covalently bound GAG side chains (22). Proteoglycans bind with fibrillar collagen and influence the interaction of collagen fibrils and their assembly (22,23). An enhanced proteoglycan depostion in the subepithelial layer of the airway wall was shown in asthmatic subjects (24) and was correlated with increased airway responsiveness, suggesting that proteoglycans may play a role in the airway wall remodeling and airway mechanics in mild and severe asthma. It has been reported that versican, biglycan, decorin, and hyaluronan were localized in airways in postmortem lung tissue from six patients who had severe asthma and for whom asthma was considered to be the cause of, or a significant contributor to, death (22). The up-regulation of proteoglycans in asthmatic airway wall may be driven by inflammatory mediators such as transforming growth factor-β (TGF-β) (25) or by mitogens such as platelet-derived growth factor (PDGF) (26). However, the exact functional role of increased proteoglycan deposition in the airway wall of asthmatics is unknown.

Collagen and proteins. In the submucosa of asthmatics, electron microscopy (EM) studies show that collagen is not completely normal. In some patients, hyperplasia of collagen fibers can be observed (20). These fibers may be irregularly disposed but the exact nature of collagen is not completely characterized. Fibronectin, laminin, and tenascin deposition in the submucosa was found in the biopsies of asthmatics but not in those of normal subject (10,27). In addition, increased collagen III and V has been found in the submucosa of the airways of asthmatic subjects. Fibronectin levels are increased in BAL fluid of asthmatics and correlate with the levels of the profibrotic growth factor TGF-β (28), which stimulates fibroblast activation and synthesis of ECM proteins. These suggest that the submucosa of the asthmatic airway contains significantly more ECM than normal controls, giving rise to the possibility that airway scar formation may have greater functional implications than has been previously believed from consideration of the RBM alone.

Although asthma has been proposed to be a fibrotic disease (29), it is important to not that the increased ECM production and deposition within the airways of asthmatics does not lead to progressive and irreversible distortion of the lung's architecture found in true fibrotic lung diseases such as interstitial lung diseases. This likely reflects differences in the mechanisms regulating ECM deposition and degradation between these two diseases.

B. Fibrogenic Growth Factors

Increased expression of insulin-like growth factor-1 (IGF-1), epidermal growth factor (EGF), and TGF-β (25,28,30–35) and fibroblast growth factor (FGF) (36) has been reported in biopsies or BAL fluid. TGF-β expression was found to correlate with the degree of subepithelial fibrosis (30) and to be significantly increased in severe asthmatics with a rich eosinophilic infiltration of the airways (31).

C. Proteases and Protease Inhibitors

Metalloproteases (MMPs) selectively degrade ECM components. They have been implicated in angiogenesis and smooth muscle hyperplasia (37,38). MMPs also play a crucial role in the trafficking of inflammatory and structural cells (39,40).

MMP-9 is the major MMP expressed in asthma (41,42). In normal subjects, MMP-9 is cosecreted with tissue inhibitor metalloprotease-1 (TIMP-1) in 1:1 stoichiometry. An overproduction of TIMP-1 over MMP-9 seems to be a characteristic of patients with stable asthma (41,43). Moreover, no activated form of MMP-9 could be detected in BAL fluid from untreated stable asthmatics, suggesting that there was enough counterinhibitor (TIMP-1) to protect the molecule against activation (41,44). However, an excess of MMP-9 is found in BAL fluid from patients with uncontrolled asthma, or during a severe exacerbation (45), suggesting that in these patients with unstable asthma, free metallogelatinolytic activity is present.

Imbalances between MMPs and their inhibitors may contribute to tissue damage and some of the remodeling features seen in asthma. MMP-9 can degrade native type IV and type V collagens, denatured collagens, entactin, proteoglycans, and elastin (46). As such, MMP-9 has been shown to play a role in the disruption of the basement membrane and in the diapedesis of monocytes/macrophages or eosinophils to inflammatory foci by increasing the migration of these cells through the basement membrane cells (39,40). On the other hand, an excess of TIMP-1 over MMP-9 in stable asthma may protect the bronchi against metalloproteinase-degrading activity (47).

Other proteases and inhibitors are released in the airways. In particular, free elastase was found to be increased in sputum of asthmatics, and there was a correlation between its levels and low FEV_1 values (43).

D. Blood Vessels

An increase in blood vessel area has been reported as part of the structural alterations observed in asthma of various severity (48–51). Furthermore, the degree of vascularity has been shown to be inversely correlated with airway caliber and airway responsiveness (52). Changes in the tissue vasculature are of great importance in repair processes and usually lead to plasma leakage and tissue edema as well as to an increase in the number of vessels. Angiogenesis has recently been proposed as one step of the complex events characterizing airway remodeling in asthma (53), but its demonstration is still unclear. In angiogenesis, two key events are required: the release of factors capable of regulating endothelial cell proliferation and the development of changes of the ECM, mainly represented by extracellular proteolysis.

The switch to an angiogenic phenotype is characterized by the presence of new vessels, usually capillaries and small venules, and depends on a net balance of "positive" factors (stimulating angiogenesis) such as aFGF (acidic fibroblast growth factor), bFGF (basic fibroblast growth factor), and VEGF (vascular endothelial growth factor), and of "negative" factors (inhibiting angiogenesis) such as thrombospondin and angiostatin (54). VEGF also acts on endothelial cells increasing microvasculature permeability, resulting in extravasation of fibrinogen and in constitution of a clot of fibrin such that incorporating other matrix molecules, such as fibronectin, could provide a provisional matrix into which fibroblasts, endothelial cells, and other cells migrate. Having a double effect of endothelial cells and on FCM, VEGF promotes transformation of extracellular space into vascularized connective tissue and the constitution of a suitable "milieu" for cell growth and migration. The antiproliferative activity of thrombospondin is correlated with its binding with heparin, inhibiting that of bFGF.

Surpisingly, very few studies have examined angiogenesis in asthma, probably because there are technical limitations. The production of VEGF has been investigated in asthma. In one study the levels of VEGF have not been found to be increased in asthmatic airways, suggesting a low degree of angiogenesis in patients with stable asthma (55). However, in another study a higher VEGF and bFGF and angiogenin immunoreactivity was found in the submucosa of asthmatics than in control subjects. In addition, numbers of angiogenic factor–positive cells within the asthmatic airways were significantly correlated with the vascular area (52).

E. Smooth Muscle

Increased accumulation of bronchial smooth muscle cells is another prominent feature of airway wall remodeling that is believed to play a fundamental role in the pathogenesis of exaggerated airway narrowing in asthma. Hypertrophy and ·hyperplasia of airway smooth muscle (56–59) have been reported in postmortem specimens of asthmatic bronchi, albeit this observation has not been invariably confirmed (60). In some patients, the muscle mass may occupy up to 20% of the bronchial wall. In patients who died from an asthma exacerbation, the increase in smooth muscle is far greater than in those who died from another cause (58), suggesting that the increase of smooth muscle mass may have a major impact on the severity of airway obstruction in asthma. This increase in muscle mass is also more important than in chronic bronchitis (57). However, the importance of these findings is not completely clear since a study in asthmatic patients who died from other causes did not reveal any hyperplasia or hypertrophy (60). It is likely that these discrepancies are due to some degree of heterogeneity of the smooth muscle thickening, as recent studies have shown (61,62).

F. Mucus Glands

Mucus glands are distributed throughtout the airways in asthma and are even present in peripheral bronchioles where normally they are absent. The mucus glands in the segmental bronchi of asthmatics are considerably enlarged, and Dunhill et al. (56) showed that their volume was twice greater in asthmatics by comparison with normal subjects. These values overlap those found in the case of chronic bronchitis. In asthma, hypertrophy of mucus glands appears to be the cause of increased volume, whereas hyperplasia of the mucus-secreting cells is usually observed in chronic bronchitis. However, animal models indicate that goblet cell hyperplasia and increased mucus production can occur in the large airways following prolonged allergen exposure, suggesting that a persistent inhalation of allergens may be an important causative factor for the development of mucus gland remodeling (63).

III. Airway Remodeling and Natural History of Asthma

The natural history of lung growth and senescence in individuals with asthma is still poorly known. Lung growth appears to be relatively normal in most children with asthma but is reduced throughout childhood and adolescence in those with severe and persistent symptoms (64). It is not known if this reflects a failure to reach full growth in relation to bronchoconstriction or congenitally small lungs (65). Little is known about the influence of the degree of bronchial obstruction and the outcome of asthma in children. Approximately 50% of children with asthma still have respiratory symptoms in adult life (66).

For decades, asthma has been considered as a completely reversible obstructive, and, in many patients, complete reversibility of long-standing abnormal spirometric measurements, such as FEV_1, may be observed after bronchodilators and/or a course of corticosteroids (67). On the other hand, many asthmatic patients, both children and adults, have evidence of residual airway obstruction. This irreversible component of airway obstruction is more prominent in patients with severe asthma and even persists after aggressive anti-inflammatory treatment. Many epidemiological studies suggest that asthma is associated with an accelerated decline of the pulmonary function, which is considered as one of the possible consequences of airway remodeling. Although there are no longitudinal studies starting in infancy, it is supposed that such a decline may start at a very early stage of the natural history of the disease (68). However, a prospective study conducted in asthmatic children did not find that there was an increased decline in FEV_1 after bronchodilation in patients receiving placebo, nedocromil sodium, or budesonide (68). This study suggests that decline in lung function is not a feature of most asthmatic children, but early effects of asthma could not be assessed in this study.

An increase in the rate of decline in FEV_1 can also occur during adult life in asthmatics, particularly in middle-aged and elderly smokers, thus making a differentiation between chronic bronchitis and asthma by means of FEV_1 (69). However, this decline, appears to be highly heterogeneous between patients; whereas it seems to be minimal in some, it is quite extensive in others, being similar to that of patients with chronic obstructive pulmonary disease. Loss of pulmonary function does not appear to constantly increase during life but may be a stepwise process. Moreover, such a functional decline is greatly influenced by the smoking habit, thus significantly increasing the decline of FEV_1 in smoking asthmatic subjects.

Another component of remodeling is nonspecific bronchial hyperresponsiveness (BHR) (70,71). Convincing mathematical models suggest that remodeling, resulting in an increased thickness of the airway wall, thickening of the smooth muscle layer, and changes in the adventitial matrix, significantly contribute to BHR. At the same time, however, other models predict that remodeling could actually protect against excessive airway narrowing, thus opposing BHR (for review, see Ref. 72).

It is still a matter of debate whether pathological features of inflammation and remodeling may occur before or concomitant with the onset of asthma. However, it seems that in some infants some structural changes of the airways can develop before the clinical manifestation of the disease (73). It is also likely that the persistent exposure to several known factors, such as allergens (74–76), viruses (77), or indoor (78,79) and outdoor pollutants (80–86), may further contribute to alter the original airway architecture and lead to airway remodeling.

IV. Cell Activation by Allergens and Possible Remodeling Effects

Increased IgE production results from B-cell differentiation under the effects of Th2 cytokines and contact-mediated signals. IgE binds to high (FcεRI) and low-affinity receptors (FcεRII, CD23) specific for the ε heavy chain, which are expressed on the surface of many cells including mast cells and other airways cells, such as epithelial cells, eosinophils, macrophages, and smooth muscle cells. Cross-linking of the Fc receptors initiates signal transduction events, leading to the release of a wide range of inflammatory mediators, some of which may play an important role in the pathogenesis of airway remodeling.

Both structural and inflammatory cells are involved directly or indirectly in the IgE inflammatory response. Epithelial and mesenchymal cells mediate bidirectional growth control creating an epithelial-mesenchymal trophic unit that may be important in asthma remodeling (87).

A. IgE-Dependent Mast Cell Activation and Fibroproliferative Response

Mast cell activation is an initiating event in asthma pathogenesis. Mast cells are found in the bronchi of normal subjects and asthmatics (88–91). These cells are activated by the cross-linking of FcεRI molecules, which occurs by the binding of multivalent antigens to the attached IgE molecules. Activation of mast cells results in three types of biological responses: secretion of the preformed contents of their granules by a regulated process of exocytosis; synthesis and secretion of lipid mediators (such as cysteinyl- leukotrienes, Cys - LTs); and secretion of cytokines, such as tumor necrosis factor-α (TNF-α) and interleukin-1 (IL-1)(92,93). Mast cell degranulation has been documented in the airways of asthmatics in both their stable phase and following allergen challenge as shown directly by EM (94,95).

Mast Cell–Derived Mediators Involved in Tissue Remodeling

Mast cell–derived mediators can modulate the inflammatory cascade at several levels. They can promote the recruitment of eosinophils and Th2 cells as well as the activation of mesenchymal cells, such as fibroblasts, myofibroblasts, and airway smooth muscle cells. This implies that activation of mast cells by an IgE-dependent mechanism can play an important role in the pathogenesis of airway inflammation and remodeling.

The potential implication of mast cells in tissue remodeling is demonstrated by their ability to contribute to the pathogenesis of pulmonary fibrosis (96–98). Mast cells lines have also been shown to release components of basement membranes such as laminin and collagen IV (99) and may potentially contribute to abnormal ECM deposition in the inflamed airways. Mast cell products can also stimulate the migration and proliferation of fibroblasts (100,101) and modulate their functional activation through the release of tryptase (102).

Tryptase and Tissue Remodeling

Tryptase has the potential to influence the remodeling response in the airways of asthmatics. This serine protease is a potent stimulant of fibroblast and smooth muscle cell proliferation and is capable of stimulating synthesis of type I collagen by human fibroblasts (103). Tryptase also induces a concentration-dependent increase in the proliferation of fibroblasts, a phenomenon mediated via the activation of protease-activated receptor-2 (PAR-2) (103). These studies suggest that the release of tryptase from activated mast cells may play an important role in the fibroproliferative response observed in asthma and chronic obstructive pulmonary disease.

Mast Cell–Derived Plasmin, Plasmin Inhibitors, and Tissue Remodeling

Another potential mechanism by which mast cells can participate to the development of airway remodeling is by the release of factors capable of influencing the degradation of proteins of the ECM and basement membranes. Among these factors, an important role is played by plasmin, an extracellular serine protease synthesized as an inactive proenzyme, plasminogen, which can be converted to plasmin by two plasminogen activators, tissue plasminogen activator (tPA) and urokinase plasminogen activator (uPA) (104). Plasmin enhances proteolytic degradation of the ECM by activating MMPs directly to degrade ECM components (104) and by inhibiting MMP inhibitors. Due to these biological properties, plasmin exerts control over MMP activity at the substrate, activation, and inhibitor levels, and is therefore capable of playing a central role in ECM homeostasis.

An important mechanism in the regulation of PA activity is the inhibition of uPA or tPA by three major inhibitors (PAI-1, PAI-2, and PAI-3) (105), with PAI-1 showing the highest inhibitory activity. Deficiency of PAI-1 in mice and humans is associated with increased fibrinolysis, whereas PAI-1 overexpression leads to abnormal deposition of ECM after bleomycin challenge (106) or hyperoxia (107).

Human mast cells are an important source of tPA (108), and it has been proposed that mast cell–derived tPA may function as a "repair molecule," preventing fibrin deposition during some pathophysiological processes (108). However, mast cells can also produce PAI whose levels may influence the amount of ECM deposition in the airways. It is interesting to note that activated human mast cells are able to release a striking amount of functionally active PAI-1. Since PAI-1 is a major inhibitor of the MMPs, it is likely that its abnormal production may block fibrinolysis and promote airway remodeling by increasing fibrin and collagen deposition (109) (Fig. 1).

Conclusions

Taken together these data support the concept that mast cells not only are crucial in the initiation of the inflammatory response in the airways of asthmatics but also may have an important role in its chronic development. It is therefore likely that a persistent functional activation of mast cells due to a chronic exposure to antigens may lead to release of mediators with the potential to affect

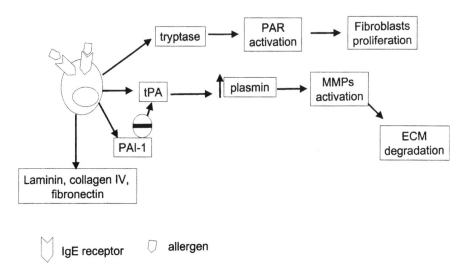

Figure 1 IgE-dependent mast cell activation and fibroproliferative response. The figure shows that mast cell activation via an IgE-dependent mechanism can potentially cause the release of mediators capable of modulating the proliferation of fibroblasts, such as tryptase, as well as the synthesis and degradation of ECM proteins, such as tPA and PAI.

the structure of the airways. If this stable functional activation of mast cells is not properly controlled, this process may increase and perpetuate the development of airway remodeling in asthma.

B. IgE-Dependent Activation of Dendritic Cells and Potential Effects on the Fibroproliferative Response

Human Langherans cells (LCs) express FcεRI (110–112). FcεRI seems to enable specific antigen uptake via receptor-mediated endocytosis in LCs.

FcεRI ligation on LCs triggers the synthesis and release of mediators that may initiate a local inflammatory reaction, as has been demonstrated for mast cells and suggested by the role of epidermal dendritic cells (DCs) in atopic dermatitis. It has been shown that murine LCs are able to synthesize and release many cytokines and exert significant polarizing influences on T-helper differentiation (113). This strongly suggests that LCs are involved in the initiation of inflammation, especially in the context of allergic reactions. Furthermore, mediators released either spontaneously or secondary to receptor ligation by LCs most probably dictate the route of differentiation that stimulated T cells will undergo in the context of antigen presentation. Thus, LCs contribute to direct T cells into the Th0, Th1, or Th2, pathways and may represent direct inflammatory cells through the secretion of cytokines such as TNF-α.

C. Epithelial Cells

Bronchial epithelial cells have an active role in the development of airway inflammation and remodeling in asthma (87). Bronchial epithelial injury initiates a complex series of repair mechanisms, one of which is reepithelialization of a denuded luminal surface. Regenerative changes are sometimes observed as demonstrated by varying stages of ciliogenesis in the nonciliated "metaplastic" surface epithelium (114). Bronchial epithelial cells initially affected by bronchial injury may be able to initiate the repair of an injured area by producing chemotactic factors for epithelial cells. Epithelial cells in asthma express several membrane markers, including adhesion molecules (115), and release a wide spectrum of molecules participating in airway repair, including fibronectin (116), growth factors (30,117,118), cytokines [IL-9, IL-16 (119), and IL-18 (120)], or chemokines such as granulocyte-macrophage colony-stimulating factor (GM-CSF) (121,122), and eotaxin (123,124).

Bronchial epithelial cells may be activated in asthma by indirect cell-to-cell interactions, but also by direct IgE activation since the expression of the FcεRI and FcεRII receptors allows these cells to respond to allergen stimulation (125). IgE-dependent activation of bronchial epithelial cells results in the release of mediators that are involved in tissue repair and remodeling, such as fibronectin and endothelin. Both of these mediators may play a major role in airway remodeling. Indeed, endothelin-1 acts in synergy with factors such as epidermal growth factor (EGF), PDGF, bFGF, TGFs, and insulin, amplifying the activation of mesenchymal cells and their effect on remodeling of the matrix (126). Endothelin-1 may also contribute significantly to the increased muscle mass and bronchial obstruction observed in asthma (127). It is therefore likely that IgE-dependent activation of bronchial epithelial cells contributes to an increased release of factors which, together with other profibrotic mediators (such as TGF-β, FGF, and EFG), can directly regulate the phenotypic and functional features of mesenchymal cells located underneath the basement membrane, such as fibroblasts and myofibroblasts (87) (Fig. 2). These cells, under the effects of epithelial-derived growth factors, produce collagen, reticular and elastic fibers, as well as proteoglycans and glycorproteins of the amorphous ECM, all likely contributing to the thickened airway wall of asthmatic subjects.

D. Eosinophils

In chronic asthma, eosinophils are found in increased numbers in bronchial biopsies (128). They are usually located in the epithelium and beneath the basement membrane, and show an enhanced state of activation. Most allergic and nonallergic asthmatics, including those with mild asthma, have eosinophils in their bronchi, and there is a significant association between the activation of eosinophils nad the severity of asthma (128) or BHR (90).

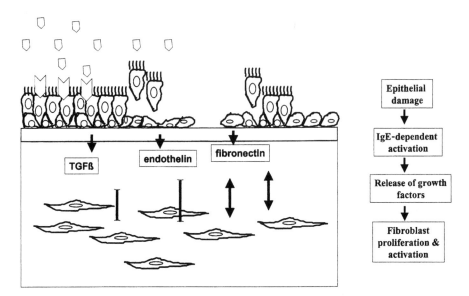

Figure 2   Activation of bronchial epithelial cells by allergens. The ability of bronchial epithelial cells of asthmatic subjects to express both the low and high receptors for IgE allow these cells to respond to allergen stimulations. Through this mechanism epithelial cells can release mediators involved in airway remodeling, such as TGF-β, endothelin, and fibronectin.

Eosinophils possess a wide array of biological properties due to their release of toxic granule proteins, oxygen free radicals, eicosanoids (Cys-leukotrienes) (129), platelet activating factor Th2 cytokines (130,131), and growth factors (132–134). Activated eosinophils may initiate contraction of human bronchial smooth muscle (135), may increase permeability (136), and may induce airway hyperresponsiveness (137).

Eosinophils can also release cytokines, growth factors (138,139), and elastase (140), which may be involved in remodeling and fibrosis. Eosinophil products stimulate fibroblasts in vitro (141,142). Eosinophils appear to be involved in pulmonary fibrosis (143–145) and are a source of TGF-β in bronchial biopsies of asthmatic subjects (25,30).

Therefore, it is believed that eosinophils can truly play a central role in the pathogenesis of asthma. However, recent observations with the anti-IL-5 blocking monoclonal antibodies administered for up to 16–20 weeks have revealed that although blood and sputum eosinophils were reduced almost to undetectable levels, no effect on the allergens EAR, LAR, BHR, or clinical outcome measures could be observed. These findings bring into question the role of the eosinophils as a proinflammatory cell in asthma, especially when similar reductions in eosinophil count are produced by exogenous IL-12 or IFN-γ without any evidence of physiological or clinical benefit (146).

Eosinophils express both FcεRI (147,148) and FcεRII (149) receptors and can be activated through an IgE-dependent mechanism (150–152). IgE-mediated activation of eosinophils is proposed as an important mechanism for host defense and in the pathophysiology of human disease, including allergic diseases. Indeed, in atopic subjects, IgE, FcεRII stimulation induces functional changes in eosinophils characterized by increased eosinophil migration associated with enhanced late function antigen-1 and Mac-1 expression (153).

E. Monocyte Macrophages

Mononuclear phagocytes have a fundamental role in specific immunity via their accessory cell function and are metabolic cells that have a major role in chronic inflammation. The spectrum of their biological activity is vast and while many of the products released are involved in inflammation, they also take part in healing and repair.

Mononuclear phagocytes are likely to be involved in the pathogenesis of asthma (154). An increased number of macrophages infiltrate the airways of asthmatics (90,155–157), particularly in non-atopic asthma (157). In addition, activated macrophages have the potential to secrete a wide variety of products, many of which play a major role in the pathogenesis of injury and repair (158–160). Alveolar macrophages can synthesize and secrete PA and a group of MMPs having the capacity to degrade various ECM macromolecules, including elastin (161). Macrophages may also be involved in the regulation of the airway remodeling through the secretion of growth factors such as PDGF, bFGF, or TGF-β (28) (Fig. 3). In interstitial lung diseases, alveolar macrophages are activated and release cytokines and growth factors (162–164).

Airway macrophages bear FcεRII and possibly FcεRI. It was shown that AM from non-atopic donors passively sensitized with allergen-specific IgE antibody from the serum of asthmatic patients (165) were able to release lysosomal β-glucuronidase after stimulation with the related allergen or with anti-human IgE antibody, in the absence of any mast cells or basophils. The cell reactivity was dependent on the interaction of macrophages with IgE. AMs from asthmatic patients behaved similarly to passively sensitized normal macrophages. Contact with the related allergen or with anti-IgE antibody induced the same percentage of enzyme release, demonstrating that these cells possess allergen-specific IgE bound on their surface. Other studies have shown that AMs sensitized with human myeloma IgE and challenged with anti-IgE were able to release LTB_4, $PGF_{2\alpha}$, TxB_2, and N-acetyl-β-glucosaminidase (166,167), IL-1β, TNF-α, or IL-6 (168–170).

AMs from asthmatics present an increased expression of FcεRII. Instillation of allergen in the asthmatic airways up-regulated FcεRII on AMs (171). Up-regulation of FcεRII in atopic individuals may therefore reflect allergen-induced exposure of mononuclear phagocytes to cytokines (IL-4, GM-CSF, IFN-γ, IFN-α, and M-CSF).

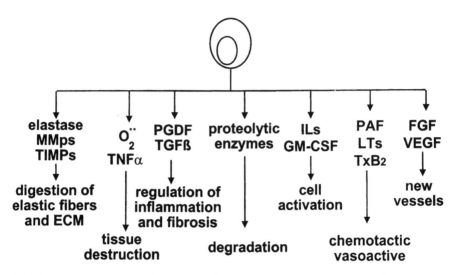

Figure 3 Alveolar macrophages can release several mediators capable of playing an important role in tissue remodeling in asthma. Release of these mediators is also regulated by the activation of macrophages through an IgE-dependent mechanism.

F. Smooth Muscle Cells and IgE-Mediated Inflammation

Smooth muscle cells have recently been involved as inflammatory cells in asthma (117,172–176). In addition to contractile responses and mitogenesis (177), airway smooth muscle cell have synthetic and secretory potential with the release of RANTES (178), other chemokines, cytokines, and MMPs. They may participate in chronic airway inflammation by interacting with both Th1- and Th2-derived cytokines to modulate chemoattractant activity for eosinophils, activated T lymphocytes, and monocytes/macrophages. Smooth muscle cells also have the potential to alter the composition of the ECM environment and orchestrate key events in the process of chronic airway remodeling (179).

Cell culture studies have disclosed a wide range of soluble factors that can promote proliferation of human airway smooth muscle cells, suggesting that, through autocrine loops, these cells can regulate their own proliferative rate. The proactivating signals for converting airway smooth muscle cells into a proliferative and secretory cell in asthma are unknown but may include viruses and IgE.

It has also been shown that EGF activates ErbB-2 and stimulates phosphatidylinositol 3-kinase in human airway cells, a mechanism that induces transcription from the cyclin D1 promoter (180,181), thereby influencing an important checkpoint of cell proliferation (for a review, see 182). An additional autocrine mechanism regulating smooth muscle proliferation is the production of MMP-2 (183). Production of MMP-2 suggests that airway smooth muscle may contribute to ECM turnover and airway remodeling. Furthermore, in vivo

MMP-2 may be produced by other airway cells including fibroblasts and macrophages, indicating that other airway cells may interact to support airway smooth muscle proliferation asthma.

It is also conceivable that abnormal smooth muscle cell proliferation may be accompanied by a failure of the antiproliferative mechanisms that may counterbalance these remodeling processes and limit the quantity of smooth muscle in the airways. Apoptosis is an important homeostatic mechanism providing a pathway by which tissues can eliminate unhealthy, harmful, or excess cells. Interestingly, it has recently been shown that Fas cross-linking induces apoptosis in cultured human smooth muscle cells, suggesting that smooth muscle cells are susceptible to undergo apoptosis (184). Whether or not this and/ or other mechanisms of cell death are functioning in asthma is still unknown.

Fc receptors may also be expressed and activated in non–bone marrow–derived cell types, including airway smooth muscle. This concept raises the hypothesis that the phenotype of airway smooth muscle cells of atopic asthmatics is associated with an altered endogenous expression and action of specific Fcε receptors present in the airway smooth muscle cells itself. This hypothesis is supported by the evidence that human airway smooth muscle tissue expresses messenger RNA and surface protein for FcεRII, as well as for all the Fcγ receptor subtypes, and that FcεRII is significantly up-regulated in inherently asthmatic airway smooth muscle cells tissue (185). Up-regulated expression of FcεRII represents, at least in part, an inducible phenomenon that is largely attributed to IgE immune complex–coupled activation of the receptor. Interestingly, the latter action has been shown to be associated with FcεRII-induced autologous production of the proinflammatory cytokine IL-1β by the atopic sensitized airway smooth muscle cells. In addition, serum from asthmatic individuals causes a significant increase in the production of fibronectin, perlecan, laminin, and chondroitin sulfate, suggesting that airway smooth muscle cells activation via an IgE-dependent mechanism may contribute to remodeling in asthma by altering ECM deposition in the airways (186).

It is also known that passive sensitization of human airways induces an increase not only in histamine but also in leukotriene responsiveness. It is likely that allergen responses in sensitized airways are affected through a combination of increased mediator release from inflammatory cells and increased responsiveness of airway smooth muscle (187,188). This raises the question of whether alterations in smooth muscle behavior may be somehow affected by allergen exposure. Indeed, it has been shown that sensitized airway smooth muscle displays increased shortening velocity, without any concomitant change in isometric force generating capability (189).

Recent evidence have shown the presence of smooth muscle mitogens in the BAL fluids from asthmatic subjects who underwent allergen challenge (180). Molecular sieving of BAL fluids demonstrates that mitogenic activity is present exclusively in the <10-kD fraction, which is compatible with a series of potential candidate factors, such as EGF, TGF-β, and PDGF (180). In vivo animal studies show that prolonged allergen exposure can increase smooth muscle thickness (63).

G. Role of T Cells in the Pathogenesis of Airway Remodeling

T lymphocytes are among the principal factors that regulate and coordinate immune responses in allergic diseases. Although a strict dichotomy is not as clear as in the murine system (190–192), two helper T-cell subsets have been identified in humans (193,194):

Th1 cells, which release predominantly IFN-γ and IL-2 and are involved
    in the delayed hypersensitivity immune reactions
Th2 cells, which release predominantly IL-4 and IL-5 and are mainly
    involved in IgE-mediated allergic inflammation

An imbalance of Th1 and Th2 cells has been proposed in various diseases. In atopy, Th2 cells are thought to predominate regulating IgE synthesis and cell recruitment at the sites of inflammation. T-cell differentiation, activation, and cytokine production are determined by several factors (195), including cytokines (196), inflammatory mediators (197), and hormones (194).

T lymphocytes are frequently found in the airway mucosa of normal individuals. They are present in increased numbers in the airways of patients with fatal asthma (198) or in asthmatics of variable asthma etiology, including occupational asthma (90,157,199–202). The majority bear CD4 receptors in asthma, whereas CD8-positive cells are more rarely identified, even during exacerbations of asthma (203). After allergen challenge there is an increase, in bronchial biopsies of asthmatics, in activated T cells and Th2 cytokines (204,205).

T cells may play a role in pulmonary fibrosis by their cytotoxic effect against lung parenchymal cell (144). Recently, an increase in the CD4/CD8 ratio has been demonstrated to be associated with asthma symptoms and airway fibrosis (206). Although it is still unknown whether T lymphocytes can directly cause tissue damage and remodeling in asthma, these cells contribute to the pathogenesis of structural changes of the airways by orchestrating the recruitment and activation of inflammatory cells (207).

Activated T lymphocytes are proinflammatory cells in their own right because they release Th2 cytokines of the IL-4 gene cluster, GM-CSF, IL-3, IL-4, IL-5, IL-9, and IL-13 (208–211), which have pronounced effects on the growth, differentiation, activation, and survival of many inflammatory cells of the airways (212). In addition to lymphocytes, cytokines of the IL-4 gene cluster are also produced by basophils, mast cells, and eosinophils (92), giving rise to a redundant and self-maintaining inflammatory response.

Th2 cytokine overexpression can have an indirect impact on airway remodeling by promoting the recruitment of inflammatory cells which, in turn, are capable of releasing mediators involved in tissue repair processes. Indeed, infiltration of the airways by increased numbers of eosinophils, neutrophils, and macrophages, and their potential to release growth factors, proteolytic enzymes, and oxygen free radicals, represent further important steps in the airway remodeling process in asthma.

In transgenic mouse models, overexpression of the Th2 cytokine IL-13 leads to profound changes of the airways, with increased eosinophilic and mononuclear inflammation, mucus cell metaplasia, subepithelial fibrosis, airway obstruction, and AHR (213). IL-4, IL-5, and IL-9 can also induce extensive mucus cell metaplasia, and IL-9 and IL-5 can cause subepithelial fibrosis and AHR (214,215).

A Th2 cytokine pattern has been found to predominate in the pulmonary interstitium of patients with cryptogenic fibrosing alveolitis (216). On the other hand, it has been demonstrated that IL-4 increases both fibroblast growth, collagen production, and adhesion molecule expression (217,218). IL-4 and IL-13 have also been found to induce the production of eotaxin by dermal fibroblasts (219–221).

These studies suggest that an abnormal Th2-derived cytokine production can have direct effect on the development of airway inflammation and remodeling.

H. Fibroblasts

Structural cells like fibroblasts play important roles in allergic inflammation through the production of an array of cytokines and chemokines such as GM-CSF (222), IL-8, RANTES (223,224), or eotaxin (225,226). They appear therefore to be essential for the recruitment of effector cells and for the growth and survival of mast cells and eosinophils (225–227). Interaction with fibroblasts results in the modulation of the proteoglycan content in mast cells.

Fibroblasts play a key role in the remodeling process. They produce collagen, reticular and elastic fibers, as well as proteoglycans and glycoproteins of the amorphous ECM (228). Their biological activity is regulated by a range of cytokines and growth factors (229). Although regarded as fixed cells of ECM, they retain the capacity for growth and regeneration and may evolve into various cell types including smooth muscle cells becoming myofibroblasts (230). Myofibroblast can potentially contribute to tissue remodeling by releasing ECM components such as elastin, fibronectin, and laminin (231). Increased numbers of myofibroblasts are found in the airways of asthmatics, and their number has been correlated with the size of the basement reticular membrane (11). It appears that the ability of myofibroblasts to promote tissue remodeling in asthma is profoundly influenced by the degree of activation and damage of bronchial epithelial cells releasing bFGF, PDGF, insulin-like growth factor-1 (IGF-1), TGF-β2, and endothelin-1 (232,233). It seems that to be effective the release of these growth factors has to occur simultaneously. Indeed, the combination of growth factors, such as endothelin-1, TGF-β, and PDGF-BB, significantly increased DNA synthesis and collagen production of bronchial fibroblasts isolated from both normal and asthmatic subjects (234).

Following bronchial allergen challenge myofibroblast numbers are increased and the cells present a differentiation process (235). Following bronchial allergen challenge an increased number of fibroblasts has been found in bronchial biospies taken from allergic asthmatic subjects. This raises the concept that mesenchymal cells are able to respond to allergen stimulation and this may lead to their increased proliferation. In addition, it seems that allergen stimulation can promote fibroblast differentiation into myofibroblast and then into smooth muscle cells (235). Indeed, in allergen-challenged airways myofibroblasts appear to share many untrastructural feature with smooth muscle cells, such as the nucleus outline and the amount of rough endoplasmic reticulum. If this hypothesis is proven correct, allergen stimulation of mesenchymal cells may be considered as a potential pathway leading to the increased smooth muscle mass in asthma. Finally, it also seems that airway allergen challenge can also lead to increased functional activation of airway fibroblasts as shown by the raise of fibronectin levels in BAL fluids of asthmatics after bronchial allergen challenge (236).

Although these studies indicate that fibroblasts respond to allergens, the mechanism by which this response is elicited is still not fully understood. For example, to date no evidence has been provided about the ability of fibroblasts to express Fc receptors for IgE.

I. Cysteinyl Leukotrienes and Tissue Remodeling

Cysteinyl leukotrienes may also alter airway remodeling since they modulate proliferation of epithelial cells and LTC_4 was shown to up-regulate collagenase expression in human lung fibroblasts (237).

Leukotrienes induce cell survival signaling in intestinal epithelial cells. LTD_4 and LTB_4, but not LTC_4, caused a time- and dose-dependent increase in expression and/or membrane accumulation of COX-2, β-catenin, and Bcl-2, as well as PGE_2 production (238). Leukotriene receptor antagonists and synthesis inhibitors reverse survival in eosinophils of asthmatics (239).

LTD_4 facilitates airway smooth muscle cell proliferation via modulation of the IGF axis (240). It induces MMP-1, which functions as an TGF-binding protein (IGFBP) protease in human airway smooth muscle cells (241). The effects of LTD_4 on human airway smooth muscle cell proliferation, matrix expression, and contraction in vitro appear to be of importance (242). LTD_4 alone had no effect on DNA synthesis in human airway smooth muscle cells. However, LTD_4 markedly augmented proliferation induced by the mitogen EGF. In the same study, LTD_4 did not increase the total messenger RNA expression of the ECM proteins (pro-alpha type I or alpha type IV collagen), elastin, biglycan, decorin, and fibronectin, and did not influence

TFG-β-induced effects on the expression of these proteins in human airway smooth muscle cells.

In animal models, the involvement of cysteinyl leukotrienes has been observed in airway smooth muscle cell DNA synthesis after repeated allergen exposure in sensitized brown Norway rats (63).

V. Airway Allergen Challenge Induces Airway Remodeling

It is likely repetitive injury to airway wall and the ensuing tissue repair process may establish, through autocrine and paracrine immune-regulatory mechanisms, highly dynamic interactions between airway cells possibly affecting the extent of airway remodeling in asthma. There are a great variety of proinflammatory inducers to which the airways are continuously exposed. These interact with allergens to induce inflammation and possibly remodeling. For example, repeated inhalation of large amounts of cold air, as occurs in ski athletes during strenuous training, has recently been shown to induce airway inflammation and remodeling (243).

A. Animal Models of Airway Remodeling

Although there is no clear animal model of airway remodeling, repeated exposures to allergens have been used since they likely lead to the maintenance of a persistent inflammatory process leading to structural airway changes. This possibility was tested using sensitized brown Norway rats. Following repeated allergen exposure for periods of 2, 4, or 12 weeks to aerosolized ovalbumin, serum IgE and the number of peribronchial eosinophils significantly increased due to the development of an inflammatory response. Of note, after 2 weeks of ovalbumin exposure, structural airway changes occurred, such as goblet cell hyperplasia, an increase in airway epithelium proliferation, increased fibronectin deposition, and thickening of the airway inner wall area (244). These changes were accompanied by AHR to aerosolized carbachol. Interestingly, all these histological alterations were not influenced by an additional 10-week period of exposure to allergen, which only caused a further increase in fibronectin and collagen deposition in the submucosa (244). In another study, repeated allergen exposure of sensitized brown Norway rats induced airway cell DNA synthesis and remodeling (63). There was increased subepithelial collagen deposition and mucus secretion along with significant eosinophil and lymphocyte recruitment to the airways. Increased rates of DNA synthesis in both airway smooth muscle and epithelial cells along with changes to the airway wall pathology may precede the establishment of smooth muscle thickening and airway remodeling after repeated allergen exposure in rats. Increase in endothelin-1 was also found in association with remodeling (63). In another set of studies, it was found that repeated allergen inhalations induce DNA synthesis in airway smooth muscle and epithelial cells in vivo (177).

In a brown Norway rat model of chronic exposure to the occupational allergen trimellitic anhydride, BHR, epithelial damage, and airway eosinophilia were observed (245). Thickness of the airway wall, airway luminal narrowing, and the number of goblet cells and eosinophils in the airway wall had increased at the end of the 9-week allergen exposure (246).

These findings suggest that structural alterations of the inner airway wall occur at a very early stage of the remodeling process and represent a sort of "first response" of the airways to external stimuli. In addition, it is likely that as soon as the exposure to inflammatory agents becomes chronic it may lead to the involvement of the submucosal structures and subsequent increase in the amount of collagen in the impaired tissue, leading to remodeling of the structure of the conducting airways. These data support the concept that remodeling of the airways is a multistep process, in which changes in the inner airway wall, and particularly in the bronchial epithelium, may play a fundamental role.

Experiments in dogs confirm that increasing airway wall thickness by infusing saline potentiates airway reactivity to inhaled histamine (247). A rat model was developed to exhibit characteristics of airway remodeling by exposing animals repeatedly over a prolonged time to aerosolized ovalbumin. This results in an increased thickness of the airway wall in both large and small airways associated with an increase in BHR. In vivo animal studies also confirm that prolonged allergen exposure can increase smooth muscle thickness (63). However, with a more prolonged exposure, scarring occurs with increased fibronectin and collagen deposition mainly in the outer airway wall and reduction in the thickness of the airway wall. At the same time, BHR wanes and even turns into a slight hyporesponsiveness (248).

These findings support the mathematically derived concepts relating BHR to wall thickness. At the same time, however, these observations also illustrate that depending on its location and extensiveness the airway wall, remodeling may not be associated with BHR and may even protect against excessive airway narrowing

Taken together these studies strongly suggest that a chronic exposure to allergens plays an important role in the development of airway remodeling. In addition, it seems that if allergen exposure becomes continuous and prolonged it can determine the development of structural changes of the entire airway wall, and not of single airway structures.

A still unanswered question is whether or not corticosteroids can affect the development of airway remodeling or at least reverse some structural alteration due to this process. This question has been addressed by evaluating the effects on airway remodeling of fluticasone propionate administered concomitantly or after repeated allergen exposure in brown Norway rats. Concomitant treatment with fluticasone propionate was found to decrease all allergen-induced structural changes (the increase in total airway wall area, the enhanced fibronectin deposition, the epithelial cell proliferation, goblet cell hyperplasia, and AHR) without being able to reverse them to normal. Interestingly, initiating the treatment after the allergen exposure had not effect on any of the structural airway changes. Although it is mandatory to reproduce these results in asthmatic subjects, it may be proposed that if a treatment with inhaled corticosteroids is introduced concomitantly to allergen exposure, then a partial inhibition of structural airway changes as well as of BHR can be observed. By contrast, post hoc treatment seems to fail to reverse established airway remodeling (249).

Although transgenic modeling or, more widely, animal models with conventional overexpression and knockout approaches have provided a highly useful approach to the better understanding of the mechanisms of airway remodeling (250–252), it is important to understand their limitations. Targeted gene disruption cannot be employed to study the importance of a protein in an adult phenotype if the same protein plays a critical role in development. The redundancy of biological processes can also allow compensatory mechanisms to appear in knockout animals that may not be relevant to the wild-type phenotype. In addition, in overexpression modeling, transgene can be initiated in utero and proceed chronically thereafter. This makes the differentiation of developmental and adult phenotypic features difficult and makes the modeling of waxing and waning diseases such as asthma problematic. Maximal insight into pathogenesis will be obtained when appropriate chronic models of remodeling and externally modulatable transgenic approaches are combined and state-of-the-art immunological, pathological, and physiological assessment techniques are utilized to address crucial issues in airway biology.

B. Effect of Allergen Exposure and Removal on Airway Remodeling in Humans

A better understanding of the potential effects of antigen exposure and removal is of great importance to provide more effective preventive and therapeutic strategies of airway remodeling in asthma. As mentioned earlier, allergen challenge has been shown to activate functionally fibroblasts in the airways of asthmatic subjects and to increase the release of fibronectin (236). It is also known that allergen exposure can promote phenotypic differentiation of fibroblasts into myofibroblasts (235). These data indicate that allergen challenge causes the activation of mesenchymal cells and the release of ECM proteins, and suggest that exposure of the airways to allergens can contribute to the development of structural changes of the airways.

Structural alterations occurring following exposure to toluene diiodocyanate (TDI) represent another good example of the potential role played by antigen exposure on airway remodeling. Pathology of airways in patients exposed to TDI resembles that of asthmatic subjects, including increased thickening of the basement membrane (202), suggesting that persistent TDI exposure may contribute to remodeling of the airways. The role played by TDI exposure on airway remodeling is also demonstrated by evidence that after cessation of TDI exposure there is a significant decrease in the number of fibroblasts as well as a reduction of the thickness of the basement membrane (253).

VI. Longstanding Asthma and Chronic Inflammation Are Likely to Increase Airway Remodeling

The airways of elderly subjects who have had persistent asthma for decades are likely candidates for airway remodeling (254). Because the duration of asthma in the elderly can range from several months to many decades, this has been considered an ideal population in which to study the consequence of long-standing asthma (255). By comparing airflow and lung volumes in a cohort of elderly asthmatic subjects, it has been shown that those with asthma of long duration had a significant lower FEV_1 than those with asthma of short duration. Interestingly, the duration of asthma was found to be inversely associated with FEV_1 and lung hyperinflation, suggesting that long-standing asthma is characterized by a greater degree of lung function decline (255). In addition, most subjects with asthma of long duration failed to achieve normal airflow after bronchodilator administration, indicating that severe decrements in pulmonary function associated with long-term asthma may become irreversible (255) and suggesting that long-standing asthma is associated with an increased duration of airway remodeling. Histopathological evidence supports this hypothesis by showing that there is an increase in airway wall area, including smooth muscle, and airway narrowing with increasing duration of severe asthma or with old age (256).

VII. Conclusions

Antigen exposure leads to the activation of many airway cells and to the subsequent release of a wide range of mediators capable of modulating airway inflammation and remodeling. It is therefore likely that repeated exposure to inhaled antigens, including allergens, may lead to the development of structural alteration of the airways and to their remodeling.

Whether or not chronic exposure to antigens may lead to an increased extent of airway remodeling in asthma is difficult to ascertain; however, if the insights provided by animal models are correct, it may be hypothesized that enhanced structural changes observed in the airways of subjects with long-standing asthma may result from the continuous and persistent activation of inflammatory and immunological processes by inhaled antigens.

References

1. Cotran R, Kumar V, Robin S. Inflammation and repair. Robbins Pathologic Basis of Disease 1989; 39–87.
2. Reid L. Sputum rheology in evaluation of anti-asthmatic drugs. Scand J Respir Dis Suppl 1979; 103:90–95.
3. Bousquet J, Chanez P, Lacoste JY, White R, Vic P, Godard P, Michel FB. Asthma: a disease remodeling the airways. Allergy 1992; 47:3–11.
4. Vignola AM, Kips J, Bousquet J. Tissue remodeling as a feature of persistent asthma. J Allergy Clin Immunol 2000; 105:1041–2053.
5. Bousquet J, Jeffery PK, Busse WW, Johnson M, Vignola AM. Asthma. From bronchoconstriction to airways inflammation and remodeling. J Allergy Clin Immunol 2000; 105:1720–1745.
6. Streuli C. Extracellular matrix remodelling and cellular differentiation. Curr Opin Cell Biol 1999; 11:634–640.
7. Murphy G, Gavrilovic J. Proteolysis and cell migration: creating a path? Curr Opin Cell Biol 1999; 11:614–621.
8. McGowan SE. Extracellular matrix and the regulation of lung development and repair. Faseb J 1992; 6:2895–2904.
9. Roche WR, Beasley R, Williams JH, Holgate ST. Subepithelial fibrosis in the bronchi of asthmatics. Lancet 1989; 1:520–524.
10. Altraja A, Laitinen A, Virtanen I, Kampe M, Simonsson BG, Karlsson SE, Hakansson L, Venge P, Sillastu H, Laitinen LA. Expression of laminins in the airways in various types of asthmatic patients: a morphometric study. Am J Respir Cell Mol Biol 1996; 15:482–488.
11. Brewster CE, Howarth PH, Djukanovic R, Wilson J, Holgate ST, Roche WR. Myofibroblasts and subepithelial fibrosis in bronchial asthma. Am J Respir Cell Mol Biol 1990; 3:507–511.
12. Jeffery PK, Wardlaw AJ, Nelson FC, Collins JV, Kay AB. Bronchial biopsies in asthma. An ultrastructural, quantitative study and correlation with hyper-reactivity. Am Rev Respir Dis 1989; 140:1745–1753.
13. Saetta M, Maestrelli P, Di-Stefano A, De-Marzo N, Milani GF, Pivirotto F, Mapp CE, Fabbri LM. Effect of cessation of exposure to toluene diisocyanate (TDI) on bronchial mucosa of subjects with TDI-induced asthma. Am Rev Respir Dis 1992; 145:169–174.
14. Chu HW, Halliday JL, Martin RJ, Leung DY, Szefler SJ, Wenzel SE. Collagen deposition in large airways may not differentiate severe asthma from milder forms of the disease. Am J Respir Crit Care Med 1998; 158:1936–1944.
15. Boulet LP, Turcotte H, Laviolette M, Naud F, Bernier MC, Martel S, Chakir J. Airway hyperresponsiveness, inflammation, and subepithelial collagen deposition in recently diagnosed versus long-standing mild asthma. Influence of inhaled corticosteroids [In Process Citation]. Am J Respir Crit Care Med 2000; 162: 1308–1313.
16. Chetta A, Foresi A, Del-Donno M, Bertorelli G, Pesci A, Olivieri D. Airways remodeling is a distinctive feature of asthma and is related to severity of disease. Chest 1997; 111:852–857.

17. Chakir J, Laviolette M, Boutet M, Laliberte R, Dube J, Boulet LP. Lower airways remodeling in nonasthmatic subjects with allergic rhinitis. Lab Invest 1996; 75:735–744.

18. Bousquet J, Lacoste J, Chanez P, Vic P, Godard P, Michel F. Bronchial elastic fibers in normal subjects and asthmatic patients. Am J Respir Crit Care Med 1996; 153:1648–1653.

19. Mauad T, Xavier AC, Saldiva PH, Dolhnikoff M. Elastosis and fragmentation of fibers of the elastic system in fatal asthma. Am J Respir Crit Care Med 1999; 160: 968–975.

20. Carroll NG, Perry S, Karkhanis A, Harji S, Butt J, James AL, Green FH. The airway longitudinal elastic fiber network and mucosal folding in patients with asthma. Am J Respir Crit Care Med 2000; 161:244–248.

21. Bousquet J, Chanez P, Lacoste JY, Enander I, Venge P, Peterson C, Ahlstedt S, Michel FB, Godard P. Indirect evidence of bronchial inflammation assessed by titration of inflammatory mediators in BAL fluid of patients with asthma. J Allergy Clin Immunol 1991; 88:649–660.

22. Roberts CR, Wight TN, Hascall VC, eds. Proteoglycans, 2nd ed. Philadelphia.: Lippincott–Raven Publishers, 1997: 757–767. (R. G. Crystal JBW, E. R. Weibel, and P. J. Barnes, eds., The Lung: Scientific Foundations)

23. Hardingham TE, Fosang AJ. Proteoglycans: many forms and many functions. FASEB J 1992; 6:861–870.

24. Huang J, Olivenstein R, Taha R, Hamid Q, Ludwig M. Enhanced proteoglycan deposition in the airway wall of atopic asthmatics. Am J Respir Crit Care Med 1999; 160:725–729.

25. Minshall EM, Leung DY, Martin RJ, Song YL, Cameron L, Ernst P, Hamid Q. Eosinophil-associated TGF-beta1 mRNA expression and airways fibrosis in bronchial asthma. Am J Respir Cell Mol Biol 1997; 17:326–333.

26. Ohno I, Nitta Y, Yamauchi K, Hoshi H, Honma M, Woolley K, O'Byrne P, Dolovich J, Jordana M, Tamura G, et al. Eosinophils as a potential source of platelet-derived growth factor B-chain (PDGF-B) in nasal polyposis and bronchial asthma. Am J Respir Cell Mol Biol 1995; 13:639–647.

27. Laitinen A, Altraja A, Kampe M, Linden M, Virtanen I, Laitinen LA. Tenascin is increased in airway basement membrane of asthmatics and decreased by an inhaled steroid. Am J Respir Crit Care Med 1997; 156:951–958.

28. Vignola A, Chanez P, Chiappara G, Merendino A, Zinnanti E, Bousquet J, Bonsignore G. Release of transforming growth factor-β and fibronectin by alveolar macrophages in airway diseases. Clin Exp Immunol 1996; 106:114–119.

29. Redington AE. Fibrosis and airway remodelling. Clin Exp Allergy 2000; 1:42–45.

30. Vignola AM, Chanez P, Chiappara G, Merendino AM, Pace E, Rizzo A, La Rocca AM, Bellia V, Bonsignore G, Bousquet J. Transforming growth factor-β expression in mucosal biopsies in asthma and chronic bronchitis. Am J Respir Crit Care Med 1997; 156:591–599.

31. Wenzel SE, Schwartz LB, Langmack EL, Halliday JL, Trudeau JB, Gibbs RL, Chu HW. Evidence that severe asthma can be divided pathologically into two inflammatory subtypes with distinct physiologic and clinical characteristics. Am J Respir Crit Care Med 1999; 160:1001–1008.

32. Ohno K, Ammann P, Fasciati R, Maier P. Transforming growth factor beta 1 preferentially induces apoptotic cell death in rat hepatocytes cultured under pericentral-equivalent conditions. Toxicol Appl Pharmacol 1995; 132:227–236.

33. Redington AE, Madden J, Frew AJ, Djukanovic R, Roche WR, Holgate ST, Howarth PH. Transforming growth factor-beta 1 in asthma. Measurement in bronchoalveolar lavage fluid. Am J Respir Crit Care Med 1997; 156:642–647.

34. Hoshino M, Takahashi M, Takai Y, Sim J. Inhaled corticosteroids decrease subepithelial collagen deposition by modulation of the balance between matrix metalloproteinase-9 and tissue inhibitor of metalloproteinase-1 expression in asthma. J Allergy Clin Immunol 1999; 104:356–363.

35. Amishima M, Munakata M, Nasuhara Y, Sato A, Takahashi T, Homma Y, Kawakami Y. Expression of epidermal growth factor and epidermal growth factor receptor immunoreactivity in the asthmatic human airway. Am J Respir Crit Care Med 1998; 157:1907–1912.

36. Redington AE, Roche WR, Madden J, Frew AJ, Djukanovic R, Holgate ST, Howarth PH. Basic fibroblast growth factor in asthma: measurement in bronchoalveolar lavage fluid basally and following allergen challenge. J Allergy Clin Immunol 2001; 107:384–387.

37. Rajah R, Nachajon RV, Collins MH, Hakonarson H, Grunstein MM, Cohen P. Elevated levels of the IGF-binding protein protease MMP-1 in asthmatic airway smooth muscle. Am J Respir Cell Mol Biol 1999; 20:199–208.

38. Stetler-Stevenson WG. Matrix metalloproteinases in angiogenesis: a moving target for therapeutic intervention. J Clin Invest 1999; 103:1237–1241.

39. Shipley JM, Wesselschmidt RL, Kobayashi DK, Ley TJ, Shapiro SD. Metalloelastase is required for macrophage-mediated proteolysis and matrix invasion in mice. Proc Natl Acad Sci USA 1996; 93:3942–3946.

40. Legrand C, Gilles C, Zahm JM, Polette M, Buisson AC, Kaplan H, Birembaut P, Tournier JM. Airway epithelial cell migration dynamics. MMP-9 role in cell–extracellular matrix remodeling. J Cell Biol 1999; 146:517–529.

41. Mautino G, Henriquet C, Oliver N, Bousquet J, Capony F. Elevated levels of tissue inhibitor of metalloproteinase-1 in bronchoalveolar lavage of asthmatic patients. Lab Invest 1999; 1:39–47.

42. Hoshino M, Nakamura Y, Sim J, Shimojo J, Isogai S. Bronchial subepithelial fibrosis and expression of matrix metalloproteinase-9 in asthmatic airway inflammation. J Allergy Clin Immunol 1998; 102:783–788.

43. Vignola AM, Riccobono L, Mirabella A, Profita M, Chanez P, Bellia V, Mautino G, D'accardi P, Bousquet J, Bonsignore G. Sputum metalloproteinase-90/tissue inhibitor of metalloproteinase-1 ratio correlates with airflow obstruction in asthma and chronic bronchitis. Am J Respir Crit Care Med 1998; 158:1945–1950.

44. Cataldo D, Munaut C, Noel A, Frankenne F, Bartsch P, Foidart JM, Louis R. MMP-2- and MMP-9-linked gelatinolytic activity in the sputum from patients with asthma and chronic obstructive pulmonary disease [In Process Citation]. Int Arch Allergy Immunol 2000; 123:259–267.

45. Lemjabbar H, Gosset P, Lechapt-Zalcman E, Franco-Montoya ML, Wallaert B, Harf A, Lafuma C. Overexpression of alveolar macrophage gelatinase B (MMP-9) in patients with idiopathic pulmonary fibrosis: effects of steroid and immunosuppressive treatment. Am J Respir Cell Mol Biol 1999; 20:903–913.

46. Shapiro SD, Senior RM. Matrix metalloproteinases. Matrix degradation and more [In Process Citation]. Am J Respir Cell Mol Biol 1999; 20:1100–1102.
47. Mautino G, Capony F, Bousquet J, Vignola AM. Balance in asthma between matrix metalloproteinases and their inhibitors [editorial]. J Allergy Clin Immunol 1999; 104:530–533.
48. Dunnill M. The pathology of asthma with special references of changes in the bronchial mucosa. J Clin Pathol 1960; 13:27–33.
49. Kuwano K, Bosken CH, Pare PD, Bai TR, Wiggs BR, Hogg JC. Small airways dimensions in asthma and in chronic obstructive pulmonary disease. Am Rev Respir Dis 1993; 148:1220–1225.
50. Li X, Wilson JW. Increased vascularity of the bronchial mucosa in mild asthma. Am J Respir Crit Care Med 1997; 156:229–233.
51. Vrugt B, Wilson S, Bron A, Holgate ST, Djukanovic R, Aalbers R. Bronchial angiogenesis in severe glucocorticoid-dependent asthma. Eur Respir J 2001; 15:1014–1021.
52. Hoshino M, Takahashi M, Aoike N. Expression of vascular endothelial growth factor, basic fibroblast growth factor, and angiogenin immunoreactivity in asthmatic airways and its relationship to angiogenesis. J Allergy Clin Immunol 2001; 107:295–301.
53. Wilson JW, Stewart AG. Airway vascularity in asthma [In Process Citation]. Clin Exp Allergy 1999; 29:1295–1297.
54. O'Reilly MS, Holmgren L, Shing Y, Chen C, Rosenthal RA, Moses M, Lane WS, Cao Y, Sage EH, Folkman J. Angiostatin: a novel angiogenesis inhibitor that mediates the suppression of metastases by a Lewis lung carcinoma [see comments]. Cell 1994; 79:315–328.
55. Demoly P, Maly FE, Mautino G, Grad S, Gougat C, Sahla H, Godard P, Bousquet J. VEGF levels in asthmatic airways do not correlate with plasma extravasation. Clin Exp Allergy 1999; 29:1390–1394.
56. Dunnill M, Massarella G, Anderson J. Comparison of the quantitative anatomy of the bronchi in normal subjects, in status asthmaticus, in chronic bronchitis, and in emphysema. Thorax 1969; 24:176–179.
57. Hossain S, BE H. Hyperplasia of bronchial muscle in chronic bronchitis. J Pathol 1970; 101:171–184.
58. Carroll N, Elloit J, Morton A, James A. The structure of large and small airways in nonfatal and fatal asthma. Am Rev Respir Dis 1993; 147:405–410.
59. Bai TR. Abnormalities in airway smooth muscle in fatal asthma. Am Rev Respir Dis 1990; 141:552–557.
60. Sobonya RE. Quantitative structural alternations in long-standing allergic asthma. Am Rev Respir Dis 1984; 130:289–292.
61. Ebina M, Yaegashi H, Takahashi T, Motomiya M, Tanemura M. Distribution of smooth muscles along the bronchial tree. A morphometric study of ordinary autopsy lungs. Am Rev Respir Dis 1990; 141:1322–1326.
62. Ebina M, Takahashi T, Chiba T, Motomiya M. Cellular hypertrophy and hyperplasia of airway smooth muscles underlying bronchial asthma. A 3-D morphometric study. Am Rev Respir Dis 1993; 148:720–726.
63. Salmon M, Walsh DA, Koto H, Barnes PJ, Chung KF. Repeated allergen exposure of sensitized Brown-Norway rats induces airway cell DNA synthesis and remodelling. Eur Respir J 1999; 14:633–641.

64. Peat JK, Woolcock AJ, Cullen K. Rate of decline of lung function in subjects with asthma. Eur J Respir Dis 1987; 70:171–179.
65. Kelly WJ, Hudson I, Raven J, Phelan PD, Pain MC, Olinsky A. Childhood asthma and adult lung function. Am Rev Respir Dis 1988; 138:26–30.
66. Gerritsen J, Koeter GH, Postma DS, Schouten JP, Knol K. Prognosis of asthma from childhood to adulthood. Am Rev Respir Dis 1989; 140:1325–1330.
67. Cade J, Pain M. Pulmonary function durign clinical remission of asthma. How reversible is asthma? Aust NZ J Med 1973; 3:545–551.
68. Long-term efects of budesonide or nedocromil in children with asthma. The Childhood Asthma Management Program Research Group [see comments]. N Engl J Med 2000; 343:1054–1063.
69. Lange P, Parner J, Vestbo J, Schnohr P, Jensen G. A 15-year follow-up study of ventilatory function in adults with asthma. N Engl J Med 1998; 339:1194–1200.
70. Sterk PJ. The place of airway hyperresponsiveness in the asthma phenotype. Clin Exp Allergy 1995; 2:8–11.
71. Woolcock AJ, Reddel H, Trevillion L. Assessment of airway responsiveness as a guide to diagnosis, prognosis, and therapy in asthma. Allergy Proc 1995; 16: 23–26.
72. Kips JC, Pauwels RA. Airway wall remodelling: does it occur and what does it mean? Clin Exp Allergy 1999; 29:1457–1466.
73. Warner JO, Pohunek P, Marguet C, Clough JB, Roche WR. Progression from allergic sensitization to asthma [In Process Citation]. Pediatr Allergy Immunol 2000; 13:12–14.
74. Reid MJ, Moss RB, Hsu, YP, Kwasnicki JM, Commerford TM, Nelson BL. Seasonal asthma in northern California: allergic causes and efficacy of immuno-therapy. J Allergy Clin Immunol 1986; 78:590–600
75. Pollart SM, Chapman MD, Fiocco GP, Rose G, Platts-Mills TA. Epidemiology of acute asthma: IgE antibodies to common inhalant allergens as a risk factor for emergency room visits. J Allergy Clin Immunol 1989; 83:875–882.
76. Suphioglu C, Singh MB, Taylor P, Bellomo R, Holmes P, Puy R, Knox RB. Mechanism of grass-pollen-induced asthma. Lancet 1992; 339:569–572.
77. Johnston SL, Pattemore PK, Sanderson G, Smith S, Lampe F, Josephs L, Symington P, O'Toole S, Myint SH, Tyrrell DA, et al. Community study of role of viral infections in exacerbations of asthma in 9–11 year old children. BMJ 1995; 310:1225–1229.
78. Evans D, Levison MJ, Feldman CH, Clark NM, Wasilewski Y, Levin B, Mellins RB. The impact of passive smoking on emergency room visits of urban children with asthma. Am Rev Respir Dis 1987; 135:567–572.
79. Ostro BD, Lipsett MJ, Mann JK, Wiener MB, Selner J. Indoor air pollution and asthma. Results from a panel study [see comments]. Am J Respir Crit Care Med 1994; 149:1400–1406.
80. Samet J, Malbury M, Spengler J. Health effects and source of indoor air pollu-tion. Part I. Am Rev Respir Dis 1987; 136:1486–1508.
81. Wardlaw AJ. The role of air pollution in asthma. Clin Exp Allergy 1993; 23: 81–96.
82. Thurston GD, Ito K, Kinney PL, Lippmann M. A multi-year study of air pol-lution and respiratory hospital admissions in three New York State metropolitan

areas: results for 1988 and 1989 summers. J Expo Anal Environ Epidemiol 1992; 2: 429–450.

83. Walters S, Phupinyokul M, Ayres J. Hospital admission rates for asthma and respiratory disease in the West Midlands: their relationship to air pollution levels. Thorax 1995; 50:948–954.

84. Schwartz J, Slater D, Larson TV, Pierson WE, Koenig JQ. Particulate air pollution and hospital emergency room visits for asthma in Seattle. Am Rev Respir Dis 1993; 147:826–831.

85. Romieu I, Meneses F, Sienra-Monge JJ, Huerta J, Ruiz-Velasco S, White MC, Etzel RA, Hernandez-Avila M. Effects of urban air pollutants on emergency visits for childhood asthma in Mexico City. Am J Epidemiol 1995; 141:546–553.

86. Castellsague J, Sunyer J, Saez M, Anto JM. Short-term association between air pollution and emergency room visits for asthma in Barcelona. Thorax 1995; 50: 1051–1056.

87. Holgate ST, Davies DE, Lackie PM, Wilson SJ, Puddicombe SM, Lordan JL. Epithelial-mesenchymal interactions in the pathogenesis of asthma. J Allergy Clin Immunol 2000; 105:193–204.

88. Djukanovic R, Wilson JW, Britten KM, Wilson SJ, Walls AF, Roche WR, Howarth PH, Holgate ST. Quantitation of mast cells and eosinophils in the bronchial mucosa of symptomatic atopic asthmatics and healthy control subjects using immunohistochemistry. Am Rev Respir Dis 1990; 142:863–871.

89. Pesci A, Foresi A, Bertorelli G, Chetta A, Oliveri D. Histochemical characteristics and degranulation of mast cells in epithelium and lamina propria of bronchial biopsies from asthmatic and normal subjects. Am Rev Respir Dis 1993; 147:684–689.

90. Bradley BL, Azzawi M, Jacobson M, Assoufi B, Collins JV, Irani AM, Schwartz LB, Durham SR, Jeffery PK, Kay AB. Eosinophils, T-lymphocytes, mast cells, neutrophils, and macrophages in bronchial biopsy specimens from atopic subjects with asthma: comparison with biopsy specimens from atopic subjects without asthma and normal control subjects and relationship to bronchial hyperresponsiveness. J Allery Clin Immunol 1991; 88:661–674.

91. Koshino T, Arai Y, Miyamoto Y, Sano Y, Takaishi T, Hirai K, Ito K, Morita Y. Mast cell and basophil number in the airway correlate with the bronchial responsiveness of asthmatics. Int Arch Allergy Immunol 1995; 107:378–379.

92. Bradding P, Feather IH, Howarth PH, Mueller R, Roberts JA, Britten K, Bews JP, Hunt TC, Okayama Y, Heusser CH, et al. Interleukin 4 is localized to and released by human mast cells. J Exp Med 1992; 176:1381–1386.

93. Bradding P, Roberts JA, Britten KM, Montefort S, Djukanovic R, Mueller R, Heusser CH, Howarth PH, Holgate ST. Interleukin-4, -5 and -6 and tumor necrosis factor-alpha in normal and asthmatic airways: evidence for the human mast cell as a source of these cytokines. Am J Respir Cell Mol Biol 1994; 10: 471–480.

94. Laitinen LA, Heino M, Laitinen A, Kava T, Haahtela T. Damage of the airway epithelium and bronchial reactivity in patients with asthma. Am Rev Respir Dis 1985; 131:599–606.

95. Beasley R, Roche WR, Roberts JA, Holgate ST. Cellular events in the bronchi in mild asthma and after bronchial provocation. Am Rev Respir Dis 1989; 139:806–817.

96. Kawanami O, Ferrans VJ, Fulmer JD, Crystal RG. Ultrastructure of pulmonary mast cells in patients with fibrotic lung disorders. Lab Invest 1979; 40:717–4734.
97. Jordana M. Mast cells and fibrosis—who's on first? Am J Respir Cell Mol Biol 1993; 8:7–8.
98. Chanez P, Lacoste JY, Guillot B, Giron J, Barneon G, Enander I, Godard P, Michel FB, Bousquet J. Mast cells' contribution to the fibrosing alvelolitis of the scleroderma lung. Am Rev Respir Dis 1993; 147:1497–1502.
99. Thompson HL, Burbelo PD, Gabriel G, Yamada Y, Metcalfe DD. Murine mast cells synthesize basement membrane components. A potential role in early fibrosis. J Clin Invest 1991; 87:619–623.
100. Ruoss SJ, Hartmann T, Caughey GH. Mast cell tryptase is a mitogen for cultured fibroblasts. J Clin Invest 1991; 88:493–499.
101. Nagata Y, Matsumura F, Motoyoshi H, Yamasaki H, Fukuda K, Tanaka S. Secretion of hyaluronic acid from synovial fibroblasts is enhanced by histamine: a newly observed metabolic effect of histamine. J Lab Clin Med 1992; 120:707–712.
102. Cairns JA, Walls AF. Mast cell tryptase stimulates the synthesis of type I collagen in human lung fibroblasts. J Clin Invest 1997; 99:1313–1321.
103. Akers IA, Parsons M, Hill MR, Hollenberg MD, Shahin S, Laurent GJ, McAnulty RJ. Mast cell tryptase stimulates human lung fibroblast proliferation via protease-activated receptor-2. Am J Physiol Cell Mol Physiol 2000; 278: L193–L201.
104. Andreasen PA, Egelund R, Petersen HH. The plasminogen activation system in tumor growth, invasion, and metastasis. Cell Mol Life Sci 2000; 57:25–40.
105. Irigoyen JP, Munoz-Canoves P, Montero L, Koziczak M, Nagamine Y. The plasminogen activator system: biology and regulation. Cell Mol Life Sci 1999; 56:104–132.
106. Hattori N, Degen JL, Sisson TH, Liu H, Moore BB, Pandrangi RG, Simon RH, Drew AF. Bleomycin-induced pulmonary fibrosis in fibrinogen-null mice. J Clin Invest 2000; 106:1341–1350.
107. Barazzone C, Belin D, Piguet PF, Vassalli JD, Sappino AP. Plasminogen activator inhibitor-1 in acute hyperoxic mouse lung injury. J Clin Invest 1996; 98:2666–2673.
108. Sillaber C, Baghestanian M, Bevec D, Willheim M, Agis H, Kapiotis S, Fureder W, Bankl HC, Kiener HP, Speiser W, Binder BR, Lechner K, Valent P. The mast cell as site of tissue-type plasminogen activator expression and fibronolysis. J Immunol 1999; 162:1032–1041.
109. Cho SH, Tam SW, Demissie-Sanders S, Filler SA, Oh CK. Production of plasminogen activator inhibitor-1 by human mast cells and its possible role in asthma. J Immunol 2000; 165:3154–3161.
110. Geiger E, Magerstaedt R, Wessendorf JH, Kraft S, Hanau D, Bieber T. IL-4 induces the intracellular expression of the alpha chain of the high-affinity receptor for IgE in in vitro–generated dendritic cells. J Allergy clin Immunol 2000; 105:150–156.
111. Oppel T, Schuller E, Gunther S, Moderer M, Haberstok J, Bieber T, Wollenberg A. Phenotyping of epidermal dendritic cells allows the differentiation between extrinsic and intrinsic forms of atopic dermatitis. Br J Dermatol 2000; 143:1193–1198.

112. Shibaki A. Fc epsilon RI on dendritic cells: a receptor, which links IgE mediated allergic reaction and T cell mediated cellular response. J Dermatol Sci 1998; 20:29–38.

113. Moser M, Murphy KM. Dendritic cell regulation of TH1-TH2 development. Nat Immunol 2000; 1:199–205.

114. Zahm JM, Chevillard M, Puchelle E. Wound repair of human surface respiratory epithelium. Am J Respir Cell Mol Biol 1991; 5:242–248.

115. Vignola AM, Campbell AM, Chanez P, Bousquet J, Paul-Lacoste P, Michel FB, Godard P. HLA-DR and ICAM-1 expression on bronchial epithelial cells in asthma and chronic bronchitis. Am Rev Respir Dis 1993; 148:689–694.

116. Campbell Am, Chanez P, Vignola AM, Bousquet J, Couret I, Michel FB, Godard P. Functional characteristics of bronchial epithelium obtained by brushing from asthmatic and normal subjects. Am Rev Respir Dis 1993; 147:529–534.

117. Chung KF, Barnes PJ. Cytokines in asthma. Thorax 1999; 54:825–857.

118. Holgate ST, Lackie PM, Davies DE, Roche WR, Walls AF. The bronchial epithelium as a key regulator of airway inflammation and remodelling in asthma. Clin Exp Allergy 1999; 2:90–95.

119. Arima M, Plitt J, Stellato C, Bickel C, Motojima S, Makino S, Fukuda T, Schleimer RP. Expression of interleukin-16 by human epithelial cells. Inhibition by dexamethasone [In Process Citation]. Am J Respir Cell Mol Biol 1999; 21: 684–692.

120. Cameron LA, Taha RA, Tsicopoulos A, Kurimoto M, Olivenstein R, Wallaert B, Minshall EM, Hamid QA. Airway epithelium expresses interleukin-18. Eur Respir J 1999; 14:553–559.

121. Cromwell O, Hamid Q, Corrigan CJ, Barkans J, Meng Q, Collins PD, Kay AB. Expression and generation of interleukin-8, IL-6 and granulocyte-macrophage colony-stimulating factor by bronchial epithelial cells and enhancement by IL-1 beta and tumour necrosis factor-alpha. Immunology 1992; 77:330–337.

122. Sousa AR, Poston RN, Lane SJ, Nakhosteen JA, Lee TH. Detection of GM-CSF in asthmatic bronchial epithelium and decrease by inhaled corticosteroids. Am Rev Respir Dis 1993; 147:1557–1561.

123. Matsukura S, Stellato C, Plitt JR, Bickel C, Miura K, Georas SN, Casolaro V, Schleimer RP. Activation of eotaxin gene transcription by NF-kappa B and STAT6 in human airway epithelial cells. J Immunol 1999; 163:6876–6883.

124. Ying S, Meng Q, Zeibecoglou K, Robinson DS, Macfarlane A, Humbert M, Kay AB. Eosinophil chemotactic chemokines (eotaxin, eotaxin-2, RANTES, monocyte chemoattractant protein-3 (MCP-3), and MCP-4), and C-C chemokine receptor 3 expression in bronchial biopsies from atopic and nonatopic (Intrinsic) asthmatics. J Immunol 1999; 163:6321–6329.

125. Campbell AM, Vachier I, Chanez P, Vignola AM, Lebel B, Kochan J, Godard P, Bousquet J. Expression of the high-affinity receptor for IgE on bronchial epithelial cells of asthmatics. Am J Respir Cell Mol Biol 1998; 19(1):92–97.

126. Takuwa N, Takuwa Y, Yanagisawa M, Yamashita K, Masaki T. A novel vasoactive peptide endothelin stimulates mitogenesis through inositol lipid turnover in Swiss 3T3 fibroblasts. J Biol Chem 1989; 264:7856–7861.

127. Luscher TF. Endothelin: systemic arterial and pulmonary effects of a new peptide with potent biologic properties. Am Rev Respir Dis 1992; 146:S56–S60.

128. Bousquet J, Chanez P, Lacoste JY, Barneon G, Ghavanian N, Enander I, Venge P, Ahlstedt S, Simony-Lafontaine J, Godard P, Michel FB. Eosinophilic inflammation in asthma. N Engl J Med 1990; 323:1033–1039.

129. Busse WW, Sedgwick JB. Eosinophil eicosanoid relations in allergic inflammation of the airways. Adv Prostaglandin Thromboxane Leukot Res 1994; 22: 241–249.

130. Ying S, Durham SR, Corrigan CJ, Hamid Q, Kay AB. Phenotype of cells expressing mRNA for TH2-type (interleukin 4 and interleukin 5) and TH1-type (interleukin 2 and interferon gamma) cytokines in bronchoalveolar lavage and bronchial biopsies from atopic asthmatic and normal control subjects. Am J Respir Cell Mol Biol 1995; 12:477–487.

131. Broide DH, Paine MM, Firestein GS. Eosinophils express interleukin 5 and granulocyte macrophage-colony-stimulating factor mRNA at sites of allergic inflammation in asthmatics. J Clin Invest 1992; 90:1414–1424.

132. Weller PF. The immunobiology of eosinophils. N Engl J Med 1991; 324: 1110–1118.

133. Gleich GJ, Adolphson CR, Leiferman KM. The biology of the eosinophilic leukocyte. Annu Rev Med 1993; 44:85–101.

134. Venge P, Hakansson L, Peterson CG. Eosinophil activation in allergic disease. Int Arch Allergy Appl Immunol 1987; 82:333–337.

135. Rabe KF, Munoz NM, Vita AJ, Morton BE, Magnussen H, Leff AR. Contraction of human bronchial smooth muscle caused by activated human eosinophils. Am J Physiol 1994; 267:L326–L334.

136. Collins DS, Dupuis R, Gleich GJ, Bartemes KR, Koh YY, Pollice M, Albertine KH, Fish JE, Peters SP. Immunoglobulin E-mediated increase in vascular permeability correlates with eosinophilic inflammation. Am Rev Respir Dis 1993; 147:677–683.

137. Leff AR. Inflammatory mediation of airway hyperresponsiveness by peripheral blood granulocytes. The case for the eosinophil. Chest 1994; 106:1202–1208.

138. Ohno I, Lea RG, Flanders KC, Clark DA, Banwatt D, Dolovich J, Denburg J, Harley CB, Gauldie J, Jordana M. Eosinophils in chronically inflamed human upper airways tissues express transforming growth factor beta 1 gene (TGF beta 1). J Clin Invest 1992; 89:1662–1668.

139. Walz TM, Nishikawa BK, Malm C, Wasteson A. Production of transforming growth factor alpha by normal human blood eosinophils. Leukemia 1993; 7:1531–1537.

140. Lungarella G, Menegazzi R, Gardi C, Spessotto P, de-Santi MM, Bertoncin P, Patriarca P, Calzoni P, Zabucchi G. Identification of elastase in human eosinophils: immunolocalization, isolation, and partial characterization. Arch Biochem Biophys 1992; 292:128–135.

141. Pincus SH, Ramesh KS, Wyler DJ. Eosinophils stimulate fibroblast DNA synthesis. Blood 1987; 70:572–574.

142. Levi-Schaffer F, Garbuzenko E, Rubin A, Reich R, Pickholz D, Gillery P, Emonard H, Nagler A, Maquart FA. Human eosinophils regulate human lung-

and skin-derived fibroblast properties in vitro: a role for transforming growth factor beta (TGF-beta). Proc Natl Acad Sci USA 1999; 96:9660–9665.

143. Noguchi H, Kephart GM, Colby TV, Gleich GJ. Tissue eosinophilia and eosinophil degranulation in syndromes associated with fibrosis. Am J pathol 1992; 140:521–528.

144. Schlick W. Current issues in the assessment of interstitial lung disease. Monaldi Arch Chest Dis 1993; 48:237–244.

145. Ottesen EA, Nutman TB. Tropical pulmonary eosinophilia. Annu Rev Med 1992; 43:417–424.

146. Bryan SA, O'Connor BJ, Matti S, Leckie MJ, Kanabar V, Khan J, Warrington SJ, Renzetti L, Rames A, Bock JA, Boyce MJ, Hansel TT, Holgate ST, Barnes PJ. Effects of recombinant human interleukin-12 on eosinophils, airway hyperreactivity and the late asthmatic response. The Lancet 2000; in press.

147. Gounni AS, Lamkhioued B, Ochiai K, Tanaka Y, Delaporte E, Capron A, Kinet JP, Capron M. High-affinity IgE receptor on eosinophils is involved in defence against parasites. Nature 1994; 367:183–186.

148. Gounni AS, Lamkhioued B, Delaporte E, Dubost A, Kinet JP, Capron A, Capron M. The high-affinity IgE receptor on eosinophils: from allergy to parasites or from parasites to allergy? J Allergy Clin Immunol 1994; 94: 1214–1216.

149. Truong MJ, Gruart V, Liu FT, Prin L, Capron A, Capron M. IgE-binding molecules (Mac-2/epsilon BP) expressed by human eosinophils. Implication in IgE-dependent eosinophil cytotoxicity. Eur J Immunol 1993; 23:3230–3235.

150. Capron M, Capron A, Dessaint JP, Torpier G, Johansson SG, Prin L. Fc receptors for IgE on human and rat eosinophils. J Immunol 1981; 126:2087–2092.

151. Capron M, Jouault T, Prin L, Joseph M, Ameisen JC, Butterworth AE, Papin JP, Kusnierz JP, Capron A. Functional study of a monoclonal antibody to IgE Fc receptor (Fc epsilon R2) of eosinophils, platelets, and macrophages. J Exp Med 1986; 164:72–89.

152. Capron M. Eosinophils: receptors and mediators in hypersensitivity. Clin Exp Allergy 1989; 19 (Suppl 1):3–8.

153. Lantero S, Alessandri G, Spallarossa D, Scarso L, Rossi GA. Stimulation of eosinophil IgE low-affinity receptor leads to increased adhesion molecule expression and cell migration. Eur Respir J 2000; 16:940–946.

154. Bousquet J, Chanez P, Arnoux B, Vignola M, Damon M, Michel F, Godard P. Monocytes and macrophages and asthma. Immunopharmacol Allergic Dis 1996; 8:263–286.

155. Poulter LW, Power C, Burke C. The relationship between bronchial immunopathology and hyperresponsiveness in asthma. Eur Respir J 1990; 3:792–799.

156. Poston RN, Chanez P, Lacoste JY, Litchfield T, Lee TH, Bousquet J. Immunohistochemical characterization of the cellular infiltration in asthmatic bronchi. Am Rev Respir Dis 1992; 145:918–921.

157. Bentley AM, Menz G, Storz C, Robinson DS, Bradley B, Jeffery PK, Durham SR, Kay AB. Identification of T lymphocytes, macrophages, and activated eosinophils in the bronchial mucosa in intrinsic asthma. Relationship to symptoms and bronchial responsiveness. Am Rev Respir Dis 1992; 146:500–506.

158. Nathan CF. Secretory products of macrophages. J Clin Invest 1987; 79:319–326.
159. Johnston R, Jr. Current concepts: immunology. Monocytes and macrophages. N Engl J Med 1988; 318:747–752.
160. Werb Z, Underwood J, Rappolee D. The role of macrophage-derived growth factors in tissue repair. In: van-Furth R, ed. Mononuclear Phagocytes. Dordrecht: Kluwer Academic, 1992: 404–409.
161. Senior RM, Connolly NL, Cury JD, Welgus HG, Campbell EJ. Elastin degradation by human alveolar macrophages. A Prominent role of metalloproteinase activity. Am Rev Respir Dis 1989; 139:1251–1256.
162. Lyberg T, Nakstad B, Hetland O, Boye NP. Procoagulant (thromboplastin) activity in human bronchoalveolar lavage fluids is derived from alveolar macrophages. Eur Respir J 1990; 3:61–67.
163. Piguet PF, Ribaux C, Karpuz V, Grau GE, Kapanci Y. Expression and localization of tumor necrosis factor-alpha and its mRNA in idiopathic pulmonary fibrosis. Am J Pathol 1993; 143:651–655.
164. Standiford TJ, Rolfe MW, Kunkel SL, Lynch Jd, Burdick MD, Gilbert AR, Orringer MB, Whyte RI, Strieter RM. Macrophage inflammatory protein-1 alpha expression in interstitial lung disease. J Immunol 1993; 151:2852–2863.
165. Joseph M, Tonnel AB, Torpier G, Capron A, Arnoux B, Benveniste J. Involvement of immunoglobulin E in the secretory processes of alveolar macrophages from asthmatic patients. J Clin Invest 1983; 71:221–230.
166. Fuller RW, MacDermot J. Stimulation of IgE sensitized human alveolar macrophages by anti-IgE is unaffected by sodium cromoglycate. Clin Allergy 1986; 16: 523–526.
167. Fuller RW, Morris PK, Richmond R, Sykes D, Varndell IM, Kemeny DM, Cole PJ, Dollery CT, MacDermot J. Immunoglobulin E-dependent stimulation of human alveolar macrophages: significance in type 1 hypersensitivity. Clin Exp Immunol 1986; 65:416–426.
168. Borish L, Mascali JJ, Rosenwasser LJ. IgE-dependent cytokine production by human peripheral blood mononuclear phagocytes. J Immunol 1991; 146:63–67.
169. Gosset P, Tsicopoulos A, Wallaert B, Vannimenus C, Joseph M, Tonnel AB, Capron A. Increased secretion of tumor necrosis factor alpha and interleukin-6 by alveolar macrophages consecutive to the development of the late asthmatic reaction. J Allergy Clin Immunol 1991; 88:561–571.
170. Gosset P, Tsicopoulos A, Wallaert B, Joseph M, Capron A, Tonnel AB. Tumor necrosis factor alpha and interleukin-6 production by human mononuclear phagocytes from allergic asthmatics after IgE-dependent stimulation. Am Rev Respir Dis 1992; 146:768–774.
171. Williams J, Johnson S, Mascali JJ, Smith H, Rosenwasser LJ, Borish L. Regulation of low affinity IgE receptor (CD23) expression on mononuclear phagocytes in normal and asthmatic subjects. J Immunol 1992; 149:2823–2829.
172. Hirst SJ, Twort CH, Lee TH. Differential effects of extracellular matrix proteins on human airway smooth muscle cell proliferation and phenotype. Am J Respir Cell Mol Biol 2000; 23:335–344.
173. Hirst SJ, Walker TR, Chilvers ER. Phenotypic diversity and molecular mechanisms of airway smooth muscle proliferation in asthma [In Process Citation]. Eur Respir J 2000; 16:159–177.

174. Fong CY, Pang L, Holland E, Knox AJ. TGF-beta1 stimulates IL-8 release, COX-2 expression, and PGE(2) release in human airway smooth muscle cells. Am J Physiol Lung Cell Mol Physiol 2000; 279:L201–207.

175. Pang L, Knox AJ. Synergistic inhibition by beta(2)-agonists and corticosteroids on tumor necrosis factor-alpha–induced interleukin-8 release from cultured human airway smooth muscle cells. Am J Respir Cell Mol Biol 2000; 23:79–85.

176. Knox AJ, Pang L, Johnson S, Hamad A. Airway smooth muscle function in asthma. Clin Exp Allergy 2000; 30:606–614.

177. Panettieri R, Jr., Murray RK, Eszterhas AJ, Bilgen G, Martin JG. Repeated allergen inhalations induce DNA synthesis in airway smooth muscle and epithelial cells in vivo. Am J Physiol 1998; 274:L417–424.

178. John M, Hirst SJ, Jose PJ, Robichaud A, Berkman N, Witt C, Twort CH, Barnes PJ, Chung KF. Human airway smooth muscle cells express and release RANTES in response to T helper 1 cytokines: regulation by T helper 2 cytokines and corticosteroids. J Immunol 1997; 158:1841–1847.

179. Hirst SJ. Airway smooth muscle cell culture: application to studies of airway wall remodelling and phenotype plasticity in asthma. Eur Respir J 1996; 9:808–820.

180. Naureckas ET, Ndukwu IM, Halayko AJ, Maxwell C, Hershenson MB, Solway J. Bronchoalveolar lavage fluid from asthmatic subjects is mitogenic for human airway smooth muscle. Am J Respir Crit Care Med 1999; 160: 2062–2066.

181. Krymskaya VP, Hoffman R, Eszterhas A, Kane S, Ciocca V, Panettieri R, Jr. EGF activates ErbB-2 and stimulates phosphatidylinositol 3-kinase in human airway smooth muscle cells. Am J Physiol 1999; 276:L246–L255.

182. Wilkinson MG, Millar JB. Control of the eukaryotic cell cycle by MAP kinase signaling pathways [In Process Citation]. FASEB J 2000; 14:2147–2157.

183. Johnson S, Knox A. Autocrine production of matrix metalloproteinase-2 is required for human airway smooth muscle proliferation. Am J Physiol 1999; 277:L1109–L1117.

184. Hamann KJ, Vieira JE, Halayko AJ, Dorscheid D, White SR, Forsythe SM, Camoretti-Mercado B, Rabe KF, Solway J. Fas cross-linking induces apoptosis in human airway smooth muscle cells. Am J Physiol Lung Cell Mol Physiol 2000; 278:L618–L624.

185. Hakansson L, Bjornsson E, Janson C, Schmekel B. Increased adhesion to vascular cell adhesion molecule-1 and intercellular adhesion molecule-1 of eosinophils from patients with asthma. J Allergy Clin Immunol 1995; 96:941–950.

186. Johnson PR, Black JL, Carlin S, Ge Q, Underwood PA. The production of extracellular matrix proteins by human passively sensitized airway smoothmuscle cells in culture: the effect of beclomethasone. Am J Respir Crit Care Med 2000; 162:2145–2151.

187. Schmidt D, Ruehlmann E, Branscheid D, Magnussen H, Rabe KF. Passive sentitization of human airways increases responsiveness to leukotriene C4. Eur Respir J 1999; 14:315–319.

188. Schmidt D, Watson N, Ruelhmann E, Magnussen H, Rabe KF. Serum immunoglobulin E levels predict human airway reactivity in vitro. Clin Exp Allergy 2000; 30:233–241.

189. Mitchell RW, Ruhlmann E, Magnussen H, Leff AR, Rabe KF. Passive sensitization of human bronchi augments smooth muscle shortening velocity and capacity. Am J Physiol 1994; 267:L218–222.

190. Mosmann TR, Bond MW, Coffman RL, Ohara J, Paul WE. T-cell and mast cell lines respond to B-cell stimulatory factor 1. Proc Natl Acad Sci USA 1986; 83:5654–5658.

191. de-Vries JE, Gauchat JF, Aversa GG, Punnonen J, Gascan H, Yssel H. Regulation of IgE synthesis by cytokines. Curr Opin Immunol 1991:3:851–858.

192. Borish L, Rosenwasser L. TH1/TH2 lymphocytes: doubt some more. J Allergy Clin Immunol 1997; 99:161–164.

193. Romagnani S. Human TH1 and TH2 subsets: doubt no more. Immunol Today 1991; 12:256–257.

194. Romagnani S. Lymphokine production by human T cells in disease states. Annu Rev Immunol 1994; 12:227–257.

195. Parronchi P, Brugnolo F, Sampognaro S, Maggi E. Genetic and environmental factors contributing to the onset of allergic disorders. Int Arch Allergy Immunol 2000; 121:2–9.

196. de-Vries JE, Gauchat J-F, Aversa G, Punnonen J, Gascan H, Yssel H. Regulation of IgE synthesis by cytokines. Curr Opin Immunol 1992; 3:851–858.

197. Snijdewint FG, Kalinski P, Wierenga EA, Bos JD, Kapsenberg ML. Prostaglandin E2 differentially modulates cytokine secretion profiles of human T helper lymphocytes. J Immunol 1993; 150:5321–5329.

198. Azzawi M, Johnston PW, Majumdar S, Kay AB, Jeffery PK. T lymphocytes and activated eosinophils in airway mucosa in fatal asthma and cystic fibrosis. Am Rev Respir Dis 1992; 145:1477–1482.

199. Azzawi M, Bradley B, Jeffery PK, Frew AJ, Wardlaw AJ, Knowles G, Assoufi B, Collins JV, Durham S, Kay AB. Identification of activated T lymphocytes and eosinophils in bronchial biopsies in stable atopic asthma. Am Rev Respir Dis 1990; 142:1407–1413.

200. Bentley AM, Maestrelli P, Saetta M, Fabbri LM, Robinson DS, Bradley BL, Jeffery PK, Durham SR, Kay AB. Activated T-lymphocytes and eosinophils in the bronchial mucosa in isocyanate-induced asthma. J Allergy Clin Immunol 1992; 89:821–829.

201. Corrigan CJ, Kay AB. Asthma. Role of T-lymphocytes and lymphokines. Br Med Bull 1992; 48:72–84.

202. Saetta M, Di-Stefano A, Maestrelli P, De-Marzo N, Milani GF, Pivirotto F, Mapp CE, Fabbri LM. Airway mucosal inflammation in occupational asthma induced by toluene diisocyanate. Am Rev Respir Dis 1992; 145:160–168.

203. Corrigan CJ, Hamid Q, North J, Barkans J, Moqbel R, Durham S, Gemou-Engesaeth V, Kay AB. Peripheral blood CD4 but not CD8 T-lymphocytes in patients with exacerbation of asthma transcribe and translate messenger RNA encoding cytokines which prolong eosinophil survival in the context of a Th2-type pattern: effect of glucocorticoid therapy. Am J Respir Cell Mol Biol 1995; 12:567–578.

204. Robinson D, Hamid Q, Bentley A, Ying S, Kay AB, Durham SR. Activation of CD4+ T cells, increased TH2-type cytokine mRNA expression, and eosinophil

recruitment in bronchoalveolar lavage after allergen inhalation challenge in patients with atopic asthma. J Allergy Clin Immunol 1993; 92:313–324.

205. Bentley AM, Meng Q, Robinson DS, Hamid Q, Kay AB, Durham SR. Increases in activated T lymphocytes, eosinophils, and cytokine mRNA expression for interleukin-5 and granulocyte/macrophage colony-stimulating factor in bronchial biopsies after allergen inhalation challenge in atopic asthmatics. Am J Respir Cell Mol Biol 1993; 8:35–42.

206. Laprise C, Laviolette M, Boutet M, Boulet LP. Asymptomatic airway hyperresponsiveness: relationships with airway inflammation and remodelling. Eur Respir J 1999; 14:63–73.

207. Kay AB. T cells as orchestrators of the asthmatic response. Ciba Found Symp 1997; 206:56–67.

208. Holgate ST. The epidemic of allergy and asthma. Nature 1999; B2–B4.

209. Kay AB. Asthma and inflammation. J Allergy Clin Immunol 1991; 87:893–910.

210. Romagnani S. The role of lymphocytes in allergic disease. J Allergy Clin Immunol 2000; 105:399–408.

211. Kay AB. Allergy and allergic diseases. First of two parts. N Engl J Med 2000; 344:30–37.

212. Holgate S. Mediator and cytokine mechanisms in asthma. Thorax 1993; 48:103–109.

213. Zhu Z, Homer RJ, Wang Z, Chen Q, Geba GP, Wang J, Zhang Y, Elias JA. Pulmonary expression of interleukin-13 causes inflammation, mucus hypersecretion, subepithelial fibrosis, physiologic abnormalities, and eotaxin production. J Clin Invest 1999; 103:779–788.

214. Temann UA, Geba GP, Rankin JA, Flavell RA. Expression of interleukin 9 in the lungs of transgenic mice causes airway inflammation, mast cell hyperplasia and bronchial hyperresponsiveness. J Exp Med 1998; 188:1307–1320.

215. Lee JJ, McGarry MP, Farmer SC, Denzler KL, Larson KA, Carrigan PE, Brenneise IE, Horton MA, Haczku A, Gelfand EW, Leikauf GD, Lee NA. Interleukin-5 expression in the lung epithelium of transgenic mice leads to pulmonary changes pathognomonic of asthma. J Exp Med 1997; 185:2143–2156.

216. Wallace WA, Ramage EA, Lamb D, Howie SE. A type 2 (Th2-like) pattern of immune response predominates in the pulmonary interstitium of patients with cryptogenic fibrosing alveolitis (CFA). Clin Exp Immunol 1995; 101:436–441.

217. Spoelstra FM, Postma DS, Hovenga H, Noordhoek JA, Kauffman HF. Interferon-gamma and interleukin-4 differentially regulate ICAM-1 and VCAM-1 expression on human lung fibroblasts. Eur Respir J 1999; 14:759–766.

218. Trautmann A, Krohne G, Brocker EB, Klein CE. Human mast cells augment fibroblast proliferation by heterotypic cell-cell adhesion and action of IL-4. J Immunol 1998; 160:5053–5057.

219. Miyamasu M, Misaki Y, Yamaguchi M, Yamamoto K, Morita Y, Matsushima K, Nakajima T, Hirai K. Regulation of human eotaxin generation by Th1-/Th2-derived cytokines. Int Arch Allergy Immunol 2000; 1:54–58.

220. Terada N, Hamano N, Nomura T, Numata T, Hirai K, Nakajima T, Yamada H, Yoshie O, Ikeda-Ito T, Konno A. Interleukin-13 and tumour necrosis factor-

alpha synergistically induce eotaxin production in human nasal fibroblasts. Clin Exp Allergy 2000; 30:348–355.

221. Mochizuki M, Schroder J, Christophers E, Yamamoto S. IL-4 induces eotaxin in human dermal fibroblasts. Int Arch Allergy Immunol 1999; 1:19–23.

222. Nonaka M, Pawankar R, Saji F, Yagi T. Distinct Expression of RANTES and GM-CSF by lipopolysaccharide in human nasal fibroblasts but not in other airway fibroblasts. Int Arch Allergy Immunol 1999; 119:314–321.

223. Maune S, Berner I, Sticherling M, Kulke R, Bartels J, Schroder JM. Fibroblasts but not epithelial cells obtained from human nasal mucosa produce the chemokine RANTES. Rhinology 1996; 34:210–214.

224. Maune S, Warner JA, Sticherling M, Schroder JM. Fibroblasts obtained from human nasal, laryngeal and tracheal mucosa produce the chemokine RANTES. Otolaryngol Pol 1997; 51:3–10.

225. Minshall EM, Hamid QA. Fibroblasts: a cell type central to eosinophil recruitment? Clin Exp Allergy 2000; 30:301–303.

226. Sato E, Nelson DK, Koyama S, Hoyt JC, Robbins RA. Inflammatory cytokines modulate eotaxin release by human lung fibroblast cell line. Exp Lung Res 2001; 27:173–183.

227. Vancheri C, Gauldie J, Bienenstock J, Cox G, Scicchitano R, Stanisz A, Jordana M. Human lung fibroblast–derived granulocyte-macrophage colony stimulating factor (GM-CSF) mediates eosinophil survival in vitro. Am J Respir Cell Mol Biol 1989; 1:289–295.

228. Sheppard MN, Harrison NK. New perspectives on basic mechanisms in lung disease. 1. Lung injury, inflammatory mediators, and fibroblast activation in fibrosing alveolitis. Thorax 1992; 47:1064–1074.

229. Rothe M, Pesce K, Falanga V. Clinical application of growth factors in cutaneous wound healing. Clin Immunother 1994; 1:282–292.

230. Low RB. Modulation of myofibroblast and smooth-muscle phenotypes in the lung. Curr Top Pathol 1999; 93:19–26.

231. Leslie KO, Mitchell J, Low R. Lung myofibroblasts. Cell Motil Cytoskeleton 1992; 22:92–98.

232. Sun G, Stacey MA, Bellini A, Marini M, Mattoli S. Endothelin-1 induces bronchial myofibroblast differentiation. Peptides 1997; 18:1449–1451.

233. Zhang S, Smartt H, Holgate ST, Roche WR. Growth factors secreted by bronchial epithelial cells control myofibroblast proliferation: an in vitro co-culture model of airway remodeling in asthma. Lab Invest 1999; 79:395–405.

234. Dube J, Chakir J, Dube C, Grimard Y, Laviolette M, Boulet LP. Synergistic action of endothelin (ET)-1 on the activation of bronchial fibroblast isolated from normal and asthmatic subjects. Int J Exp Pathol 2001; 81:429–437.

235. Gizycki MJ, Adelroth E, Rogers AV, O'Byrne PM, Jeffery PK. Myofibroblast involvement in the allergen-induced late response in mild atopic asthma. Am J Respir Cell Mol Biol 1997; 16:664–673.

236. Meerschaert J, Kelley EA, Mosher DF, Busse WW, Jarjour NN. Segmental antigen challenge increases fibronectin in bronchoalveolar lavage fluid. Am J Respir Crit Care Med 1999; 159:619–625.

237. Medina L, Perez-Ramos J, Ramirez R, Selman M, Pardo A. Leukotriene C4 upregulates collagenase expression and synthesis in human fibroblasts. Biochim Biophys Acta 1994; 1224:168–174.

238. Ohd JF, Wikstrom K, Sjolander A. Leukotrienes induce cell-survival signaling in intestinal epithelial cells. Gastroenterology 2000; 119:1007–1018.

239. Lee E, Robertson T, Smith J, Kilfeather S. Leukotriene receptor antagonists and synthesis inhibitors reverse survival in eosinophils of asthmatic individuals. Am J Respir Crit Care Med 2000; 161:1881–1886.

240. Cohen P, Noveral JP, Bhala A, Nunn SE, Herrick DJ, Grunstein MM. Leukotriene D4 facilitates airway smooth muscle cell proliferation via modulation of the IGF axis. Am J Physiol 1995; 269:L151–L157.

241. Rajah R, Nunn SE, Herrick DJ, Grunstein MM, Cohen P. Leukotriene D4 induces MMP-1, which functions as an IGFBP protease in human airway smooth muscle cells. Am J Physiol 1996; 271:L1014–L1022.

242. Panettieri RA, Tan EM, Ciocca V, Luttmann MA, Leonard TB, Hay DW. Effects of LTD4 on human airway smooth muscle cell proliferation, matrix expression, and contraction in vitro: differential sensitivity to cysteinyl leukotriene receptor antagonists. Am J Respir Cell Mol Biol 1998; 19:453–461.

243. Karjalainen EM, Laitinen A, Sue-Chu M, Altraja A, Bjermer L, Laitinen LA. Evidence of airway inflammation and remodeling in ski athletes with and without bronchial hyperresponsiveness to methacholine. Am J Respir Crit Care Med 2000; 161:2086–2091.

244. Palmans E, Kips JC, Pauwels RA. Prolonged allergen exposure induces structural airway changes in sensitized rats. Am J Respir Crit Care Med 2000; 161:627–635.

245. Cui ZH, Skoogh BE, Pullerits T, Lotvall J. Bronchial hyperresponsiveness and airway wall remodeling induced by exposure to allergen for 9 weeks. Allergy 1999; 54:1074–1082.

246. Cui ZH, Sjostrand M, Pullerits T, Andius P, Skoogh BE, Lotvall J. Bronchial hyperresponsiveness, epithelial damage, and airway eosinophilia after single and repeated allergen exposure in a rat model of anhydride-induced asthma. Allergy 1997; 52:739–746.

247. Brown RH, Zerhouni EA, Mitzner W. Airway edema potentiates airway reactivity. J Appl Physiol 1995; 79:1242–1248.

248. Palmans E, Kips JC, Pauwels RA. The effect of chronic allergen exposure on airway structure and responsiveness in rats. Am J Respir Crit Care Med 2000; 161(2):.

249. Vanacker NJ, Palmans E, Kips JC, Pauwels RA. Fluticasone inhibits but does not reverse allergen-induced structural airway changes. Am J Respir Crit Care Med 2001; 163:674–679.

250. Elias JA, Zhu Z, Chupp G, Homer RJ. Airway remodeling in asthma. J Clin Invest 1999; 104:1001–1006.

251. Zheng T, Zhu Z, Wang Z, Homer RJ, Ma B, Riese RJ, Chapman HJ, Shapiro SD, Elias JA. Inducible targeting of IL-13 to the adult lung causes matrix metalloproteinase- and cathepsin-dependent emphysema [In Process Citation]. J Clin Invest 2000; 106:1081–1093.

252. Kuhn Cr, Homer RJ, Zhu Z, Ward N, Flavell RA, Geba GP, Elias JA. Airway hyperresponsiveness and airway obstruction in transgenic mice. Morphologic

correlates in mice overexpressing interleukin (IL)-11 and IL-6 in the lung. Am J Respir Cell Mol Biol 2000; 22:289–295.

253. Saetta M, Maestrelli P, Turato G, Mapp CE, Milani G, Pivirotto F, Fabbri LM, Di-Stefano A. Airway wall remodeling after cessation of exposure to isocyanates in sensitized asthmatic subjects. Am J Respir Crit Care Med 1995; 151:489–494.

254. Grol MH, Gerristen J, Vonk JM, Schouten JP, Koeter GH, Rijcken B, Postma DS. Risk factors for growth and decline of lung function in asthmatic individuals up to age 42 years. A 30-year follow-up study. Am J Respir Crit Care Med 1999; 160:1830–1837.

255. Cassino C, Berger KI, Goldring RM, Norman RG, Kammerman S, Ciotoli C, Reibman J. Duration of asthma and physiologic outcomes in elderly nonsmokers [In Process Citation]. Am J Respir Crit Care Med 2000; 162:1423–1428.

256. Bai TR, Cooper J, Koelmeyer T, Pare PD, Weir TD. The effect of age and duration of disease on airway structure in fatal asthma. Am J Respir Crit Care Med 2000; 162:663–669.

21

Immunomodulatory Aspects of Current Asthma Therapy

PETER J. BARNES

National Heart and Lung Institute
Imperial College School of Medicine
London, England

I. Introduction

Current asthma therapy is highly effective in controlling the majority of symptoms if the treatment is taken correctly. As asthma is characterized by abnormal immunological regulation (1), it is likely that this therapy exerts immunomodulatory effects on the airways. However, relatively little is understood about the effect of current antiasthma therapies on immune function and regulation, although the anti-inflammatory actions of some antiasthma therapies are well described at a clinical level. Understanding more about the immunomodulatory actions of currently used antiasthma treatment is important in developing new therapies for asthma in the future (2,3).

II. Current Asthma Therapy

The management of asthma has changed dramatically over the last 10 years, and many patients are now treated according to internationally agreed guidelines for therapy (4).

A. Controllers

As inflammation of the airways is present even in patients with mild asthma, inhaled corticosteroids have become the mainstay of treatment for patients with persistent symptoms (5). They are highly effective in controlling symptoms, preventing exacerbations of asthma, and preventing asthma death (6).

There is increasing evidence that they may also reduce the development of irreversible changes in lung function in adults and children. Other controller drugs are less effective and appear to have less effect on inflammation in the airways. Both theophylline and antileukotrienes are currently used as add-on therapies to improve asthma control in patients still symptomatic on inhaled corticosteroids but are far less effective than inhaled corticosteroids for first-line therapy in controlling asthma. Cromones (cromolyn sodium and nedocromil sodium) are only weakly effective compared to low-dose inhaled corticosteroids, and a recent meta-analysis shows that there is little benefit even in children (7). Other controller drugs include methotrexate, oral gold compounds, and cyclosporin A, but in view of the toxicity of these drugs they are only used in patients with very severe asthma who have problems with side effects of oral corticosteroids and are not very effective (8).

Current specific immunotherapy has little or no place in the modern management of asthma because it is less effective that inhaled corticosteroids but has a risk of serious adverse effects, including death (9). However, more effective and safer immunotherapeutic approaches are very likely in the future (see Chap. 23).

Several novel treatments now in development for asthma therapy may target the abnormal immune mechanisms in asthma, and these are discussed in other chapters in this volume. They will not be discussed further as they are not currently available.

B. Bronchodilators

Bronchodilators play an important role in asthma management, and β_2 agonists are by far the most effective (10). Short-acting inhaled β_2 agonists, such as albuterol and terbutaline, are used as needed for symptom relief. Both are safe and highly effective but do not give good control of the disease as they have no effects on the underlying inflammatory process. The long-acting inhaled β_2 agonists salmeterol and formoterol have proved to be more effective than short-term β_2 agonists in symptom control and are now used as the add-on therapy of choice in patients whose disease is not controlled on inhaled corticosteroids. It is unlikely that long-acting β_2 agonists have any anti-inflammatory actions and their beneficial effect is therefore likely to be due to some other, as-yet-unidentified mechanism(s). Theophylline was once considered to be a bronchodilator but is currently used in lower doses that are more likely to be anti-inflammatory or immunomodulatory (11); it is now used mainly as an add-on therapy. Anticholinergic bronchodilators are less effective than β_2 agonists and are used largely as additional bronchodilators in elderly patients with severe asthma, particularly when there is an element of fixed airway obstruction. There is no evidence or rationale for any immunomodulatory effect of anticholinergics, as muscarinic receptors do not appear to have a role in the immune system.

Fixed-combination inhalers with corticosteroids and long-acting β_2 agonists (fluticasone/salmeterol, budesonide/formoterol) are particularly effective in long-term control of asthma and are likely to become the gold standard for future management (12,13). They are more convenient for patients and prescribers and appear to be even more effective than when the components are given separately.

III. Corticosteroids

Inhaled corticosteroids are the mainstay of modern asthma management, and it is likely that their beneficial effect is due to their anti-inflammatory action. Many studies have demonstrated that inhaled corticosteroids suppress the eosinophilic inflammation in the airways that is characteristic of asthma (6). This action of steroids includes immunomodulatory effects, although it is likely to be the broad spectrum of anti-inflammatory actions that is important for clinical efficacy.

A. Molecular Mechanisms

There have been important advances in our understanding of the molecular mechanisms involved in the anti-inflammatory actions of corticosteroids (14).

Glucocorticoid Receptors

Corticosteroids bind to a single class of glucocorticoid receptor (GR) that is localized to the cytoplasm of target cells. Corticosteroids bind at the C-terminal end of the receptor, whereas the N-terminal end of the receptor is involved in gene transcription. Between these domains is the DNA binding domain which has two finger-like projections formed by a zinc molecule bound to four cysteine residues that bind to the DNA double helix. The inactive GR is bound to a protein complex that includes two molecules of 90-kD heat-shock protein (hsp90) and various other proteins that act as "molecular chaperones" to prevent the unoccupied GR from moving into the nuclear compartment. Once corticosteroids bind to GR, conformational changes in the receptor structure result in dissociation of these chaperone molecules, thereby exposing nuclear localization signals on GR, resulting in rapid nuclear localization of the activated GR–corticosteroid complex and its binding to DNA. Two GR molecules bind to DNA as a dimer, resulting in changed transcription. A splice variant of GR, termed GR-β, has been identified that does not bind corticosteroids, but binds to DNA and may theoretically interfere with the action of corticosteroids by blocking glucocorticoid response element binding (15).

Increased Gene Transcription

Corticosteroids produce their effect on responsive cells by activating GR to directly or indirectly regulate the transcription of certain target genes (16). The number of genes per cell *directly* regulated by corticosteroids is estimated to be between 10 and 100, but many genes are indirectly regulated through an interaction with other transcription factors. GR dimers bind to DNA at consensus sites termed glucocorticoid response elements (GREs) in the 5' upstream promoter region of steroid-responsive genes. This interaction changes the rate of transcription, resulting in either induction or repression of the gene. Interaction of the activated GR homodimer with GRE usually increases transcription, resulting in increased protein synthesis. GR may increase transcription by interacting with a large coactivator molecule, CREB-binding protein (CBP). CBP is bound at the start site of transcription, and this leads via a series of linking proteins to the binding and activation of RNA polymerase II, resulting in formation of messenger RNA (mRNA) and subsequent synthesis of protein. Binding of activated GR to CBP results in increased acetylation of core histones around which DNA is wound within the chromosomal structure (17), and this is critical for the subsequent activation of RNA polymerase II. For example, high concentrations of corticosteroids increase the secretion of the antiprotease secretory leukoprotease inhibitor (SLPI) from epithelial cells. This is associated with a selective acetylation of lysine residues 5 and 16 on histone 4, resulting in increased gene transcription.

Decreased Gene Transcription

In controlling inflammation, the major effect of corticosteroids is to inhibit the synthesis of inflammatory proteins. This was originally believed to be through interaction of GR with negative GREs, resulting in repression of transcription. However, negative GREs have only very rarely been demonstrated and are not a feature of the promoter region of inflammatory genes that are suppressed by steroids in the treatment of allergic diseases.

Interaction with Transcription Factors

Activated GRs may bind directly with several other activated transcription factors in a protein–protein interaction. This could be an important determinant of corticosteroid responsiveness and is a key mechanism whereby corticosteroids switch off inflammatory genes. Most of the inflammatory genes that are activated in asthma do not appear to have GREs in their promoter regions yet are repressed by corticosteroids. There is persuasive evidence that corticosteroids inhibit the effects of transcription factors that regulate the expression of genes that code for inflammatory proteins, such as cytokines, inflammatory enzymes, adhesion molecules, and inflammatory receptors. These "inflammatory" transcription factors include activator protein-1 (AP-1) and nuclear factor-κB (NF-κB), which may regulate many of the inflammatory genes that are switched on in asthmatic airways (18,19). The interaction of GR with DNA requires dimerization of the receptors, but GR monomers interact with transcription factors and other proteins. Mutant forms of GR that do not dimerize, and that therefore fail to bind to GREs in the promoters of genes, nevertheless maintain the ability to mediate the anti-inflammatory effects of corticosteroids (16), supporting the view that DNA binding is not needed for the anti-inflammatory action of corticosteroids.

It was once believed that the activated GR interacted directly with activated transcription factors through a protein–protein interaction, but thus may be a feature of transfected cells rather than what happens in primary cells. Thus, in a chronically transfected epithelial cell line with an NF-κB-driven reporter gene, there is relatively little effect of corticosteroids on transcription (20). Furthermore, treatment of asthmatic patients with high doses of inhaled corticosteroids that suppress airway inflammation is not associated with any reduction in NF-κB binding to DNA (21). This suggests that corticosteroids are acting downstream of the binding of proinflammatory transcription factors to DNA, and attention has now focused on their effects on chromatin structure and histone acetylation.

Effects on Chromatin Structure

There is increasing evidence that corticosteroids may have effects on the chromatin structure. DNA in chromosomes is wound around histone molecules in the form of nucleosomes (22,23). Several transcription factors, including AP-1, NF-κB, STATs, and GR, interact with large coactivator molecules, such as CBP and the related molecule p300, which bind to the basal transcription factor apparatus (24,25) (Fig. 1). At a microscopic level that chromatin may become dense or opaque due to the winding or unwinding of DNA around the histone core. Coactivator molecules, including CBP and the related p300, have histone acetylation activity that is stimulated by the binding of transcription factors, such as AP-1 and NF-κB. Acetylation of lysine residues in the N-terminal tails of core histones results in unwinding of DNA that is tightly coiled around the histone core of the resting gene, thus opening up the chromatin structure. This allows transcription factors and RNA polymerase to bind more readily, thereby switching on or increasing transcription.

Repression of genes reverses this process by deacetylation of the acetylated histone residues (26). Deacetylation of histones increases the winding of DNA round histone residues, resulting in dense chromatin structure and reduced access of transcription factors and RNA polymerase to their binding sites, thereby leading to repressed transcription of inflammatory genes. Activated GR may bind to several transcription corepressor molecules that associate with proteins that have histone deacetylase (HDAC) activity, resulting in deacetylation of histones, increased winding of DNA round histone

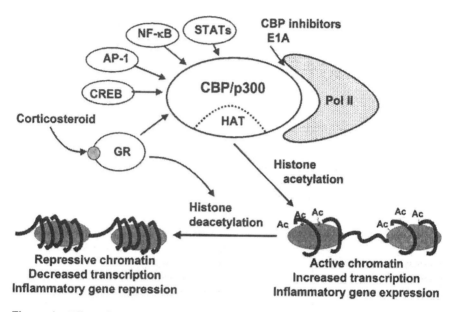

Figure 1 Effect of corticosteroids on chromatin structure. Transcription factors, such as STATs, AP-1, and NF-κB, bind to coactivator molecules, such as CREB binding protein (CBP) or p300, which have intrinsic histone acetyltransferase (HAT) activity, resulting in acetylation (-Ac) of histone residues. This leads to unwinding of DNA and this allows increased binding of transcription factors resulting in increased gene transcription. Glucocorticoid receptors (GRs) after activation by corticosteroids bind to a glucocorticoid receptor coactivator that is bound to CBP. This results in deacetylation of histone, with increased coiling of DNA around histone, thus preventing transcription factor binding leading to gene repression.

residues, reduced access of transcription factors to their binding sites, and thus repression of inflammatory genes. In addition, activated GR recruits HDACs to the transcription start site, resulting in deacetylation of histones and a decrease in inflammatory gene transcription (17,27). Several distinct HDACs are now recognized, and these are differentially expressed and regulated in different cell types (28). This may contribute to the differences in responsiveness to corticosteroids between different genes and cells.

Nontranscriptional Effects

It is increasingly recognized that GR may also affect the synthesis of some proteins by reducing the stability of mRNA through effects on ribonucleases that break down mRNA (29). Some inflammatory genes, such as the gene encoding granulocyte-macrophage colony-stimulating factor (GM-CSF), produce mRNA that has a sequence rich in AU nucleotides at the 3′ untranslated end.

It is this region that interacts with ribonucleases that break down mRNA, thus switching off protein synthesis (30).

B. Immunomodulatory Effects

Corticosteroids have several effects on immune mechanisms, and part of their anti-inflammatory actions may be mediated through immunosuppression.

Effect on Inflammatory Cytokines

The inhibitory effect of corticosteroids on cytokine synthesis is likely to be of particular importance in the control of inflammation in asthma, as cytokines play a critical role in the chronic inflammatory process (31). Corticosteroids inhibit the transcription of many cytokines and chemokines that are relevant in asthmatic inflammation (Table 1). These inhibitory effects are due, at least in part, to an inhibitory effect on the transcription factors that regulate induction of these cytokine genes, including AP-1 and NF-κB. For example, production of eotaxin, which is important in selective attraction of eosinophils from the circulation into the airways, is regulated in part by NF-κB and its expression in airway epithelial cells is inhibited by corticosteroids (32). Many transcription factors are likely to be involved in the regulation of inflammatory genes in asthma, in addition to AP-1 and NF-κB. IL-4 and IL-5 expression in T lymphocytes plays a critical role in allergic inflammation, but NF-κB does not play

Table 1 Effect of GCs on Gene Transcription

Increased transcription
Lipocortin-1 (phospholipase A_2 inhibitor)
β_2 Adrenoceptor
Secretory leukoprotease inhibitor
Clara cell protein (CC10, phospholipase A_2 inhibitor)
IL-1 receptor antagonist
IL-1R2 (decoy receptor)
IκB-α (inhibitor of NF-κB)

Decreased transcription
Cytokines (IL-1, IL-2, IL-3, IL-4, IL-5, IL-6, IL-9, IL-11, IL-12, IL-13, IL-16, IL-17, IL-18, TNF-α, GM-CSF, SCF)
Chemokines (IL-8, RANTES, MIP-1α, MCP-1, MCP-3, MCP-4, eotaxins)
Inducible nitric oxide synthase (iNOS)
Inducible cyclooxygenase (COX-2)
Cytoplasmic phospholipase A_2 (cPLA$_2$)
Endothelin-1
NK$_1$ receptors, NK$_2$ receptors
Bradykinin B$_1$ and B$_2$ receptors
Adhesion molecules (ICAM-1, E-selectin)

a role, whereas the transcription factor nuclear factor of activated T cells (NF-AT) is important (33). AP-1 is a component of the NF-AT transcription complex, so that corticosteroids inhibit IL-5, at least in part, by inhibiting the AP-1 component of NF-AT.

Effect on Anti-Inflammatory Cytokines

Corticosteroids may also increase anti-inflammatory mechanisms that may be defective in asthma (34,35). Thus, inhaled corticosteroids increase the production of IL-10 by macrophages in patients with asthma in whom secretion of this anti-inflammatory cytokine is reduced (36).

Effect on T Lymphocytes

T-helper 2 (Th2) lymphocytes have an important orchestrating role in asthma through the release of the cytokines IL-4, IL-5, IL-9, and IL-13 and may be an important target for corticosteroids in asthma therapy. The effects of corticosteroid on T-cell survival are complex as corticosteroids induce apoptosis (37), but may also inhibit apoptosis induced by other stimuli; both effects appear to involve gene induction (38).

Effect on Dendritic Cells and Antigen Presentation

Dendritic cells in the epithelium of the respiratory tract appear to play a critical role in antigen presentation in the lung as they have the capacity to take up allergen, process it into peptides, and present it via major histocompatibility complex (MHC) molecules on the cell surface for presentation to uncommitted T lymphocytes. In experimental animals the number of dendritic cells is markedly reduced by systemic and inhaled corticosteroids, thus dampening the immune response in the airways (39). A reduction in airway dendritic cells is also seen after treatment with inhaled steroids in patients with asthma (40). Corticosteroids inhibit the uptake of antigen by dendritic cells, but not the presentation of antigen to T cells (41).

Corticosteroids inhibit the transcription of IL-4, IL-5, and IL-13, and it is likely that switching off these key cytokines contributes importantly to their efficacy in controlling allergic diseases. Surprisingly, corticosteroids tip the balance toward Th2 cell predominance. This may be through suppression of interferon-γ (IFN-γ), which normally inhibits Th2 differentiation in response to IL-4 (42), or by suppression of IL-12 production and IL-12 receptor function, which promote expression of Th1 cytokines (43). Corticosteroids might therefore be expected to help polarize the immune response to the proinflammatory Th2 pattern, were it not for the overriding inhibitory effects of these agents on the secretion of IL-4, IL-5, and IL-13. Another apparently detrimental effect of corticosteroids involves the IL-4-stimulated production of IgE that is seen in B lymphocytes treated with hydrocortisone (44) and in vivo in asthmatic patients after one week of treatment with oral prednisolone (45). This observation explains why treatment with corticosteroids, even at high systemic doses, fails to inhibit responsiveness to common allergens in the skin prick test (46).

The molecular basis for these paradoxical effects of corticosteroids may be due to effects on IgE synthesis (47). Corticosteroid-induced IgE synthesis, in the presence of IL-4, depends on increased expression of the costimulatory molecule CD40 ligand (CD40L), a transmembrane glycoprotein belonging to the tumor necrosis factor (TNF) superfamily. CD40L is normally expressed on activated T lymphocytes, where it interacts with CD40, a surface glycoptotein related to TNF receptors that is expressed on all B lymphocytes (Fig. 2). The interaction between CD40L and CD40 is critical to the induction of IgE synthesis by IL-4 and IL-13 (48). Interestingly, the gene for CD40L, which maps to the X chromosome, is mutated in patients with X-linked hyper-IgM syndrome (49). Such individuals have low levels of secreted immunoglobulins,

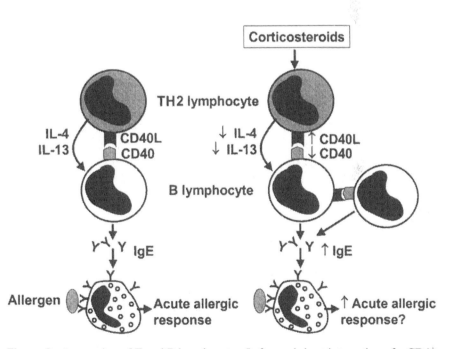

Figure 2   Interaction of T and B lymphocytes. Left panel show interaction of a CD4$^+$ T helper-2 (Th2) cell with a B lymphocytes, with release of cytokines IL-4 and IL-13. Interactions between CD40 and its ligand CD40L induce IgE synthesis and thus sensitize mast cells, which can then be triggered by allergen to activate an acute allergic response. The right panel shows the complex effects of corticosteroids, which increase the expression of CD40L in T and B cells (thereby increasing IgE formation and, potentially, acute allergic responses), but which also decrease expression of CD40L and the synthesis of IL-4 and IL-5, thus counteracting these effects.

and they fail to induce IgE synthesis in response to corticosteroids. A blocking CD40-Ig fusion protein inhibits the effects of hydrocortisone on IgE synthesis in normal B cell (47). The effect of corticosteroids on CD40L is mediated by GR, as it is blocked by the GR antagonist mifepristone (RU 486). However, corticosteroids inhibit CD40L expression in human peripheral blood $CD4^+$ lymphocytes (50), suggesting that the response to steroids differs between cell types or in the absence or presence of IL-4. Although corticosteroids increase CD40L in B lymphocytes, other studies show that in the same cells they suppress the expression of CD40, which acts as a receptor for CD40L, thus potentially diminishing any functional effect of corticosteroids on IgE production (51). Furthermore, corticosteroids suppress the synthesis of IL-4 and IL-13, which are necessary for IgE production. The suppressive effects of corticosteroids on inflammatory genes, such as IL-4 and CD40, are seen at lower concentrations than the effects that involve increased transcription, such as the increase in CD40L.

IV. Theophylline

Theophylline was previously considered to be bronchodilator, but because it is relatively weak high doses are needed to achieve relaxation of airway smooth muscle. The mechanisms for bronchodilator action is likely to be inhibition of cyclic AMP phosphodiesterases (PDEs) in airway smooth muscle, resulting in an increase in cyclic AMP (52). Unfortunately, PDE inhibition also results in side effects, such as nausea, headaches, and cardiac arrhythmias, which limit the dose of theophylline that can be used. This led to a fall in the use of theophylline, particularly as β_2 agonists are more effective bronchodilators and do not have significant side effects. However, there is now growing evidence that theophylline may have some anti-inflammatory or immunomodulatory effects and that these may be seen at doses of theophylline that are lower than those needed for bronchodilator responses (53). The molecular mechanism for these anti-inflammatory actions is uncertain; inhibition of PDE4 has anti-inflammatory and immunomodulatory effects (54,55), but the degree of inhibition of PDEs at the low concentrations of theophylline that are clinically effective (5–10 mg/L) is trivial and unlikely to account for these effects. Recently, a novel mechanism based on interaction with HDACs has been proposed, and this predicts a synergistic interaction with corticosteroids (56).

Clinically, low-dose theophylline is an effective add-on therapy in patients whose symptoms are not controlled with low- or high-dose inhaled corticosteroids (57–59).

A. Immunomodulatory Effects

A low dose of theophylline has anti-inflammatory effects in asthma, with a reduction in airway eosinophils (60,61). This may be secondary to a reduction in Th2 cytokines, particularly IL-5, suggesting an immunomodulatory effect (62). Theophylline also promotes apoptosis in eosinophils in vitro (63), which is associated with a reduction in the anti-apoptotic protein bcl-2 (64).

For many years theophylline has been shown to have several actions on T-lymphocyte function, suggesting that it might have an immunomodulatory effect in asthma. Theophylline has a stimulatory effect on suppressor ($CD8^+$) T lymphocytes that may be relevant to the control of chronic airway inflammation (65,66), and it has an inhibitory effect on graft rejection (67). In vitro theophylline inhibits IL-2 synthesis in human T lymphocytes, an effect that is secondary to a rise in intracellular cyclic AMP concentration (68,69). At high concentrations theophylline inhibits proliferation in $CD4^+$ and $CD8^+$ cells, an effect that is mediated via inhibition of PDE4 (55). Theophylline also inhibits the chemotactic response of T lymphocytes, an effect that is also mediated through PDE inhibition (70). In allergen-induced airway inflammation in guinea pigs, theophylline has a significant inhibitory effect on eosinophil infiltration (71), suggesting that it may inhibit the T-cell-derived cytokines responsible for this eosinophilic response. Theophylline has been reported to decrease circulating concentrations of IL-4 and IL-5 in asthmatic patients (72). In asthmatic patients, low-dose theophylline treatment results in an increase in activated circulating $CD4^+$ and $CD8^+$ T cells but a decrease in these cells in the airways, suggesting that it may reduce the trafficking of activated T cells to the airways (73). This is supported by studies in allergen challenge, where low-dose theophylline decreases the number of activated $CD4^+$ and $CD8^+$ T cells in bronchoalveolar lavage fluid after allergen challenge and this is mirrored by an increase in these cells in peripheral blood (74). These effects are seen even in patients treated with high does of inhaled corticosteroids, indicating that the molecular effects of theophylline are likely to be different from those of corticosteroids. Theophylline induces apoptosis of T lymphocytes, thus reducing their survival (75). This effect may be mediated via PDE4 inhibition, so may not be relevant to clinical doses of theophylline.

V. Antileukotrienes

Antileukotrienes are the first new class of drug to be introduced in asthma therapy in over 30 years. The cysteinyl-leukotriene receptor antagonists zafirlukast, montelukast, and pranlukast significantly improve lung function and reduce symptoms of asthma (76). However, they are far less effective than a low dose of inhaled corticosteroids (77,78) but have an add-on effect when added to inhaled corticosteroids (79,80). The improvement provided by these drugs has an immediate onset and is largely explained by reversal of the bronchoconstrictor effect of cysteinyl-leukotrienes. However, there is some evidence for a weak anti-inflammatory effect. There is a small reduction in circulating eosinophils and in eosinophils in induced sputum and bronchial biopsies (80–82). The mechanism of this effect is uncertain, but in animal models antileukotrienes appear to reduce the expression of IL-5 (83), suggesting a possible immunomodulatory effect. Antileukotrienes reduce eosinophil survival induced by cysteinyl-leukotrienes and GM-CSF (84).

In turn, immune mechanism may regulate the synthesis of cysteinyl-leukotrienes. Thus, IL-4 has a marked effect on the expression of LTC_4 synthase in human mast cells (85), suggesting that immunomodulation may inhibit the increased leukotriene production in asthma.

VI. β_2-Agonists

In contrast to corticosteroids, inhaled β_2-agonists have no effect on the chronic inflammation of asthma (86–88). However, β_2-agonists have inhibitory effects on several inflammatory cells in vitro (89), and the lack of effects in vivo may be accounted for by desensitisation of β_2-receptors after repeated administration of β_2-agonists.

Peripheral blood lymphocytes express β_2-receptors and β_2-agonists increase cyclic AMP concentrations (90) and are expressed equally on both B and T lymphocytes. Helper ($CD4^+$) T cells are reported to have a lower density of β_2-receptors than suppressor ($CD8^+$) T cells (91). The β_2 agonists inhibit synthesis and release of GM-CSF, IFN-γ, and IL-3 but have no effect on expression of IL-4 (92). However, the β-receptor on lymphocytes is rapidly tachyphylactic; therefore, any effect on lymphocyte function may not be relevant in vivo.

VII. Steroid-Sparing Therapies

Several treatments have been used in asthma in an attempt to reduce the requirement for oral corticosteroids in patients with steroid-dependent asthma, but these treatments have serious side effects of their own and are therefore not widely used. The clinical effectiveness of these treatments, including methotrexate, oral gold, troleandomycin, and cyclosporin, are minimal (93–96). All of these treatments may have immunomodulatory effects, although these are poorly understood in the case of methotrexate, gold, and troleandomycin. Cyclosporin A is a more specific modulator of T cells and inhibits the production of Th2 cytokines (97). In clinical studies cyclosporin A has a small steroid-sparing effect (98) and inhibits allergen-induced late responses (99). However, in clinical practice it is not very effective (95). This suggests that T lymphocytes do not have an important clinical role in patients with severe asthma and that the patients whose symptoms are not controlled on oral steroids have some other mechanism contributing to their pathophysiology. It is possible that inhaled delivery might be more effective as this may have fewer toxic effects, allowing higher local concentrations and in a broader range of patients.

VIII. Specific Immunotherapy

Specific immunotherapy using extracts of allergens has some beneficial effect in asthma in highly selected patients with single allergy responses (100,101) but is not very effective in patients with multiple sensitivities, which is the usual case (102). There is also a risk of adverse local and systemic reactions, particularly in patients with asthma. However, immunotherapy, may have immunomodulatory effects and has the potential for long-term modification of the allergic inflammatory response, as demonstrated in the treatment of hay fever (103). Specific immunotherapy may alter the balance of the immune response, tipping the balance from Th2 predominance to Th1 predominance, as evidenced by a reduction in IL-4 and IL-5 and an increase in IFN-γ (104). This may be due to increased local production of IL-12 (105) and increased production of the anti-inflammatory cytokine IL-10 (106).

IX. Future Prospects

Although several currently used antiasthma therapies have immunomodulatory effects in patients with asthma, it is still uncertain how important these are in contributing to their clinical benefit. The disappointing clinical effect of cyclosporin A, a relatively pure immunomodulator, suggests that immune mechanisms may not be so critical in patients with established asthma, at least in those patients with severe disease. However, more specific and less toxic immunomodulators are now in clinical development, as discussed elsewhere in this volume. It is possible that some patients might benefit more than others from this approach or that immunomodulators might be more useful at particular times in the natural history of asthma.

References

1. Busse WW, Lemanske RF. Asthma. N Engl J Med 2001; 344:350–362.
2. Barnes PJ. Therapeutic strategies for allergic diseases. Nature 1999;402:B31–B38.
3. Barnes PJ. New treatments for asthma. Eur J Intern Med 2000;11:9–20.
4. Global Initiative for Asthma. Global strategy for asthma management and prevention. NHLBI/WHO Workshop Report, Publication 95-3659, 1995.
5. Barnes PJ. Inhaled glucocorticoids for asthma. Engl J Med 1995;332:868–875.
6. Barnes PJ, Pedersen S, Busse WW. Efficacy and safety of inhaled corticosteroids: an update. Am J Respir Crit Care Med 1998;157:S1–S53.
7. Tasche MJ, Uijen JH, Bernsen RM, de Jongste JC, van Der W. Inhaled disodium cromoglycate (DSCG) as maintenance therapy in children with asthma: a systematic review. Thorax 2000;55:913–920.
8. Hill SJ, Tattersfield AE. Corticosteroid sparing agents in asthma. Thorax 1995;50:577–582.

9. Barnes PJ. Is there a role for immunotherapy in the treatment of asthma? No [editorial]. Am J Respir Crit Care Med 1996; 154:1227–1228.
10. Nelson HS. Beta-adrenergic bronchodilators. N Engl J Med 1995;333:499–506.
11. Barnes PJ, Pauwels RA. Theophylline in asthma: time for reappraisal? Eur Respir J 1994; 7:579–591.
12. Nelson HS. Advair: combination treatment with fluticasone propionate/salmeterol in the treatment of asthma. J Allergy Clin Immunol 2001; 107:398–416.
13. Zetterstrom O, Buhl R, Mellem H, Perpiña M, Hedman J, O'Neill S, Ekström T. Improved asthma control with budesonide/formoterol in a single inhaler, compared with budesonide alone. Eur Respir Dis 2001; 18, 254–261.
14. Barnes PJ. Anti-inflammatory actions of glucocorticoids: molecular mechanisms. Clin Sci 1998; 94:557–572.
15. Bamberger CM, Bamberger AM, de Castr M, Chrousos GP. Glucocorticoid receptor β, a potential endogenous inhibitor of glucocorticoid action in humans. J Clin Invest 1995; 95:2435–2441.
16. Reichardt HM, Kaestner KH, Tuckermann J, Kretz O, Wessely O, Bock R, Gass P, Schmid W, Herrlich P, Angel P, Schutz G. DNA binding of the glucocorticoid receptor is not essential for survival. Cell 1998; 93:531–541.
17. Ito K, Barnes PJ, Adcock IM. Glucocorticoid receptor recruitment of histone deacetylase 2 inhibits IL-1b-induced histone H4 acetylation on lysines 8 and 12. Mol Cell Biol 2000; 20:6891–6903.
18. Barnes PJ, Karin M. Nuclear factor-κB: a pivotal transcription factor in chronic inflammatory diseases. N Engl J Med 1997; 336:1066–1071.
19. Barnes PJ, Adcock IM. Transcription factors and asthma. Eur Respir J 1998; 12:221–234.
20. Newton R, Hart LA, Stevens DA, Bergmann M, Donnelly LE, Adcock IM, Barnes PJ. Effect of dexamethasone on interleukin-1β (IL-1β)–induced nuclear factor-κB (NF-κB) and κB-dependent transcription in epithelial cells. Eur J Biochem 1998; 254:81–89.
21. Hart L, Lim S, Adcock I, Barnes PJ, Chung KF. Effects of inhaled corticosteroid therapy on expression and DNA-binding activity of nuclear factor-κB in asthma. Am J Respir Crit Care Med 2000; 161:224–231.
22. Wolffe AP, Hayes JJ. Chromatin disruption and modification. Nucl Acids Res 1999; 27:711–720.
23. Grunstein M. Histone acetylation in chromatin structure and transcription. Nature 1997; 389:349–352.
24. Kamei Y, Xu L, Heinzel T, Torchia J, Kurokawa R, Gloss B, Lin SC, Heyman RA, Rose DW, Glass CK, Rosenfeld MG. A CBP integrator complex mediates transcriptional activation and AP-1 inhibition by nuclear receptors. Cell 1996; 85:403–414.
25. Ogryzko VV, Schiltz RL, Russanova V, Howard BH, Nakatani Y. The transcriptional coactivators p300 and CBP are histone acetyltransferases. Cell 1996; 87:953–959.
26. Imhof A, Wolffe AP. Transcription: gene control by targeted histone acetylation. Curr Biol 1998; 8:R422–424.

27. Ito K, Jazwari E, Cosio B, Barnes PJ, Adcock IM. p65-activated histone acetyltransferase activity is repressed by glucocorticoids: mifepristone fails to recruit HDAC2 to the p65/HAT complex. J Biol Chem 2001; 276: 30208–30215.

28. Kuo MH, Allis CD. Roles of histone acetyltransferases and deacetylases in gene regulation. Bioessays 1998; 20:615–626.

29. Newton R, Staples KJ, Hart L, Barnes PJ, Bergmann M. GM-CSF expression in pulmonary epithelial cells is regulated negatively by post-transcriptional mechanisms. Biochem Biophys Res Commun 2001 (in press).

30. Bergmann M, Barnes PJ, Newton R. Molecular regulation of granulocyte macrophage colony-stimulating factor in human lung epithelial cells by interleukin (IL)-1β, IL-4, and IL-13 involves both transcriptional and post-transcriptional mechanisms. Am J Respir Cell Mol Biol 2000; 22:582–589.

31. Chung KF, Barnes PJ. Cytokines in asthma. Thorax 1999; 54:825–857.

32. Lilly CM, Nakamura H, Kesselman H, Nagler Anderson C, Asano K, Garcia Zepeda EA, Rothenberg ME, Drazen JM, Luster AD. Expression of eotaxin by human lung epithelial cells: induction by cytokines and inhibition by glucocorticoids. J Clin Invest 1997; 99:1767–1773.

33. Rao A, Luo C, Hogan PG. Transcription factors of the NFAT family: regulation and function. Annu Rev Immunol 1997; 15:707–747.

34. Barnes PJ. Endogenous inhibitory mechanisms in asthma. Am J Respir Crit Care Med 2000; 161:S176–S181.

35. Barnes PJ, Lim S. Inhibitory cytokines in asthma. Mol Med Today 1998;4:452–458.

36. John M, Lim S, Seybold J, Robichaud A, O'Connor B, Barnes PJ, Chung KF. Inhaled corticosteroids increase IL-10 but reduce MIP-1α, GM-CSF and IFN-γ release from alveolar macrophages in asthma. Am J Respir Crit Care Med 1998; 157:256–262.

37. Evans-Storms RB, Cidlowski JA. Regulation of apoptosis by steroid hormones. J Steroid Biochem Mol Biol 1995; 53:1–8.

38. Riccardi C, Cifone MG, Migliorati G. Glucocorticoid hormone-induced modulation of gene expression and regulation of T-cell death: role of GITR and GILZ, two dexamethasone-induced genes. Cell Death Differ 1999; 6:1182–1189.

39. Nelson DJ, McWilliam AS, Haining S, Holt PG. Modulation of airway intraepithelial dendritic cells following exposure to steroids. Am J Respir Crit Care Med 1995; 151:475–481.

40. Hoogsteden HC, Verhoeven GT, Lambrecht BN, Prins JB. Airway inflammation in asthma and chronic obstructive pulmonary disease with special emphasis on the antigen-presenting dendritic cell: influence of treatment with fluticasone propionate. Clin Exp Allergy 1999; 29 Suppl 2:116–124.

41. Holt PG, Thomas JA. Steroids inhibit uptake and/or processing but not presentation of antigen by airway dendritic cells. Immunology 1997; 91:145–150.

42. Ramirez F. Glucocorticoids induce a Th2 response in vitro. Dev Immunol 1998; 6:233–243.

43. Wu CY, Wang K, McDyer JF, Seder RA. Prostaglandin E$_2$ and dexamethasone inhibit IL-12 receptor expression and IL-12 responsiveness. J Immunol 1998; 161:2723–2730.

44. Jabara HH, Ahern DJ, Vercelli D, Geha RS. Hydrocortisone and IL-4 induce IgE isotype switching in human B cells. J Immunol 1991; 147:1557–1560.

45. Zieg G, Lack G, Harbeck RJ, Gelfand EW, Leung DY. In vivo effects of glucocorticoids on IgE production. J Allergy Clin Immunol 1994; 94:222–230.
46. Barnes PJ. Corticosteroids, IgE, and atopy. J Clin Invest 2001; 107:265–266.
47. Jabara HH, Brodeur SR, Geha RS. Glucocorticoids upregulate CD40 ligand (CD40L) expression and induce CD40L dependent immunoglobulin isotype switching. J Clin Invest 2001; 107:371–378.
48. Spriggs MK, Armitage RJ, Strockbine L, Clifford KN, Macduff BM, Sato TA, Maliszewski CR, Fanslow WC. Recombinant human CD40 ligand stimulates B cell proliferation and immunoglobulin E secretion. J Exp Med 1992; 176:1543–1550.
49. Aruffo A, Farrington M, Hollenbaugh D, Li X, Milatovich A, Nonoyama S, Bajorath J, Grosmaire LS, Stenkamp R, Neubauer M. The CD40 ligand, gp39, is defective in activated T cells from patients with X-linked hyper-IgM syndrome. Cell 1993; 72:291–300.
50. Bischof F, Melms A. Glucocorticoids inhibit CD40 ligand expression of peripheral CD4+ lymphocytes. Cell Immunol 1998; 187:38–44.
51. Jirapongsananuruk O, Leung DY. The modulation of B7.2 and B7.1 on B cells by immunosuppressive agents. Clin Exp Immunol 1999; 118:1–8.
52. Rabe KF, Magnussen H, Dent G. Theophylline and selective PDE inhibitors as bronchodilators and smooth muscle relaxants. Eur Respir J 1995; 8:637–642.
53. Barnes PJ, Pauwels RA. Theophylline in asthma: time for reappraisal? Eur Respir J 1994,7:579–591.
54. Torphy TJ. Phosphodiesterase isoenzymes. Am J Respir Crit Care Med 1998; 157:351–370.
55. Giembycz MA, Corrigan CJ, Seybold J, Newton R, Barnes PJ. Identification of cyclic AMP phosphodiesterases 3, 4 and 7 in human CD4+ and CD8+ T-lymphocytes. Br J Pharmacol 1996; 118:1945–1958.
56. Ito K, Lim S, Caramori G, Cosio B, Chung KF, Adcock JM, Barnes PJ. A molecular mechanism of action of theophylline: induction of histone deacetylase activity to decrease inflammatory gene expression. Proc Natl Acad Sci USA 2002; 99:8921–8926.
57. Evans DJ, Taylor DA, Zetterstrom O, Chung KF, O'Connor BJ, Barnes PJ. A comparison of low-dose inhaled budesonide plus theophylline and high-dose inhaled budesonide for moderate asthma. N Engl J Med 1997; 337:1412–1418.
58. Ukena D, Harnest U, Sakalauskas R, Magyar P, Vetter N, Steffen H, Leichtl S, Rathgeb F, Keller A, Steinijans VW. Comparison of addition of theophylline to inhaled steroid with doubling of the dose of inhaled steroid in asthma [In Process Citation]. Eur Respir J 1997; 10:2754–2760.
59. Lim S, Jatakanon A, Gordon D, Macdonald C, Chung KF, Barnes PJ. Comparison of high dose inhaled steroids, low dose inhaled steroids plus low dose theophylline, and low dose inhaled steroids alone in chronic asthma in general practice. Thorax 2000; 55:837–841.
60. Sullivan P, Bekir S, Jaffar Z, Page C, Jeffery P, Costello J. Anti-inflammatory effects of low-dose oral theophylline in atopic asthma. Lancet 1994; 343:1006–1008.
61. Lim S, Tomita K, Carramori G, Jatakanon A, Oliver B, Keller A, Adcock I, Chung KF, Barnes PJ. Low-dose theophylline reduces eosinophilic inflammation but not exhaled nitric oxide in mild asthma. Am J Respir Crit Care Med 2001; 16:273–276.

62. Finnerty JP, Lee C, Wilson S, Madden J, Djukanovic R, Holgate ST. Effects of theophylline on inflammatory cells and cytokines in asthmatic subjects: a placebo-controlled parallel group study. Eur Respir J 1996; 9:1672–1677.

63. Yasui K, Hu B, Nakazawa T, Agematsu K, Komiyama A. Theophylline accelerates human granulocyte apoptosis not via phosphodiesterase inhibition. J Clin Invest 1997; 100:1677–1684.

64. Chung IY, Nam-Kung EK, Lee NM, Chang HS, Kim DJ, Kim YH, Park CS. The down regulation of bcl-2 expression is necessary for theophylline-induced apoptosis of eosinophil. Cell Immunol 2000; 203:95–102.

65. Shohat B, Volovitz B, Varsano I. Induction of suppressor T cells in asthmatic children by theophylline treatment. Clin Allergy 1983; 13:487–493.

66. Fink G, Mittelman M, Shohat B, Spitzer SA. Theophylline-induced alterations in cellular immunity in asthmatic patients. Clin Allergy 1987; 17:313–316.

67. Guillou PJ, Ramsden C, Kerr M, Davison AM, Giles GR. A prospective controlled clinical trial of aminophylline as an adjunct immunosuppressive agent. Transplant proc 1984; 16:1218–1220.

68. Didier M, Aussel C, Ferrua B, Fehlman M. Regulation of interleukin 2 synthesis by cAMP in human T cells. J Immunol 1987; 139:1179–1184.

69. Mary D, Aussel C, Ferrua B, Fehlmann M. Regulation of interleukin 2 synthesis by cAMP in human T cells. J Immunol 1987; 139:1179–1184.

70. Hidi R, Timmermans S, Liu E, Schudt C, Dent G, Holgate ST, Djukanovic R. Phosphodiesterase and cyclic adenosine monophosphate-dependent inhibition of T-lymphocyte chemotaxis. Eur Respir J 2000; 15:342–349.

71. Sanjar S, Aoki S, Kristersson A, Smith D, Morley J. Antigen challenge induces pulmonary eosinophil accumulation and airway hyperreactivity in sensitized guinea pigs: the effect of anti-asthma drugs. Br J Pharmacol 1990; 99:679–686.

72. Kosmas EN, Michaelides SA, Polychronaki A, Roussou T, Toukmatzi S, Polychronopoulos V, Baxevanis CN. Theophylline induces a reduction in circulating interleukin-4 and interleukin-5 in atopic asthmatics. Eur Respir J 1999; 13: 53–58.

73. Kidney J, Dominguez M, Taylor PM, Rose M, Chung KF, Barnes PJ. Immunomodulation by theophylline in asthma: demonstration by withdrawal of therapy. Am J Respir Crit Care Med 1995; 151:1907–1914.

74. Jaffar ZH, Sullivan P, Page C, Costello J. Low-dose theophylline modulates T-lymphocyte activation in allergen-challenged asthmatics. Eur Respir J 1996; 9:456–462.

75. Ohta K, Yamashita N. Apoptosis of eosinophils and lymphocytes in allergic inflammation. J Allergy Clin Immunol 1999; 104:14–21.

76. Drazen JM, Israel E, O'Byrne PM. Treatment of asthma with drugs modifying the leukotriene pathway. N Engl J Med 1999; 340:197–206.

77. Busse W, Raphael GD, Galant S, Kalberg C, Goode-Sellers S, Srebro S, Edwards L, Rickard K. Low-dose fluticasone propionate compared with montelukast for first-line treatment of persistent asthma: a randomized clinical trial. J Allergy Clin Immunol 2001; 107:461–468.

78. Kim KT, Ginchansky EJ, Friedman BF, Srebro S, Pepsin PJ, Edwards L, Stanford RH, Rickard K. Fluticasone propionate versus zafirlukast: effect in

patients previously receiving inhaled corticosteroid therapy. Ann Allergy Asthma Immunol 2000; 85:398–406.

79. Lofdahl CG, Reiss TF, Leff JA, Israel E, Noonan MJ, Finn A, Seidenberg BC, Capizzi T, Kundu S, Godard P. Randomised, placebo controlled trial of effect of a leukotriene receptor antagonist, montelukast, on tapering inhaled corticosteroids in asthmatic patients. Br Med J 1999; 319:87–90.

80. Malmstrom K, Rodriguez-Gomez G, Guerra J, Villaran C, Pineiro A, Wei LX, Seidenberg BC, Reiss TF. Oral montelukast, inhaled beclomethasone, and placebo for chronic asthma. A randomized, controlled trial. Ann Intern Med 1999; 130:487–495.

81. Pizzichini E, Leff JA, Reiss TF, Hendeles L, Boulet LP, Wei LX, Efthimiadis AE, Zhang J, Hargreave FE. Montelukast reduces airway eosinophilic inflammation in asthma: a randomized, controlled trial. Eur Respir J 1999; 14:12–18.

82. Nakamura Y, Hoshino M, Sim JJ, Ishii K, Hosaka K, Sakamoto T. Effect of the leukotriene receptor antagonist pranlukast on cellular infiltration in the bronchial mucosa of patients with asthma. Thorax 1998; 53:835–841.

83. Hojo M, Suzuki M, Maghni K, Hamid Q, Powell WS, Martin JG. Role of cysteinyl leukotrienes in CD4(+) T cell-driven late allergic airway responses. J Pharmacol Exp Ther 2000; 293:410–416.

84. Lee E, Robertson T, Smith J, Kilfeather S. Leukotriene receptor antagonists and synthesis inhibitors reverse survival in eosinophils of asthmatic individuals. Am J Respir Crit Care Med 2000; 161:1881–1886.

85. Hsieh FH, Lam BK, Penrose JF, Austen KF, Boyce JA. T helper cell type 2 cytokines coordinately regulate immunoglobulin E-dependent cysteinyl leukotriene production by human cord blood-derived mast cells: profound induction of leukotriene C(4) synthase expression by interleukin 4. J Exp Med 2001; 193: 123–133.

86. Laitinen LA, Laitinen A, Haahtela T. A comparative study of the effects of an inhaled corticosteroid, budesonide, and of a β_2-agonist, terbutaline, on airway inflammation in newly diagonised asthma. J Allergy Clin Immunol 1992; 90: 32–42.

87. Gardiner PV, Ward C, Booth H, Allison A, Hendrick DJ, Walters EH. Effect of eight weeks of treatment with salmeterol on bronchoalveolar lavage inflammatory indices in asthmatics. Am J Respir Crit Care Med 1994; 150:1006–1011.

88. Howarth PH, Beckett P, Dahl R. The effect of long-acting beta2-agonists on airway inflammation in asthmatic patients. Respir Med 2000; 94 Suppl F:S22–S25.

89. Barnes PJ. Effect of beta agonists on inflammatory cells. J Allergy Clin Immunol 1999; 104:10–17.

90. Kariman K. β-Adrenergic receptor binding in lymphocytes from patients with asthma. Lung 1980; 158:41–51.

91. Maisel AS, Fowler P, Rearden A, Motulsky HJ, Michel MC. A new method for isolation of human lymphocyte-subsets reveals differential regulation of β-adregergic receptors by terbutaline treatment. Clin Pharmacol Ther 1989; 46:429–439.

92. Borger P, Hoekstra Y, Esselink MT, Postma DS, Zaagsma J, Vellenga E, Kauffman HF. Beta-adrenoceptor-mediated inhibition of IFN-γ, IL-3, and GM-

CSF mRNA accumulation in activated human T lymphocytes is solley mediated by the beta2-adrenoceptor subtype. Am J Respir Cell Mol Biol 1998; 19:400–407.

93. Davies H, Olson L, Gibson P. Methotrexate as a steroid sparing agent for asthma in adults. Cochrane Database Syst Rev 2000; 2:CD000391.

94. Evans DJ, Cullinan P, Geddes DM. Gold as an oral corticosteroid sparing agent in stable asthma (Cochrane Review). Cochrane Database Syst Rev 2001; 2:CD002985.

95. Evans DJ, Cullinan P, Geddes DM. Cyclosporin as an oral corticosteroid sparing agent in stable asthma (Cochrane Review). Cochrane Database Syst Rev 2001; 2:CD002993.

96. Evans DJ, Cullinan P, Geddes DM. Troleandomycin as an oral corticosteroid steroid sparing agent in stable asthma (Cochrane Review). Cochrane Database Syst Rev 2001; 2:CD002987.

97. Corrigan CJ, Brown PH, Barnes NC, Tsai J-J, Frew AJ, Kay AB. Peripheral blood T lymphocyte activation and comparison of the T lymphocyte inhibitory effects of glucocorticoids and cyclosporin A. Am Rev Respir Dis 1991; 144:1026–1032.

98. Lock SH, Kay AB, Barnes NC. Double-blind, placebo-controlled study of cyclosporin A as a corticosteroid-sparing agent in corticosteroid-dependent asthma [see comments]. Am J Respir Crit Care Med 1996; 153:509–514.

99. Sihra BS, Kon OM, Durham SR, Walker S, Barnes NC, Kay AB. Effect of cyclosporin A on the allergen-induced late asthmatic reaction. Thorax 1997; 52:447–452.

100. Creticos PS, Reed CE, Norman PS, Khoury J, Adkinson NF, Buncher R, Busse WW, Bush RK, Gaddie J, Li JT, Richerson HB, Rosenthal RR, Solomon WR, Steinberg P, Yunginger JW. Ragweed immunotherapy in adult asthma. N Engl J Med 1996; 334:501–506.

101. Abramson MJ, Puy RM, Weiner JM. Allergen immunotherapy for asthma. Cochrane Database Syst Rev 2000;2:CD001186.

102. Adkinson NF, Jr., Eggleston PA, Eney D, Goldstein EO, Schuberth KC, Bacon JR, Hamilton RG, Weiss ME, Arshad H, Meinert CL, Tonascia J, Wheeler B. A controlled trial of immunotherapy for asthma in allergic children. N Engl J Med 1997; 336:324–331.

103. Durham SR, Walker SM, Varga EM, Jacobson MR, O'Brien F, Noble W, Till SJ, Hamid QA, Nouri-Aria KT. Long-term clinical efficacy of grass-pollen immunotherapy. N Engl J Med 1999; 341:468–475.

104. Durham SR, Till SJ. Immunologic changes associated with allergen immunotherapy. J Allergy Clin Immunol 1998; 102:157–164.

105. Hamid QA, Schotman E, Jacobson MR, Walker SM, Durham SR. Increases in IL-12 messenger RNA+ cells accompany inhibition of allergen-induced late skin responses after successful grass pollen immunotherapy. J Allergy Clin Immunol 1997; 99:254–260.

106. Akdis CA, Blesken T, Akdis M, Wuthrich B, Blaser K. Role of interleukin 10 in specific immunotherapy. J Clin Invest 1998; 102:98–106.

22

Immunomodulators in the Treatment of Asthma

MARTIN J. PLUMMERIDGE

Frenchay Hospital
Bristol, England

ANTHONY J. FREW

University of Southampton School of Medicine
Southampton General Hospital
Southampton, England

I. Introduction

For many years glucocorticosteroids (GCS) have been acknowledged as effective agents in the control of asthma in the majority of patients. As our understanding of the central role of the pulmonary immune response and its dysregulation in the pathophysiology of asthma has increased, we have come to comprehend the reasons for their efficacy. The cellular changes associated with the inflammatory process of asthma and the role of cell-derived products such as cytokines are discussed elsewhere in this volume. In the half-century since the introduction of systemic GCS in the treatment of asthma, their unacceptable long-term side effects have been increasingly appreciated. The introduction of inhaled GCS in the 1970s and of high-dose inhaled GCS in the 1980s allowed the effective use of GCS by many asthmatics without the need for systemic treatment.

Unfortunately, a significant number of asthmatics do not achieve adequate control of their disease with inhaled GCS and often require treatment with systemic GCS (see Table 1). The search for acceptable treatments for this group of asthmatics has led to an interest in the use of nonsteroidal immunomodulators in the treatment of asthma. The aims of this treatment are twofold: to provide better control of the symptoms of asthma and, where possible, to allow the withdrawal of systemic GCS or a clinically significant reduction in the dose. The aim of this chapter is to discuss the use of these immunomodulators in the treatment of asthma, and to examine the available evidence for their use and potential problems associated with them. Newer immunomodulatory agents of potential interest will also be considered.

Table 1   Characteristics of Patients with Difficult-to-Manage Asthma

Persistent symptoms in spite of maximal therapy
Sudden unpredictable and catastrophic deterioration
Frequent exacerbations
High doses of steroids required for adequate control

II. Cyclosporin A

Cyclosporin A (CyA) is a fungal cyclic undecapeptide with potent immuno-
supressive actions. It is particularly active against T lymphocytes. CyA inhibits
cytokine gene transcription in activated T cells via inhibition of the calcineurin/
NAFT pathway. It also blocks the activation of JNK and p38 signaling pathways, which are activated by antigen recognition (1). Cytokines inhibited
include interleukins (IL)-2, -3, -4, and -5 and tumor necrosis factor (TNF) (2).
In addition, CyA inhibits other cells of potential importance in asthma, including monocytes, B lymphocytes, mast cells, basophils, and neutrophils (3,4). The
recognition of the importance of the role of the T cell and the concept of asthma
as a T-cell-driven disorder led to an interest in the use of CyA in its treatment.
Among specific effects of CyA in asthma is a reduction in airway hyperresponsiveness (AHR) (5). Moreover, CyA blocks the late asthmatic response (LAR)
and inhibits eosinophil-associated cytokine release after allergen challenge
(6,7). These effects are consistent with the drug exerting its main action on
T lymphocyte function.
     Apart from anecdotal reports and uncontrolled studies, there have been
three controlled trials with CyA in asthma. In these trials, both the efficacy of
CyA in the control of the disease and its role as a steroid-sparing agent have
been studied. The major criticisms of each of these trials are that they have
involved small numbers of patients and that, in the context of both asthma as a
chronic disease and the mode of action of CyA, they have been relatively short
term. Alexander et al. conducted a placebo-controlled cross-over trial asses-
sing the efficacy of CyA in asthma (8). After 12 weeks, CyA treatment resulted in
an improvement in both forced expiratory volume in 1 (FEV_1) and peak
expiratory flow rate (PEFR) and a reduction in exacerbations of asthma
requiring oral GCS treatment. There was no significant change in respiratory
symptoms or in bronchodilator use. Although this trial was not designed to
assess the steroid-sparing properties of CyA, this was demonstrated in another
study by Lock et al., who examined the steroid-sparing effects of CyA in 39
patients and found a significant (25%) reduction in GCS does in the actively
treated group (9). Lowest achieved steroid doses during the study period were
compared between treated and placebo group. While there were no significant
improvements in FEV_1, forced vital capacity (FVC), or symptom scores,
morning PEFR did improve. The reduction in GCS dose was statistically

significant but the actual daily dose reduction in the CyA-treated group did not appear to be of clinical importance. In contrast, Nizankowska et al. studied the effect of CyA in a group of 34 asthmatics, all of whom were steroid dependent. No significant differences in either steroid-sparing effect or lung function were observed between the CyA and placebo-treated groups (10).

The adverse effects of CyA are well recognized and potentially serious. Renal impairment is an important side effect that makes adequate assessment and monitoring of renal function mandatory. Other recognized side effects include hypertrichosis, hypertension, gingival hyperplasia, tremor, and neuropathy in combination with nonspecific flu-like symptoms. In addition, immunosuppression may increase the risk of infection. Thus while CyA is theoretically attractive as an immunomodulator in the treatment of asthma, the potential risks at present appear to outweigh the possible benefits for the majority of patients. After careful consideration and assessment, individual patients with particularly difficult steroid-dependent disease may benefit, but if no improvement is seen after 3 months there is little point in continuing therapy (11). The development of an inhaled CyA formula may appear a more attractive option in the future.

III. Antimetabolites

A number of antimetabolites are used in the treatment of both malignancies and chronic inflammatory conditions. Their general action is via inhibition of cellular function, the cells affected including those of relevance in asthma. Two agents have been investigated in the treatment of asthma, methotrexate and azathioprine.

A. Methotrexate

Methotrexate (MTX) is the most widely studied of the nonsteroidal immunomodulators used in the treatment of asthma. It is a folic acid antagonist, inhibiting dihydrofolate reductase and consequently thymidine synthesis, hence blocking the DNA synthesis and cell division. In addition to its antimetabolic effects, MTX also appears to act as an anti-inflammatory agent when used in lower doses. It inhibits histamine release from basophils, cytokine production by mononuclear cells, and neutrophil chemotaxis (12,13). Moreover, MTX increases the sensitivity of lymphocytes to the inhibitory effects of GCS when given to asthmatic subjects (14). Thus there are valid reasons for interest in MTX as an immunomodulator in asthma.

In 1988, Mullarkey and colleagues carried out a double-blind placebo-controlled trial of the use of MTX in systemic GCS-dependent asthmatic patients. This trial reported significant reduction in oral GCS dose in asthmatics using MTX (15). However, the study was both short term and rather small (13 subjects completed the trial). More significantly, no attempt was undertaken before the trial to reduce oral GCS doses to a minimum. Since this trial, subsequent controlled trials have reported various results (16–24). The largest, by Shiner et al., reported a significant decrease in steroid requirement in the MTX group with a significant reduction in the number of exacerbations of asthma requiring an increase in oral GCS dosage. There were no significant differences in lung function. However, the trial included subjects with significant smoking histories and did not attempt tapering of the steroid dose prior to commencement of the trial.

There is still no consensus on the use of MTX in asthma. Meta-analysis of 11 controlled studies has indicated a definite steroid-sparing effect in patients dependent on oral GCS (25). The overall effect on prednisolone usage was a reduction of less than 5 mg per day. The greatest effect was seen in those subjects using MTX for more than 24 weeks in whom oral GCS had been reduce at baseline. Conversely, a meta-analysis of 12 randomized double-blind placebo-controlled trials involving 250 patients concluded that the reduction in systemic steroid dose was insignificant, at slightly over 3 mg per day, and achieved at the expense of significantly more side effects (26).

Although the possible reduction in oral GCS dose may be statistically significant, its clinical significance is highly debatable. There is no effect on symptom control and no consistent effect on airflow. MTX has predictable effects on bone marrow, inhibiting neutrophil production. It can cause nausea, anorexia, diarrhea, and hair loss. Abnormalities of liver function and hepatic fibrosis are well-recognized complications of treatment, as in pulmonary toxicity. Death from *Pneumocystis carinii* pneumonia has been reported in a patient taking MTX for asthma (18). Careful consideration should be given before a therapeutic trial of MTX is undertaken. Regular testing of liver function and blood-count monitoring are required and some authorities advocate periodic measurement of gas transfer and liver biopsy. Certainly oral GCS dose should be tapered to a minimum prior to commencing MTX therapy to minimize the risk of opportunistic infection. Effect on oral GCS dose may not be seen for 3 or 4 months and if no benefit is seen by 12 months of treatment MTX should be stopped.

B. Azathioprine

Less information is available about the use of this antimetabolite in the treatment of asthma, although it is a useful steroid-sparing agent in other chronic inflammatory diseases. Two short-term studies have failed to show any benefit either in terms of symptom control or steroid-sparing properties. The duration of these trials may have been insufficient to allow potential benefits to be detected (27,28).

IV. Other Immunomodulators

There are a number of other immunomodulators with a variety of actions whose effect in other chronic inflammatory disease has resulted in interest in their potential benefit in asthma.

A. Gold Salts

Gold is used successfully in the treatment of rheumatoid arthritis. It is useful both as a steroid-sparing agent and to modify the course of the disease. In vitro studies show gold to be active in the inhibition of histamine release from basophils and mast cells, the inhibition of mast-cell leukotriene production, and the inhibition of smooth muscle contraction and antibody production, all properties of potential value in the treatment of asthma (29,30). Initially parenteral gold therapy was studied (31). In a study, 79 patients not all requiring oral steroid therapy, were treated for 30 weeks in a double-blind placebo-controlled trial. The gold-treated group had fewer symptoms and needed less concomitant antiasthma treatment, including oral GCS. This trial was followed by a study comparing gold treatment ($+/-$ immunotherapy) with "conventional" pharmacological therapy. Bronchial hyperreactivity tended to reduce in gold-treated patients and more demonstrated complete remission of symptoms. The groups treated, however, were small (32). Another small study of intramuscular gold showed only a nonsignificant steroid-sparing effect (33).

Gold therapy can also be given orally, with obvious potential advantages over parenteral treatment. In a study, 28 steroid-dependent patients achieved a significantly greater reduction in both the GCS dose and asthma exacerbations along with an increase in FEV_1 and a decrease in symptoms (34). As with the other immunomodulators discussed above, the clinical significance of these changes is debatable. The use of oral gold in a larger (136 patients) multicenter study showed that, after 28 weeks, 41.2% of those treated with gold were able to reduce their dose of oral GCS by at least 50%, compared with 26.6% of patients in the placebo group. There was no difference in either symptoms or lung function, but there was a marked improvement in subjective self-assessment in the treated group. It has been suggested that this effect was secondary to reduced systemic GCS intake (35).

Gold is not without significant side effects. Significant numbers of participants in the above studies withdrew because of dermatitis, gastrointestinal upset, and proteinuria. Neutropenia and thrombocytopenia are also recognized problems. In selected patients, oral gold may be successful but it cannot be recommended as a routine immunomodulator in the treatment of asthma.

B. Troleandomycin

This compound is a macrolide antibiotic, an oleandomycin derivative first produced in the 1950s. At one time it was used quite widely in the treatment of exacerbations of asthma. It has a number of actions including the inhibition of the hepatic metabolism of methyl prednisolone (36). It may also act via inhibition of neutrophil chemotaxis, reduction of mucus secretion, and reduction in basophil histamine release. Lymphocyte proliferation is inhibited (37,38). There is no convincing evidence of any effect on airway hyperresponsiveness.

There are no consistent conclusions from clinical trials of troleandomycin. Improvement in FEV_1, symptom control, and a reduced oral GCS requirement were seen in one trial using a placebo-controlled cross-over design (39). Conversely, a parallel group design trial found no significant difference in the potential to withdraw oral GCS over 2 years (40). Open trials suggest benefits in terms of both steroid-sparing and improved pulmonary function (41). However, side effects are potentially serious. They include increased steroid-related side effects, consistent with the effect of the drug on steroid metabolism, gastrointestinal symptoms and deranged liver function. Reduced bone mineral content and increased blood glucose have also been reported, again presumably related to alteration in steroid metabolism (41). Hence, interest in troleandomycin has diminished in the past decade, partly because of its side-effect profile and partly because of the introduction of high-dose ICS. Review of the previous data suggests there is little to justify the use of troleandomycin as an immunomodulator.

C. Dapsone

Dapsone acts via sulfone inhibition of neutrophil function. It is used in the treatment of leprosy (where its antibacterial action is also exploited) and has been used for the treatment of rheumatoid-type diseases. Its use in steroid-dependent asthma has been examined in an open trial (42). Although the trial was neither controlled nor blinded, the results showed a significant reduction in oral GCS doses. The nature and size of the trial make it impossible to ascribe this effect to dapsone alone. Recognized side effects included malaise, rashes, and hemolytic anemia. Thrombocytopenia and psychosis were observed. Drug interactions resulted in theophylline toxicity. Further trials are required before the use of dapsone as an immunomodulator in asthma can be recommended.

D. Colchicine

Colchicine is an inhibitor of neutrophil function used in the treatment of acute hyperuricemic gout. Initial studies suggested that it may be of value in asthma, but subsequent studies have suggested both a lack of effect and an unacceptable level of side effects (43,44).

E. Hydroxychloroquine

Used primarily as an antimalarial drug, hydroxychloroquine is also exploited as a disease-modifying agent for rheumatoid arthritis and other collagen diseases. It inhibits phospholipase A2, decreasing leukotriene and prostaglandin production, which makes it of potential value in the treatment of asthma (45). Initially reported as having no effect in asthma (46), hydroxychloroquine has subsequently been reported to improve symptom scores and lung function when given for 6 months. It has subsequently been shown to exert beneficial effects on airflow and serum IgE levels (47). Now that newer, more specific leukotriene receptor antagonists are available, it is unlikely that hydroxy-chloroquine has any additive value in asthma.

F. Leukotriene Modulators

In the last two decades, drugs modifying the 5-lipoxygenase (5-LO) pathway have been developed and currently two types have been registered in various countries worldwide: 5-lipoxygenase inhibitors and leukotriene receptor antagonists (LTRAs) (48). Currently, only one compound has been registered from the first category, being the 5-LO inhibitor zileuton (Zyflo®, in the USA only), whereas several LTRAs have been introduced into clinical practice (pranlukast: Ultair/Onon® [in Japan only]; zafirlukast: Accolate®; and mon-telukast: Singulair®). 5-LO inhibitors block the synthesis of all leukotrienes, while the LTRAs block the effects of the cysteinyl leukotrienes at the CysLT1 receptor. This novel class of oral antiasthma therapy has a dual mechanism of action: both (mild) bronchodilator and anti-inflammatory (mainly anti-eosinophil); both effects being superimposed on those of β_2-agonists and inhaled corticosteroids (ICS), respectively (49,50). The clinical effectiveness of the novel class is mainly based on their additive effects to ICS, which even in high oral doses could not reduce the leukotriene release in asthma (51,52). Currently, in most countries, LTRAs have been registered as additive therapy to low and moderate doses of ICS (53).

G. Intravenous Immunoglobulin

In addition to its value as replacement therapy in humoral immunodeficiency, intravenous immunoglobulin (IVIG) exerts multiple effects on the immune system and has been used to treat a variety of disorders. Its use as an immuno-modulator in asthma was also supported by the observation of low serum levels of IgG subclasses in some children with asthma (54). Asthmatics treated with IVIG have been shown to exhibit reduced lymphocyte infiltration in the air-ways and altered lymphocyte responsiveness to steroids (55,56). Initial open studies suggested benefit from IVIG both in terms of steroid-sparing effect and symptom reduction (57,58). However, subsequent double-blind controlled stud-ies have yielded conflicting results (59,60). Any improvement seen appears to be transient and ceases following cessation of therapy. On the basis of current data, the cost-benefit ratio and the possible risks of disease transmission do not jus-tify the use of IVIG in asthma.

V. The Future of Immunomodulators in the Treatment of Asthma

As has been discussed, there is only a limited role for the use of the majority of the currently available immunomodulators in asthma. Their benefits, if any, tend to be small and their side effects significant (except for leukotriene modulators). The risk:benefit ratio may be acceptable for specific patients when immunomodulators may be used under specialist supervision. Appropriate monitoring for complications is essential. Our increased understanding of the pathophysiology of asthma, together with new techniques in drug design and manufacture and in molecular biology, have already allowed us to develop promising new immunomodulators aimed more specifically at the treatment of asthma. Most of these newer treatments have been designed to target specific components of the inflammatory process found in asthmatic airways. These targets include IgE antibodies, specific cytokines and various components of the cellular recruitment process such as chemokines and vascular adhesion molecules. While large-scale placebo-controlled trials have not yet been completed, initial findings are encouraging in many cases.

A. Anti-IgE

The role of B lymphocytes and immunoglobulin in asthma is discussed in detail elsewhere in this volume. It is well established that IgE triggers mast-cell release of inflammatory mediators via attachment to high-affinity IgE receptors and subsequent cross-linking. It also plays a role in antigen presentation and in T and B lymphocyte development. The serum concentration of free IgE is significantly reduced by treatment with humanized monoclonal anti-IgE antibodies, as is the response to inhaled antigen (61,62). Initial clinical trials suggest that anti-IgE treatment may allow significant reduction of GCS dose (63). It has also been suggested that anti-IgE may affect the way that antigens are captured and presented to lymphocytes, by disrupting the IgE-focused presentation of antigens by dendritic cells. It remains to be proven whether this is a biologically important effect of anti-IgE.

B. Anticytokine Therapy

Several cytokines have been implicated in the development and expression of allergic asthma. In particular, IL-4 plays a critical role in regulating B-cell switching to make IgE, but also has effects on mucus production and endothelial adhesion molecule expression. IL-5 has a key role (64) in the development, recruitment and activation of eosinophils and some have suggested it may be more relevant to asthma, whereas IL-4 may be the cytokine relevant to allergy. IL-13 can substitute for IL-4 in B-cell switching, but has also been implicated in some aspects of airways remodeling (65). Anti-IL-5 antibodies block the development of airway eosinophilia and allergen-induced airway hyper-responsiveness in animal models (66,67). In clinical trials of monoclonal anti-IL-5 antibody, the eosinophilic response during the late phase after allergen inhalation was reduced. Interestingly, however, allergen-induced airway responses were not affected (68).

Interleukin-4 (IL-4) affects IgE class switching and endothelial adhesion molecule expression (69). IL-4 inhalation causes increased sputum eosinophilia and increases airway hyperresponsiveness in patients with asthma (70). The inhibition of IL-4 with synthesized soluble IL-4 receptor (sIL-4R) molecules results in inhibition of eosinophil recruitment and of mucus production in animal models. Preliminary clinical trials have been promising (71) and further work will be watched with interest.

C. Cytokine Therapy

Several cytokines have "antiallergic" properties, either by promoting the TH1 pattern of response, or by opposing TH2 development. In particular IFN-γ opposes the actions of IL-4, while IL-12 works upstream, influencing antigen-presenting cells so that they are biased toward the TH1 phenotype (72).

D. Interferon-Gamma

The administration of parenteral interferon-gamma to steroid-dependent asthmatic patients resulted only in a reduction in blood eosinophil numbers. There was no improvement in lung function or reduction in oral GCS requirements (73).

E. Interleukin-12

Interleukin-12 (IL-12) is a proinflammatory cytokine whose key role is to regulate the balance between TH1 and TH2 lymphocytes away from a TH2 response. There are reduced concentrations of IL-12 in the blood of patients with allergic asthma and alveolar macrophages from asthmatic subjects are deficient in IL-12 production (74,75).

In animal models, airway hyperresponsiveness and airway eosinophilia are inhibited by IL-12 (76). The administration of IL-12 to patients with mild allergic asthma resulted in a reduction in blood eosinophil count and in sputum eosinophil count following allergen challenge. There was no statistical improvement in airway hyperresponsiveness nor was the late asthmatic reaction affected. The trial was complicated by significant side effects in over 20% of the patients (77). The potentially dangerous proinflammatory properties of cytokines may limit their use as immunomodulators is asthma.

F. Anti-CD4 Monoclonal Antibody Therapy

As an alternative to targeting individual cytokines, it is possible to target CD4$^+$ T cells. Ideally, this should take out T cells responding to current stimulating antigens without damaging the T cells needed for defense against future pathogens. This anti-T-cell strategy has been used in rheumatoid arthritis and investigated in severe corticosteroid-dependent asthma (78). Significant improvement was observed in morning and evening PEFR and improvements in symptom scores were seen in a randomized double-blind placebo-controlled trial involving 22 patients. No serious adverse effects were seen.

VI. T-Cell-Specific Immunosuppressive Drugs

There are a number of newer T-cell specific drugs that may be useful in the treatment of asthma, although as yet remain untried. These include tacrolimus, rapamycin, mycophenolate mofetil, and deoxysperguanolin. These have multiple actions, including inhibition of cytokine production and IgE-dependent histamine release and blocking of T-cell stimulation via CD28 pathway and T-cell differentiation and proliferation (79).

VII. Targeting Cellular Recruitment

Monoclonal antibodies against adhesion molecules have been developed and their effects in animal models of asthma investigated. There are concerns that blocking these molecules may critically affect antigen presentation and recognition involved in normal host defense mechanisms. In animal studies, anti-ICAM-1 and anti-E-selectin have been shown to block both airway hyperresponsiveness and airway eosinophilia following allergen challenge (80,81). The action of the former was most clear cut in the noninflamed, sensitized airway, whereas the latter was more effective following allergen challenge to an inflamed airway. No trials of antiadhesion molecule therapy have been undertaken in humans as yet.

VIII. Antichemokine Strategies

Chemokines play a vital role in the recruitment and activation of inflammatory cells in asthma (82). Neutralization of RANTES results in reduced lymphocyte and eosinophil infiltration in animal models; airway hyperresponsiveness and inflammation are reduced by neutralizing MCP1 (83). The development of selective antagonists to the various chemokines may provide way of blocking cellular recruitment and controlling the pulmonary inflammatory response in asthma.

IX. Conclusions

Although existing antiasthma therapies are effective, there still remains a need for new drugs, both to assist those patients who are not controlled by existing treatment and to explore the possibility of reversing or abolishing the inflammatory and immunological processes found in asthma. Existing immunomodulatory treatments have limited value, but some have a place in the management of selected cases. Several new immunomodulatory treatments are currently going through tests and show promise. Further work needs to determine the value of these treatments, the patients who are most likely to benefit, and the parameters that should guide their use in clinical settings.

References

1. Matsuda S, Koyasu S. Mechanisms of action of cyclosporine. Immunopharmacology 2000; 47:119–135.
2. Kaufman Y, Chang AE, Robb RJ, Rosenberg SA. Mechanism of action of cyclosporin A; inhibition of lymphokine secretion studied with antigen-simulated T cell hybridomas. J Immunol 1984; 153:3107–3111.
3. Calderon E, Lockey RF, Bukantz SC, Coffey RG, Ledford DK. Is there a role for cyclosporin in asthma? J Allergy Clin Immunol 1992; 89(2):629–635.
4. Mosby J. Cyclosporin A in asthma therapy; a pharmacological rationale. J autoimmunity 1992; 5(suppl A): 265–269.
5. Fukada T, Asakawa J, Motojima S, Makino S. Cyclosporin A reduces T lymphocyte activity and improves airway hyperresponsiveness in corticosteroid dependent chronic severe asthma. Ann Allergy Asthma Immunol 1995; 75:65–72.
6. Sihra BS, Kon OM, Durham SR, Walker S, Barnes NC, Kay AB. Effect of Cyclosporin A on the allergen-induced late asthmatic reaction. Thorax 1997; 52:447–452.
7. Khan LN, Kon OM, MacFarlane, A Meng Q, Ying S, Barnes NC, Kay AB. Attenuation of the late asthmatic reaction by Cyclosporin A is associated with inhibition of bronchial eosinophils, interleukin-5, granulocyte macrophage colony-stimulating factor and eotaxin. Am J Respir Crit Care Med 2000; 162:1377–1382.
8. Alexander AG, Barnes NC, Kay AB. Trial of cyclosporin in corticosteroid-dependent chronic severe asthma. Lancet 1992; 339:324–328.
9. Lock SH, Kay AB, Barnes NC. Double-blind, placebo-controlled study of cyclosporin A as a corticosteroid-sparing agent in corticosteroid-dependent asthma. Am J Respir Crit Care Med 1996; 153:509–514.
10. Nizankowska E, Soja J, Pinis G, Szczeklik A. Treatment of steroid-dependent bronchial asthma with cyclosporin. Eur Resp J 1995; 8:1091–1099.
11. Kon OM, Kay AB. Anti-T cell strategies in asthma. Inflamm Res 1999; 48:516–523.
12. Hu S, Mitcho YL, Oronsky AL, Kerwar SS. Studies on the effect of methotrexate on macrophage function. J Rheumatol 1988; 15:206–209.
13. Nolte H, Skov PS. Inhibition of basophil methotrexate release by methotrexate. Agents Actions 1988; 23:173–176.
14. Vrugt B, Wilson S, Bron A, Shute J, Holgate ST, Djukanovic R, Aalbers R. Low dose methotrexate treatment in severe glucocorticoid dependent treatment asthma: effect on mucosal inflammation and in vitro sensitivity to glucocorticoids of mitogen-induced T-cell proliferation. Eur Resp J 2000; 15:478–485.
15. Mullarkey MF, Blumenstein BA, Andrade WP, Bailey GA, Olasen I, Wetzel CE. Methotrexate in the treatment of corticosteroid-dependent asthma. N Engl J Med 1988; 318:603–607.
16. Shiner RJ, Nunn AJ, Chung KF, Geddes DM. Randomised double-blind placebo-controlled trial of methotrexate in steroid-dependent asthma. Lancet 1990; 336:137–140.
17. Dyer PD, Vaughan TR, Weber RW. Methotrexate in the treatment of steroid-dependent asthma. J Allergy Clin Immunol 1991; 88:208–212.

18. Erzurum SC, Leff JC, Cochran JE, Ackerson LM, Szefler SJ, Martin RJ, Cott GR. Lack of benefit of methotrexate in severe steroid-dependent asthma. A double blind, placebo-controlled study. Ann Intern Med 1991; 114:353–360.

19. Trigg CJ, Davies RJ. Comparison of methotrexate 30 mg/week with placebo in chronic steroid-dependent asthma: a 12 week double-blind crossover study. Respir Med 1993; 87:211–216.

20. Coffey MJ, Sanders G, Eschenbacher WL, Tsien A, Ranesh S, Weber RW, Toews GB, McCunes WJ. The role of methotrexate in the management of steroid dependent asthma. Chest 1994; 105:117–121.

21. Shiner RJ, Katz I, Shulimzon T, Silkoff P, Benzary S. Methotrexate in steroid dependent asthma: long term results. Allergy 1994; 49:565–568.

22. Stewart GE, Diaz JD, Lockey RF, Seleznick MJ, Trudeau WL, Ledford DK. Comparison of oral pulse methotrexate with placebo in the treatment of severe glucocorticoid-dependent asthma. J Allergy Clin Immunol 1994; 94:482–489.

23. Ogirala RG, Sturm TM, Aldrich TK, Meller FF, Pacia EB, Keane AM, Finkel RI. Single high dose intramuscular triamcinolone acetate versus weekly oral methotrexate in life-threatening asthma: a double blind study. Am J Respir Crit Care Med 1995; 152:1461–1466.

24. Hedman J, Seideman P, Albertioni F, Stenius-Aarniala B. Controlled trial of methotrexate in patients with chronic severe asthma. Eur J Clin Pharmacol 1996; 49:347–349.

25. Marin MG. Low dose methotrexate spares steroid usage in steroid-dependent asthmatic patients: a meta-analysis. Chest 1997; 112:29–33.

26. Aaron SD, Dales RE, Phan B. Management of steroid-dependent asthma with methotrexate; a meta-analysis of randomised clinical trials. Respir Med 1998; 92:1059–1065.

27. Admundsson T, Kilburn KH, Lazzlo J, Krock CJ. Immunosuppressive therapy of asthma. J Allergy 1971; 47:136–147.

28. Hodges NG, Brewis RAL, Howell JBL. An evaluation of azathioprine in severe chronic asthma. Thorax 1971; 26:734–739.

29. Marone G, Columbo M, Galeone D, Guidi G, Kagey G, Sobotka A, Lichtenstein LM. Modulation of the release of histamine and arachadonic acid metabolites from human basophils and mast cells by auranofin. Agents Actions 1986; 18:100–102.

30. Malo PE, Wasserman M, Parris D, Pfeiffer D. Inhibition by auranofin on pharmacologic and antigen-induced contractions of the isolated guinea pig trachea. J Allergy Clin Immunol 1986; 77:371–376.

31. Muranaka MM, Miyamoto T, Shida T, Kabe J, Makino S, Okumara H. Gold salt in the treatment of asthma—a double-blind study. Ann Allergy 1978; 40:132–137.

32. Muranaka MM, Nakajima K, Suzuki S. Bronchial responsiveness to acetyl choline in patients with bronchial asthma after long-term treatment with gold salt. J Allergy Clin Immunol 1981; 67:350–354.

33. Klaustermeyer WB, Noritake DT, Kwong FK. Chrysotherapy in the treatment of corticosteroid-dependent asthma. J Allergy Clin Immunol 1987; 79:720–725.

34. Nierop G, Gijzel WP, Bel EH, Zwinderman AH, Dijkman JH. Auranofin in the treatment of steroid-dependent asthma: a double-blind study. Thorax 1992; 47:349–354.

35. Bernstein IL, Bernstein DI, Dubb JW, Faiferman I, Wallin B. A placebo-controlled multicenter study of auranofin in the treatment of corticosteroid-dependent chronic severe asthma. J Allergy Clin Immunol 1996; 98:317–324.

36. Szefler SJ, Brenner M, Jusko WJ, Spector SL, Flesher KA, Ellis EF. Dose and time-related effect of troleandomycin on methyl prednisolone elimination. Clin Pharmacol Ther 1982; 32:166–171.

37. Ong KS, Grieco MH, Rosner W. Enhancement by oleandomycin of the inhibitory effect of methylprednisolone on phyto haemaglutinin-stimulated lymphocytes. J Allergy Clin Immunol 1978; 62:115–118.

38. Goswami SK, Kivity S, Marom Z. Erythromycin inhibits respiratory glyconjugate secretion from human airways in vitro. Am Rev Respir Dis 1990; 141:72–78.

39. Spector SL, Katz FH, Farr RS. Troleandomycin: effectiveness in steroid-dependent asthma and bronchitis. J Allergy Clin Immunol 1974; 54:367–379.

40. Nelson HS, Hamilos DL, Corsello PR, Levesque NV, Buchmeier AD, Bucher BL. A double-blind study of troleandomycin and methyl prednisolone in asthmatic subjects who require daily corticosteroids. Am Rev Respir Dis 1993; 47:398–404.

41. Siracuna A, Brugnami G, Fiordi T, Areni S, Severini C. Troleandomycin in the treatment of difficult asthma. J Allergy Clin Immunol 1993; 92:677–682.

42. Berlow BA, Liebhaber MI, Dyer Z. The effect of dapsone in steroid-dependent asthma. J Allergy Clin Immunol 1991; 81:710–715.

43. Schwarz YA, Kivity S, Ilfeld DN, Schlesinger M, Greif J, Topilsky M, Garty MS. A clinical and immunologic study of colchicines in asthma. J Allergy Clin Immunol 1990; 85:578–582.

44. Newman K, Mason UG, Buchmeier A, Schmaling KB, Nelson HS. Failure of colchicines to reduce inhaled triamcinolone dose in patients suffering with asthma. J Allergy Clin Immunol 1997; 90:176–178.

45. Kench JB, Seal JP, Temple DM, Tennant C. The effect of non-steroidal inhibitors of phospholipase A2 on leukotriene and histamine release from human and guinea pig lung. Prostaglandins 1985; 30:199–206.

46. Roberts JA, Gunneberg A, Elloitt JA, Thomson NC. Hydroxychloroquine in steroid dependent asthma. Pulm Pharmacol 1988; 1:59–61.

47. Charous BL, Halpern EF, Steven GC. Hydroxychloroquine improves airflow and lowers circulating IgE levels in subjects with moderate symptomatic asthma. J Allergy Clin Immunol 1998; 102:198–203.

48. Drazen JM, Israel E, O'Byrne PM. Treatment of asthma with drugs modifying the leukotriene pathway. N Engl J Med 1999; 340:197–206.

49. Diamant Z, Sampson AP. Anti-inflammatory mechanisms of leukotriene modulators. Clin Exp Allergy 1999; 29:1449–1453.

50. Laviolette M, Malmstrom K, Lu S et al. Montelukast added to inhaled beclomethasone in treatment of asthma. Am J Respir Crit Care Med 1999; 160:1862–1868.

51. Dworski R, Fitzgerald GA, Oates JA et al. Effect of oral prednisone on airway inflammatory mediators in atopic asthma. Am J Respir Crit Care Med 1994; 149:953–959.

52. O'Shaughnessy KM, Wellings R, Gillies B et al. Differential effects of flucticasone propionate on allergen-evoked bronchoconstriction and increased urinary leukotriene E_4 excretion. Am Rev Respir Dis 1993; 147:1472–1476.

53. National Institutes of Health. Global Initiative for Asthma: global strategy for asthma management and prevention. NHBLI/WHO Workshop, NIH publication, 1998.
54. Smith TF, Morris EC, Bain RP. IgG subclasses in non allergic children with chronic chest symptoms. J Paediatrics 1984; 105:896–900.
55. Vrugt B, Wilson S, van Velzen E, Bron A, Shute JK, Holgate ST, Djukanovic R, Aalbers R. Effects of high dose intravenous immunoglobulin in two severe corticosteroid-insensitive asthmatic patients. Thorax 1997; 52:662–664.
56. Spahn JD, Leung DYM, Chan MTS Szefler SJ, Gelfand EW. Mechanisms of glucocorticoid reduction in asthmatic subjects treated with intravenous immunoglobulin. J Allergy Clin Immunol 1999; 103:421–426.
57. Mazere BD, Gelfand EW. An open study of high dose intravenous immunoglobulin in severe childhood asthma. J Allergy Clin Immunol 1991; 87:976–983.
58. Jakobsson T, Croner S, Kjellman MPA, Vassella C, Bjoksten B. Slight steroid-sparing effect of intravenous immunoglobulin in children and adolescents with moderately severe bronchial asthma. Allergy 1994; 49:413–420.
59. Salmun LM, Barlan I, Wolf HM, Eibl M, Twarog FJ, Geha RS, Schneider LC. Effect of intravenous immunoglobulin on steroid consumption in patients with severe asthma: a double-blind, placebo-controlled, randomised trial. J Allergy Clin Immunol 1999; 103:810–815.
60. Valacer DJ, Kishima JL, Com MD. A multicenter, randomised placebo-controlled trial of high dose intravenous gammaglobulin for oral corticosteroid-dependent asthma. J Appl Biometer 1999; 91:126–133.
61. Boulet LP, Chapman KR, Cote J et al. Inhibitory effects of an anti-IgE antibody E25 on allergen-induced early asthmatic response. Am J Respir Crit Care Med 1997; 155:1835–1840.
62. Fahy J, Fleming HE, Wong HH et al. The effect of an anti-IgE monoclonal antibody on the early and late-phase responses to allergen inhalation in asthmatic subjects. Respir Crit Care Med 1997; 155:1828–1834.
63. Milgrom H, Fick RB, Su JQ, Reimann JD, Bush RK, Watrous ML, Metzger WJ. Treatment of allergic asthma with monoclonal anti IgE. N Eng J Med 1999; 341:1966–1973.
64. Sanderson C, Warren DJ, Strath M. Identification of a lymphokine that stimulates eosinophil differentiation in vitro. J Exp Med 1985; 162:60–74.
65. Wills-Karp M, Luyimbazi J, Xu X, Schofield B, Neben TY, Karp C, Donaldson DD. IL-13: central mediator of allergic asthma. Science 1998; 282:2258–2261.
66. Mauser PJ, Pitman AM, Fernandez X et al. Effects of an antibody to IL-5 in a monkey model of asthma. Am J Respir Crit Care Med 1995; 152:467–472.
67. Mauser PJ, Pitman AM, Witt A et al. Inhibitory effect of the TRFK-5 anti-IL-5 antibody in a guinea pig model of asthma. Am Rev Respir Dis 1993; 148:1623–1627.
68. Leckie MJ, ten Brinke A, Khan J et al. Effects of an IL-5 blocking monoclonal antibody on eosinophils, airway hyperresponsiveness and the response to allergen in patients with asthma. Lancet 2000; 356:2144–2148.
69. Finkelman FD, Katona IM, Urban JF, Holmes J, Tung AS, Sample JG, Paul WE. IL-4 is required to generate and sustain in vivo IgE responses. J Immunol 1988; 141:2335–2341.

70. Shi H-Z, Deng JM, Xu H, Nong ZXH, Xiao CQ, Liu ZM, Qin SM, Jiang HX, Liu GN, Chen YQ. Effect of inhaled IL-4 on airway hyperreactivity in asthmatics. Am J Respir Crit Care Med 1998; 157:1818–1821.

71. Borish L, Nelson HS, Lanz MJ, Claussen L, Whitmore JB, Agosti JM, Garrison L. IL-4 receptor in moderate atopic asthma: a phase 1/2 randomised placebo-controlled trial. Am J Respir Crit Care Med 1999; 160:1816–1823.

72. Trinchieri G. Interleukin-12 and its role in the generation of TH1 cells. Immunol Today 1993; 14:335–338.

73. Boguniewicz M, Schneider LC, Milgrom H, Newell D, Kelly N, Tam P, Izu AE, Jaf HS, Bucalo LR, Leung DY. Treatment of steroid-dependent asthma with recombinant interferon-gamma. Clin Exp Allergy 1993; 23:785–790.

74. Van der Pouw Kraan TCTM, Boeije LCM, de Groot ER, Stapel SO, Snijders A, Kapsenberg ML, van der Zee JS, Aarden LA. Reduced production of IL-12 and IL-12 dependent IFN-gamma release in patients with allergic asthma. J Immunol 1997; 158:5560–5565.

75. Plummeridge MJ, Armstrong L, Birchall MA, Millar AB. Reduced production of interleukin 12 by interferon gamma primed alveolar macrophages from atopic asthmatic subjects. Thorax 2000; 55:842–847.

76. Schwarze J, Hamelmann E, Cieslewicz G et al. Local treatment with IL-12 is an effective inhibitor of airway hyperresponsiveness and lung eosinophilia after airway challenge in sensitised mice. J Allergy Clin Immunol 1998; 102:86–93.

77. Bryan SA, O'Connor BJ, Matti S, Leckie MJ, Kanabar V, Khan J, Warrington SJ, Renzetti L, Rames A, Bock JA, Boyce MJ, Hansel TT, 1 Holgate ST, Barnes PJ. Effects of recombinant human interleukin-12 on eosinophils, airway hyper-responsiveness, and the late asthmatic response. Lancet 2000; 356:2149–2153.

78. Kon OM, Shira BD, Compton CH, Leonard TB, Kay AB, Barnes NC. Rando-mised dose-ranging placebo-controlled study of chimeric antibody to CD4 (Keliximab) in chronic severe asthma. Lancet 1998; 352:1109–1113.

79. Kon Oml, Kay AB. Anti-T cell strategies in asthma. Inflamm Res 1999; 48:516–523.

80. Wegner CD, Gundel RH, Reilly HN, Letts GL, Rothlein R. Intercellular adhesion molecule-1 (ICAM-1) in the pathogenesis of asthma. Science 1990; 247:416–418.

81. Gundel RH, Wegner CD, Torcellini CA, Clarke CC, Haynes N, Rothlein R, Letts LG. Endothelial leukocyte adhesion molecule-1 mediates antigen-induced acute airway inflammation and late-phase obstruction in monkeys. J Clin Invest 1991; 88:1407–1411.

82. Nickel R, Beck LA, Stellato C, Schleimer RP. Chemokines and allergic disease. J Allergy Clin Immunol 1999; 104:723–742.

83. Gonzalo JA, Lloyd CM, Wen D, Albar JP, Wells TNC, Proudfoot A, Martinez A, Dorf M, Bjerke T, Coyle AJ, Gutierrez-Ramos JC. The co-ordinated action of CC chemokines in the lung orchestrates allergic inflammation and airway hyper-responsiveness. J Exp Med 1998; 188:157–167.

23

Immunotherapy of Asthma
Prospects for a Vaccine?

GISELA WOHLLEBEN and KLAUS J. ERB

University of Würzburg
Würzburg, Germany

I. Introduction

Allergic-type immune responses to common environmental antigens lead to clinical disorders such as allergic asthma, hay fever, eczema, and allergic rhinitis. Asthma is the most severe atopic disorder, affecting up to 20% of the population in developed countries. It is characterized by chronic inflammation of the airways, bronchial hyperresponsiveness (BHR), reversible airway obstruction, and infiltration of eosinophils and T cells into the mucosa of the airways. Although it is still not understood why some individuals but not others develop asthma, it is clear that the etiological process involves both genetic and environmental factors leading to the production of interleukin-4 (IL-4). IL-4 acts on naive T cells [activated by antigen-presenting cells (APCs)] through IL-4 receptor/STAT6–mediated signaling and the activation of specific downstream transcription factors such as c-Maf, GATA-3, NIP45, and NFATc, resulting in the development of allergen-specific T-helper (Th2) cells in the lymph nodes or spleen (1,2). Once generated, effector Th2 cells migrate to the submucosa of the lung where they interact with allergen-derived peptides associated with major histocompatibility complex class II (MHC class II) molecules expressed on APC. The interaction of the allergen-specific Th2 cells with the APCs leads to the activation of the T cell [via T-cell receptor (TCR), CD28, and CD40 ligand-mediated signaling] resulting in the secretion of IL-4, IL-5, and IL-13. The secretion of these cytokines induces the production of allergen-specific IgE by B cells (IL-4 and IL-13), the development of airway eosinophilia (IL-5), and airway smooth muscle contraction (IL-13). Degranulation of eosinophils and mast cells (via IgE cross-linking) in turn are two of the major primary events leading to chronic airway inflammation and asthma. Although relatively much is known about the immunological processes leading to the development of asthma, thus far no effective prevention measure exists. Furthermore, over the past decade the incidence, severity, and mortality rates of asthma have steadily increased, despite the widespread use of inhaled corticosteroids and bronchodilators. For these reasons it is very important to develop novel therapeutic approaches and effective prevention measures.

Recent animal experiments using live bacteria, bacterial components, or DNA give rise to the hope that it may be possible to develop novel vaccines protecting atopic-prone humans from developing asthma in their lifetime. The basis of these vaccinations is to induce Th1 immune responses leading to the production of interferon-γ (IFN-γ), IL-12, and IL-18. The presence of these cytokines during Th cell development have been shown to inhibit the development of allergen-specific Th2 cells both in vitro and in vivo (3,4). Two approaches may prove successful. First, it has been suggested that the neonatal immune response of non-atopics is biased toward Th2 responses, which subsequently shift toward Th1 responses during the first few years of life. Children who become atopic do not lose the tendency to develop Th2 responses, thus developing allergen-specific Th2 cells after being exposed to inhaled allergens (this process is called the atopic march). The idea is to treat children at an early age with reagents that cause a shift from the residual neonatal Th2 response to a more Th1-biased immune status. This could be achieved by unspecific immunizations inducing local or systemic Th1 immune responses. It is hoped that this would protect children from developing allergen-specific Th2-type cells during the first months and years of life. A second approach is based on the hypothesis that non-atopic individuals are protected from the development of asthma because they have developed allergen-specific Th1 responses. The secretion of IFN-γ by Th1 cells during the encounter with allergen is sufficient to suppress allergen-specific Th2 cell development and thus the development of asthma, without causing any major immunopathology usually associated with Th1 immune responses directed against, for example, viruses or bacteria. The proposed vaccination regimes are aimed at establishing allergen-specific Th1 memory immune responses against certain allergens. This could be achieved by immunizing children with allergens in conjunction with adjuvants or DNA vaccines inducing strong Th1 responses. This chapter focuses on the possible future use of attenuated live or killed bacteria, CpG oligonucleotides, and plasmid DNA as vaccines (or vaccine adjuvants) protecting against asthma in humans. Alternative methods are also briefly reviewed. Furthermore, possible side effects of the proposed vaccination strategies will also be discussed.

II. Potential Use of Live or Killed Bacteria as an Asthma Vaccine

The incidence and severity of asthma is steadily increasing in developed but not developing countries. It has been speculated that this discrepancy between industrialized nations and third-world countries may be at least in part due to the steady decline of infectious diseases in the developed world (3,4). Recent epidemiological studies demonstrating an inverse relationship between atopy and infection with *Mycobacterium tuberculosis*, measles, or hepatitis A (5–7) support this hypothesis. This theory is also referred to as the "hygiene hypothesis." The rationale behind this theory is that infectious diseases (or exposure to antigens derived from pathogens) induce the production of IFN-γ and IL-12, during the immediate postnatal period or early childhood. This early IFN-γ/IL-12 production then shifts the immune response of children with an allergic predisposition away from Th2 toward Th1 responses, thus protecting from the development of asthma. Supporting this view is the finding that the lack of Th2 response suppression in atopic children was linked to the inability of these children to produce sufficient amounts of IFN-γ as neonates (8).

Although this is a very compelling hypothesis, clear scientific data proving or disproving it are still lacking since susceptibility toward asthma and certain infectious diseases may be mutually inclusive or exclusive. However, experiments in animals have provided clear evidence that certain types of infections can inhibit the development of asthma. For example, infection of the lung with live *Mycobacterium bovis* bacillus Calmette-Guerin (BCG) suppressed allergen-induced airway eosinophilia and the development of AHR in mice (9,10). Interestingly, BCG does not have to be alive to mediate this effect, since the application of heat-killed BCG into the lung of mice also inhibited the development of allergen-induced airway eosinophilia (Fig. 1). Furthermore, the application of killed *Mycobacterium vaccae* and killed *Listeria monocytogenes* has also been shown to suppress the induction of allergen-specific IgE in mice (11,12). There is also some evidence suggesting that the intradermal application of BCG to children may help to reduce the risk of developing atopy. A recent report attributed lower atopy rates among children living in Guinea-Bissau to a history of vaccination with BCG (as vaccine against *M. tuberculosis*) early in life (13). This suggests that a simple and widely used BCG vaccination could also reduce the risk of developing asthma. However, two other epidemiological studies found no protective effect of a BCG vaccination on the development of atopy in children (14,15).

Can bacteria or their products be used in humans to protect against the development of asthma? Two potential uses are conceivable. First, attenuated bacteria or their products could be used as adjuvants together with allergens to vaccinate children subcutaneously or intramuscularly. The goal of this vaccination regime would be to establish a long-lasting Th1 memory response against the allergen by inducing IL-12 and IFN-γ production by the bacterial products

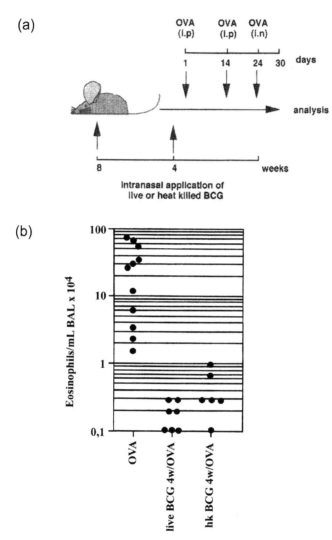

Figure 1 Intranasal application of live and heat-killed BCG strongly inhibits the development of allergen-induced airway eosinophilia. (a) Experimental design used to investigate the influence of live and heat-killed (hk) BCG on ovalbumin (OVA)–induced eosinophilia in the lung. Mice were subjected to an OVA immunization scheme consisting of two intraperitoneal injections of $2\,\mu g$ OVA mixed in $200\,\mu L$ of aluminum hydroxide followed by an intranasal application of $50\,\mu g$ OVA in PBS. Four weeks prior to OVA airway challenge mice were treated intranasally with either 2×10^6 colony-forming units (CFU) of live or heat-killed ($2 \times 1\,h\ 80°C$) BCG. (b) Six days following OVA airway challenge, bronchoalveolar lavages (BAL) were performed and the cells counted, stained with hematoxylin–eosin, and the different cell types identified microscopically. Shown are the numbers of eosinophils present in the BALs of individual mice. Control mice only subjected to the OVA immunization protocol were also included in the analysis.

at the site of allergen-specific Th-cell priming. It is hoped that the encounter of Th1 cells with the respective allergen later in life will lead to the secretion of IFN-γ in the lung, suppressing the generation of asthma-promoting Th2 responses. Second, one could envision the application of attenuated bacteria or their products directly into the lung of young children, inducing a Th1 immune response in the lung. This early and possible first strong Th1 immune response could then bias all further immune responses in the lung toward Th1 and away from Th2. However, it is likely that strong Th1 immune responses will be needed for both approaches to lead to the inhibition of subsequent Th2 responses. This may basically rule out the use of live bacteria because relatively large amounts of bacteria may have to be used to induce the appropriate Th1 response, resulting in severe immunopathology. Furthermore, the consequences of treating young children with live bacteria may lead to disseminated bacterial disease during the treatment or possibly more importantly later in life during permanent or transient immune suppression. Using killed bacteria (or defined bacterial products), in contrast to live bacteria, seems a more promising approach. The challenge, in respect to human use, will be to develop an immunization scheme where sufficient amounts of dead bacteria (or bacterial products) can be given alone or together with an allergen leading to the suppression of asthma without causing serious side effects.

III. Development of an Asthma Vaccine Using CpG Oligodeoxynucleotides

A. Structure and Mechanism of Action

The immunostimulatory CpG motifs are noncoding DNA sequences, which are common and very frequent in bacterial DNA (about 6% of total DNA). They are also found in some viral and invertebrate DNA but at a lower percentage. In mammalian genomes these sequences are rare (1–2% of total DNA) and not mitogenic because of the methylation at specific positions (16–18). Essential for the mitogenic effect are sequences with a central C-G dinucleotide, flanked at the 5' end by two purines and at the 3' end by two pyrimidines for optimal efficiency (19). Exchange or reversal of the CpG dinucleotides stops the stimulatory effects. The effects of bacterial DNA containing CpG motifs were first described by Yamamoto et al., showing limited antitumor activity of *M. bovis* by activating IFN-γ-producing NK cells (20–22). In the meantime, mostly synthetic oligodeoxynucleotides (ODNs), containing these immune-stimulatory sequences (ISS-ODNs), are used because they can be produced in large quantities and in high purity without lipopolysaccharide (LPS) contamination.

The CpG-ODNs activate the cells of the innate and adaptive immune system in vitro and in vivo by signaling "infectious danger" in different ways (23–25). Dendritic cells (DCs) and macrophages are directly stimulated by

CpG-DNA, leading to increased expression of surface MHC class II molecules and the costimulatory molecules CD80, CD86, and CD40, resulting in improved antigen presentation (26–28). Furthermore, the production of the cytokines IL-1, IL-6, IL-12, IL-18, tumor necrosis factor-α (TNF-α), and IFN-α is also induced. Under the influence of CpG-DNA, immature DCs can differentiate into mature DCs, thus enhancing the antigen presenting function further (29). For resting and activated B cells CpG-DNA is a very potent mitogen leading to proliferation; up-regulation of the costimulatory molecules MHC class II, CD80, and CD86, and secretion of IL-6, which is necessary for IgM production (17,30). Furthermore, the treatment of B cells with CpG-ODN rescues the cells from anti-Ig-induced apoptosis (31,32). While DC, macrophages, and B cells are directly activated by CpG-DNA, NK cells and T cells are not. Under the influence of CpG-DNA, NK cells show cytolytic activity and produce IFN-γ, which feeds back on the macrophages and DCs stimulating them further (33,34). But this effect depends strongly on the preceding secretion of IL-12, TNF-α, and IFN-α by the CpG-ODN-stimulated APCs (35). T cells are also activated by CpG-DNA in an indirect way. After ligation of their receptor T cells become sensitive of CpG-DNA. This costimulation leads to T-cell activation, IL-2 secretion, and differentiation into cytolytic effector cells (36,37). Furthermore, secretion of IL-12 and IL-18 by the APCs create a milieu that favors the differentiation of naive Th cells into Th1 and not Th2 cells. Figure 2 summarizes the effects of CpG-ODN on innate and adaptive immune responses.

While the effects of CpG-DNA are well known, the molecular mechanisms are not completely understood. Recently published data show that the cells react to CpG-DNA by using the toll-like receptor (TLR) 9 (38). Mice deficient in this receptor show no response to CpG-ODN administration. It appears that CpG-DNA binds to the TLR9 expressed on APCs and B cells, leading to the activation of the cells. It is assumed that CpG-ODNs are internalized into the cells because immobilization of CpG-DNA abolished the immune-stimulatory effect (39). It has also been suggested that CpG-ODNs bind to intracellular receptors, leading to the activation of the MAP kinase and NF-κB signaling pathways, possibly by interfering with the function of Iκ kinase (26,40,41).

B. CpG-ODNs as Vaccine in Murine Asthma

Since CpG-ODNs induce the production of the cytokines IL-12 and IFN-γ, several studies have addressed the question of whether CpG-ODNs can be used as a vaccine against asthma. Using a similar ovalbumin (OVA) immunization protocol as described in Fig. 1a, Broide et al. showed that intranasal and intraperitoneal administration of CpG-ODNs reduced airway eosinophilia (by 93%) and BHR (42). Furthermore, blood eosinophilia and production of eosinophils in the bone marrow were also suppressed in the CpG-ODN-treated animals.

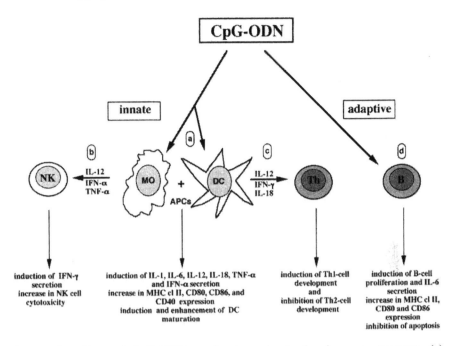

Figure 2 Effects of CpG-ODN on innate and adaptive immune responses. (a) Dendritic cells (DCs) and macrophages (MOs) are directly stimulated by CpG-DNA. This activation leads to increased expression of surface MHC class II molecules and of the costimulatory molecules CD80, CD86, and CD40. This secretion of IL-1, IL-6, IL-12, IL-18, TNF-α, and IFN-α by the antigen-presenting cells (APCs) is also enhanced. (b) The secretion of IL-12, TNF-α, and IFN-α by the activated APC leads to the secretion of IFN-γ by natural killer (NK) cells and increases NK cell cytotoxicity. (c) Production of IL-12, IFN-γ, and L-18 by the CpG-ODN-activated APCs induces the development of Th1 cells and inhibits Th2 cell development. (d) CpG-DNA is also a very potent mitogen for B cells leading to proliferation, up-regulation of the costimulatory molecules MHC class II, CD80, CD86, and secretion of IL-6. CpG-ODN treatment also rescues B cells from anti-Ig induced apoptosis.

Spleen cells from those mice secreted less IL-5 and more IFN-γ after in vitro stimulation with OVA in comparison with the mice treated with allergen only. These results clearly show that the application of CpG-DNA strongly suppressed the development of allergen-induced asthma in mice, suggesting that this effect was achieved by diverting the allergen-specific Th2 to a Th1 response. This was confirmed by two other studies in which the intraperitoneal or intranasal application of CpG-ODNs also clearly inhibited the development of allergic asthma in mice (43,44).

One of the most important factors governing the potential use of CpG-DNA for the vaccination of humans is the question of the duration of the inhibitory effect. While Broide et al. (42) and Kline et al. (43) showed only short-term effects, Sur et al. (44) demonstrated for the first time a longer lasting effect. Mice presensitized with ragweed (ragweed antigen in alum given intraperitoneally) and rechallenged with the allergen three times intratracheally showed reduced lung inflammation and bronchial BHR even 6 weeks after the last CpG-ODN administration. Furthermore, CpG-ODN-treated mice developed a ragweed antigen-specific Th1 memory response in the spleen and lung, characterized by increased numbers of antigen-specific IFN-γ-producing cells and decreased numbers of IL-4-producing cells. Under the influence of CpG-ODNs the mice also showed an increase in allergen-specific IgG$_{2a}$ and decrease in allergen-specific-IgE and IgG$_1$ producing B cells. The switch from a ragweed-specific Th2 response to a Th1 response was not observed in mice deficient in IFN-γ. This clearly identifies IFN-γ as one of the major mediators in CpG-ODN-induced suppression of allergic Th2 responses. Taken together the current view is that CpG-DNA acts on the cells of the innate immune system, inducing the secretion of IFN-α, IFN-β, IFN-γ, and IL-12. These cytokines (particularly IL-12) have positive effects on Th1 cell development and differentiation, finally resulting in the development of antigen-specific Th1 cells. Simultaneously the cytokines also have a negative influence on the generation of allergen-specific Th2 cells, thereby inhibiting the development of asthma. While these effects are mediated by the innate immune system shortly after CpG-ODN administration (within a few hours), immunological memory is mediated by the antigen-specific Th1 cells (secreting IFN-γ) and takes longer to be established. This event is believed to be one of the most important features of CpG-ODN treatments, leading to the inhibition of asthma upon subsequent encounters with allergen by suppressing the development of allergen-specific Th2 cells.

C. CpG-ODNs as Vaccine in Human Studies

In vitro experiments have clearly shown that human cells also react strongly to CpG-DNA. Macrophages and DCs produce IL-12 and TNF-α, and PBM cells secrete IL-18, IL-12, and IFN-γ after CpG-ODN treatment (45). Furthermore, the expression of costimulatory molecules is also up-regulated (46–48). These findings suggest that the encounter of CpG-activated APCs with naive T cells should lead to the development of Th1-type cells in vivo. Furthermore, this view is supported by the observation that human NK cells produce IFN-γ after exposure to CpG-DNA (33). Taken together it appears that human and murine cells react in similar ways to CpG-DNA, suggesting that the treatment of humans with CpG-ODNs could also be very effective in inhibiting the development of asthma.

What would an asthma vaccine using CpG-DNA look like? Basically, the same approaches may be used as described for bacteria (see above). CpG-DNA could be coadministered together with the allergen as an adjuvant, establishing long-lasting allergen-specific Th1 memory responses. Alternatively, CpG-ODN could be directly given into the lung of young children hoping to bias all further immune responses in the lung to Th1 and away from Th2 responses. Based on the published data in animal models it is likely that these approaches may also be successful in humans helping to reduce the development of asthma. However, CpG-ODNs similar to live or dead bacteria rely on Th1 immune responses to inhibit Th2 responses. Therefore, possible harmful effects after CpG-ODN treatment need to be ruled out. Besides the potential problem of inducing strong Th1 responses in the lung leading to immunopathology, use of CpG-DNA could also have other serious side effects. CpG-ODN directly induces the production of TNF-α by macrophages. This could result in septic shock as was reported to occur in mice (49). Furthermore, patients suffering from infections with gram-negative bacteria (endotoxin producers) could be especially vulnerable to CpG-ODN-mediated side effects. The LPS-mediated TNF-α release (as a consequence of the infection) may be increased by CpG-ODN application, leading to toxic effects normally not associated with the bacterial infection. Moreover, the production of IFN-γ by human NK cells after CpG treatment could also increase the toxicity of LPS in humans, a finding reported in an appropriate animal model (34). However unlikely, the occurrence of these possible side effects cannot be completely ruled out.

D. CpG-ODNs and the Risk of Inducing Autoimmunity

A greater problem concerning the use of CpG-ODNs could be the development of autoimmune diseases after the application of CpG-ODNs as an asthma vaccine. Immune responses in humans need to be tightly regulated to suppress the development of autoimmune disease. Normally most autoreactive T and B cells are negatively selected and deleted in the thymus and bone marrow, respectively. However, some autoreactive T and B cells remain. The unresponsiveness of these cells to self-antigens is ensured by different peripheral tolerance mechanisms. The basis of this control is that autoreactive T and B cells are not sufficiently activated to cause harm. Usually sufficient costimulation either by cytokines or costimulatory molecules is lacking, leading to apoptosis or anergy of the autoreactive cells. Since CpG-DNA is such a strong trigger of innate immune responses leading to the up-regulation of costimulatory molecules and the secretion of proinflammatory cytokines, it may be possible that autoreactive T and B cells may become sufficiently activated resulting in autoimmune disease. The observation that CpG-ODN treatment exacerbated autoimmune myocarditis (50), transient inflammatory arthritis (51), and experimental autoimmune encephalomyelitis (52) in different animal models supports this view. Thus far, it is totally unclear if this could also occur in humans. However, it is important to keep in mind that autoimmune disorders may develop at a much later time point after the initial CpG-ODN treatment.

The challenge will be to design a vaccine using sufficient amounts of CpG-ODN to inhibit the development of asthma, without causing any serious side effects. Supporting the use of CpG-DNA as a component of a vaccine against asthma is the finding that 100-fold less CpG-ODN could be used to inhibit allergen-induced eosinophilia in mice when the CpG-DNA was directly conjugated to the allergen, in comparison to using an CpG-ODN/allergen mix (53). This suggest that by using CpG-ODN/allergen conjugates instead of CpG-ODN alone or in a mix with protein may rule out possible negative side effects normally associated with CpG-ODN.

IV. Plasmid DNA Immunization as a Basis for an Efficient Asthma Vaccine

A. Structure and Mechanisms of Action

DNA vaccination, also named gene vaccination, is a relatively new immunization method, first published in the early 1990s. By injection of plasmid (p) DNA encoding for a defined antigen, a strong and long-lived cellular and humoral immune response is elicited lasting in part for more than a year (54–56). The cell-mediated immune response is characterized by the induction of antigen-specific Th1 cells and cytotoxic T lymphocytes (CTLs). After pDNA inoculation, antigen is continuously synthesized in the transfected cells, which serve as an "antigen reservoir." This way the immune system is permanently stimulated without the need of booster immunizations. While this mechanism explains the persistent memory response by gene vaccination, it does not explain why the response is so strongly biased toward Th1. The current view is that CpG motifs in the noncoding regions of the pDNA mediate this effect and influence the efficiency of DNA vaccination by acting as intrinsic adjuvants (57–59). The CpG motifs also enhance the activation of APCs and stimulate DCs in the draining lymph nodes, as shown recently (60,61). Therefore, DNA vaccines are considered to be two-component systems (62). The first component is the antigen-coding transcription unit, including a eukaryotic promoter and polyadenylation terminator sequences, responsible for protein synthesis. The second component consists of CpG motifs in the plasmid backbone, mediating the Th1-directed response and the adjuvant activity, leading to a very strong response to very little antigen. Gene gun experiments (gold particles coated with pDNA are "shot" into the skin by using pressurized air) confirm the suggestion that the Th1-biased immune response is mediated through DNA containing CpG-ODN. By transfecting cells with 100-fold less pDNA and therefore less CpG motif, Th2 and not Th1 responses were induced (63).

In most studies pDNA is administrated by injection, either intradermally or intramuscularly (64–66). Both routes lead to antigen processing and peptide loading onto MHC class I and MHC class II molecules. For this effect, professional APCs are needed, which are found especially in the dermis of the skin in great numbers (67). While CD4$^+$ T-helper cells recognize antigen derived from exogenous antigen in the context of MHC class II molecules, CD8$^+$ T cells (CTLs) recognize endogenous antigen in combination with MHC class I molecules. Thus, DNA vaccination has the great advantage over most conventional vaccines because it induces both CD4$^+$ and CD8$^+$ T-cell-mediated responses.

B. Use as Vaccine in Animal Models of Asthma

Successful DNA vaccination was carried out in different animal species, including nonhuman primates, using a variety of antigens such as hepatitis B virus surface antigen (68), human immunodeficiency virus type 1 (HIV-1), gp120 and gp160 (69,70), or influenza virus antigen (71), to mention a few. Furthermore, whether DNA vaccination could be used to protect against the development of allergic disorders was also investigated. It could be shown that gene vaccination with pDNA, coding for the house dust mite allergen Der p5, inhibited specific IgE synthesis, BHR, and histamine release in the airways after allergen challenge in rats (65). Another report demonstrated the efficiency of gene vaccination in mice presensitized to a latex allergen (Hev b5). After onset of the allergy, injection of pDNA, coding for Hev b5, decreased the antigen-specific IgE response significantly (72). Very convincing results were also obtained in an OVA model of asthma in the mouse. After intradermal injection of pDNA encoding for OVA, the OVA immunization protocol was started by intraperitoneal application of OVA in aluminum hydroxide followed by subsequent OVA airway inhalation. The DNA vaccination resulted in a shift toward an OVA-specific Th1-biased immune response (increase in OVA-specific IgG$_{2a}$ and IFN-γ secretion by T cells; decrease in OVA-specific IgE and IgG$_1$) and the inhibition of airway eosinophilia in the OVA-immunized animals (73). Moreover, a recent study showed enhanced efficiency of DNA vaccination by using a pDNA construct, containing the cDNA of OVA fused to the cDNA of IL-18 (74). In contrast to the OVA construct given alone, injection of this fusion construct to unsensitized mice not only protected mice from allergen-induced AHR but also reversed preexisting BHR. The suppressive effect on the allergen-specific Th2 response was dependent on IFN-γ and CD8$^+$ T cells. Furthermore, the use of this fusion construct was also more efficient in inhibiting allergen-specific Th2 responses than a mixture of OVA pDNA coadministered with IL-18 pDNA. Interestingly, the negative side effects associated with application of IL-18 protein in vivo (75,76) were not observed using the pDNA containing the IL-18 cDNA. The plasmids used in the studies discussed so far always contained the cDNA of an allergen (or parts of it). However, pDNA can also be used to inhibit the development of asthma when the plasmid only contains the cDNA for IFN-γ. This was shown in mice, where mucosal IFN-γ gene transfer led to the inhibition of pulmonary allergic responses (77).

C. Use as Vaccines in Human Asthma?

The results obtained in the different animal models have led to the suggestion that DNA vaccination might be a very promising method for prevention and management of asthma in humans. However, gene vaccination trials, started in humans management of malaria (78) and of infections with HIV-1 (79,80), show only low levels of humoral and cellular immune responses against the respective antigens. The reason could be that the CpG motifs currently used are not optimal for humans. Therefore, the efficiency of pDNA might be improved by modifying the CpG motifs or by enhancing their numbers. However, this may result in the opposite effect because large numbers of CpG motifs can down-regulate expression of the encoded gene (81). Other approaches to enhance the effects of DNA vaccines containing cDNA to allergens include cDNA encoding for cytokines, chemokines, or costimulatory molecules known to be involved in the suppression of Th2 responses or enhancement of Th1 responses (82–84). Furthermore, combining DNA vaccines with a subsequent vaccinia virus infection may also lead to a stronger Th1 immune response against the plasmid-encoded antigen. This effect was observed in mice, where a DNA vaccination followed by a vaccinia virus infection (pDNA and vaccinia virus contained the same malaria antigen) induced complete protection from an infection with *Plasmodium berghei* (85). Neither the pDNA nor the vaccinia virus infection had any protective effect administered alone. Taken together, DNA vaccination is very efficient and safe in protecting animals from developing asthma. However, it is also clear that a prospective DNA vaccine, protecting humans from the development of asthma needs to be further optimized and tested for safety. This is especially true when the cDNA encoding for cytokine, chemokine, or costimulatory molecules is incorporated into the pDNA used as a vaccine or when vaccinia virus is used as a booster imunization.

V. Additional Approaches Leading to the Discovery of a Potential Asthma Vaccine

Thus far we have discussed the use of bacteria, CpG-ODN, and pDNA as prospective vaccines against asthma. The reason we have focused on these reagents is that their efficiency has been clearly established in different animal models. In the following section, we will discuss the use of other approaches possibly also leading to an asthma vaccine.

Besides using the above-discussed vaccination strategies to induce the production of IL-12, IL-18, or IFN-γ in humans, these cytokines could be directly applied with or without allergen to suppress Th2 responses. In an animal model of asthma, it was clearly shown that administration of nebulized IFN-γ inhibited allergen-induced BHR, cutaneous reactivity, and secondary OVA-specific IgE production (86,87). Furthermore, a similar effect was seen when IL-12 was given into the lung at the time of antigen airway challenge (88). This was accompanied by a decrease in IL-4 and IL-5 secretion and an increase in IFN-γ production in the lung. However, another study failed to confirm this result, where IL-12 had to be given together with IL-18 to have an inhibitory effect on allergen-specific Th2 cell responses (89). Interestingly, although IL-18 induces the production of IFN-γ, it was reported that the administration of IL-18 alone into the lung of mice enhanced antigen-induced recruitment of eosinophils into the airways and exacerbated airway inflammation (75). This result was confirmed by Wild et al., suggesting that IL-18 application exacerbates rather than suppresses allergic asthma (76). Taken together, there is some evidence suggesting that the application of IL-12, IL-18 and IFN-γ alone or in combination with allergen could help in reducing the risk of developing asthma in humans. However, due to the generally poor track record of cytokine therapy and the reported morbidity and mortality associated with the use of IL-12 in clinical trials (90), other approaches to an asthma vaccine seem more promising.

A further approach protecting humans from asthma may be administration of allergen-specific Th1 cell lines. After their establishment in vitro (by culturing PBM cells from the patients in the presence of APCs, allergen, IL-12, and anti-IL-4), a defined amount of allergen-specific Th1 cells could be applied back into the patient. It is hoped that these cells could then prevent the development of asthma at a later time when the patient is naturally exposed to the allergen. This approach has been used successfully in an animal model of asthma (91,92). However, other groups failed to confirm these results (93,94), also making this approach an unlikely candidate for a human asthma vaccine.

A better strategy for the development of an asthma vaccine may be the use of allergen pulsed DCs. DCs can easily be obtained from progenitors present in the blood of patients (95,96). Animals vaccinated with DCs pulsed with antigen showed very efficient protection against infectious diseases (97) or cancer (98,99). First clinical trials in humans, based on DC vaccination, have already started in patients with cancer. However, it remains to be seen in humans if DCs pulsed with allergen induce predominantly allergen-specific Th1 responses, leading to the inhibition of asthma, or Th2 responses, exacerbating the allergic response. In the mouse, administration of myeloid DCs clearly leads to Th2 priming, exacerbating the airway eosinophilia (see Chap. 15).

Possibly one of the most attractive vaccination strategies against asthma could be the induction of allergen-specific CD4$^+$ T regulatory (T$_{reg}$) cells. These are characterized by the secretion of transforming growth factor-β (TGF-β) only (called Th3) or by secretion of a combination of TGF-β and/or IL-10 and/or IL-4 (called Tr1). Regardless of the exact cytokine pattern produced by T$_{reg}$ cells, they all have in common that they secrete anti-inflammatory and immunosuppressive cytokines in an antigen-specific context. Animal studies have shown that T$_{reg}$ cells can inhibit both Th1 and Th2 cell

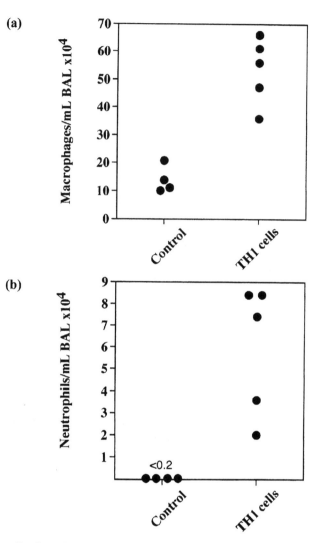

Figure 3 Application of allergen-specific Th1 cells induces an influx of macrophages and neutrophils into the lung of allergen-challenged mice. OVA-specific Th1 cells were obtained by incubating purified CD4$^+$ T cells from transgenic mice expressing the DO11.10 T cell receptor (TCR) in vitro with APC, IL-12, OVA-peptide, and anti-IL-4 antibodies for 6 days. The cells were then washed and restimulated with APCs and mitogen. 24 h later 5×10^6 Th1-type cells (produce only IFN-γ and no IL-4 or IL-5 after in vitro restimulation) were intravenously injected into mice. One and three days after the application of the Th1 cells the mice were treated with 50 µg of OVA in PBS intranasally. Three days after the last OVA airway challenge a BAL was performed and cells identified as described in Figure 1. Shown are the amounts of macrophages (a) and neutrophils (b) present in the lung of individual mice treated with OVA-specific Th1 cells. The amount of macrophages and neutrophils present in untreated mice is also shown.

development during autoimmune disease and asthma. By oral administration of antigen, autoimmune encephalomyelitis (Th3 cells) (100) and experimental colitis (Th1 cells) (101) were inhibited by the induction of T_{reg} cells. Furthermore, inhibition of experimental tracheal eosinophilia was also due to the induction of TGF-β-secreting CD4$^+$T cells (102). The most convincing evidence that the induction of T_{reg} cells could be used as a vaccination strategy protecting against asthma are the reports of Hansen et al. (103,104) and Cottrez et al. (105). They could show that application of in vitro engineered allergen-specific T_{reg} cell lines (secreting TGF-β or IL-10) protected mice from developing asthma.

In summary, a vaccine that induces allergen-specific T_{reg} cells seems very desirable, since Th2 cell development can be inhibited without inducing potentially proinflammatory Th1 cells. However, it is still unclear how a vaccine must be applied to induce sufficient numbers of T_{reg} cells and no Th1 or Th2 cells in humans. Thus far, almost all animal experiments point to oral vaccination as the key to the successful induction of T_{reg} cells. Furthermore, the use of immature DCs pulsed with antigen has also been suggested to selectively induce T_{reg} cells (106). It remains to be seen if it will be possible to induce allergen-specific T_{reg} cells in humans, leading to the protection against asthma.

VI. Conclusions

Asthma continues to be a major health hazard in the developed countries of the world despite the widespread use of inhaled corticosteroids and bronchodilators. Furthermore, no effective prevention measure exists to date. However, recent studies have clearly shown that animals could be protected against the development of asthma by using different vaccination approaches. These results suggest that it may now also be possible to develop an asthma vaccine for human use. Two approaches seem the most promising. Young children could be treated with reagents that induce the production of IL-12, IL-18, and IFN-γ leading to Th1 immune responses in the lung. This could protect children from developing allergen-specific Th2-type cells during the first months and years of life, which are believed to be the most critical for the development of asthma later in life. Alternatively, vaccinations could be used that selectively induce allergen-specific Th1 responses. It is hoped that the secretion of IFN-γ by Th1 cells during the subsequent encounter with allergen is sufficient to continuously suppress allergen-specific Th2 cell development. This could be achieved by immunizing children with allergens in conjunction with adjuvants or DNA vaccines inducing strong Th1 responses. Both approaches may work because adjuvants inducing Th1 responses are readily available and have been shown to be effective in animal models of asthma. They include attenuated live or killed bacteria, CpG oligonucleotides,

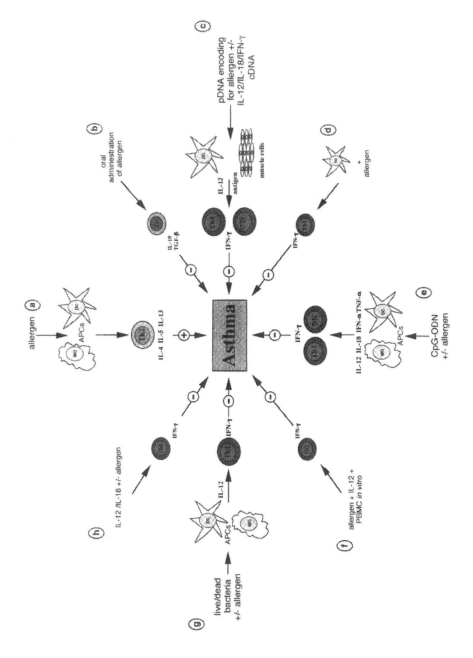

◀───

Figure 4   Prospective vaccination strategies possibly leading to the protection against asthma. Allergens are taken up by APCs. Environmental and genetic factors then determine if naive T cells develop into allergen-specific Th2 cells. These Th2 cells then secrete IL-4, IL-5, and IL-13 leading to the development of asthma (a), Oral administration of allergen leads to the development of allergen-specific regulatory T (Tr) cells. These cells inhibit the development of allergen-specific Th2 responses through the secretion of the immunosuppressive cytokines IL-10 and TGF-β. (b), Development of asthma can also be inhibited by inducing allergen-specific Th1 memory cells. After exposure to allergen these Th1 cells secrete IFN-γ and IL-18 leading to the suppression of allergen-specific Th2 cell development. Different vaccination strategies may be used to induce allergen-specific Th1 cells. These include the use of DNA vaccines (c), dendritic cells (DCs) pulsed with allergen in vitro (d), CpG-ODN alone or together with allergen (e), allergen-specific Th1 cell lines established in vitro from PBMC stimulated with allergen and IL-12 (f), live or dead bacteria alone or together with allergen (g), and allergen together with recombinant IL-12 or IL-18 (h).

plasmid DNA, or cytokines. However, all proposed approaches harbor the potential to cause serious side effects. A particular problem may be the induction of allergen-specific Th1 cells, since they may lead to airway inflammation and subsequent tissue damage upon encountering inhaled allergen. Supporting this view is the finding that allergen-specific Th1 cells adaptively transferred into naive mice induce the recruitment of macrophages and neutrophils into the lung after allergen airway challenge (Fig. 3). Taken together the data obtained in animal models for asthma clearly give rise to the hope that it may also be possible to develop an effective vaccine against asthma in humans. However, the safety aspect of a vaccine cannot be overemphasized, especially because the most promising targets for an efficient vaccination are young children. The induction of allergen-specific T_{reg} cells in contrast to Th1 cells may be a safer approach. Figure 4 shows a summary of possible vaccination strategies protecting against asthma.

References

1. O'Garra A. Cytokines induce the development of functionally heterogeneous T helper cell subsets (Review). Immunity 1998; 8:275–283.
2. Glimcher LH, Sing H. Transcription factors in lymphocyte development—T and B cells get together. Cell 1999; 96:13–23.
3. Erb KJ. Atopic disorders: a default pathway in the absence of infection (Review)? Immunol Today 1999; 20:317–322.
4. Herz U, Lacy P, Renz H, Erb K. The influence of infections on the development and severity of allergic disorders (Review). Curr Opin Immunol 2000; 12:632–640.
5. Shirakawa T, Enomoto T, Shimazu S, Hopkin JM. The inverse association between tuberculin responses and atopic disorder. Science 1997; 275:77–79.

6. Shaheen SO, Aaby P, Hall AJ, Barker DJ, Heyes CB, Shiell AW, Goudiaby A. Measles and atopy in Guinea-Bissau. Lancet 1996; 347:1792–1796.

7. Matricardi PM, Rosmini F, Riondino S, Fortini M, Ferrigno L, Rapicetta M, Bonini S. Exposure to foodborne and orofecal microbes versus airborne viruses in relation to atopy and allergic asthma: epidemiological study. Br Med J 2000; 320: 412–417.

8. Prescott SL, Macaubas C, Smallacombe T, Holt BJ, Sly PD, Holt PG. Development of allergen-specific T-cell memory in atopic and normal children. Lancet 1999; 353:196–200.

9. Herz U, Gerhold K, Gruber C, Braun A, Wahn U, Renz H, Paul K. BCG infection suppresses allergic sensitization and development of increased airway reactivity in an animal model. J Allergy Clin Immunol 1998; 102:867–874.

10. Erb KJ, Holloway JW, Sobeck A, Moll H, Le Gros G. Infection of mice with *Mycobacterium bovis*-bacillus Calmette-Guerin (BCG) suppresses allergen-induced airway eosinophilia. J Exp Med 1998; 187:561–569.

11. Yeung VP, Gieni RS, Umetsu DT, DeKruyff RH. Heat-killed Listeria monocytogenes as an adjuvant converts established murine Th2-dominated immune responses into Th1-dominated responses. J Immunol 1998; 161:4146–4152.

12. Wang CC, Rook GA. Inhibition of an established allergic response to ovalbumin in BALB/c mice by killed *Mycobacterium vaccae*. Immunology 1998; 93:307–313.

13. Aaby P, Shaheen SO, Heyes CB, Goudiaby A, Hall AJ, Shiell AW, Jensen H, Marchant A. Early BCG vaccination and reduction in atopy in Guinea-Bissau. Clin Exp Allergy 2000; 30:644–650.

14. Alm JS, Lilja G, Pershagen G, Scheynius A. BCG vaccination does not seem to prevent atopy in children with atopic heredity. Allergy 1998; 53:537.

15. Strannegard IL, Larsson LO, Wennergren G, Strannegard O. Prevalence of allergy in children in relation to prior BCG vaccination and infection with atypical mycobacteria. Allergy 1998; 53:249–254.

16. Bird AP. DNA methylation and the frequency of CpG in animal DNA. Nucleic Acids Res 1980; 8:1499–1504.

17. Krieg AM, Yi AK, Matson S, Waldschmidt TJ, Bishop GA, Teasdale R, Koretzky GA, Klinman DM. CpG motifs in bacterial DNA trigger direct B-cell activation. Nature 1995; 374:546–549.

18. Heeg K, Zimmermann S. CpG DNA as a Th1 trigger (Review). Int Arch Allergy Immunol 2000; 121:87–97.

19. Yamamoto S, Yamamoto T, Kataoka T, Kuramoto E, Yano O, Tokunaga T. Unique palindromic sequences in synthetic oligonucleotides are required to induce IFN and augment IFN-mediated natural killer activity. J Immunol 1992; 148:4072–4076.

20. Yamamoto S, Kuramoto E, Shimada S, Tokunaga T. In vitro augmentation of natural killer cell activity and production of interferon-alpha/beta and -gamma with deoxyribonucleic acid fraction from *Mycobacterium bovis* BCG. Jpn J Cancer Res 1988; 79:866–873.

21. Yamamoto S, Yamamoto T, Shimada S, Kuramoto E, Yano O, Kataoka T, Tokunaga T. DNA from bacteria, but not from vertebrates, induces interferons, activates natural killer cells and inhibits tumor growth. Microbiol Immunol 1992; 36:983–997.

22. Tokunaga T, Yamamoto H, Shimada S, Abe H, Fukuda T, Fujisawa Y, Furutani Y, Yano O, Kataoka T, Sudo T, et al. Antitumor activity of deoxyribonucleic acid fraction from *Mycobacterium bovis* BCG. I. Isolation, physicochemical characterization, and antitumor activity. J Natl Cancer Inst 1984; 72:955–962.

23. Krieg AM. The role of CpG motifs in innate immunity. Curr Opin Immunol 2000; 12:35–43.

24. Heeg K, Zimmermann S. CpG DNA as a Th1 trigger (Review). Int Arch Allergy Immunol 2000; 121:87–97.

25. Lipford GB, Heeg K, Wagner H. Bacterial DNA as immune cell activator (Review). Trends Microbiol 1998; 6:496–500.

26. Stacey KJ, Sweet MJ, Hume DA. Macrophages ingest and are activated by bacterial DNA. J Immunol 1996; 157:2116–2122.

27. Sparwasser T, Miethke T, Lipford G, Erdmann A, Hacker H, Heeg K, Wagner H. Macrophages sense pathogens via DNA motifs: induction of tumor necrosis factor-alpha-mediated shock. Eur J Immunol 1997; 27:1671–1679.

28. Martin-Orozco E, Kobayashi H, Van Uden J, Nguyen MD, Kornbluth RS, Raz E. Enhancement of antigen-presenting cell surface molecules involved in cognat interactions by immunostimulatory DNA sequences. Int Immunol 1999; 11:1111–1118.

29. Sparwasser T, Koch ES, Vabulas RM, Heeg K, Lipford GB, Ellwart JW, Wagner H. Bacterial DNA and immunostimulatory CpG oligonucleotides trigger maturation and activation of murine dendritic cells. Eur J Immunol 1998; 28:2045–2054.

30. Sun S, Beard C, Jaenisch R, Jones P, Sprent J. Mitogenicity of DNA from different organisms for murine B cells. J Immunol 1997; 159:3119–3125.

31. Yi AK, Hornbeck P, Lafrenz DE, Krieg AM. CpG DNA rescue of murine B lymphoma cells from anti-IgM-induced growth arrest and programmed cell death is associated with increased expression of c-myc and bcl-xL. J Immunol 1996; 157:4918–4925.

32. Yi AK, Chang M, Peckham DW, Krieg AM, Ashman RF. CpG oligodeoxyribonucleotides rescue mature spleen B cells from spontaneous apoptosis and promote cell cycle entry. J Immunol 1998; 160:5898–5906.

33. Ballas ZK, Rasmussen WL, Krieg AM. Induction of NK activity in murine and human cells by CpG motifs in oligodeoxynucleotides and bacterial DNA. J Immunol 1996; 157:1840–1845.

34. Cowdery JS, Chace JH, Yi AK, Krieg AM. Bacterial DNA induces NK cells to produce IFN-gamma in vivo and increases the toxity of lipopolysaccharides. J Immunol 1996; 156:4570–4575.

35. Chace JH, Hooker NA, Mildenstein KL, Krieg AM, Cowdery JS. Bacterial DNA-induced NK cell IFN-gamma production is dependent on macrophage secretion of IL-12. Clin Immunol Immunopathol 1997; 84:185–193.

36. Bendigs S, Salzer U, Lipford GB, Wagner H, Heeg K. CpG-oligodeoxynucleotides co-stimulate primary T cells in the absence of antigen-presenting cells. Eur J Immunol 1999; 29:1209–1218.

37. Heeg K. CpG DNA co-stimulates antigen-reactive T cells (Review). Curr Top Microbiol Immunol 2000; 247:93–105.

38. Hemmi H, Takeuchi O, Kawai T, Kaisho T, Sato S, Sanjo H, Matsumoto M, Hoshino K, Wagner H, Takeda K, Akira S. A Toll-like receptor recognizes bacterial DNA. Nature 2000; 408:740–745.

39. Manzel L, Macfarlane DE. Lack of immune stimulation by immobilized CpG-oligodeoxynucleotide. Antisense Nucleic Acid Drug Dev 1999; 9:459–464.

40. Yi AK, Krieg AM. Rapid induction of mitogen-activated protein kinases by immune stimulatory CpG DNA. J Immunol 1998; 161:4493–4497.

41. Hacker H, Mischak H, Miethke T, Liptay S, Schmid R, Sparwasser T, Heeg K, Lipford GB, Wagner H. CpG-DNA-specific activation of antigen-presenting cells requires stress kinase activity and is preceded by non-specific endocytosis and endosomal maturation. EMBO J 1998; 17:6230–6240.

42. Broide D, Schwarze J, Tighe H, Gifford T, Nguyen MD, Malek S, Van Uden J, Martin-Orozco E, Gelfand EW, Raz E. Immunostimulatory DNA sequences inhibit IL-5, eosinophilic inflammation, and airway hyperresponsiveness in mice. J Immunol 1998; 161:7054–7062.

43. Kline JN, Waldschmidt TJ, Businga TR, Lemish JE, Weinstock JV, Thorne PS, Krieg AM. Modulation of airway inflammation by Cpg oligodeoxynucleotides in a murine model of asthma. J Immunol 1998; 160:2555–2559.

44. Sur S, Wild JS, Choudhury BK, Sur N, Alam R, Klinman DM. Long term prevention of allergic lung inflammation in a mouse model of asthma by CpG oligodeoxynucleotides. J Immunol 1999; 162:6284–6293.

45. Bohle B, Jahn-Schmid B, Maurer D, Kraft D, Ebner C. Oligodeoxynucleotides containing CpG motifs induce IL-12, IL-18 and IFN-gamma production in cells from allergic individuals and inhibit IgE synthesis in vitro. Eur J Immunol 1999; 29:2344–2353.

46. Bauer M, Heeg K, Wagner H, Lipford GB. DNA activates human immune cells through a CpG sequence–dependent manner. Immunology 1999; 97:699–705.

47. Hartmann G, Weiner GJ, Krieg AM. CpG DNA: a potent signal for growth, activation, and maturation of human dendritic cells. Proc Natl Acad Sci USA 1999; 96:9305–9310.

48. Hartmann G, Krieg AM. CpG DNA and LPS induce distinct patterns of activation in human monocytes. Gene Ther 1999; 6:893–903.

49. Sparwasser T, Miethke T, Lipford G, Borschert K, Hacker H, Heeg K, Wagner H. Bacterial DNA causes septic shock. Nature 1997; 386:336–337.

50. Bachmaier K, Neu N, de la Maza LM, Pal S, Hessel A, Penninger JM. Chlamydia infections and heart disease linked through antigenic mimicry. Science 1999; 283:1335–1339.

51. Deng GM, Nilsson IM, Verdrength M, Collins LV, Tarkowski A. Intra-articularly localized bacterial DNA containing CpG motifs induces arthritis. Nat Med 1999; 5:702–705.

52. Tsunoda I, Tolley ND, Theil DJ, Whitton JL, Kobayashi H, Fujinami RS. Exacerbation of viral and autoimmune animal models for multiple sclerosis by bacterial DNA. Brain Pathol 1999; 9:481–493.

53. Shirota H, Sano K, Kikuchi T, Tamura G, Shirato K. Regulation of murine airway eosinophilia and Th2 cells by antigen-conjugated CpG oligodeoxynucleotides as a novel antigen-specific immunomodulator. J Immunol 2000; 164:5575–5582.

54. Wolff JA, Ludtke JJ, Acsadi G, Williams P. Jani A. Long-term persistence of plasmid DNA and foreign gene expression in mouse muscle. Hum Mol Genet 1992; 1:363–369.

55. Davis HL, Mancini M, Michel ML, Whalen RG. DNA-mediated immunization to hepatitis B surface antigen: longevity of primary response and effect of boost. Vaccine 1996; 14:910–915.

56. Deck RR, De Witt CM, Donnelly JJ, Liu MA, Ulmer JB. Characterization of humoral immune responses induced by an influenza hemagglutinin DNA vaccine. Vaccine 1997; 15:71–78.

57. Klinman DM, Yamshchikov G, Ishigatsubo Y. Contribution of CpG motifs to the immunogenicity of DNA vaccines. J Immunol 1997; 158:3635–3639.

58. Wloch MK, Pasquini S, Ertl HC, Pisetsky DS. The influence of DNA sequence on the immunostimulatory properties of plasmid DNA vectors. Hum Gene Ther 1998; 9:1439–1447.

59. Sato Y, Roman M, Tighe H, Lee D, Corr M, Nguyen MD, Silverman GJ, Lotz M, Carson DA, Raz E. Immunostimulatory DNA sequences necessary for effective intradermal gene immunization. Science 1996; 273:352–354.

60. Akbari O, Panjwani N, Garcia S, Tascon R, Lowrie D, Stockinger B. DNA vaccination: transfection and activation of dendritic cells as they events for immunity. J Exp Med 1999; 189:169–178.

61. Krieg AM, Yi AK, Schorr J, Davis HL. The role of CpG dinucleotides in DNA vaccines (Review). Trends Microbiol 1998; 6:23–27.

62. Donnelly JJ, Ulmer JB, Shiver JW, Liu MA. DNA vaccines (Review). Annu Rev Immunol 1997; 15:617–648.

63. Feltquate DM, Heaney S. Webster RG, Robinson HL. Different T helper cell types and antibody isotypes generated by saline and gene gun DNA immunization. J Immunol 1997; 158:2278–2284.

64. Raz E, Tighe H, Sato Y, Corr M, Dudler JA, Roman M, Swain SL, Spiegelberg HL, Carson DA. Preferential induction of a Th1 immune response and inhibition of specific IgE antibody formation by plasmid DNA immunization. Proc Natl Acad Sci USA 1996; 93:5141–5145.

65. Hsu CH, Chua KY, Tao MH, Lai YL, Wu HD, Huang SK, Hsieh KH. Immunoprophylaxis of allergen-induced immunoglobulin E synthesis and airway hyperresponsiveness in vivo by genetic immunization. Nat Med 1996; 2:540–544.

66. Manickan E, Rouse RJ, Yu Z, Wire WS, Rouse BT. Genetic immunization against herpes simplex virus. Protection is mediated by CD4+ T lymphocytes. J Immunol 1995; 155:259–265.

67. Raz E, Carson DA, Parker SE, Parr TB, Abai AM, Aichinger G, Gromkowski SH, Singh M, Lew D, Yankauckas MA et al. Intradermal gene immunization: the possible role of DNA uptake in the induction of cellular immunity to viruses. Proc Natl Acad Sci USA 1994; 91:9519–9523.

68. Davis HL, McCluskie MJ, Gerin JL, Purcell RH. DNA vaccine for hepatitis B: evidence for immunogenicity in chimpanzees and comparison with other vaccines. Proc Natl Acad Sci USA 1996; 93:7213–7218.

69. Wang B, Boyer J, Srikantan V, Coney L, Carrano R, Phan C, Merva M, Dang K, Agadjanan M, Gilbert L et al. DNA inoculation induces neutralizing immune responses against human immunodeficiency virus type 1 in mice and nonhuman primates. DNA Cell Biol 1993; 12:799–805.

70. Boyer JD, Ugen KE, Wang B, Agadjanyan M, Gilbert L, Bagarazzi ML, Chattergoon M, Frost P, Javadian A, Williams WV, Refaeli Y, McCallus D,

Coney L, Weiner DB. Protection of chimpanzees from high-dose heterologous HIV-1 challenge by DNA vaccination. Nat Med 1997; 3:526–532.

71. Ulmer JB, Donnely JJ, Parker SE, Rhodes GH, Felgner PL, Dwarki VJ, Gromkowski SH, Deck RR, DeWitt CM, Friedman A, et al. Heterologous protection against influenza by injection of DNA encoding a viral protein. Science 1993; 259:1745–1749.

72. Slater JE, Paupore E, Zhang YT, Colberg-Poley AM. The latex allergen Hev b5 transcript is widely distributed after subcutaneous injection in BALB/c mice of its DNA vaccine. J Allergy Clin Immunol 1998; 102:469–475.

73. Broide D, Orozco EM, Roman M, Carson DA, Raz E. Intradermal gene vaccination down-regulates both arms of the allergic response (abstr). J Allergy Clin Immunol 1997; 99:129.

74. Maecker HT, Hansen G, Walter DM, DeKruyff RH, Levy S, Umetsu DT. Vaccination with allergen-IL-18 fusion DNA protects against, and reverses established, airway hyperreactivity in a murine asthma model. J Immunol 2001; 166:959–965.

75. Kumano K, Nakao A, Nakajima H, Hayashi F, Kurimoto M, Okamura H, Saito Y, Iwamoto I. Interleukin-18 enhances antigen-induced eosinophil recruitment into the mouse airways. Am J Respir Crit Care Med 1999; 160:873–878.

76. Wild JS, Sigounas A, Sur N, Siddiqui MS, Alam R, Kurimoto M, Sur S. IFN-gamma-inducing factor (IL-18) increases allergic sensitization, serum IgE, Th2 cytokines, and airway eosinophilia in a mouse model of allergic asthma. J Immunol 2000; 164:2701–2710.

77. Li XM, Chopra RK, Chou TY, Schofield BH, Wills-Karp M, Huang SK. Mucosal IFN-gamma gene transfer inhibits pulmonary allergic responses in mice. J Immunol 1996; 157:3216–3239.

78. Wang R, Doolan DL, Le TP, Hedstrom RC, Coonan KM, Charoenvit Y, Jones TR, Hobart P, Margalith M, Ng J, Weiss WR, Sedegah M, de Taisne C, Norman JA, Hoffman SL. Induction of antigen-specific cytotoxic T lymphocytes in humans by a malaria DNA vaccine. Science 1998; 282:476–480.

79. Calarota S, Bratt G, Nordlund S, Hinkula J, Leandersson AC, Sandstrom E, Wahren B. Cellular cytotoxic response induced by DNA vaccination in HIV-1-infected patients. Lancet 1998; 351:1320–1325.

80. MacGregor RR, Boyer JD, Ugen KE, Lacy KE, Gluckman SJ, Bagarazzi ML, Chattergoon MA, Baine Y, Higgins TJ, Ciccarelli RB, Coney LR, Ginsberg RS, Weiner DB. First human trial of a DNA-based vaccine for treatment of human immunodeficiency virus type 1 infection; safety and host response. J Infect Dis 1998; 178:92–100.

81. Krieg AM, Wu T, Weeratna R, Efler SM, Love-Homan L, Yang L, Yi Ak, Short D, Davis HL. Sequence motifs in adenoviral DNA block immune activation by stimulatory CpG motifs. Proc Natl Acad Sci USA 1998; 95:12631–12636.

82. Tsuji T, Hamajima K, Fukushima J, Xin KQ, Ishii N, Aoki I, Ishigatsubo Y, Tani K, Kawamoto S, Nitta Y, Miyazaki J, Koff WC, Okubo T, Okuda K. Enhancement of cell-mediated immunity against HIV-1 induced by coinnoculation of plasmid-encoded HIV-1 antigen with plasmid expressing IL-12. J Immunol 1997; 158:4008–4013.

83. Svanholm C, Lowenadler B, Wigzell H. Amplification of T-cell and antibody responses in DNA-based immunization with HIV-1 Nef by co-injection with a GM-CSF expression vector. Scand J Immunol 1997; 46:298–303.

84. Iwasaki A, Stiernholm BJ, Chan AK, Berinstein NL, Barber BH. Enhanced CTL responses mediated by plasmid DNA immunogens encoding costimulatory molecules and cytokines. J Immunol 1997; 158:4591–4601.

85. Schneider J, Gilbert SC, Blanchard TJ, Hanke T, Robson KJ, Hannan CM, Becker M, Sinden R, Smith GL, Hill AV. Enhanced immunogenicity for CD8+ T cell induction and complete protective efficacy of malaria DNA vaccination by boosting with modified vaccinia virus Ankara. Nat Med 1998; 4:397–402.

86. Lack G, Renz H, Saloga J, Bradley KL, Loader J, Leung DY, Larsen G, Gelfand EW. Nebulized but not parenteral IFN-gamma decreases IgE production and normalizes airways function in a murine model of allergen sensitization. J Immunol 1994; 152:2546–2554.

87. Lack G, Bradley KL, Hamelmann E, Renz H, Loader J, Leung DY, Larsen G, Gelfand EW. Nebulized INF-gamma inhibits the development of secondary allergic responses in mice. J Immunol 1996; 157:1432–1439.

88. Gavett SH, O'Hearn DJ, Li X, Huang SK, Finkelman FD, Wills-Karp M. Interleukin 12 inhibits antigen-induced airway hyperresponsiveness, inflammation, and Th2 cytokine expression in mice. J Exp Med 1995; 182:1527–1536.

89. Hofstra CL, Van Ark I, Hofman G, Kool M, Nijkamp FP, Van Oosterhout AJ. Prevention of Th2-like cell responses by coadministration of IL-12 and IL-18 is associated with inhibition of antigen-induced airway hyperresponsiveness, eosinophilia, and serum IgE levels. J Immunol 1998; 161:5054–5060.

90. Marshall E. Cancer trial of interleukin-12 halted. Science 1995; 268:1555.

91. Cohn L, Homer RJ, Niu N, Bottomly K. T helper 1 cells and interferon gamma regulate allergic airway inflammation and mucus production. J Exp Med 1999; 190:1309–1318.

92. Huang TJ, MacAry PA, Eynott P, Moussavi A, Daniel KC, Askenase PW, Kemeny DM, Chung KF. Allergen-specific Th1 cells counteract efferent Th2 cell-dependent bronchial hyperresponsiveness and eosinophilic inflammation partly via IFN-gamma. J Immunol 2001; 166:207–217.

93. Hansen G, Berry G, DeKruyff RH, Umetsu DT. Allergen-specific Th1 cells fail to counterbalance Th2 cell-induced airway hyperreactivity but cause severe airway inflammation. J Clin Invest 1999; 103:175–183.

94. Randolph DA, Carruthers CJ, Szabo SJ, Murphy KM, Chaplin DD. Modulation of airway inflammation by passive transfer of allergen-specific Th1 and Th2 cells in a mouse model of asthma. J Immunol 1999; 162:2375–2383.

95. Reddy A, Sapp M, Feldman M, Subklewe M, Bhardwaj N. A monocyte conditioned medium is more effective than defined cytokines in mediating the terminal maturation of human dendritic cells. Blood 1997; 90:3640–3646.

96. Romani N, et al. Generation of mature dendritic cells from human blood: An improved method with special regard to clinical applicability. J Immunol Meth 1996; 196:137–151.

97. Reis e Sousa C, Sher A, Kaye P. The role of dendritic cells in the induction and regulation of immunity to microbial infection. Currr Opin Immunol 1999; 11:392–399. Review.

98. Fong L, Engleman EG. Dendritic cells in cancer immunotherapy (Review). Annu Rev Immunol 2000; 18:245–273.
99. Timmerman JM, Levy R. Dendritic cell vaccines for cancer immunotherapy. Annu Rev Med 1999; 50: 507–529.
100. Chen Y, Kuchroo VK, Inobe J, Hafler DA, Weiner HL. Regulatory T cell clones induced by oral tolerance: suppression of autoimmune encephalomyelitis. Science 1994; 265:1237–1240.
101. Groux H, O'Garra A, Bigler M, Rouleau M, Antonenko S, de Vires JE, Roncarolo MG. A CD4+ T-cell subset inhibits antigen-specific T-cell responses and prevents colitis. Nature 1997; 389:737–742.
102. Haneda K, Sano K, Tamura G, Shirota H, Ohkawara Y, Sato T, Habu S, Shirato K. Transforming growth factor-beta secreted from CD4(+) T cells ameliorates antigen-induced eosinophilic inflammation. A novel high-dose tolerance in the trachea. Am J Respir Cell Mol Biol 1999; 21:268–274.
103. Hansen G, McIntire JJ, Yeung VP, Berry G, Thorbecke GJ, Chen L, DeKruyff RH, Umetsu DT. CD4(+) T helper cells engineered to produce latent TGF-beta1 reverse allergen-induced airway hyperreactivity and inflammation. J Clin Invest 2000; 105:61–70.
104. Thorbecke GJ, Umetsu DT, deKruyff RH, Hansen G, Chen LZ, Hochwald GM. When engineered to produce latent TGF-beta1, antigen specific T cells down regulate Th1 cell-mediated autoimmune and Th2 cell–mediated allergic inflammatory processes (Review). Cytokine Growth Factor Rev 2000; 11:89–96.
105. Cottrez F, Hurst SD, Coffman RL, Groux H. T regulatory cells 1 inhibit a Th2-specific response in vivo. J Immunol 2000; 165:4:848–853.
106. Yang JS, Xu LY, Huang YM, Van Der Meide PH, Link H, Xiao BG. Adherent dendritic cells expressing high levels of interleukin-10 and low levels of interleukin-12 induce antigen-specific tolerance to experimental autoimmune encephalomyelitis. Immunology 2000; 101:397–403.

24

Adenovirus-Mediated Gene Therapy for Asthma

RYAN E. WILEY, DAVID ALVAREZ, and MANEL JORDANA

McMaster University
Hamilton, Ontario, Canada

I. Introduction

Applications of gene therapy for asthma, though the enticing consideration of numerous reviews both hopeful and tepid, remain at an early stage of investigation (1–7). Even less is understood about the particular contribution adenoviral constructs might play in the management of asthma, as a heterogeneous body of often tangential research into asthma gene therapy has emerged from a diverse cross-section of genetic vectors. Nonetheless, experimental work in animal models of antigen-induced airways inflammation has afforded compelling insight into the prospects for the short-term intervention, long-term management, and even reversal of asthma pathophysiology through the delivery of therapeutic genetic vectors, although translation of this progress to the clinical setting is only now receiving serious consideration. Emerging from this profusion of experimental strategies, however, are two basic conceptualizations of gene-based therapeutic modalities: to attenuate the expression of key effector mediators of asthmatic inflammation through, for example, the inhibition of gene transcription or translation; and to subvert allergic sensitization through genetic immunotherapy with or without the concurrent provision of genes encoding immunomodulatory signals. This chapter surveys the gene-based therapeutic modalities that have been proposed for asthma and considers these in the context of the advantages and limitations of potential adenovirus (Ad)–mediated applications.

II. Prospects for Adenoviral Gene Therapy

When considering gene therapy for asthma, one can conceive any number of potential molecular targets—including cell adhesion molecules (VCAM-1, ICAM-1) (8), proinflammatory cytokines (IL-1, IL-6, TNF-α) (9,10), Th2-affiliated cytokines (IL-4, IL-5, IL-13) (10), and costimulatory molecules (11)—or therapeutic interventions, such as the provision of anti-inflammatory or immunomodulatory cytokines (IL-10, TGF-β) (12) (Table 1). The design of an adenoviral construct, therefore, reflects both an understanding of the pathophysiology of asthma and a strategic conceptualization of asthma therapy: is the object of the intervention to manage asthma exacerbations transiently or to reprogram the immunological underpinnings of the disease? For instance, interference with specific molecular targets is conceptually consonant with the conventional asthma armamentarium of brochodilators and corticosteroids, which preempt or abort the expression of a persistent asthmatic phenotype but do not cure disease; conversely, the provision of allergen in the context of appropriate immunomodulatory signals might best be described as an attempt to modify or eradicate the underlying pathology permanently. The sections that follow explore these therapeutic paradigms for asthma in the context of various adenoviral applications. We shall begin by considering some of the molecular targets that may prove particularly relevant to asthma therapy.

A. Potential Molecular Targets

Cytokine Networks

Over the last decade, the exponential proliferation of knowledge about the importance of cytokine networks in the pathogenesis of allergic asthma has propagated a therapeutic mission that aims to interfere *selectively* with the biological activity of cytokines. Descriptive findings in human asthmatics have

Table 1 Potential Molecular Targets for Therapeutic Intervention in Allergic Asthma

Category	Examples
Cytokine networks	Proinflammatory (GM-CSF, TNF-α) Th2-associated (IL-4, IL-5) Immunoregulatory (IL-10, TGF-β)
Chemokine networks	Ligands (MCP-1, eotaxin, TARC) Receptors (CCR2, CCR3, CCR4)
Intracellular signaling molecules	Jak/STAT pathway Transcription factors (NF-κB)
Costimulatory molecules	APC-associated (B7 family) T-cell-associated (CD28, ICOS)

identified several cytokines pertinent to disease pathogenesis, including the proimmune cytokine GM-CSF, proinflammatory cytokines (IL-1, IL-6, IL-11, and TNF-α), the helper T-cell type 2 (Th2)–derived cytokines (IL-3, IL-4, IL-5, IL-9, and IL-13), and, to some extent, cytokines with anti-inflammatory or immunoregulatory properties (IL-1RA, IL-10, IL-12, TGF-β and IFN-γ) (10,13,14). Indeed, the majority of such cytokines have been evaluated experimentally in animal models of allergic airways inflammation. Despite encouraging experimental data for many of these cytokines, only a few have advanced to the clinical setting.

Most attention has been focused on blockade of IL-4 or IL-5, either through antibodies against receptors, receptor antagonists, soluble receptors, or neutralizing antibodies. Initial studies in human asthmatics reported that IL-5 neutralization reduced blood eosinophilia and prevented eosinophil infiltration into the airways following allergen provocation. However, blockade of IL-5 in humans showed little to no impact on the early- or late-phase response to allergen or on airway hyperresponsiveness (AHR) (15). A more recent phase I trial with a humanized anti-IL-5 antibody in severe persistent asthmatics resulted in long-lasting reduction in peripheral blood eosinophilia and a trend toward improvement in FEV_1 (16). Similarly, recent clinical studies have reported some benefit associated with nebulized soluble IL-4 receptor treatment in moderate asthmatics (17,18). As of yet, long-term clinical studies are still required to evaluate fully the therapeutic potential of anti-IL-5 and anti-IL-4 therapy in human asthmatics (19).

Chemokines and Chemokine Receptors

Leukocyte trafficking and homing in health and disease are regulated by a family of small chemoattractant cytokines and their receptors. Important advances in the field of chemoakine biology warrant the development of selective inhibitors of chemokine function, particularly in the form of chemokine receptor antagonists. Several chemokines (eotaxin, RANTES, MCP-1, TARC, MIP-1α, MIP-3α) and chemokine receptors (CCR1-4, -8, and CXCR1-2) have been shown to play important roles in the recruitment of specific cells, such as eosinophils, basophils, macrophages, monocytes, mast cells, and Th2 lymphocytes, and have therefore prompted research into a new generation of exciting drug targets for asthma (20,21). Debate over whether small-molecule antagonists of chemokine receptors could ever be efficacious has been prompted by the apparent redundancy of chemokine networks, which suggests that disruption of specific ligand–receptor interactions may offer limited benefit for a given inflammatory disease. Although experimental data in animal models of allergic airways disease utilizing chemokine receptor antibodies or chemokine/chemokine receptor–deficient mouse strains are promising, the recently patented small-molecule chemokine receptor antagonists still await evaluation in human clinical trials (20).

Intracellular Signaling Molecules

Several signal transduction pathways have been described for specific immune events implicated in acute and chronic inflammatory responses in asthma. Intracellular signaling cascades for cytokine receptors, G-protein-coupled chemokine receptors, and antibody Fc receptors have unveiled a wide spectrum of potential novel targets for drug design. New therapeutic agents now under development include phosphodiesterase (PDE_4) inhibitors, receptor-coupled protein kinase (Jak/STAT pathway) inhibitors, nonreceptor protein tyrosine kinase (Syk and Lyk) inhibitors, MAP kinase inhibitors, and inhibitors of the transcription factor NF-κB (22). Among these various strategies, the newest generation PDE_4 inhibitors have proven the most promising and have reached their final phase of clinical evaluation. Although tyrosine kinase inhibition appears to be a very attractive strategy for drug development, the ponderous family of kinases of multiple subtypes presents a significant obstacle to the design of highly specific inhibitors with limited side effects. That the transcription factor NF-κB functions downstream of the tyrosine kinase signaling cascade and seems to be responsible for the transcription of various proinflammatory genes implicated in asthma renders it an especially promising target for pharmacological manipulation (23,24). The next few years should witness the evaluation of their efficacy in human patients.

Costimulatory Molecules

Cognate interactions between naive T cells and antigen-presenting cells initiate a series of molecular interactions that can result in T-cell activation and the establishment of antigen-specific immunity. There is some support for the notion that the nature of the interaction between B7 costimulatory molecules and their counterligands CD28 and CTLA-4 may determine the extent to which T cells become polarized to a Th2-associated phenotype (11). Indeed, blocking antibodies to B7-2 or CD28 have been shown to inhibit pulmonary eosinophilia and AHR in models of allergic airway disease (25). Moreover, blockade of the B7–CD28 interaction with soluble CTLA-4 fusion protein has effectively prevented AHR in murine models of asthma (26). In the last few years, the family of costimulatory molecules has grown to include such members as inducible costimulator (ICOS) and the B7-related proteins 1 and 2 (27–33). Further experimental support for the involvement of such molecules in optimal T-cell activation and effective T-cell-dependent immune responses will shed light on the promise of costimulatory molecules as potential therapeutic targets for asthma.

B. Adenoviral Constructs: Potential Therapeutic Modalities

Antisense Strategies: Techniques and Targets

Antisense oligonucleotides (ASOs) directed against mRNA species or DNA sequences of pathophysiological interest represent a vigorously contemplated

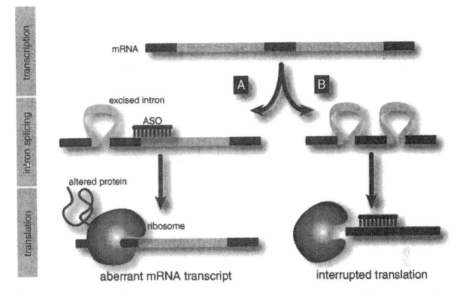

Figure 1 Schematic representation of antisense oligonucleotide (ASO) therapy. (A) ASO directed against intron–exon boundaries can promote differential excision of introns and exons, yielding an aberrant mRNA transcript and a therapeutically modified translated peptide. (B) ASO directed against processed mRNA can interrupt translation and ablate production of intact protein.

genetic therapy for asthma (34). By hybridizing with complementary mRNA transcripts in the cell, ASO can interrupt the translation of targeted immune-inflammatory genes that potentiate disease (Fig. 1). Although most experimental antisense therapies for asthma have been delivered in the context of native oligonucleotides, Ad-mediated expression of regulatory DNA or RNA sequences is certainly not without precedent (35–37) and, in a single instance, has even been described in an experimental model of allergic airways inflammation (38). With the circumspection advised by Stein's recent critique (39) that ASO studies historically have been improperly controlled and their results likely overinterpreted, we shall consider the range of experimental antisense genetic therapies for asthma that have been investigated to date, regardless of vector identity (Table 2).

Given its prominent role in the differentiation, degranulation, and survival of eosinophils, IL-5 has been a logical and particularly robust target of experimental (and, by extension, Ad-mediated) ASO intervention in asthma (40). Karras et al. (41), in both a murine model of ovalbumin (OVA)–induced allergic airways inflammation and a model of allergic peritonitis, have demonstrated that intravenous administration of ASO specifically targeted to IL-5 mRNA suppresses eosinophilia in the target organ. In the lung, this inhibition

Table 2 Experimental ASO Strategies Attempted in Animal Models

Target	Functional role	Effect of ASO intervention	Ref.
IL-5, IL-5 receptor	Eosinopoiesis	↓(?) Eosinophilia ↓ Th2 cytokines	41–45
IL-4	Th2 differentiation	↓ Eosinophilia ↓ Late-phase response	45
SCF	Eosinophil/basophil activation/chemotaxis	↓ Inflammation ↓IL-4 production	46
Syk PTK	Leukocyte signaling	↓ Inflammation	47
Lyn	IL-5 signaling	↓ Eosinophilia	48
GATA-3	IL-5 transcription factor	↓ Inflammation ↓ AHR	50
gob-5	Mucus production	↓ Mucus production ↓ AHR	38
Adenosine receptor	Airway hypersensitivity	Allergen desensitization	57

conferred prolonged protection, persisting for up to 17 days following termination of anti-IL-5 ASO treatment, and was associated with improvement in antigen-mediated late-phase AHR. This group has also presented some pioneering work in the development of chemically modified ASOs that, rather than inhibit translation, promote therapeutic splicing of their mRNA targets. In particular, they have manufactured an ASO that preferentially deletes individual exons from the subunit of IL-5 receptor mRNA and promotes translation of the soluble form of this receptor; unlike the membrane-bound variant, the soluble form of the IL-5 receptor inhibits IL-5 signaling and may represent a naturally occurring negative regulator of IL-5 activity (42,43). Corroborating these data is the complementary finding that ASO directed against the IL-5 receptor inhibited eosinopoiesis in a murine model of ragweed-induced allergic peritonitis (44). Of note, however, are the conflicting—but potentially promising—results of Molet et al. (45) who, employing a model of allergic asthma involving intraperitoneal transfer of OVA-primed CD4$^+$ T cells to brown Norway rats, have shown that ASO directed against IL-4, but not IL-5, mRNA attenuates Th2 cytokine production, BAL eosinophilia and late airways responses after OVA aerosol challenge. Whether the difference in the efficacy of these two IL-5-directed ASO interventions simply reflects nuanced idiosyncracies in ASO design or underscores substantive limitations of IL-5 mRNA as a tractable therapeutic target has yet to be elucidated fully. Finally, Finotto et al. (46) have reported that intrapulmonary delivery of ASO targeted to the c-kit ligand stem cell factor (SCF), a key activation and chemotactic signal for eosinophils and basophils, attenuates airway inflammation and IL-4 production in a murine model of asthma.

Prospective ASO therapy for asthma may also include targeting the intracellular signaling molecules or transcription factors that regulate cytokine production. For instance, ASO directed against Syk protein tyrosine kinase (PTK), a molecule involved in leukocyte signaling, depresses Syk PTK expression and inhibits antigen-induced pulmonary inflammation in rats (47). In this light, the IL-5 signaling molecule Lyn—whose inactivation by a peptide inhibitor has been shown to block eosinophil differentiation, survival, and airway eosinophilic inflammation in a mouse model of allergic asthma (48)—and the transcription factor GATA-3 whose ASO-mediated silencing in cultured Th2 cells specifically inhibits IL-5 promoter activation (49) and, in mice, attenuates experimental allergic airway inflammation and hyperresponsiveness (50)—may represent highly tailored therapeutic targets. In a similar vein, the work of McKinlay et al. (51), who were able to repress the activity of the GM-CSF reporter in cultured mast cells by administering an ASO targeting the transcription factor Ets-1, may ultimately find application in the therapeutic regulation of GM-CSF's hematopoietic and immunostimulatory activities—activities that have particular relevance to the evolution of the allergic phenotype (52).

Alternatively, ASO may be designed to interrupt cardinal physiological manifestations of asthma. For example, an ASO against the mucin gene has been shown to inhibit retinoic acid–induced mucus mRNA production and mucus secretion in rabbit tracheal epithelial cells in vitro (53); and Nakanishi et al. (38), employing recombinant Ad to express antisense RNA against *gob-5* (a member of the calcium-activated chloride channel family) in the airway, reported suppression of AHR and mucus overproduction in a murine model of asthma. The proliferation of smooth muscle and activation of its contractile apparatus, whose dysregulation accounts for the chest tightness and dyspnea characteristic of the asthmatic response, furnish another promising target for antisense gene therapy (54). To this end, Lee et al. (55) have demonstrated that ASO species against extracellular signal–regulated kinases (ERK), which play a key role in the signal transduction pathways that induce cell proliferation, inhibit the expansion of human airway smooth muscle cells in vitro and may represent a viable therapeutic option for the reversal of smooth muscle hyperplasia endemic to the pathological presentation of asthma. Finally, Nyce and Metzger (56) have documented allergen desensitization in dust mite–allergic rabbits treated with ASOs targeting the A1 receptor, whose ligand, the endogenous purine adenosine, has been implicated in the airway hypersensitivity characteristic of bronchial asthma (57).

Immunomodulation

Ad-based cytokine therapy for asthma is not restricted to strategies that inhibit endogenous cytokine production and thereby prevent the expression of a pathological allergic phenotype. Indeed, several investigators have explored the *delivery* of exogenous cytokine genes whose expression might modulate the immunological profile of allergic asthma. To this end, Kang et al. (58) have documented the repolarization of the OVA-specific immunoglobulin profile—from IgE to IgG_{2a}—following intramuscular injection of the cDNA for IFN-γ in mice concurrently sensitized to OVA in the context of aluminum hydroxide. Interestingly, parallel treatment with the cDNA for IL-4 also inhibited expression of IgE, although this intervention did not simultaneously potentiate Th1-polarized immunoglobulin production. Corroborating these findings in a more relevant murine model of allergic asthma—and elaborating data initially reported by Li et al. (59)—Dow et al. (60) describe the inhibition of AHR, airways eosinophilia, and serum IgE in OVA-sensitized mice following intravenous (and to a lesser extent intratracheal) IFN-γ gene delivery (as a lipid–DNA complex) at the time of OVA challenge. Moreover, the therapeutic benefits of IFN-γ gene delivery far exceeded those elicited by treatment with recombinant IFN-γ. Finally, airway gene transfer of vaccinia virus–encoded IL-12—the paradigmatic Th1-polarizing cytokine—has been shown to prevent the development of allergic disease and AHR, to suppress the expression of established allergy, and to restore antiviral cell-mediated immunity in the lungs of mice (61).

Informing each of these approaches to cytokine gene transfer is the notion that immune deviation (i.e., the elaboration of competing Th1 phenomena) is therapeutically advantageous for Th2-polarized disorders such as allergic asthma (62). However, the inflammation associated with Th1-privileged immune modulation can be just as pathological as the allergic phenotype. Indeed, Ad-mediated airway gene transfer of IL-12 (63) or the Th1-affiliated chemokine IP-10 (64) to mice undergoing mucosal allergic sensitization to OVA elicits robust mononuclear cell inflammation, cytokine expression, and immunoglobulin production, and conditions a Th1-polarized inflammatory memory response upon OVA recall in vivo. In this light, genetic delivery of immunomodulatory cytokines such as IL-10, which conveys anti-inflammatory properties and has been implicated in the development of immunological tolerance, may represent a more appropriate therapeutic modality (65–67). Indeed, airway gene transfer of IL-10, unlike IL-12 and IP-10, to mice mucosally sensitized to OVA completely abrogated allergic airways inflammation and rendered mice persistently nonresponsive to subsequent OVA challenge (68). Critical to the consideration of IL-10 as a candidate for asthma immunomodulation, however, are recent data implicating IL-10 in the expression of AHR in allergic mice (69).

Allergen Immunotherapy

Allergen gene transfer has emerged as one of the most promising therapeutic modalities for allergic diseases (70–75). This genetic incarnation of conventional allergen immunotherapy, typically involving the prophylactic or therapeutic administration of naked DNA encoding or presented in the context of allergen peptides, has been associated in animal models with the induction of allergen "tolerance" (76) and with IgG antibodies supplanting the allergic IgE response (77–80). While these immunological changes are credited with the amelioration of respiratory sequelae, including immediate hypersensitivity, histamine content in bronchoalveolar lavage (BAL), pulmonary eosinophilic inflammation, and AHR (77,80), this association must be interpreted cautiously because antigen-specific AHR and airway eosinophilia can develop in mice via IgE-independent mechanisms (81). With respect to the mechanism underlying these phenomena, experimental evidence suggests that immunization with plasmid DNA sequences, which encode immunostimulatory CpG motifs, elicits Th1-polarized immunological phenomena, which effectively deviate or subvert the development of the cardinal Th2-affiliated features of allergy (78,80,82–84). Theoretically, however, any genetic instrument, such as a recombinant Ad vector, that induces a Th1 response could have the same immunomodulatory effect; indeed, immunization of mice with recombinant BCG vaccine, modified to express a surrogate allergen, elaborated elevated levels of IFN-γ and inhibited the production of IL-5 and antigen-specific IgE compared with mice inoculated with antigen alone (85). In this light, it may also be germane to consider combination genetic strategies that deliver allergen in conjunction with an explicit immunomodulatory signal. An adenoviral construct whose genome encodes an allergenic sequence and, for instance, the gene for IL-10 or IL-12 could conceivably potentiate an allergen-specific immune response designed to subvert or reeducate prevailing Th2-associated immunopathology.

Context

While expounding the prospects for asthma gene therapy, one must be cognizant of the limitations that attend this technology. For example, the identity of the recombinant genetic vector and the route of administration have important implications for the magnitude and duration of transgene expression. While adenoviral vectors offer superior transduction efficiency compared with, for example, plasmid DNA, the relatively high antigenicity of Ad vectors would predispose them to therapeutic applications that require only transient modulation of immune microenvironment. In addition, while *airway* gene transfer is certainly alluring for asthma therapy, the intrinsic resistance of the airway lumen to adenoviral infection represents a significant barrier to gene delivery by Ad constructs. Moreover, the immune response initiated by the vector itself is an important therapeutic consideration which, ironically, may obviate the need for genetic engineering of the vector and insertion of an immunomodulatory transgene. Both intramuscular (86) and intranasal (87) administration of replication-deficient adenovirus have been shown to inhibit OVA-specific allergic airway responses in mice, possibly through the endogenous upregulation of Th1 cytokines. These and other limitations of Ad-mediated gene transfer will be considered systematically in the sections that follow.

III. Inherent Limitations of the Adenoviral Vector

Among the panoply of gene transfer technologies, replication-deficient recombinant adenoviruses offer distinct mechanical and biological advantages: they have an almost ubiquitous infectious tropism, resulting in efficient transduction of a diverse range of cell types irrespective of differentiation status; they are stably rendered replication deficient; they can be produced at high titer; and their genomes are readily manipulated to accommodate relatively large transgenes (88,89) (Fig. 2). However, as a prospective therapeutic instrument, adenoviruses present important obstacles that merit consideration and redress (Table 3). Perhaps chief among these limitations is the attendant antiviral immune-inflammatory response, which dampens and abbreviates transgene expression, and potentially precludes efficacious readministration of the vector. Indeed, premature silencing of *cftr* (cystic fibrosis transmembrane conductance regulator) transgene expression in humans has been the rejoinder to prospects for sustained amelioration of cystic fibrosis by recombinant adenoviruses (90–97). Admittedly, a transient therapeutic effect—while incompatible with cystic fibrosis, a congenital disease necessitating uninterrupted correction—may befit episodic syndromes, such as milder manifestations of asthma, that are characterized by periodic exacerbations. Therefore, while the therapeutic objectives of gene delivery for asthma may be strategically and conceptually different from those necessitated by cystic fibrosis, research into gene therapy for cystic fibrosis has afforded valuable insight into the immunology of adenoviral vectors and the options for mitigating the potentially confounding immune-inflammatory responses they elicit.

A. Vector-Induced Immune-Inflammatory Responses: Mechanisms and Implications

The Ad-induced cytotoxic T lymphocyte (CTL) response, whose targeted deletion of virus-infected cells ultimately aborts expression of the transgene, has been an area of intense investigation. Dependent on the induction of Th1 cells and the up-regulation of MHC class I by IFN-γ (98,99)—possibly by a mechanism that supplants the conventional requirement for professional

Table 3 Advantages and Disadvantages of Recombinant Adenovirus as a Therapeutic Vector

Advantages	Disadvantages
– Transduces a diverse variety of cell types	– Elicits immune-inflammatory response
– Stably rendered replication deficient	– Transgene expression is transient
– Genome accommodates large transgenes	– Multiple administrations hampered by preexisting anti-Ad immunity

antigen-presenting cells (APCs) (100)—the CTL response in rodents has conventionally been associated with expression of viral genes by virus-infected cells (101). However, it is equally apparent that both native viral structural proteins (102–104) and the therapeutic transgene itself can serve as MHC class I–restricted targets of CTL activity (105). Indeed, intratracheal immunization of mice with genetically incomplete or inactivated viral particles elicits an inflammatory response comparable to infection by intact virus (102), and cells infected ex vivo with genetically inert viral particles are efficiently lysed by splenocytes from virus-infected mice (103). Moreover, it has been demonstrated that the progressive deletion of the adenoviral genome may not be sufficient to extend the in vivo persistence of transduced cells or to subvert the anti-Ad immune response (104). Alternatively, CTL activity against *foreign* transgene–encoded proteins may in fact provide the principal explanation for the instability of gene expression following Ad administration to mice, a problem that, experimentally, is readily circumvented by the judicious incorporation of autologous transgene sequences into the recombinant virus (105).

While the role of *adaptive* CTL-mediated immunity in the surveillance of Ad and the termination of transgene expression has been compellingly documented in several experimental settings, other studies have implicated *innate* inflammatory mechanisms in the disruption of Ad-mediated gene transfer. The delayed-type hypersensitivity response to replication-deficient adenovirus (RDA) in the footpad of immunized mice, for example, is MHC class I independent (106); and immunodeficient (athymic) mice evolve inflammatory responses to recombinant RDA that diminish the efficiency of gene transfer (107). In the lung, the precursor to this nonspecific inflammation is likely the up-regulation of the proinflammatory cytokines TNF-α and IL-6 (108), possibly by alveolar macrophages which have been shown to internalize Ad rapidly following acute respiratory infection (109). Moreover, RDA infection of human lung–derived epithelial (A549) cells enhances the expression of the neutrophilic chemokine IL-8 (110), the cell adhesion molecule ICAM-1 (111), and the CD-18-dependent adhesion of activated neutrophils (112) in vitro. Combined, these data indicate that innate and adaptive inflammatory processes preclude sustained expression of Ad-delivered transgenes.

Corroborating these experimental findings, clinical experience with cystic fibrosis has consistently suggested that acute inflammatory responses attenuate the efficiency and duration of Ad-mediated *cftr* gene expression in the lung (90–97). As the episodic nature of allergy and mild asthma does not necessitate sustained genetic correction, one could therefore conceive a therapeutic regimen involving, for instance, the seasonal administration of recombinant adenovirus to alleviate asthmatic symptoms prophylactically or as they arise. However, it is evident that the viability of this strategy may be complicated by the humoral component of the anti-Ad immune response

(91,92,96,113). Indeed, the $CD4^+$ T-cell-dependent elaboration of neutralizing antibodies that associate with adenoviral capsid proteins and prohibit infection could effectively restrict the use of adenovirus to a single therapeutic application. It bears mentioning, however, that anti-Ad immunoglobulin production and resistance to subsequent vector exposure are not exquisitely commensurate. Zabner et al. (114) were able to detect CFTR protein in rhesus monkeys after repeated administration of Ad-encoded *cftr* to nasal epithelia; and Harvey et al. (115) did not detect any change in baseline anti-Ad neutralizing antibody levels in normal subjects after aerosol delivery of RDA, although these researchers have also demonstrated that the progressive diminution of transgene expression upon multiple administration of recombinant Ad does not strictly correlate with the induction of systemic anti-Ad neutralizing antibodies (94). However, the fact that adenoviral vectors do not invariably evoke anti-Ad neutralizing antibody responses in human recipients may be moot given that a significant fraction of individuals have already evolved a potent anti-Ad antibody repertoire through virtually unavoidable prior contact with adenovirus (91); moreover, the magnitude of this preemptive humoral immunity has been shown to predict the extent of the response to preparations of recombinant RDA (116). Therefore, these caveats aside, the conundrum for nonintegrating, nonreplicating adenoviral vectors is their intrinsic transience: acute inflammatory responses abbreviate transgene expression, while humoral immunity precludes the extension of therapy through repetitive vector administration.

B. Circumventing Anti-Ad Immunity

In an effort to subvert therapeutically prohibitive anti-Ad immunity, several researchers have considered options to modify the immunological context in which adenovirus is delivered to the lung (Table 4). To this end, the interaction between T cells and APCs has been a particularly robust target of experimental intervention. In mice, for instance, systemic administration of CTLA4 fusion protein (CTLA4-Ig)—which blocks the B7/CD28 costimulatory pathway—has been shown to impair the development of neutralizing antibodies to Ad during primary infection in the lung and, concomitantly, to permit efficient transgene expression upon secondary exposure to the vector in the absence of concurrent immunomodulatory therapy (117). Although this strategy did not have an appreciable effect on the duration of transgene expression, cotreatment with CTLA4-Ig and a monoclonal antibody against the activated T-cell marker CD40 ligand, whose interaction with CD40 on APCs regulates immunoglobulin production and the expression of costimulatory molecules, mitigated acute inflammation and permitted persistent transgene expression in the airways and alveoli of mice treated intratracheally with a recombinant adenoviral vector (118). Comparably encouraging results have been documented in parallel experimental systems with anti-CD4 (119) and anti-T-cell receptor

Table 4 Strategies to Circumvent Anti-Ad Immunity

Target	Examples
Immune-inflammatory response	Pre-empt the development of anti-Ad adaptive immunity by impairing costimulatory pathways (e.g., B7/CD28, CD40/CD40L)
	Attenuate the inflammatory response by neutralizing proinflammatory cytokines and chemokines (e.g., TNF-α, IL-1, IL-8)
Vector immunogenicity	Delete additional genes (e.g., E2, E4) from first-generation Ad vectors
	Utilize helper-dependent Ad whose genome has been denuded of virtually all endogenous viral sequences

(120) antibody preparations. Even administration of the Th1-affiliated immunomodulatory cytokine IL-12 (or its inducible counterpart IFN-γ) to the airways of mice aborts the development of Th2-dependent blocking IgA antibodies to adenovirus and facilitates repeated introduction of vector to the lung (121); intuitively, however, one must be wary of an intervention strategy that *promotes* Th1 phenomena and cell-mediated immunity. Importantly, in none of these instances was there any evidence of bonafide induction of immunological tolerance of adenovirus; that is, the vector, though persistent, was not necessarily rendered indefinitely benign. Ilan et al. (122), on the other hand, have demonstrated that instillation of adenoviral protein extracts via gastroduodenostomy achieves adoptively transferable "oral" tolerance of viral antigens and, in their model system, efficaciously permits repetitive intravenous administration of RDA to rats.

Although these studies point to the possibility of attenuating the inconvenient immune response to adenoviral vectors, their therapeutic potential must be anticipated with guarded optimism. Each of these strategies is predicated on modifying the context in which adenovirus is initially presented—when, for instance, costimulation is especially relevant—in order to condition a less vigorous immune response against the vector. Unfortunately, this premise belies the clinical reality that established adenoviral immunity is extraordinarily common and may be impervious to interventions that address incipient events in the adaptive response to adenovirus. A more viable approach, therefore, might be to interrupt inflammatory processes directly rather than to reprogram the immune response substantively. For example, administration of a soluble receptor for TNF-α, a proinflammatory cytokine implicated in the manifestation of cellular and humoral immunity induced by adenovirus-mediated airway gene transfer (123), dramatically reduced the inflammatory response to intranasally delivered RDA and, predictably, prolonged transgene expression in the airways of mice (124). Likewise, inhibition of IL-1 activity by an IL-1 receptor antagonist impairs the production of IL-8 by cultured airway epithelial cells stimulated with recombinant adenovirus and, by extension, may provide a means to manage the Ad-induced inflammatory response in vivo (125). Moreover, Minter et al. (126) have suggested that compartmentalized airway expression of an Epstein-Barr virus–derived IL-10 analogue, whose affinity for the IL-10 receptor is at least 1000-fold greater than that for endogenous IL-10, may counteract vector-induced immune-inflammatory responses. Alternatively, general immunosuppression with either cyclophosphamide (127) or cyclosporine, azathioprine, and methylprednisolone (128) have proven effective in ablating neutralizing antibody production or prolonging transgene expression upon adenoviral vector delivery to the lungs of mice, although the clinical side effects of nonspecific immunosuppression may outweigh the benefits of extended adenoviral transgene expression.

Though meritorious, these attempts to rescue replication-deficient adenoviral vectors from their therapeutically retrograde immunogenicity are possibly ill conceived; first-generation recombinant adenoviruses may simply be irremediably poor vectors for sustained transgene expression in the human airway. Moreover, and ironically, the anti-inflammatory nature of each of these rescue strategies may even obviate to some extent the need for therapeutic gene transfer to control asthmatic inflammation. Acknowledging these limitations, a number of investigators have directed their attention to the construction of second-generation and helper-dependent (or "gutless") Ad vectors in which the E1/E3-deleted adenoviral genome has been denuded of additional immunogenic sequences otherwise essential for virus propagation in vitro (88). Systems for the generation of recombinant Ad vectors with deletions in E2 (129–132) or E4 (133–135) have been described. However, the theoretically reduced immunogenicity and enhanced efficacy of these constructs, whose expression of late viral proteins is impaired in vitro (130,136), have yet to be validated conclusively in vivo, particularly in the context of airway gene transfer—although it is known that airway instillation of an adenoviral vector with a temperature-sensitive mutation in the E2a region stabilizes transgene expression and attenuates the inflammatory response in comparison with a conventional first-generation vector (137). Perhaps more promising is the helper-dependent Ad (HDA), the *cause célèbre* of adenoviral gene therapy, whose genome is devoid of virtually all viral sequences and whose in vitro derivation, therefore, requires provision of viral proteins in *trans* by an intact helper Ad (88,138). Although the therapeutic potential of these constructs is potentially complicated by intrinsic vector instability (139) and contamination of vector preparations with helper Ad, preliminary data indicate that impressively pure preparations of recombinant HDA can achieve high levels of transgene expression for a protracted period (about 1 year) in vivo (140–143). These promising findings have yet to be translated to pulmonary gene transfer applications.

The advent of helper-dependent adenovirus has predictably renewed enthusiasm for the therapeutic potential of Ad vectors for management of chronic disease. However, though dramatically enfeebled, these constructs are not immunologically silent. In particular, that viral capsid proteins per se can elicit a humoral response may still preclude potentially necessary read-ministration of HDA (102–104). In this instance, it may be possible to alter-nate the administration of unique adenoviral serotypes from dissimilar (144) or identical (145) subgroups, a stealth tactic that can circumvent anti-Ad neutralizing antibodies and facilitate repetitive gene transfer. And there remains one further consideration: while second-generation Ad and gutless HDA are distinguished by the systematic excision of the virus's genetic iden-tity to minimize immune detection, bonafide immune evasion may actually *benefit* from the expression of certain viral proteins. It is well established that the 19K glycoprotein (gp19K) encoded in the E3 region of the adenoviral genome blocks cell surface expression of MHC class I antigens (146); more recently, Bruder et al. (147) documented comparatively sustained transgene expression in the lungs and livers of mice treated with a gp19K-sufficient recombinant Ad. Likewise, other peptides arising from E3 (148) and E4 (149) have been implicated in the dampening of antiviral immunity and transgene persistence. Even E1a, whose expression is essential for viral propagation and is therefore critically excised from the genome of replication-deficient Ad, can interact directly with STAT1 and suppress the IFN-α-driven, STAT1-dependent gene activation involved in the immunological management of viral infection (150).

IV. Therapeutic Gene Transfer: Targeting the Lung

A significant barrier to Ad-mediated gene transfer to the lung, to which *cftr* gene therapy trials for cystic fibrosis attest, is the intrinsic resistance of the airway epithelium to adenoviral infection. The preeminent conceptualization of ade-noviral entry into cells is described by a biphasic model: initial attachment of the Ad fiber-knob protein to the high-affinity coxsackie B and adenovirus receptor (CAR) (151,152), followed by coated-pit internalization and translo-cation of the virus into the cell cytoplasm, a process attributable to the inter-action of $\alpha_{v3/5}$ integrins with an RGD sequence in the viral penton base (153). That expression of both the CAR (154–156) and $\alpha_{v3/5}$ integrins (157,158) is essentially restricted to the basolateral surface of airway epithelial cells—an interface effectively inaccessible to vectors administered to the airway lumen—renders the apical surface of well-differentiated airway epithelium particularly refractory to viral transduction. However, deficient receptor expression does not account exhaustively for epithelial resistance to vector internalization (159). Notably, modified Ad lacking the $\alpha_{v3/5}$-binding RGD motif are able to transduce human epithelia (160); and the airway epithelial cells from mice unable to express α_{v5} integrins are as susceptible to Ad infection as cells from α_{v5}-sufficient mice (161). Moreover, van Heeckren et al. (162) have demonstrated that *Pseudomonas*-induced bronchopulmonary inflammation diminishes the efficiency of Ad-mediated airway gene transfer, a finding whose implications may be relevant to an airway inflammatory condition such as asthma.

A. Receptor-Mediated Targeting of Airway Epithelium

Given the accessibility of the airway lumen for pulmonary gene transfer—an interface that, with the possible exception of allergen immunotherapy, represents the most logical route for therapeutic gene delivery to asthmatics—substantial research attention has been devoted to overcoming intrinsic epithelial cell resistance to Ad infection. To this end, a number of strategies, ranging from manipulation of adenoviral tropism to selection of an appropriate vector delivery vehicle, have been contemplated (Table 5). Among the most conceptually appealing of these approaches is *adenoviral targeting*: the reorientation of the fiber knob or penton base components of the viral capsid to receptors typically expressed on the apical surface of epithelial cells (163). Typically, this requires disruption of the Ad vector's native receptor affinity and the introduction of novel, tissue-specific ligands through (1) the coadministration of a bispecific liaison molecule that tethers Ad to the target cell; or (2) the genetic reconstruction of adenoviral coat proteins to modify their target cell specificity (163).

Wickham et al. (164) and Haisma et al. (165) have characterized bispecific antibodies that efficiently target Ad to the α_v integrin expressed by otherwise impervious endothelial and smooth muscle cells, or to the EpCAM antigen on malignant cells refractory to Ad infection. However, though conceptually elegant, the translation of this instrument to the in vivo setting is complicated by the potential detection of the vector by the Fc receptor or engagement of the complement system. Immunologically, a more tenable approach may be development of penton base (166,167) or, perhaps more likely, fiber protein (166,168–171) Ad chimeras with therapeutically tractable cell specificities. Indeed, in a

Table 5 Strategies to Increase Adenoviral Gene Transfer

Receptor-specific targeting	Nonspecific targeting
Coadministration of a bispecific liaison molecule (e.g., antibody) that tethers adenovirus to receptors on the target cell	Introduction of adenovirus in the context of a vehicle that enhances distribution or prolongs contact time with target cells
Genetic reconstruction of adenoviral coat proteins to modify their target cell specificity	Administration of a chelating agent that temporarily disrupts intercellular junctions at the epithelial border

seminal paper, Michael et al. (172) proposed the addition of short, receptor-targeted peptide ligands to the carboxy terminus of the adenoviral fiber protein, at once ablating native specificity and dispatching the vector to CAR-deficient tissue. Experimentally, the incorporation of a heparan-binding domain into the fiber coat protein has been shown to enhance adenoviral tropism for heparan sulfate cellular receptors, which are expressed by a diverse spectrum of tissues including fibroblasts, macrophages, smooth muscle, endothelium, and T lymphocytes (170). Likewise, the duplication of an RGD motif (which is native to the penton base) in the fiber knob improves adenoviral transduction of α_v integrin–sufficient smooth muscle and endothelial cells (171) or primary tumor cells in the absence of CAR expression (168).

Moreover, these techniques have been successfully introduced to gene transfer applications directed at the airway epithelium. Zabner et al. (173), for instance, have demonstrated that replacement of the type 2 Ad fiber, which is generally excluded by airway epithelial cells, with an infection-permissive fiber from the type 17 Ad serotype enhances gene transfer to human airway epithelia in vitro. Other molecular targets might include the glycosylphosphatidylinositol-linked urokinase plasminogen activator receptor (174) or G-protein-coupled receptors (175), which reside in abundance on the apical surface of the airway epithelium. Notably, it may *not* be necessary to engineer a chimeric Ad with novel cell-surface receptor selectivity, or to introduce a potentially immunostimulatory bispecific antibody, in order to manipulate adenoviral tropism. For example, the tethering of Ad to a homing ligand through a bifunctional polyethylene glycol bridge has been shown to facilitate gene transfer to cultured airway epithelial cells (174), and may also partially camouflage the vector to evade detection by neutralizing antibodies (176). And in an intriguing inversion of the Ad targeting premise, Lee et al. (177) document the amelioration of adenoviral transduction of cultured cells engineered to express a novel cell surface receptor; by metabolically incorporating a synthetic monosaccharide (ManLev, a modified mannosamine with a levulinate group substituted for the acetyl group) into cell-surface glycoconjugates, cell were bedecked with a functional ketone group to which surrogate adenoviral receptors could be covalently attached.

B. Nonspecific Targeting of Airway Epithelia

It may also be possible to improve the *nonspecific* (i.e., receptor-independent) association of Ad with airway epithelium in order to enhance the efficiency of gene transfer (Table 5). Indeed, data from Zabner et al. (178) and Kitson et al. (159) intimate that Ad delivery strategies that prolong contact time of the vector with epithelia may remedy chronically low transduction rates. For example, complexes of Ad with cationic polymers and cationic lipids increase Ad uptake and transgene expression in differentiated human airway epithelia in vitro and in the nasal epithelium of mice with cystic fibrosis; it has been speculated that the cationic molecules neutralize the intrinsic negative charge of Ad thereby facilitating its attachment to and internalization by the negatively charged epithelial cell membrane (179). Though enticing in its simplicity, this technique is fraught with physiological and immunological complications: cationic lipids are associated with cell toxicity (180,181), activation of complement (182), and may even serve as an adjuvant to augment the transgene-silencing immune response against coadministered Ad (183). A safer alternative might include the transmission of Ad in the context of free cholesterol (184) or a calcium phosphate coprecipitate (185). This latter approach, in particular, enhances CAR- and integrin-independent gene transfer by decorating the epithelial surface with Ad complexes that enter the cell via normal endocytotic mechanisms (186) without introducing additional toxicity or increasing inflammation (187).

Alternatively, the intrinsic resistance of the luminal surface of airway epithelium to Ad infection may be circumvented by selecting an appropriate medium for vector delivery. While pulmonary surfactant, for example, serves as a barrier to gene transfer by nonviral genetic instruments, such as naked plasmid DNA (188,189), the provision of exogenous surfactant (Survanta beractant) actually enhances the distribution and efficiency of Ad-mediated transgene delivery to the lungs of rats, especially when administered at low volumes (190). Similarly, perfluorochemical liquids, which improve gas exchange and lung compliance in models of lung injury, may also serve to convey Ad vectors more uniformly throughout the lungs of rats, thereby optimizing transgene recovery, especially in the distal airways and alveolar epithelium (191). However, the option of enhancing Ad transduction through pervasive pulmonary distribution of the vector must be evaluated in the context of relevant clinical objectives and considerations. Indeed, therapeutic applications of Ad-mediated gene transfer for asthma—for which localized aerosol delivery of the vector to the upper airway should prove most efficacious—may be incompatible with pharmacological vehicles that facilitate diffuse vector deposition throughout the alveoli (192,193). A more tenable solution might involve the temporary disruption of epithelial junctions—and the concomitant admission of Ad to the CAR-competent basal surface of epithelial cells—through the administration of Ca^{2+} chelators such as EGTA, which has been shown to enhance Ad-mediated gene transfer to rabbit tracheal epithelia in vivo (194).

V. Context

What this body of evidence overwhelmingly asserts is that adenovirus, as a vector for therapeutic gene transfer to the airway (especially the lower airway), is at a nascent stage of experimental valuation. Researchers have exhaustively documented the limitations of adenoviral vectors in the context of pulmonary gene transfer and have begun to devise promising strategies to circumvent these challenges, but the addition of recombinant RDA to the asthma armamentarium—particularly given that experimental consideration of therapeutic gene delivery for asthma has primarily addressed nonviral genetic instruments—is premature indeed. Certainly, second-generation and gutless Ad vectors are recommended by an impressive dossier of strategically important gene transfer advantages, but it is not clear to what extent these credentials can be translated to the clinical management or reversal of the asthma phenotype.

Moreover, this discussion of the prospects of adenoviral gene therapy for asthma begs more strategic questions about what constitutes a bonafide, meritorious gene transfer strategy for allergic airways diseases. Should the object of genetic intervention be to interrupt a single molecular pathway or to modulate an immunological program? What molecular targets or genetic constructs hold the most promise? The extensive knowledge compiled over the last decade on the relevance of cytokine, chemokine, costimulatory, and intracellular signaling networks in the pathogenesis of allergic asthma has impelled researchers in academia and, particularly, the pharmaceutical industry to investigate a variety of strategies to interfere with the biological actions of these immune mediators and, ultimately, to develop novel asthma therapeutics. The ponderous number of studies that have been reported to date impart, in our opinion, two main conclusions: first, that the actual testing of intervention strategies has, irrespective of outcome, clearly advanced our understanding of the role of these molecules in the pathogenesis of asthma; and second, that none of these interventions appears to promise to become an important addition to, or replacement for, the existing therapeutic armamentarium. It may be informative to speculate and elaborate on the reasons underlying this admittedly argumentative second conclusion.

If a strategy is developed as a *therapeutic*, which implies an ability to ameliorate clinical features of an *already established* allergic phenotype, then the candidate therapy must face, and survive, the challenge of comparison with currently available medicines. That short- and long-acting bronchodilators and, especially, inhaled corticosteroids introduce a rather outstanding "therapeutic index" makes this challenge particularly steep. It is conceivable, however, that gene transfer could be employed to enhance the activity of corticosteroids. In corticosteroid-resistant asthma, for example, the pharmacologically deleterious accumulation of c-fos, the inducible component of activating peptide-1 (AP-1), diminishes the binding of glucocorticoid receptor–corticosteroid complexes to transcription regulatory elements on DNA; however, Lane et al. (195) have demonstrated that pretreatment of PBMCs from steroid-resistant patients with ASO targeted to c-fos mRNA enhanced the binding of glucocorticoid receptors to DNA.

In light of our appreciation of molecular networks and, notably, of molecular redundancy, the notion that interference with a single effector molecule will confer a profound and sustained effect on the expression of the asthmatic phenotype is tenuous. Indeed, the overlapping functions of proinflammatory cytokines such as IL-1, IL-6, and TFN-α, or of the Th2-affliated cytokines IL-4, IL-9, and IL-13, in the development and presentation of allergy weave a complex, highly resilient immunological fabric. Intuitively, a more compelling approach would be no intervene simultaneously with several targets or to interrupt shared intracellular signaling molecules, as proposed by ASO-mediated blockade of the Th2-affiliated transcription factor GATA-3 (50).

We also suggest that a fundamental element in the appraisal of novel therapeutics is to consider the intrinsic heterogeneity of asthma. For example, there is increasing consensus that AHR can be elicited by several mechanisms, some IgE-dependent, others IgG_1-dependent, and yet others altogether independent of immunoglobulins. This suggests that a given genetic construct engineered for the selective inhibition of IgE (through, for instance, the provision of antagonistic cytokines or the immobilization of costimulatory pathways) will likely have a sectarian impact on the correction of AHR and its associated symptoms.

Moreover, asthma is not a static disease. There is a history of progression that can be affected by numerous etiological factors, including smoking, environmental exposure, and treatment. We suggest that underlying this diversity of clinical progressions is an equally diverse cellular and molecular network. In other words, the incipient trigger of the allergic phenotype is not necessarily what maintains or perpetuates this phenotype at later stages of disease. The clinical ramifications of this proposition are clear: the therapeutic impact of a given cytokine-targeted ASO strategy in an asthmatic whose near-normal pulmonary function necessitates only occasional use of bronchodilators will likely be vastly different in an asthmatic whose FEV_1 is 65% and who requires regular, low-dose, inhaled steroids to control symptoms.

Where does this rather complicated perspective leave us? It forces us to consider strategically the kinds of adenovirus-based modalities that afford *the best chance of supplanting existing pharmacopoeia*. In particular, inhaled steroids and bronchodilators, while therapeutically unimpeachable, do not cure asthma: that is, they do not permanently reverse the immunological and pathophysiological phenomena that account for the persistence of disease. It is in this light that treatments with adenoviral constructs encoding allergens and/or immunomodulatory signals, rather than treatments to neutralize effector cytokines or their molecular pathways, introduce a unique therapeutic tangent: to modify the very nature of allergen-initiated and, even, allergen-perpetuated events, in all likelihood by conditioning the context in which the allergen is presented by APCs to T cells. Admittedly, this prospect is tricky, especially considering that such therapy would be implemented in asthmatics who, by definition, have already been sensitized; nonetheless, this reeducation of the immune system is conceptually plausible given that conventional allergen immunotherapy, though cumbersome, protracted, and poorly standardized, is a remarkably effective treatment in some patients. However, to contemplate such therapies renders one vulnerable to the same limitations to which other genetic

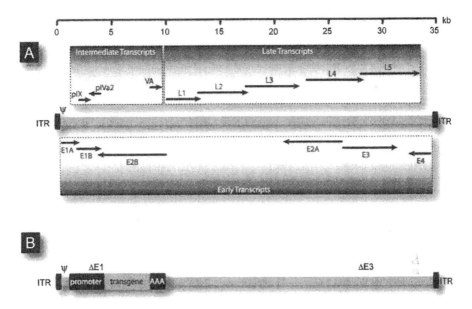

Figure 2 (A) Map of the adenoviral genome and transcription units illustrating early, intermediate, and late genes and the direction of transcription. (B) Map of a first-generation Ad vector, indicating the location of the promoter/transgene insert, the polyadenylation signal (denoted by AAA), and the sites of E1 and E3 deletion (denoted by E1 and E3, respectively). ψ designates the packaging signal, and ITR indicates the inverted terminal repeats flanking the genome.

modalities have succumbed: the reductionist tendency to simplify the molecular underpinnings of allergic sensitization. In other words, if the goal is therapeutic reeducation of the immune response to allergens, the design of the genetic vector must be informed by an integrated conceptualization of immune function—both molecularly and topographically. However, with these caveats in mind, we argue that it is in the manipulation of allergen-specific immunity— the conversion of an inflammatory response to a persistently inert response upon recognition of allergen—where the greatest promise of novel, genetically based therapies for asthma rests.

Acknowledgments

Research from our laboratory cited in this manuscript has been funded in part by the Canadian Institutes for Health Research (CIHR). REW and DA hold CIHR Doctoral Research Awards. The authors also gratefully acknowledge the support of Hamilton Health Sciences and St. Joseph's Hospital (Hamilton). The authors also thank Dr. Mary Hitt for assistance with the figures.

References

1. Alton EW, Griesenbach U, Geddes DM. Gene therapy for asthma: inspired research or unnecessary effort? Gene Ther 1999; 6:155–156.
2. Barnes PJ. Therapeutic strategies for allergic diseases. Nature 1999; 402:B31–38.
3. Bryan SA, Leckie MJ, Hansel TT, Barnes PJ. Novel therapy for asthma. Expert Opin Invest Drugs 2000; 9:25–42.
4. Crystal RG. Research opportunities and advances in lung disease. JAMA 2001; 285:612–618.
5. Demoly P, Mathieu M, Curiel DT, Godard P, Bousquet J, Michel FB. Gene therapy strategies for asthma. Gene Ther 1997; 4:507–516.
6. Fuloria M, Rubin BK. Evaluating the efficacy of mucoactive aerosol therapy. Respir Care 2000; 45:868–873.
7. Hedley ML. Gene therapy of chronic inflammatory disease. Adv Drug Deliv Rev 2000; 44:195–207.
8. Curley GP, Blum H, Humphries MJ. Integrin antagonists. Cell Mol Life Sci 1999; 56:427–441.
9. Evans CH, Robbins PD. The interleukin-1 receptor antagonist and its delivery by gene transfer. Receptor 1994; 4:9–15.
10. Alvarez D, Wiley RE, Jordana M. Cytokine therapeutics for asthma: an appraisal of current evidence and future prospects. Curr Pharm Des 2001; 7:1059–1081.
11. Djukanovic R. The role of co-stimulation in airway inflammation. Clin Exp Allergy 2000; 30 (Suppl 1):46–50.
12. Hansen G. McIntire JJ, Yeung VP, Berry G, Thorbecke GJ, Chen L, Dekruyff RH, Umetsu DT. CD4(+) T helper cells engineered to produce latent TGF-β1 reverse allergen-induced airway hyperractivity and inflammation. J Clin Invest 2000; 105:61–70.
13. Chung KF, Barnes PJ. Cytokines in asthma. Thorax 1999; 54:825–857.
14. Zangrilli JP, Peters SP. Cytokines in allergic airway disease. In: Busse W, Holgate ST, eds. Asthma and Rhinitis, Vol. 1. Oxford: Blackwell Science, 2000:577–596.
15. Leckie MJ, ten Brinke A, Khan J, Diamant Z, O'Connor BJ, Walls CM, Mathur AK, Cowley HC, Chung KF, Djukanovic R, Hansel TT, Holgate ST, Sterk PJ, Barnes PJ. Effects of an interleukin-5 blocking monoclonal antibody on eosinophils, airway hyper-responsiveness, and the late asthmatic response. Lancet 2000; 356:2144–2148.
16. Kips JC, O'Connor BJ, Langley SJ, Woodcock A, Kerstjens HAM, Postma DS, Danzig M, Cuss F, Pauwels RA, Kenilworth NJ. Results of a phase I clinical trial with SCH55700, a humanized anti-IL-5 antibody, in severe persistent asthma. American Thoracic Society/American Lung Association (ATS/ALA) Conference, Toronto, Canada, May, 2000. Abstract 624.
17. Borish LC, Nelson HS, Lanz MJ, Claussen L, Whitemore JB, Agosti JM, Garrison L. Interleukin-4 receptor in moderate atopic asthma. A phase I/II randomized, placebo-controlled trial. Am J Respir Crit Care Med 1999; 160: 1816–1823.
18. Borish LC, Nelson HS, Corren J, Bensch G, Busse WW, Whitemore JB, Agosti JM. Efficacy of soluble IL-4 receptor for the treatment of adults with asthma. J Allergy Clin Immunol 2001; 107:963–970.

19. Kips JC, Tournoy KG, Pauwels RA. New anti-asthma therapies: suppression of the effect of interleukin (IL)-4 and IL-5. Eur Respir J 2001; 17:499–506.

20. Owen C. Chemokine receptors in airway disease: which receptors to target? Pulm Pharmacol Ther 2001; 14:193–202.

21. Wells TN, Proudfoot AE. Chemokine receptors and their antagonists in allergic lung disease. Inflamm Res 1999; 48:353–362.

22. Wong WS, Koh DS. Advances in immunopharmacology of asthma. Biochem Pharmacol 2000; 59:1323–1335.

23. Christman JW, Sadikot RT, Blackwell TS. The role of nuclear factor-κB in pulmonary diseases. Chest 2000; 117:1482–1487.

24. Das J, Chen CH, Yang L, Cohn L, Ray P, Ray A. A critical role for NF-κB in GATA3 expression and Th2 differentiation in allergic airway inflammation. Nat Immunol 2001; 2:45–50.

25. Haczku A, Takeda K, Redai I, Hamelmann E, Cieslewicz G, Joetham A, Loader J, Lee JJ, Irvin C, Gelfand EW. Anti-CD86 (B7.2) treatment abolishes allergic airway hyperresponsiveness in mice. Am J Respir Crit Care Med 1999; 159:1638–1643.

26. Van Oosterhout AJ, Hofstra CL, Shields R, Chan B, Van Ark I, Jardieu PM, Nijkamp FP. Murine CTLA4-IgG treatment inhibits airway eosinophilia and hyperresponsiveness and attenuates IgE upregulation in a murine model of allergic asthma. Am J Respir Cell Mol Biol 1997; 17:386–392.

27. Dong C, Juedes AE, Temann UA, Shresta S, Allison JP, Ruddle NH, Flavell RA. ICOS co-stimulatory receptor is essential for T-cell activation and function. Nature 2001; 409:97–101.

28. Gonzalo JA, Delaney T, Corcoran J, Goodearl A, Gutierrez-Ramos JC, Coyle AJ. Cutting edge: the related molecules CD28 and inducible costimulator deliver both unique and complementary signals required for optimal T cell activation. J Immunol 2001; 166:1–5.

29. Gonzalo JA, Tian J, Delaney T, Corcoran J, Rottman JB, Lora J, Al-garawi A, Kroczek R, Gutierrez-Ramos JC, Coyle AJ. ICOS is critical for T helper cell–mediated lung mucosal inflammatory responses. Nat Immunol 2001; 2:597–604.

30. Guo J, Stolina M, Bready JV, Yin S, Horan T, Yoshinaga SK, Senaldi G. Stimulatory effects of B7-related protein-1 on cellular and humoral immune responses in mice. J Immunol 2001; 166:5578–5584.

31. Ozkaynak E, Gao W, Shemmeri N, Wang C, Gutierrez-Ramos JC, Amaral J, Qin S, Rottman JB, Coyle AJ, Hancock WW. Importance of ICOS-B7RP-1 costimulation in acute and chronic allograft rejection. Nat Immunol 2001; 2: 591–596.

32. Tafuri A, Shahinian A, Bladt F, Yoshinaga SK, Jordana M, Wakeham A, Boucher LM, Bouchard D, Chan VS, Duncan G, Odermatt B, Ho A, Itie A, Horan T, Whoriskey JS, Pawson T, Penninger JM, Ohashi PS, Mak TW. ICOS is essential for effective T-helper-cell responses. Nature 2001; 409:105–109.

33. Tesciuba AG, Subudhi S, Rother RP, Faas SJ, Frantz AM, Elliot D, Weinstock J, Matis LA, Bluestone JA, Sperling AI. Inducible costimulator regulates Th2-mediated inflammation, but not Th2 differentiation, in a model of allergic airway disease. J Immunol 2001; 167:1996–2003.

34. Metzger WJ, Nyce JW. Oligonucleotide therapy of allergic asthma. J Allergy Clin Immunol 1999; 104:260–266.

35. Eizema K, Fechner H, Bezstarosti K, Schneider-Rasp S, van der Laarse A, Wang H, Schulthesis HP, Poller WC, Lamers JM. Adenovirus-based phospholamban antisense expression as a novel approach to improve cardiac contractile dysfunction: comparison of a constitutive viral versus an endothelin-1-responsive cardiac promoter. Circulation 2000; 101:2193–2199.

36. Mohuczy D, Tang X, Phillips MI. Delivery of antisense DNA by vectors for prolonged effects in vitro and in vivo. Meth Enzymol 2000; 314: 32–51.

37. Potter PM, McKenzie PP, Hussain N, Noonberg S, Morton CL, Harris LC. Construction of adenovirus for high level expression of small RNAs in mammalian cells. Application to a Bcl-2 ribozyme. Mol Biotechnol 2000; 15:105–114.

38. Nakanishi A, Morita S, Iwashita H, sagiya Y, Ashida Y, Shirafuji H, Fujisawa Y, Nishimura O, Fujino M. Role of gob-5 in mucus overproduction and airway hyperresponsiveness in asthma. Proc Natl Acad Sci USA 2001; 10:10.

39. Stein CA. The experimental use of antisense oligonucleotides: a guide for the perplexed. J Clin Invest 2001; 108:641–644.

40. Weltman JK, Karim AS. Interleukin-5: a proeosinophil cytokine mediator of inflammation in asthma and a target for antisense therapy. Allergy Asthma Proc 1998; 19:257–261.

41. Karras JG, McGraw K, McKay RA, Cooper SP, Lerner D, Lu T, Walker C, Dean NM, Monia BP. Inhibition of antigen-induced eosinophilia and late phase airway hyperresponsiveness by an IL-5 antisense oligonucleotide in mouse models of asthma. J Immunol 2000; 164:5409–5415.

42. Karras JG, McKay RA, Lu T, Dean NM, Monia BP. Antisense inhibition of membrane-bound human interleukin-5 receptor-α chain does not affect soluble receptor expression and induces apoptosis in TF-1 cells. Antisense Nucleic Acid Drug Dev 2000; 10:347–357.

43. Karras JG, McKay RA, Dean NM, Monia BP. Deletion of individual exons and induction of soluble murine interleukin-5 receptor-α chain expression through antisense oligonucleotide-mediated redirection of pre-mRNA splicing. Mol Pharmacol 2000; 58:380–387.

44. Lach-Trifilieff E, McKay RA, Monia BP, Karras JG, Walker C. In vitro and in vivo inhibition of interleukin (IL)-5-mediated eosinopoiesis by murine IL-5Rα antisense oligonucleotide. Am J Respir Cell Mol Biol 2001; 24:116–122.

45. Molet S, Ramos-Barbon D, Martin JG, Hamid Q. Adoptively transferred late allergic response is inhibited by IL-4, but not IL-5, antisense oligonucleotide. J Allergy Clin Immunol 1999; 104:205–214.

46. Finotto S, Buerke M, Lingnau K, Schmitt E, Galle PR, Neurath MF. Local administration of antisense phosphorothioate oligonucleotides to the c-kit ligand, stem cell factor, suppresses airway inflammation and IL-4 production in a murine model of asthma. J Allergy Clin Immunol 2001; 107:279–286.

47. Stenton GR, Kim MK, Nohara O, Chen CF, Hirji N, Wills FL, Gilchrist M, Hwang PH, Park JG, Finlay W, Jones RL, Befus AD, Schreiber AD. Aerosolized Syk antisense suppresses Syk expression, mediator release from macrophages, and pulmonary inflammation. J Immunol 2000; 164:3790–3797.

48. Adachi T, Stafford S, Sur S, Alam R. A novel Lyn-binding peptide inhibitor blocks eosinophil differentiation, survival, and airway eosinophilic inflammation. J Immunol 1999; 163:939–946.

49. Zhang DH, Yang L, Ray A. Differential responsiveness of the IL-5 and IL-4 genes to transcription factor GATA3. J Immunol 1998; 161:3817–3821.

50. Finotto S, De Sanctis GT, Lehr HA, Herz U, Buerke M, Schipp M, Bartsch B, Atreya R, Schmitt E, Galle PR, Renz H, Neurath MF. Treatment of allergic airway inflammation and hyperresponsiveness by antisense-induced local blockade of GATA3 expression. J Exp Med 2001; 193:1247–1260.

51. McKinlay LH, Tymms MJ, Thomas RS, Seth A, Hasthorpe S, Hertzog PJ, Kola I. The role of Ets-1 in mast cell granulocyte-macrophage colony-stimulating factor expression and activation. J Immunol 1998; 161:4098–4105.

52. Stampfli MR, Wiley RE, Neigh GS, Gajewska BU, Lei XF, Snider DP, Xing Z, Jordana M. GM-CSF transgene expression in the airway allows aerosolized ovalbumin to induce allergic sensitization in mice. J Clin Invest 1998; 102:1704–1714.

53. Manna B, Ashbaugh P, Bhattacharyya SN. Retinoic acid–regulated cellular differentiation and mucin gene expression in isolated rabbit tracheal-epithelial cells in culture. Inflammation 1995; 19:489–502.

54. Solway J, Forsythe SM, Halayko AJ, Vieira JE, Hershenson MB, Camoretti-Mercado B. Transcriptional regulation of smooth muscle contractile apparatus expression. Am J Respir Crit Care Med 1998; 158:S100–108.

55. Lee JH, Johnson PR, Roth M, Hunt NH, Black JL. ERK activation and mitogenesis in human airway smooth muscle cells. Am J Physiol Lung Cell Mol Physiol 2001; 280:L1019–1029.

56. Nyce JW, Metzger WJ. DNA antisense therapy for asthma in an animal model. Nature 1997; 385:721–725.

57. Van Schoor J, Joos GF, Pauwels RA. Indirect bronchial hyperresponsiveness in asthma: mechanisms, pharmacology and implications for clinical research. Eur Respir J 2000; 16:514–533.

58. Kang KW, Kim TS, Kim KM. Interferon-γ- and interleukin-4-targeted gene therapy for atopic allergic disease. Immunology 1999; 97:462–465.

59. Li XM, Chopra RK, Chou TY, Schofield BH, Wills-Karp M, Huang SK. Mucosal IFNγ gene transfer inhibits pulmonary allergic responses in mice. J Immunol 1996; 157:3216–3219.

60. Dow SW, Schwarze J, Health TD, Potter TA, Gelfand EW. Systemic and local interferon γ gene delivery to the lungs for treatment of allergen-induced airway hyperresponsiveness in mice. Hum Gene Ther 1999; 10:1905–1914.

61. Hogan SP, Foster PS, Tan X, Ramsay AJ. Mucosal IL-12 gene delivery inhibits allergic airways disease and restores local antiviral immunity. Eur J Immunol 1998; 28:413–423.

62. Huang TJ, MacAry PA, Eynott P, Moussavi A, Daniel KC, Askenase PW, Kemeny DM, Chung KF. Allergen-specific Th1 cells counteract efferent Th2 cell–dependent bronchial hyperresponsiveness and eosinophilic inflammation partly via IFNγ. J Immunol 2001; 166:207–217.

63. Stampfli MR, Scott Neigh G, Wiley RE, Cwiartka M, Ritz SA, Hitt MM, Xing Z, Jordana M. Regulation of allergic mucosal sensitization by interleukin-12 gene transfer to the airway. Am J Respir Cell Mol Biol 1999; 21:317–326.

64. Wiley R, Palmer K, Gajewska B, Stampfli M, Alvarez D, Coyle A, Gutierrez-Ramos J, Jordana M. Expression of the Th1 chemokine IFNγ-inducible protein

10 in the airway alters mucosal allergic sensitization in mice. J Immunol 2001; 166:2750–2759.

65. Chun S, Daheshia M, Lee S, Rouse BT. Immune modulation by IL-10 gene transfer via viral vector and plasmid DNA: implication for gene therapy. Cell Immunol 1999; 194:194–204.

66. Chun S, Daheshia M, Lee S, Eo SK, Rouse BT. Distribution fate and mechanism of immune modulation following mucosal delivery of plasmid DNA encoding IL-10. J Immunol 1999; 163: 2393–2402.

67. Meng X, Sawamura D, Tamai K, Hanada K, Ishida H, Hashimoto I. Keratinocyte gene therapy for systemic diseases. Circulating interleukin-10 released from gene-transferred keratinocytes inhibits contact hypersensitivity at distant areas of the skin. J Clin Invest 1998; 101:1462–1467.

68. Stampfli MR, Cwiartka M, Gajewska BU, Alvarez D, Ritz SA, Inman MD, Xing Z, Jordana M. Interleukin-10 gene transfer to the airway regulates allergic mucosal sensitization in mice. Am J Respir Cell Mol Biol 1999; 21:586–596.

69. Makela MJ, Kanehiro A, Borish L, Dakhama A, Loader J, Joetham A, Xing Z, Jordana M, Larsen GL, Gelfand EW. IL-10 is necessary for the expression of airway hyperresponsiveness but not pulmonary inflammation after allergic sensitization. Proc Natl Acad Sci USA 2000; 97:6007–6012.

70. Becker AB. Is primary prevention of asthma possible? Pediatr Pulmonol 2000; 30:63–72.

71. Campbell D, Dekruyff RH, Umetsu DT. Allergen immunotherapy: novel approaches in the management of allergic diseases and asthma. Clin Immunol 2000; 97:193–202.

72. Chiang BL. Molecular mechanisms of allergen-specific immunotherapy for atopic diseases. Zhonghua Min Guo Xiao Er Ke Yi Xue Hui Za Zhi 1998; 39:293–296.

73. Huang SK, Chua KY, Hsieh KH. Allergen gene transfer. Curr Opin Immunol 1997; 9:800–804.

74. Rolland JM, Douglass J, O'Hehir RE. Allergen immunotherapy: current and new therapeutic strategies. Expert Opin Invest Drugs 2000; 9:515–527.

75. TePas EC, Umetsu DT. Immunotherapy of asthma and allergic diseases. Curr Opin Pediatr 2000; 12:574–578.

76. Hackett CJ, Dickler HB. Immunologic tolerance for immune system-mediated diseases. J Allergy Clin Immunol 1999; 103:362–370.

77. Hsu CH, Chua KY, Tao MH, Lai YL, Wu HD, Huang SK, Hsieh KH. Immunoprophylaxis of allergen-induced immunoglobulin E synthesis and airway hyperresponsiveness in vivo by genetic immunization. Nat Med 1996; 2:540–544.

78. Kohama Y, Akizuki O, Hagihara K, Yamada E, Yamamoto H. Immunostimulatory oligodeoxynucleotide induces Th1 immune response and inhibition of IgE antibody production to cedar pollen allergens in mice. J Allergy Clin Immunol 1999; 104:1231–1238.

79. Raz E, Spiegelberg HL. Deviation of the allergic IgE to an IgG response by gene immunotherapy. Int Rev Immunol 1999; 18:271–289.

80. Spiegelberg HL, Broide D, Tighe H, Roman M, Raz E. Inhibition of allergic inflammation in the lung by plasmid DNA allergen immunization. Pediatr Pulmonol Suppl 1999; 18:118–121.

81. Mehlhop PD, van de Rijn M, Goldberg AB, Brewer JP, Kurup VP, Martin TR, Oettgen HC. Allergen-induced bronchial hyperreactivity and eosinophilic inflammation occur in the absence of IgE in a mouse model of asthma. Proc Natl Acad Sci USA 1997; 94:1344–1349.

82. Broide D, Raz E. DNA-Based immunization for asthma. Int Arch Allergy Immunol 1999; 118:453–456.

83. Kline JN. Effects of CpG DNA on Th1/Th2 balance in asthma. Curr Top Microbiol Immunol 2000; 247:211–225.

84. Weiner GJ. The immunobiology and clinical potential of immunostimulatory CpG oligodeoxynucleotides. J Leukoc Biol 2000; 68:455–463.

85. Kumar M, Behera AK, Matsuse H, Lockey RF, Mohapatra SS. A recombinant BCG vaccine generates a Th1-like response and inhibits IgE synthesis in BALB/c mice. Immunology 1999; 97:515–521.

86. Stampfli MR, Ritz SA, Neigh GS, Sime PJ, Lei XF, Xing Z, Croitoru K, Jordana M. Adenoviral infection inhibits allergic airways inflammation in mice. Clin Exp Allergy 1998; 28:1581–1590.

87. Suzuki M, Suzuki S, Yamamoto N, Komatsu S, Inoue S, Hashiba T, Nishikawa M, Ishigatsubo Y. Immune responses against replication-deficient adenovirus inhibit ovalbumin-specific allergic reactions in mice. Hum Gene Ther 2000; 11:827–838.

88. Hitt MM, Gauldie J. Gene vectors for cytokine expression in vivo. Curr Pharm Des 2000; 6:613–632.

89. Look DC, Brody SL. Engineering viral vectors to subvert the airway defense response. Am J Respir Cell Mol Biol 1999; 20:1103–1106.

90. Boucher RC. Status of gene therapy for cystic fibrosis lung disease. J Clin Invest 1999; 103:441–445.

91. Chirmule N, Propert K, Magosin S, Qian Y, Qian R, Wilson J. Immune responses to adenovirus and adeno-associated virus in humans. Gene Ther 1999; 6:1574–1583.

92. Zeitlin PL. Cystic fibrosis gene therapy trials and tribulations. Mol Ther 2000; 1:5–6.

93. Zuckerman JB, Robinson CB, McCoy KS, Shell R, Sferra TJ, Chirmule N, Magosin SA, Propert KJ, Brown-Parr EC, Hughes JV, Tazelaar J, Baker C, Goldman MJ, Wilson JM. A phase I study of adenovirus-mediated transfer of the human cystic fibrosis transmembrane conductance regulator gene to a lung segment of individuals with cystic fibrosis. Hum Gene Ther 1999; 10:2973–2985.

94. Harvey BG, Leopold PL, Hackett NR, Grasso TM, Williams PM, Tucker AL, Kaner RJ, Ferris B, Gonda I, Sweeney TD, Ramalingam R, Kovesdi I, Shak S, Crystal RG. Airway epithelial CFTR mRNA expression in cystic fibrosis patients after repetitive administration of a recombinant adenovirus. J Clin Invest 1999; 104:1245–1255.

95. West J, Rodman DM. Gene therapy for pulmonary diseases. Chest 2001; 119:613–617.

96. Yang Y, Li Q, Ertl HC, Wilson JM. Cellular and humoral immune responses to viral antigens create barriers to lung-directed gene therapy with recombinant adenoviruses. J Virol 1995; 69:2004–2015.

97. Knowles MR, Hohneker KW, Zhou Z, Olsen JC, Noah TL, Hu PC, Leigh MW, Engelhardt, JF, Edwards LJ, Jones KR et al. A controlled study of adenoviral-vector-mediated gene transfer in the nasal epithelium of patients with cystic fibrosis. N Engl J Med 1995; 333:823–831.

98. Geginat G, Ruppert T, Hengel H, Holtappels R, Koszinowski UH. IFNγ is a prerequisite for optimal antigen processing of viral peptides in vivo. J Immunol 1997; 158:3303–3310.

99. Yang Y, Xiang Z, Ertl HC, Wilson JM. Upregulation of class I major histocompatibility complex antigens by interferon gamma is necessary for T-cell-mediated elimination of recombinant adenovirus-infected hepatocytes in vivo. Proc Natl Acad Sci USA 1995; 92:7257–7261.

100. Prasad SA, Norbury CC, Chen W, Bennink JR, Yewdell JW. Cutting edge: Recombinant adenoviruses induce CD8 T cell responses to an inserted protein whose expression is limited to nonimmune cells. J Immunol 2001; 166:4809–4812.

101. Yang Y, Jooss KU, Su Q, Ertl HC, Wilson JM. Immune responses to viral antigens versus transgene product in the elimination of recombinant adenovirus-infected hepatocytes in vivo. Gene Ther 1996; 3:137–144.

102. McCoy RD, Davidson BL, Roessler BJ, Huffnagle GB, Janich SL, Laing TJ, Simon RH. Pulmonary inflammation induced by incomplete or inactivated adenoviral particles. Hum Gene Ther 1995; 6:1553–1560.

103. Kafri T, Morgan D, Krahl T, Sarvetnick N, Sherman L, Verma I. Cellular immune response to adenoviral vector infected cells does not require de novo viral gene expression: implications for gene therapy. Proc Natl Acad Sci USA 1998; 95:11377–11382.

104. Lusky M, Christ M, Rittner K, Dieterle A, Dreyer D, Mourot B, Schultz H, Stoeckel F, Pavirani A, Mehtali M. In vitro and in vivo biology of recombinant adenovirus vectors with E1, E1/E2A, or E1/E4 deleted. J Virol 1998; 72:2022–2032.

105. Tripathy SK, Black HB, Goldwasser E, Leiden JM. Immune responses to transgene-encoded proteins limit the stability of gene expression after injection of replication-defective adenovirus vectors. Nat Med 1996; 2:545–550.

106. Russi TJ, Hirschowitz EA, Crystal RG. Delayed-type hypersensitivity response to high doses of adenoviral vectors. Hum Gene Ther 1997; 8:323–330.

107. Otake K, Ennist DL, Harrod K, Trapnell BC. Nonspecific inflammation inhibits adenovirus-mediated pulmonary gene transfer and expression independent of specific acquired immune responses. Hum Gene Ther 1998; 9:2207–2222.

108. Thorne PS, McCray PB, Howe TS, O'Neill MA. Early-onset inflammatory responses in vivo to adenoviral vectors in the presence or absence of lipopoly-saccharide-induced inflammation. Am J Respir Cell Mol Biol 1999; 20:1155–1164.

109. Zsengeller Z, Otake K, Hossain SA, Berclaz PY, Trapnell BC. Internalization of adenovirus by alveolar macrophages initiates early proinflammatory signaling during acute respiratory tract infection. J Virol 2000; 74:9655–9667.

110. Amin R, Wilmott R, Schwarz Y, Trapnell B, Stark J. Replication-deficient adenovirus induces expression of interleukin-8 by airway epithelial cells in vitro. Hum Gene Ther 1995; 6:145–153.

111. Nicolis E, Tamanini A, Melotti P, Rolfini R, Berton G, Cassatella MA, Bout A, Pavirani A, Cabrini G. ICAM-1 induction in respiratory cells exposed to a

replication-deficient recombinant adenovirus in vitro and in vivo. Gene Ther 1998; 5:131–136.

112. Stark JM, Amin RS, Trapnell BC. Infection of A549 cells with a recombinant adenovirus vector induces ICAM-1 expression and increased CD-18-dependent adhesion of activated neutrophils. Hum Gene Ther 1996; 7:1669–1681.

113. Zabner J, Ramsey BW, Meeker DP, Aitken ML, Balfour RP, Gibson RL, Launspach J, Moscicki RA, Richards SM, Standaert TA, et al. Repeat administration of an adenovirus vector encoding cystic fibrosis transmembrane conductance regulator to the nasal epithelium of patients with cystic fibrosis. J Clin Invest 1996; 97:1504–1511.

114. Zabner J, Petersen DM, Puga AP, Graham SM, Couture LA, Keyes LD, Lukason MJ, St George JA, Gregory RJ, Smith AE, et al. Safety and efficacy of repetitive adenovirus-mediated transfer of CFTR cDNA to airway epithelia of primates and cotton rats. Nat Genet 1994; 6:75–83.

115. Harvey BG, Hackett NR, Ely S, Crystal RG. Host responses and persistence of vector genome following intrabronchial administration of an E1-E3-adenovirus gene transfer vector to normal individuals. Mol Ther 2001; 3:206–215.

116. Harvey BG, Hackett NR, Ed-Sawy T, Rosengart TK, Hirschowitz EA, Lieberman MD, Lesser ML, Crystal RG. Variability of human systemic humoral immune responses to adenovirus gene transfer vectors administered to different organs. J Virol 1999; 73:6729–6742.

117. Jooss K, Turka LA, Wilson JM. Blunting of immune responses to adenoviral vectors in mouse liver and lung with CTLA4Ig. Gene Ther 1998; 5:309–319.

118. Wilson CB, Embree LJ, Schowalter D, Albert R, Aruffo A, Hollenbaugh D, Linsley P, Kay MA. Transient inhibition of CD28 and CD40 ligand interactions prolongs adenovirus-mediated transgene expression in the lung and facilitates expression after secondary vector administration. J Virol 1998; 72:7542–7550.

119. Lei D, Lehmann M, Shellito JE, Nelson S, Siegling A, Volk HD, Kolls JK. Nondepleting anti-CD4 antibody treatment prolongs lung-directed E1-deleted adenovirus-mediated gene expression in rats. Hum Gene Ther 1996; 7:2273–2279.

120. Zsengeller ZK, Boivin GP, Sawchuk SS, Trapnell BC, Whitsett JA, Hirsch R. Anti-T cell receptor antibody prolongs transgene expression and reduces lung inflammation after adenovirus-mediated gene transfer. Hum Gene Ther 1997; 8:935–941.

121. Yang Y, Trinchieri G, Wilson JM. Recombinant IL-12 prevents formation of blocking IgA antibodies to recombinant adenovirus and allows repeated gene therapy to mouse lung. Nat Med 1995; 1:890–893.

122. Ilan Y, Prakash R, Davidson A, Jona, Droguett G, Horwitz MS, Chowdhury NR, Chowdhury JR. Oral tolerization to adenoviral antigens permits long-term gene expression using recombinant adenoviral vectors. J Clin Invest 1997; 99:1098–1106.

123. Minter RM, Rectenwald JE, Fukuzuka K, Tannahill CL, La Face D, Tsai V, Ahmed I, Hutchins E, Moyer R, Copeland EM III, Moldawer LL. TNFα receptor signaling and IL-10 gene therapy regulate the innate and humoral immune responses to recombinant adenovirus in the lung. J Immunol 2000; 164:443–451.

124. Zhang HG, Zhou T, Yang P, Edwards CK III, Curiel DT, Mountz JD. Inhibition of tumor necrosis factor α decreases inflammation and prolongs adenovirus gene expression in lung and liver. Hum Gene Ther 1998; 9:1875–1884.

125. Schwarz YA, Amin RS, Stark JM, Trapnell BC, Wilmott RW. Interleukin-1 receptor antagonist inhibits interleukin-8 expression in A549 respiratory epithelial cells infected in vitro with a replication-deficient recombinant adenovirus vector. Am J Respir Cell Mol Biol 1999; 21:388–394.

126. Minter RM, Ferry MA, Rectenwald JE, Bahjat FR, Oberholzer A, Oberholzer C, La Face D, Tsai V, Ahmed CM, Hutchins B, Copeland EM III, Ginsberg HS, Moldawer LL. Extended lung expression and increased tissue localization of viral IL-10 with adenoviral gene therapy. Proc Natl Acad Sci USA 2001; 98:277–282.

127. Jooss K, Yang Y, Wilson JM. Cyclophosphamide diminishes inflammation and prolongs transgene expression following delivery of adenoviral vectors to mouse liver and lung. Hum Gene Ther 1996; 7:1555–1566.

128. Cassivi SD, Liu M, Boehler A, Pierre A, Tanswell AK, O'Brodovich H, Mullen JB, Slutsky AS, Keshavjee SH. Transplant immunosuppression increases and prolongs transgene expression following adenoviral-mediated transfection of rat lungs. J Heart Lung Transplant 2000; 19:984–994.

129. Amalfitano A, Hauser MA, Hu H, Serra D, Begy CR, Chamberlain JS. Production and characterization of improved adenovirus vectors with the E1, E2b, and E3 genes deleted. J Virol 1998; 72:926–933.

130. Gorziglia MI, Kadan MJ, Yei S, Lim J, Lee GM, Luthra R, Trapnell BC. Elimination of both E1 and E2 from adenovirus vectors further improves prospects for in vivo human gene therapy. J Virol 1996; 70:4173–4178.

131. Schaack J, Guo X, Langer SJ. Characterization of a replication-incompetent adenovirus type 5 mutant deleted for the preterminal protein gene. Proc Natl Acad Sci USA 1996; 93:14686–14691.

132. Zhou H, O'Neal W, Morral N, Beaudet AL. Development of a complementing cell line and a system for construction of adenovirus vectors with E1 and E2a deleted. J Virol 1996; 70:7030–7038.

133. Armentano D, Sookdeo CC, Hehir KM, Gregory RJ, St George JA, Prince GA, Wadsworth SC, Smith AE. Characterization of an adenovirus gene transfer vector containing an E4 deletion. Hum Gene Ther 1995; 6:1343–1353.

134. Gao GP, Yang Y, Wilson JM. Biology of adenovirus vectors with E1 and E4 deletions for liver-directed gene therapy. J Virol 1996; 70:8934–8943.

135. Yeh P, Dedieu JF, Orsini C, Vigne E, Denefle P, Perricaudet M. Efficient dual transcomplementation of adenovirus E1 and E4 regions from a 293-derived cell line expressing a minimal E4 functional unit. J Virol 1996; 70:559–565.

136. Dedieu JF, Vigne E, Torrent C, Jullien C, Mahfouz I, Caillaud JM, Aubailly N, Orsini C, Guillaume JM, Opolon P, Delaere P, Perricaudet M, Yeh P. Long-term gene delivery into the livers of immunocompetent mice with E1/E4-defective adenoviruses. J Virol 1997; 71:4626–4637.

137. Engelhardt JF, Litzky L, Wilson JM. Prolonged transgene expression in cotton rat lung with recombinant adenoviruses defective in E2a. Hum Gene Ther 1994; 5:1217–1229.

138. Kochanek S. High-capacity adenoviral vectors for gene transfer and somatic gene therapy. Hum Gene Ther 1999; 10:2451–2459.

139. Parks RJ, Graham FL. A helper-dependent system for adenovirus vector production helps define a lower limit for efficient DNA packaging. J Virol 1997; 71:3293–3298.

140. Chen HH, Mack LM, Kelly R, Ontell M, Kochanek S, Clemens PR. Persistence in muscle of an adenoviral vector that lacks all viral genes. Proc Natl Acad Sci USA 1997; 94:1645–1650.

141. Morsy MA, Gu M, Motzel S, Zhao J, Lin J, Su Q, Allen H, Franlin L, Parks RJ, Graham FL, Kochanek S, Bett AJ, Caskey CT. An adenoviral vector deleted for all viral coding sequences results in enhanced safety and extended expression of a leptin transgene. Proc Natl Acad Sci USA 1998; 95:7866–7871.

142. O'Neal WK, Zhou H, Morral N, Langston C, Parks RJ, Graham FL, Kochanek S, Beaudet AL. Toxicity associated with repeated administration of first-generation adenovirus vectors does not occur with a helper-dependent vector. Mol Med 2000; 6:179–195.

143. Parks RJ, Chen L, Anton M, Sankar U, Rudnicki MA, Graham FL. A helper-dependent adenovirus vector system: removal of helper virus by Cre-mediated excision of the viral packaging signal. Proc Natl Acad Sci USA 1996; 93:13565–13570.

144. Mastrangeli A, Harvey BG, Yao J, Wolff G, Kovesdi I, Crystal RG, Falck-Pedersen E. "Sero-switch" adenovirus-mediated in vivo gene transfer: circumvention of anti-adenovirus humoral immune defenses against repeat adenovirus vector administration by changing the adenovirus serotype. Hum Gene Ther 1996; 7:79–87.

145. Mack CA, Song WR, Carpenter H, Wickham TJ, Kovesdi I, Harvey BG, Magovern CJ, Isom OW, Rosengart T, Falck-Pedersen E, Hackett NR, Crystal RG, Mastrangeli A. Circumvention of anti-adenovirus neutralizing immunity by administration of an adenoviral vector of an alternate serotype. Hum Gene Ther 1997; 8:99–109.

146. Burgert HG, Maryanski JL, Kvist S. "E3/19K" protein of adenovirus type 2 inhibits lysis of cytolytic T lymphocytes by blocking cell-surface expression of histocompatibility class I antigens. Proc Natl Acad Sci USA 1987; 84:1356–1360.

147. Bruder JT, Jie T, McVey DL, Kovesdi I. Expression of gp19K increases the persistence of transgene expression from an adenovirus vector in the mouse lung and liver. J Virol 1997; 71:7623–7628.

148. Harrod KS, Hermiston TW, Trapnell BC, Wold WS, Whitsett JA. Lung-specific expression of adenovirus E3-14.7K in transgenic mice attenuates adenoviral vector–mediated lung inflammation and enhances transgene expression. Hum Gene Ther 1998; 9:1885–1898.

149. Armentano D, Zabner J, Sacks C, Sookdeo CC, Smith MP, St George JA, Wadsworth SC, Smith AE, Gregory RJ. Effect of the E4 region on the persistence of transgene expression from adenovirus vectors. J Virol 1997; 71:2408–2416.

150. Look DC, Roswit WT, Frick AG, Gris-Alevy Y, Dickhaus DM, Walter MJ, Holtzman MJ. Direct suppression of Stat1 function during adenoviral infection. Immunity 1998; 9:871–880.

151. Bergelson JM, Cunningham JA, Droguett G, Kurt-Jones EA, Krithivas A, Hong JS, Horwitz MA, Crowell RL, Finberg RW. Isolation of a common receptor for Coxsackie B viruses and adenoviruses 2 and 5. Science 1997; 275:1320–1323.

152. Tomko RP, Xu R, Philipson L. HCAR and MCAR: the human and mouse cellular receptors for subgroup C adenoviruses and group B coxsackieviruses. Proc Natl Acad Sci USA 1997; 94:3352–3356.

153. Wickham TJ, Mathias P, Cheresh DA, Nemerow GR. Integrins αvβ3 and αvβ5 promote adenovirus internalization but not virus attachment. Cell 1993; 73: 309–319.

154. Pickles RJ, McCarty D, Matsui H, Hart PJ, Randell SH, Boucher RC. Limited entry of adenovirus vectors into well-differentiated airway epithelium is responsible for inefficient gene transfer. J Virol 1998; 72:6014–6023.

155. Walters RW, Grunst T, Bergelson JM, Finberg RW, Welsh MJ, Zabner J. Basolateral localization of fiber receptors limits adenovirus infection from the apical surface of airway epithelia. J Biol Chem 1999; 274:10219–10226.

156. Zabner J, Freimuth P, Puga A, Fabrega A, Welsh MJ. Lack of high affinity fiber receptor activity explains the resistance of ciliated airway epithelia to adenovirus infection. J Clin Invest 1997; 100:1144–1149.

157. Goldman MJ, Wilson JM. Expression of αvβ5 integrin is necessary for efficient adenovirus-mediated gene transfer in the human airway. J Virol 1995; 69:5951–5958.

158. Goldman M, Su Q, Wilson JM. Gradient of RGD-dependent entry of adenoviral vector in nasal and intrapulmonary epithelia: implications for gene therapy of cystic fibrosis. Gene Ther 1996; 3:811–818.

159. Kitson C, Angel B, Judd D, Rothery S, Severs NJ, Dewar A, Huang L, Wadsworth SC, Cheng SH, Geddes DM, Alton EW. The extra- and intracellular barriers to lipid and adenovirus-mediated pulmonary gene transfer in native sheep airway epithelium. Gene Ther 1999; 6:534–546.

160. Freimuth P. A human cell line selected for resistance to adenovirus infection has reduced levels of the virus receptor. J Virol 1996; 70:4081–4085.

161. Huang X, Griffiths M, Wu J, Farese RV Jr, Sheppard D. Normal development, wound healing, and adenovirus susceptibility in β5-deficient mice. Mol Cell Biol 2000; 20:755–759.

162. van Heeckeren A, Ferkol T, Tosi M. Effects of bronchopulmonary inflammation induced by *Pseudomonas aeruginosa* on adenovirus-mediated gene transfer to airway epithelial cells in mice. Gene Ther 1998; 5:345–351.

163. Wickham TJ. Targeting adenovirus. Gene Ther 2000; 7:110–114.

164. Wickham TJ, Segal DM, Roelvink PW, Carrion ME, Lizonova A, Lee GM, Kovesdi I. Targeted adenovirus gene transfer to endothelial and smooth muscle cells by using bispecific antibodies. J Virol 1996; 70:6831–6838.

165. Haisma HJ, Pinedo HM, Rijswijk A, der Meulen-Muileman I, Sosnowski BA, Ying W, Beusechem VW, Tillman BW, Gerritsen WR, Curiel DT. Tumor-specific gene transfer via an adenoviral vector targeted to the pan-carcinoma antigen EpCAM. Gene Ther 1999; 6:1469–1474.

166. Einfeld DA, Brough DE, Roelvink PW, Kovesdi I, Wickham TJ. Construction of a pseudoreceptor that mediates transduction by adenoviruses expressing a ligand in fiber or penton base. J Virol 1999; 73:9130–9136.

167. Wickham TJ, Carrion ME, Kovesdi I. Targeting of adenovirus penton base to new receptors through replacement of its RGD motif with other receptor-specific peptide motifs. Gene Ther 1995; 2:750–756.

168. Dmitriev I, Krasnykh V, Miller CR, Wang M, Kashentseva E, Mikheeva G, Belousova N, Curiel DT. An adenovirus vector with genetically modified fibers demonstrates expanded tropism via utilization of a coxsackievirus and adenovirus receptor-independent cell entry mechanism. J Virol 1998; 72:9706–9713.

169. van Beusechem VW, van Rijswijk AL, van Es HH, Haisma HJ, Pinedo HM, Gerritsen WR. Recombinant adenovirus vectors with knobless fibers for targeted gene transfer. Gene Ther 2000; 7:1940–1946.

170. Wickham TJ, Roelvink PW, Brough DE, Kovesdi I. Adenovirus targeted to heparan-containing receptors increases its gene delivery efficiency to multiple cell types. Nat Biotechnol 1996; 14:1570–1573.

171. Wickham TJ, Tzeng E, Shears LL, II, Roelvink PW, Li Y, Lee GM, Brough DE, Lizonova A, Kovesdi I. Increased in vitro and in vivo gene transfer by adenovirus vectors containing chimeric fiber proteins. J Virol 1997; 71:8221–8229.

172. Michael SI, Hong JS, Curiel DT, Engler JA. Addition of a short peptide ligand to the adenovirus fiber protein. Gene Ther 1995; 2:660–668.

173. Zabner J, Chillon M, Grunst T, Moninger TO, Davidson BL, Gregory R, Armentano D. A chimeric type 2 adenovirus vector with a type 17 fiber enhances gene transfer to human airway epithelia. J Virol 1999; 73:8689–8695.

174. Drapkin PT, O'Riordan CR, Yi SM, Chiorini JA, Cardella J, Zabner J, Welsh MJ. Targeting the urokinase plasminogen activator receptor enhances gene transfer to human airway epithelia. J Clin Invest 2000; 105:589–596.

175. Kreda SM, Pickles RJ, Lazarowski ER, Boucher RC. G-protein-coupled receptors as targets for gene transfer vectors using natural small-molecule ligands. Nat Biotechnol 2000; 18:635–640.

176. Romanczuk H, Galer CE, Zabner J, Barsomian G, Wadsworth SC, O'Riordan CR. Modification of an adenoviral vector with biologically selected peptides: a novel strategy for gene delivery to cells of choice. Hum Gene Ther 1999; 10:2615–2626.

177. Lee JH, Baker TJ, Mahal LK, Zabner J, Bertozzi CR, Wiemer DF, Welsh MJ. Engineering novel cell surface receptors for virus-mediated gene transfer. J Biol Chem 1999; 274:21878–21884.

178. Zabner J, Zeiher BG, Friedman E, Welsh MJ. Adenovirus-mediated gene transfer to ciliated airway epithelia requires prolonged incubation time. J Virol 1996; 70:6994–7003.

179. Fasbender A, Zabner J, Chillon M, Moninger TO, Puga AP, Davidson BL, Welsh MJ. Complexes of adenovirus with polycationic polymers and cationic lipids increase the efficiency of gene transfer in vitro and in vivo. J Biol Chem 1997; 272:6479–6489.

180. Fasbender AJ, Zabner J, Welsh MJ. Optimization of cationic lipid-mediated gene transfer to airway epithelia. Am J Physiol 1995; 269:L45–51.

181. Yagi K, Noda H, Kurono M, Ohishi N. Efficient gene transfer with less cytotoxicity by means of cationic multilamellar liposomes. Biochem Biophys Res Commun 1993; 196:1042–1048.

182. Plank C, Mechtler K, Szoka FC Jr, Wagner E. Activation of the complement system by synthetic DNA complexes: a potential barrier for intravenous gene delivery. Hum Gene Ther 1996; 7:1437–1446.

183. Hunter R, Strickland F, Kezdy F. The adjuvant activity of nonionic block polymer surfactants. I. The role of hydrophile-lipophile balance. J Immunol 1981; 127:1244–1250.

184. Worgall S, Worgall TS, Kostarelos K, Singh R, Leopold PL, Hackett NR, Crystal RG. Free cholesterol enhances adenoviral vector gene transfer and expression in CAR-deficient cells. Mol Ther 2000; 1:39–48.

185. Fasbender A, Lee JH, Walters RW, Moninger TO, Zabner J, Welsh MJ. Incorporation of adenovirus in calcium phosphate precipitates enhances gene transfer to airway epithelia in vitro and in vivo. J Clin Invest 1998; 102:184–193.

186. Walters R, Welsh M. Mechanism by which calcium phosphate coprecipitation enhances adenovirus-mediated gene transfer. Gene Ther 1999; 6:1845–1850.

187. Lee JH, Zabner J, Welsh MJ. Delivery of an adenovirus vector in a calcium phosphate coprecipitate enhances the therapeutic index of gene transfer to airway epithelia. Hum Gene Ther 1999; 10:603–613.

188. Ernst N, Ulrichskotter S, Schmalix WA, Radler J, Galneder R, Mayer E, Gersting S, Plank C, Reinhardt D, Rosenecker J. Interaction of liposomal and polycationic transfection complexes with pulmonary surfactant. J Gene Med 1999; 1:331–340.

189. Raczka E, Kukowska-Latallo JF, Rymaszewski M, Chen C, Baker JR Jr. The effect of synthetic surfactant Exosurf on gene transfer in mouse lung in vivo. Gene Ther 1998; 5:1333–1339.

190. Katkin JP, Husser RC, Langston C, Welty SE. Exogenous surfactant enhances the delivery of recombinant adenoviral vectors to the lung. Hum Gene Ther 1997; 8:171–176.

191. Weiss DJ, Strandjord TP, Jackson JC, Clark JG, Liggitt D. Perfluorochemical liquid–enhanced adenoviral vector distribution and expression in lungs of spontaneously breathing rodents. Exp Lung Res 1999; 25:317–333.

192. Cipolla DC, Gonda I, Shak S, Kovesdi I, Crystal R, Sweeney TD. Coarse spray delivery to a localized region of the pulmonary airways for gene therapy. Hum Gene Ther 2000; 11:361–371.

193. Lerondel S, Le Pape A, Sene C, Faure L, Bernard S, Diot P, Nicolis E, Mehtali M, Lusky M, Cabrini G, Pavirani A. Radioisotopic imaging allows optimization of adenovirus lung deposition for cystic fibrosis gene therapy. Hum Gene Ther 2001; 12:1–11.

194. Wang G, Zabner J, Deering C, Launspach J, Shao J, Bodner M, Jolly DJ, Davidson BL, McCray PB Jr. Increasing epithelial junction permeability enhances gene transfer to airway epithelia In vivo. Am J Respir Cell Mol Biol 2000; 22:129–138.

195. Lane SJ, Adcock IM, Richards D, Hawrylowicz C, Barnes PJ, Lee TH. Corticosteroid-resistant bronchial asthma is associated with increased c-fos expression in monocytes and T lymphocytes. J Clin Invest 1998; 102:2156–2164.

AUTHOR INDEX

E

Mink J, 250, *259*
Minkwitz MC, 479, *509*
Minnicozzi M, 369, 386, 387, *394, 404,*
    495, *527*
Minshall E, 195, *210,* 353, *362,* 368, 387,
    388, *394,* 537, *542*
Minshall EM, 102, *116,* 221, 232, *234,*
    323, *338,* 353, 354, 358, 359, *362,*
    364, 441, 445, 447, 452, *455, 458,*
    545, 546, 553, 559, *566, 572, 579*
Minter RM, 655, 656, *671, 672*
Minty A, 95, *112,* 349, *361*
Miotto D, 487, 488, 491, *519*
Mirabella A, 481, 482, *512, 513*
Miranda KM, 198, *214*
Misaki Y, 559, *578*
Mischak H, 624, *638*
Mishima K, 329, *342*
Mishra A, 122, 123, *135,* 148, 171, 172,
    175, 186
Mishra VS, 11, *16*
Missotten M, 487, *518*
Mistretta A, 485, 489, 494, 496, *516, 521*
Mitchell DB, 472, *501, 502*
Mitchell J, 559, *579*
Mitchell JA, 470, 494, *500, 526*
Mitchell MI, 474, *504*
Mitchell RW, 557, *577*
Mitcho YL, 605, *613*
Mitsui Y, 491, *523*
Mitsuyasu H, 89, *111*
Mittelman M, 593, *599*
Mitzer W, 298, *306*
Mitzner W, 562, *580*
Miura K, 59, *76,* 553, *572*
Miura M, 319, *336,* 479, 488, 491, 494,
    509, 520, 523, 526
Miura O, 96, *113*
Miura T, 391, *407*
Miura Y, 153, 154, *176*
Miyagawa H, 469, *499*
Miyajima I, 126, 133, *139*
Miyake K, 8, *15,* 29, *46*
Miyamasu M, 59, *76,* 159, *179,* 196, *212,*
    416, 417, *432,* 559, *578*
Miyamoto T, 607, *614*
Miyamoto Y, 121, *135,* 550, *570*
Miyao N, 301, *307*
Miyasaka M, 223, *235,* 293, *304*
Miyata A, 301, *307*

Miyatake S, 266, *278*
Miyazaki J, 630, *640*
Mizel DR, 226, *237*
Mizoguchi A, 391, *407,* 471, *501*
Mizushima S, 98, *114*
Mizutani H, 389, *406*
Mochizuki M, 59, *75, 76,* 559, *579*
Moderer M, 552, *571*
Modlin RL, 8, *15,* 29, *46*
Moereels H, 468, *497*
Moffatt JD, 198, *214*
Mohamadzadeh M, 21, *43*
Mohanty JG, 123, *137*
Mohapatra SS, 651, *669*
Mohrs M, 63, *79,* 368, 377, 385, *394, 403*
Mohuczy D, 647, *666*
Moilanen E, 153, *177*
Moldawer LL, 655, 656, *671, 672*
Molet S, 149, *175,* 195, *210,* 302, *308,*
    368, 387, 388, *394,* 447, *458,* 648,
    666
Molimard M, 485, 487, *515, 519*
Molina HA, 163, *181*
Moll H, 377, *397,* 621, *636*
Moller A, 124, 125, *145*
Moller GM, 32, 39, *48,* 380, *400*
Moloney ED, 32, *48*
Mon L, 249, *257*
Monaco A, 42, *51*
Mondino A, 229, *239*
Monia BP, 386, *403,* 647, 648, *666*
Monick MM, 191, *210,* 474, 477, *503*
Moninger TO, 659, 660, *675, 676*
Monocada S, 494, *525*
Mons H, 489, *520*
Monsma FJ, 468, *497*
Montefort S, 204, *218,* 302, *308,* 352,
    362, 441, *455,* 550, *570*
Monteiro RC, 159, *179*
Montero L, 551, *571*
Monticelli S, 60, *77*
Montjovent MO, 427, *437*
Moody CT, 99, *115*
Moore AM, 27, *45*
Moore BB, 551, *571*
Moore K, 23, *43,* 474, *505*
Moore KA, 322, *337*
Moore MA, 99, *114*
Moore PE, 71, *81,* 446, *457*
Moore PS, 428, *437*

SUBJECT INDEX